CANINE AND FELINE

NUTRITION

A Resource for Companion Animal Professionals

SECOND EDITION

LINDA P. CASE, MS
Lecturer, Companion Animals
Department of Animal Sciences
College of ACES
University of Illinois
Urbana, Illinois

DANIEL P. CAREY, DVM
Director
Technical Communications Department
The Iams Company
Lewisburg, Ohio

DIANE A. HIRAKAWA, PhD
Vice President
Research and Development
The Iams Company
Lewisburg, Ohio

LEIGHANN DARISTOTLE, DVM, PhD
Manager
Communications Department
The Iams Company
Lewisburg, Ohio

with 57 illustrations

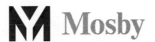 Mosby

A Harcourt Health Sciences Company

St. Louis   London   Philadelphia   Sydney   Toronto

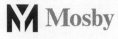

A Harcourt Health Sciences Company

Editor-In-Chief: John A. Schrefer
Editorial Manager: Linda L. Duncan
Developmental Editor: Teri Merchant
Project Manager: Catherine Jackson
Production Editor: Clay S. Broeker
Book Design Manager: Judi Lang
Interior Design: Michael Warrell
Cover Design: Michael Warrell

SECOND EDITION

Mosby, Inc.
A Harcourt Health Sciences Company
11830 Westline Industrial Drive
St. Louis, Missouri 63146

Printed in the United States of America

LIBRARY OF CONGRESS CATALOGING IN PUBLICATION DATA

Canine and feline nutrition : a resource for companion animal professionals / Linda P. Case . . . [et al.].—2nd ed.
    p. cm.
    Rev. ed. of: Canine and feline nutrition / Linda P. Case, Daniel P. Carey, Diane A. Hirakawa. c1995.
    Includes bibliographical references.
    ISBN 0-323-00443-1
    1. Dogs—Nutrition. 2. Cats—Nutrition. 3. Dogs—Food. 4. Cats—Food. 5. Dogs—Diseases—Nutritional aspects. 6. Cats—Diseases—Nutritional aspects.
    I. Case, Linda P. II. Case, Linda P. Canine and feline nutrition.

SF427.4.C37 2000
636.7'0852—dc21   00-033863

00 01 02 03 04 GW/MV 9 8 7 6 5 4 3 2 1

DEDICATED TO

Clay Mathile…a leader and visionary whose integrity and commitment to enhancing the health and well-being of companion animals is only surpassed by his unique ability to inspire and encourage others to develop talents, stretch imaginations, and believe that the impossible can become reality.

DPC, DAH, and LD

and

My parents, Jean and Bob Palas; my husband Mike (my best friend always); and the companion animals who bring such joy to our lives: the dogs Roxie, Gusto, and Nike, and the cats Nipper, Tara, and Pumpkin Joe.

In memory of Sparks: co-teacher, running companion, fan of funny noises, and lover of blueberry scones. You brought laughter and joy to so many, and will forever be in my heart.

LPC

PREFACE

Man has a long and very complex history of association with dogs and cats. This relationship has its roots in the early domestication of companion animals and has evolved to exist in today's society in a vast variety of forms. Both the dog and the cat were originally domesticated to serve a number of functions for mankind. While some dogs and cats still fulfill these roles, the primary reason that most people in today's society share their lives with dogs and cats is companionship. In recent years, scientific studies of human-animal interactions have revealed that these relationships are very strong and enduring components of many pet owners' lives. Pet ownership has also been shown to provide numerous physiological and psychological benefits. Keeping companion animals has become a national pastime, and taking proper care of dogs and cats is of great interest and concern to the many pet owners and professionals who work with these animals.

Along with proper health care and medical attention, nutrition is an important component in the care of all dogs and cats. An understanding of basic nutrition and the nutrient requirements of healthy dogs and cats is integral to the understanding of practical feeding practices. Such knowledge enables pet professionals to provide optimal nutritional care throughout life, which contributes to lasting health and longevity. This new edition of *Canine and Feline Nutrition: A Resource for Companion Animal Professionals* provides a thorough examination of the science of companion animal nutrition and practical feeding management information for dogs and cats. Information provided in this book is of value to veterinarians, animal scientists, nutritionists, breeders, exhibitors, judges, trainers, and hobbyists. The book also continues to serve as a resource for companion animal management and nutrition courses in the fields of animal science and veterinary medicine. It is the authors' intent that this book complement general animal nutrition textbooks by providing current and comprehensive information about the two most popular companion animal species, the dog and the cat.

As in the first edition, *Canine and Feline Nutrition* is organized into six sections. These address basic principles of nutrition; nutrient requirements of dogs and cats; pet food production and selection; feeding management throughout all stages of life; feeding problems; fads and fallacies; and dietary management of nutritionally responsive diseases. Current research is reviewed, and balanced discussions of controversial issues of dietary management are presented. Differences between the nutrient requirements and feeding practices of dogs and cats are addressed throughout the book. To facilitate use by readers with a wide range of backgrounds and interests, illustrative tables and boxes are included; these present technical material at a level that can be of practical use.

Section 1 is written as a basic introduction to the science of nutrition, without any application to specific species. Chapters within the section are arranged according each of the basic nutrients and the processes of digestion and absorption. These chapters will be of value to students and professionals who require introductory information about the science of nutrition. Section 2 addresses the specific nutrient requirements of dogs and cats and includes chapters that examine energy balance in companion animals, comparative nutrient requirements, and the metabolic idiosyncrasies of the cat. Recent research examining differences in growth rates and energy needs of large and small breeds of dog and the practical application of this knowledge to feeding management is included. Updated information regarding the cat's taurine requirement and the influence of diet type on taurine homeostasis is also reviewed. Section 3 provides a detailed overview of the formulation, production, and use of pet foods. Chapters include information about the history, regulation, and marketing of commercial foods; nutrient content and types of foods; and procedures for evaluating the diets of dogs and cats. Practical information about the selection of appropriate pet foods is included for pet owners. The new edition includes an expanded section describing the pet food label, with detailed information regarding the AAFCO's regulations, interpretation of terms, and current label guidelines. Section 4 includes feeding and diet recommendations for nutritional care throughout various stages of life. This new edition includes recent research that has focused on the nutrient needs of neonatal puppies and kittens, milk composition in queens and bitches, and development of optimal weaning procedures. Similarly, the importance of proper feeding management throughout growth, especially for large and giant breeds of dogs is examined in detail. New information regarding the nutritional needs and feeding of geriatric dogs and cats and the feeding of hard-working animals is included in the final two chapters of the section. Section 5 addresses nutritional and dietary misconceptions commonly reported by pet owners and professionals. The chapters examine the problems of overfeeding and obesity, supplementation with specific nutrients, nutrient imbalances that occur as a result of improper feeding practices, and a variety of currently popular nutritional fads and fallacies. Detailed therapeutic programs for the treatment of companion animal obesity have been developed and thoroughly tested in recent years. This new edition provides an in-depth overview of these studies, as well as recommendations for the successful treatment of overweight and obese pets. Finally, Section 6 deals with nutritionally responsive diseases in dogs and cats. This section has been extensively revised and expanded in the new edition. Chapters dealing with inherited disorders of metabolism, diabetes mellitus, urolithiasis, nutritionally manageable dermatoses, chronic kidney disease, and feline hepatic lipidosis all include updated reviews of research and recommendations for appropriate diets and feeding protocols. In addition, three new chapters are included; these address diet and dental health, nutritional management of gastrointestinal diseases, and nutritional care of cancer patients. The chapters in this section continue to provide an important resource for veterinarians, nutritionists, and breeders who are involved in the treatment or study of these diseases.

ACKNOWLEDGMENTS

Many colleagues and friends were instrumental in the preparation of the completed manuscript for this book. Several nutritionists with acclaimed expertise in the nutrition, feeding management, and therapeutic nutritional care of companion animals reviewed and edited all 38 chapters of this new edition. Collectively, they provided valuable advice and recommendations for updating early chapters and creating new chapters for the second edition. The authors express sincere gratitude to Marcie J. Campion, PhD; Gary M. Davenport, PhD; Michael G. Hayek, PhD; Allan J. Lepine, PhD; Gregory A. Reinhart, PhD; Gregory D. Sunvold, PhD; and Mark A Tetrick, DVM, PhD, for their help and support. The authors also thank Jill Cline, PhD, who created all of the original tables and diagrams, and Pat Norris, who provided editing support for the first edition. Many thanks to the outstanding group of editors and staff at Mosby, who provided editorial expertise and exceptional attention to detail for both editions of this book. Special appreciation goes to Linda Duncan, Editorial Manager, who has provided continuous support and enthusiasm for this project from the early days of its inception. Finally, thanks to Dr. Robert Easter, Professor and Head, Department of Animal Sciences, University of Illinois, for his continued support of the Companion Animal Program as well as his dedication to the pursuit of knowledge and understanding of all aspects of animal nutrition.

Linda P. Case

CONTENTS

NUTRIENT REQUIREMENTS OF DOGS AND CATS

SECTION 6

NUTRITIONALLY RESPONSIVE DISORDERS

1

BASICS OF NUTRITION

In recent years researchers have been able to explain why humans bond so strongly to their pets, and they have also discovered that the relationship between humans and animals is often beneficial to human health. It is not surprising that the strong emotional attachment that people feel for their pets is coupled with a concern for providing them with the best in health care and nutrition. Advances in veterinary medicine have resulted in vaccination programs that protect dogs and cats from many life-threatening diseases and in medical procedures that contribute to lengthened lifespans. Likewise, progress in the field of nutrition has generated an improved understanding of canine and feline dietetics and led to the development of well-balanced pet foods that contribute to long-term health and aid in the prevention of chronic disease.

Today's competitive market contains a vast array of foods, snacks, and nutritional supplements for dogs and cats. These products are sold in grocery stores, feed stores, pet shops, and veterinary hospitals. Products vary significantly in nutrient composition, availability, digestibility, palatability, physical form, flavor, and texture. Some foods are formulated to provide adequate nutrition throughout a pet's lifespan, while other foods have been marketed specifically for a particular stage of life or a specific disease state. This large selection of commercial products, combined with the periodic propagation of popular nutritional fads and fallacies, has resulted in much confusion among pet owners and companion animal professionals regarding the nutritional care of dogs and cats.

A basic understanding of the fundamentals of nutrition is a necessary prerequisite for evaluating pet foods and making decisions about a pet's nutritional status. The term *nutrition* refers to the study of food and the nutrients and other components that it contains. This includes an examination of the actions of specific nutrients, their interactions with each other, and their balance within a diet. In addition, the science of nutrition includes an examination of the way in which an animal ingests, digests, absorbs, and uses nutrients. This section provides an overview of each of the essential nutrients. Energy, water, carbohydrates, fats, proteins, vitamins, and minerals are examined in detail. An examination of the normal digestive and absorptive processes in dogs and cats is also provided. Subsequent sections address the specific nutrient requirements of dogs and cats, the types and compositions of pet foods, feeding management throughout the life cycle, feeding problems, and the management of nutritionally-responsive diseases. Information contained in this book will enable pet owners, students, and companion animal professionals to make informed decisions about the diets and nutritional health of dogs and cats throughout all stages of life.

1

Energy and Water

Like all living animals, dogs and cats require a balanced diet to grow normally and maintain health once they are mature. *Nutrients* are components in the diet that have specific functions within the body and contribute to growth, body-tissue maintenance, and optimal health. *Essential nutrients* are those components that cannot be synthesized by the body at a rate that is adequate to meet the body's needs. Therefore essential nutrients must be supplied in the diet. *Nonessential nutrients* can be synthesized by the body and obtained either through de novo synthesis or from the diet. Along with a requirement for energy, all animals require six major categories of nutrients. These categories are water, carbohydrates, proteins, fats, minerals, and vitamins. Energy, although not a nutrient per se, is required by the body for normal growth, maintenance, reproductive performance, and physical work. Approximately 50% to 80% of the dry matter (DM) of a dog's or cat's diet is used for energy.

With the exception of water, energy is the most critical component that must be considered in a diet. Like all animals, companion animals require a constant source of dietary energy in order to survive. Plants obtain energy from solar radiation and convert it to energy-containing nutrients. Animals consume plants and use them either directly for energy or to convert plant nutrients into other energy-containing molecules. The primary form of stored energy in plants is carbohydrate; the main form of stored energy in animals is fat. Energy is necessary for the performance of the body's metabolic work, which includes maintaining and synthesizing body tissues, engaging in physical work, and regulating normal body temperature. Given its importance, it is not surprising that energy is always the first requirement to be met by an animal's diet. Regardless of a dog's or cat's needs for essential amino acids from dietary protein or essential fatty acids (EFAs) from dietary fat, the energy-yielding nutrients of the diet are first used to satisfy energy needs. Once energy needs are met, nutrients become available for other metabolic functions.

Animals are capable of regulating their energy intake to accurately meet their daily caloric requirements. When allowed free access to a balanced, moderately palatable diet, most dogs and cats will consume enough food to meet, but not exceed, their daily energy needs.[1,2,3] *Energy density* or *caloric density* refers to the concentration of energy in a given quantity of food (see p. 8). When the energy density of a diet is decreased, animals respond by increasing the quantity of food they consume, which results in a relatively constant energy intake.[3,4] If an animal's food intake is regulated by total energy intake, the composition of all other nutrients in the diet must be balanced with respect to the diet's energy density. This balance should be calculated to ensure that when a dog or cat consumes a quantity of food adequate to meet its caloric needs, all other nutrient requirements will be met at the same time.

Contrary to popular belief, dogs and cats are unable to self-regulate their intake of most other essential nutrients. Although there is some evidence that adult dogs will select a diet that is moderately high in protein, this effect has been observed only when neither energy nor protein were limited in the experimental diets.[5] Factors such as palatability and the ratio of dietary fat to carbohydrates may have significantly affected the dogs' dietary selections in this study. Moreover, there is no evidence indicating that dogs or cats will overconsume a diet that is high in energy but low in protein in an attempt to meet their protein needs. Companion animals that are deficient in a particular vitamin, mineral, or essential amino acid will not seek foods that contain the nutrient or preferentially select a diet that is abundant in the deficient nutrient. In contrast, dogs and cats that are deficient in energy will spontaneously increase their caloric intake until energy balance is achieved.[1,2]

Although all dogs and cats have the ability to properly regulate their energy intake, this natural tendency can be overridden by environmental factors. A diet of pet foods that are both highly palatable and energy-dense leads to chronic overconsumption in some companion animals. Today's competitive pet food market includes many foods that are high in both palatability and caloric density. Coupled with this fact is a decline in physical activity among many pets in today's society. Many companion animals now lead happy but relatively sedentary lives exclusively as house pets. In recent years many cats have moved from the barnyard into the house, where their working role as mousers and pest-controllers has been effectively eliminated. Likewise, dogs have evolved from working companions to unemployed house dogs that lack adequate daily exercise. These two changes have led to an epidemic of overeating and obesity among dogs and cats in the United States; surveys have shown that obesity is the most common nutritional problem observed by practicing veterinarians.[6] These changes indicate that it may no longer be wise to rely on the inherent abilities of dogs and cats to regulate energy intake. Although companion animals certainly have this ability, many do not self-regulate because of the nature of the food they eat and the type of lifestyle they lead. In most cases, portion-controlled feeding is the best way to control a pet's energy balance, growth rate, and weight status (see Section 4, pp. 220-224).

MEASUREMENT OF ENERGY IN THE DIET

Energy has no measurable mass or dimension, but the chemical energy contained in foods is ultimately transformed by the body into heat, which can be measured. Nutrients that provide energy in an animal's diet include carbohydrates, fats, and

FIGURE **1-1**

Partitioning of dietary energy.

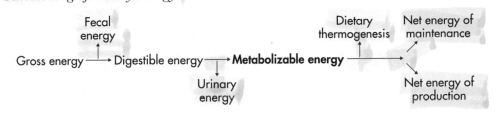

proteins. The chemical energy of foods is most often expressed in units of calories or kilocalories (kcal). A *calorie* refers to the amount of heat energy necessary to raise the temperature of 1 gram (g) of water from 14.5° Celsius (C) to 15.5° C. Because a calorie is a very small unit, it is not of practical use in the science of animal nutrition. The kcal, which is equal to 1000 calories, is the most commonly used unit of measure. A second unit of measurement for energy is the kilojoule (kJ), which is a metric unit. A *kilojoule* is defined as the amount of mechanical energy required for a force of 1 newton (N) to move a weight of 1 kilogram (kg) by a distance of 1 meter (m). To convert kcal to kJ, the number of kcal is multiplied by 4.18.

The caloric value of foods can be measured using direct calorimetry. This process involves the complete combustion (oxidation) of a premeasured amount of food in a bomb calorimeter, resulting in the release and measurement of the food's total chemical energy. This energy is called the food's *gross energy* (GE). Animals cannot use all of a food's GE because energy losses occur during digestion and assimilation. *Digestible energy* (DE) signifies the amount of energy available for absorption across the intestinal mucosa. Apparent DE can be calculated by subtracting the indigestible energy excreted in the feces from the GE of the food. Additional energy losses occur as a result of the production of combustible gases and the excretion of urea in the urine. The incomplete oxidation of absorbed dietary protein by the body results in the production of urea. Because the production of combustible gases in dogs and cats is minimal, only urinary losses are typically accounted for. *Metabolizable energy* (ME) is the amount of energy ultimately available to the tissues of the body after losses in the feces and urine have been subtracted from the GE of the food. ME is the value that is most often used to express the energy content of pet food ingredients and commercial diets. Similarly, the energy requirements of dogs and cats are usually expressed as kcal of ME. ME can be subdivided to calculate net energy and the energy lost to dietary thermogenesis. *Dietary thermogenesis,* also called the *specific dynamic action of food,* refers to the energy needed by the body to digest, absorb, and assimilate nutrients. *Net energy* is the energy available to an animal for the maintenance of body tissues and for production needs such as physical work, growth, gestation, and lactation (Figure 1-1).

The ME of a diet or food ingredient depends on both the nutrient composition of the food and the animal that is consuming it. For example, because of the length and structure of its gastrointestinal tract, a nonruminant herbivore such as a horse

FIGURE **1-2**

Calculation and example of metabolizable energy.

Calculation
Metabolizable energy = $(GE_{food}) - (GE_{feces} + GE_{urine})$

Example
1100 kcal = 3600 (food) − 2500 (feces + urine)

can derive a greater amount of energy from grass than can a dog or cat. Therefore the ME value of grass for a horse is higher than the ME value of grass for a companion animal. Three possible methods can be used to estimate the ME values of a food ingredient or diet for a given species. These methods are direct determination using feeding trials and total collection procedures; calculation from analyzed levels of protein, carbohydrate, and fat in the diet; and extrapolation of data collected from other species.

Direct Determination in Feeding Trials

Data collected in actual feeding trials with the species in question are the most accurate method for determining a food's ME content. The diet or food ingredient is fed to a number of test animals, and feces and urine are collected throughout a predesignated time period. Determination of the energy content of the food, feces, and urine allows direct calculation of ME (Figure 1-2). However, direct measurement of ME values in dogs and cats can be extremely time-consuming and costly and requires access to large numbers of test animals. To date, many of the ME values for commonly used pet food ingredients have not been directly measured. However, the manufacturers of some of the premium pet foods routinely measure the ME of their formulated pet foods and ingredients through the use of controlled feeding trials.

Calculation Method

ME values can also be determined using mathematical formulas that estimate a food's ME from its analyzed carbohydrate, protein, and fat content. The formulas that have been derived for dog and cat diets include constants that account for fecal and urinary losses of energy. The GE values, which represent total energy content, for mixed carbohydrate, fat, and protein are 4.15, 9.40, and 5.65 kcal/g, respectively.[7] However, as mentioned earlier, animals are incapable of using all of the energy present in food nutrients. The inefficiency of digestion, absorption, and assimilation result in energy losses. In human foods, the *Atwater factors* of 4-9-4 kcal/g are commonly used to estimate ME values for carbohydrate, fat, and protein. These factors are calculated using estimated digestibility coefficients of 96% for fat and carbohydrate and 91% for protein.[8] A *digestibility coefficient* is the proportion of the consumed nutrient that is actually available for absorption and use

6

TABLE **1-1**

Digestibility Coefficients and Factors

Nutrient	Human Food Digestibility Coefficient	Atwater Factor	Pet Food Digestibility Coefficient	Modified Atwater Factor
Carbohydrate	96%	4 kcal/g	85%	3.5 kcal/g
Protein	91%	4 kcal/g	80%	3.5 kcal/g
Fat	96%	9 kcal/g	90%	8.5 kcal/g

by the body. The ME value of protein was further reduced to account for urinary losses of urea.

Although it appears reasonable to use Atwater factors to determine the ME content of dog and cat foods, digestibility data collected in these two species indicate that Atwater factors tend to overestimate the ME values of most pet foods. This miscalculation occurs because the digestibility of many pet food ingredients is lower than the digestibility of most foods consumed by humans. Digestibility data collected in dogs from 106 samples of dry, semimoist, and canned commercial dog foods showed that the average digestibility coefficients for crude protein, acid-ether extract (a measure of fat content), and nitrogen-free extract (a measure of soluble carbohydrate content) were 81%, 85%, and 79%, respectively.[9] The fact that typical pet food ingredients are generally lower in digestibility than the foods consumed by humans causes the Atwater factors to be inaccurate for use in estimating the ME of pet foods. The National Research Council's (NRC's) 1985 recommendations for dogs suggested that digestibility coefficients of 80%, 90%, and 85% be used for the protein, fat, and carbohydrate in commercial dog foods.[6] When GE values are readjusted for digestibility and urinary losses, ME values of 3.5, 8.5, and 3.5 kcal/g are assigned to protein, fat, and carbohydrate, respectively (Table 1-1). These values are referred to as *modified Atwater factors*. Although these values provide a better estimate of ME values for pet foods than do the Atwater factors, they may still underestimate the ME values of high-quality dog foods that contain highly digestible protein sources and low levels of indigestible fiber. Conversely, the ME value of those foods that contain high amounts of plant fiber and/or poor quality meat sources are slightly overestimated by these factors.[7]

Several formulas for estimation of the ME in cat foods have been derived from digestibility data collected in direct feeding trials and from studies of the correlations between analyzed values and values of ME measured in vivo.[9,10] However, little data are available on the DE of specific cat foods or cat food ingredients. Moreover, this information is usually not readily available. In general, calculation of ME from analyzed levels of carbohydrate, fat, and protein in the diet using modified Atwater factors provides a reasonably accurate estimate of the ME for cat foods, as long as crude fiber is used to estimate the total fiber in the food.[10] A recent study of 14 commercial cat foods produced in the United States found that the minimum percentage of fat reported on the guaranteed analysis panel of the pet food label can also be used to estimate the food's ME. The equation ME = 3.075 + 0.066 (fat) provides a quick and simple method of estimating ME from information that is readily available on all pet food labels.[10]

Data from Other Species

The lack of direct data measuring DE and ME in cat food ingredients and the inadequacy of mathematical formulas for use with many types of foods have resulted in the use of data from other species. The NRC assigned ME values from swine data to ingredients commonly used in cat foods whenever direct data on the cat were not available.[11] This information was included in the 1986 edition of the NRC's publication *Nutrient Requirements of Cats.* Although this third method of estimating ME values of a food is not as accurate as direct measurement, data collected in swine experiments have been reported to correlate well with values from other animals with simple stomachs.[11]

ENERGY DENSITY

The *energy density* of a pet food refers to the number of calories provided by the food in a given weight or volume. In the United States, energy density is expressed as kcal of ME per kg or pound (lb) of diet. In most European countries, the unit kJ/kg is used. The importance of energy density in companion animal nutrition cannot be overemphasized. It is the principal factor that determines the quantity of food that is eaten each day and therefore directly affects the amount of all other essential nutrients that an animal ingests. A diet's energy density must be high enough to allow the pet to consume a sufficient amount of food to meet its energy needs. If the energy density is too low, food intake will be restricted by the physical limitations of the gastrointestinal tract, resulting in an energy deficit. In other words, the animal would not be physically able to consume enough of the low-energy diet to meet its caloric requirements. Such a diet is said to be "bulk-limited." If levels of the essential nutrients in such a diet are not balanced relative to energy density, multiple nutrient deficiencies could also occur.

When the caloric density of a pet food is high enough for an animal to consume a sufficient quantity to meet its daily energy needs, energy density will be the primary factor that determines the quantity of food that is consumed each day. There is an inverse relationship between energy density and the volume of food that is consumed. As a food's energy density increases, the total volume of food that is consumed decreases. However, feeding a highly palatable pet food can override a pet's tendency to correctly regulate intake. The sale of pet foods that are energy dense and highly palatable has led many owners to the use of portion-controlled feeding to manage their pet's daily food intake. Maintenance of normal body weight and growth rate are the criteria most often used to determine the appropriate quantity of food. Therefore, even when under the pet owner's control, a

TABLE **1-2**

Sample Calculation to Convert Percentage of Weight to Percentage of Energy in the Diet

Food Type	Protein (%)		Modified Atwater Factor		Kcal/100 g of Food	× 100%
Dry	27	×	3.5	÷	380	24.8
Canned	7	×	3.5	÷	98	25.0

pet's level of energy intake is still the primary factor that affects the quantity of food that is fed.

Because energy intake determines total food intake, it is important that diets are properly balanced so that requirements for all other nutrients are met at the same time that energy needs are satisfied. For this reason, it is more appropriate to express levels of energy-containing nutrients in the food in terms of ME rather than in terms of percentage of the food's weight. Expressing nutrient content as units per 1000 kcal of ME, which is called *nutrient density,* is a standardized format that can be used to compare all types of food. Actual nutrient intake can be readily determined from a pet's daily energy requirement, and foods of dissimilar energy content can quickly be compared based upon this requirement. This is consistent across moisture and fiber content unless these components make up such a large component of the diet that they prevent adequate intake of calories. A second method of comparing foods is to use the percentage of total ME contributed by each of the three energy contributing nutrients: protein, fat, and carbohydrate. This is called the *caloric distribution* of a food and can be used to compare foods with differing moisture or energy contents. It is somewhat limited when compared to the use of nutrient density because caloric distribution only considers the energy-containing nutrients of the food (see Section 3, pp. 172-174).

Using nutrient density or caloric distribution, values can be compared in any type of food or diet, regardless of water, nutrient, or energy content. For example, a complete and balanced dry dog food contains 27% protein (as a percentage of weight) and supplies 3800 kcal of ME/kg. Modified Atwater factors can be used to estimate the proportion of energy that protein contributes to the food. The calculations in Table 1-2 show that 24.8% of the food's energy is contributed by protein. These figures can be compared with a canned dog food that contains 7% protein on a weight basis and supplies 980 kcal of ME/kg. When expressed as a percentage of calories, the protein in the canned food also supplies approximately 25% of the food's calories (Table 1-2). If expressed as nutrient density, the g of protein per 1000 kcal ME are 71 g of protein per 1000 kcal of food.

These two foods that appear enormously different when compared in terms of percentage of protein on a weight basis actually contain the same amount of protein when expressed as a percentage of total calories. Differences in the water content and energy density of the two foods account for the drastic differences in

TABLE 1-3

Determination of Energy Density from Guaranteed Analysis

Nutrient	Percentage in Diet		Modified Atwater Factor		Kcal/100 g of Food
Protein	26	×	3.5	=	91
Carbohydrate	47	×	3.5	=	164.5
Fat	15	×	8.5	=	127.5
			Total Calories	=	348

383 kcal/100 g × 1000 g/kg = 3830 kcal/kg (energy density)
3830 kcal/kg × 1 kg/2.2 lb = 1740.9 kcal/lb food (energy density)

nutrient content when expressed as a percentage of weight. Attempting to compare the two foods when protein is expressed as a percentage of weight can be very confusing. Conversion to units of energy allows an accurate comparison of levels of the energy-containing nutrients in different pet foods. Because dogs and cats are fed to meet their caloric requirements, these two foods will supply an equal quantity of protein when fed at the correct level.

The energy density of a food must be known in order to estimate the quantity of food necessary to meet a pet's energy requirement. The Association of American Feed Control Officials (AAFCO), a regulating group responsible for the standards governing commercially prepared pet foods, requires that the energy value of a pet food be expressed in kcal of ME. If ME information is not included on a pet food label, it can be estimated using the proximate analysis of the food. If the proximate analysis is not available, the guaranteed analysis provided on the label of all pet foods can be used as a rough estimate of nutrient content. The modified Atwater factors provided earlier are used to calculate the amount of energy contributed by carbohydrate, protein, and fat. For example, the guaranteed analysis on a bag of a dry dog food reads as follows:

- Crude protein: not less than 26%
- Crude fat: not less than 15%
- Crude fiber: not more than 5%

An estimate of the mineral content of the food, commonly called ash, must then be made. High-quality dry pet foods generally contain between 5% and 8% ash. The food's carbohydrate content can then be estimated by subtraction:

- 100% − % protein − % fat − % fiber − % ash = % carbohydrate
- 100% − 26% − 15% − 5% − 7% = 47%

The calories provided by each nutrient in 100 g of food can then be estimated (Table 1-3). The total calories in 100 g of food is 383, or 3830 kcal/kg of food. This

BOX **1-1**

Sample Calculation to Estimate Amount of Food Required Daily

Energy requirement of an adult dog: 1100 kcal/day
Energy density of the diet: 1582 kcal/lb

Step 1
1100 kcal/day ÷ 1740 kcal/lb = 0.63 lb of food

Step 2
0.63 lb × 16 oz/lb = 10.11 oz

If an 8 oz cup of dry dog food weighs 3 oz, then:

Step 3
10 oz of dry pet food ÷ 3 oz/cup ≈ 3.3 or 3⅓ cups of dry pet food per day.

figure can also be divided by 2.2 to convert to energy density per lb of food. The quantity of food to feed can be estimated by dividing the pet's daily energy requirement by the energy density of the diet. For example, if an adult dog requires 1100 kcal/day and is fed a diet containing 1740 kcal/lb, approximately 10 ounces (oz) of food should be fed each day. An 8-oz cup of dry pet food might weigh 3 oz. Therefore this dog would require approximately 3⅓ cups of this food per day (Box 1-1). It is important to be aware that each dog and cat is an individual and that these calculations provide only a guideline or starting point when determining a pet's daily needs. The amount of food should be adjusted to attain optimal growth in young animals and optimal body weight and condition in adult animals. Adult pets in optimal condition are well-muscled and lean. Although their ribs cannot be readily seen, they should easily be felt when palpated.

ENERGY IMBALANCE

Energy imbalance occurs when an animal's daily energy consumption is either greater or less than its daily requirement, leading to changes in growth rate, body weight, and body composition. Excess energy intake is much more common in dogs and cats than is energy deficiency. Overconsumption of energy has been shown to have several detrimental effects on dogs during their growth, especially those of the large and giant breeds. When an excess amount of a balanced, high-energy pet food is fed to growing puppies, maximal growth rate and weight gain can be achieved. However, studies with growing dogs have indicated that maximal growth rate is not compatible with healthy bone growth and development.[12] Feeding growing puppies to attain maximal growth rate appears to be a significant contributing factor in the development of skeletal disorders such as osteochondrosis and hip dysplasia[12,13,14,15,16] (see Section 5, pp. 333-337).

A second problem associated with an energy surplus during growth involves fat cell hyperplasia. Studies with laboratory animals have shown that the generation of an excessive number of fat cells in the body as a result of overfeeding at a young age can predispose an animal to obesity later in life.[16,17] Although research on fat cell hyperplasia during growth has not been conducted in the dog or cat, it is possible that these species are affected in a similar manner. In adult dogs and cats, surplus energy intake leads to obesity and its medical complications (see Section 5, pp. 305-312).

Inadequate energy intake results in reduced growth rate and compromised development in young dogs and cats and in weight loss and muscle wasting in adult pets. In healthy animals this condition is most commonly seen in hard-working dogs or pregnant or lactating females that are being fed a diet that is too low in energy density.

WATER

In terms of survivability, water is the single most important nutrient for the body. Although animals can live after losing almost all of their body fat and more than half of their protein, a loss of only 10% of body water results in death.[18] Approximately 70% of lean adult body weight is water, and many tissues in the body are composed of between 70% and 90% water. Intracellular fluid is approximately 40% to 45% of the body's weight, and extracellular fluid accounts for 20% to 25%. The presence of an aqueous medium within cells and in many tissues is essential for the occurrence of most metabolic processes and chemical reactions.

Within the body, water functions as a solvent that facilitates cellular reactions and as a transport medium for nutrients and the end products of cellular metabolism. Because of its high specific heat, water is able to absorb the heat generated by metabolic reactions with a minimal increase in temperature. This property allows the many heat-generating reactions within the body to continue with a minimal change in body temperature. Water further contributes to temperature regulation by transporting heat away from the working organs through the blood and, in some species, by evaporating in the form of sweat on the outer surface of the body. Water is an essential component in normal digestion because it is necessary for *hydrolysis,* the splitting of large molecules into smaller molecules through the addition of water. The digestive enzymes of the gastrointestinal tract are secreted in solution. This aqueous medium facilitates the interaction of food components with the digestive enzymes. Elimination of waste products from the kidneys also requires a large amount of water, which acts as both a solvent for toxic metabolites and a carrier medium.

All animals experience daily water losses. Urinary excretion accounts for the greatest loss of volume in most animals. *Obligatory loss* from the kidneys is the minimum required for the body to rid itself of the daily load of urinary waste products. A certain quantity of water is necessary to act as a solvent for these end products. The remaining portion of urinary water loss, called *facultative loss,* is excreted in response to the normal water reabsorption rate of the kidneys and to mechanisms responsible for maintaining proper water balance in the body. Fecal water accounts for a much smaller portion of water excretion. The amount of water that actually appears in the feces is very low compared to the amount that is absorbed across the gastrointestinal tract and returned to the body during digestion. Fecal water loss becomes substantial only when aberrations in the intestines' capacity to absorb water occur. A third route of water loss is evaporation from the lungs during respiration. In dogs and cats this water loss is very important for the regulation of normal body temperature during hot weather. Panting substantially increases respiratory water loss and thus heat loss. Because of these mechanisms of temperature regulation, water losses from respiration and evaporation during hot weather can be very high in both dogs and cats.

Daily water consumption must compensate for these continual fluid losses. A pet's total water intake comes from three possible sources: water present in food, metabolic water, and drinking water. The quantity of water present in the food depends on the type of diet. Commercial, dry pet food may contain as little as 7% water, but some canned rations contain up to 84% water.[19,20] Within limits, increasing the water content of pet foods increases the diet's acceptability. Many owners are able to increase their pet's consumption of a dry food by adding a small amount of water to it immediately before feeding. Studies have shown that both dogs and cats are able to maintain water balance with no source of drinking water when fed diets containing more than 67% moisture.[21,22,23] Dogs appear to be able to readily compensate for changes in the amount of water present in food by increasing or decreasing voluntary water intake. Cats also have this ability, but they seem to be less precise in their adjustment.[19,24,25]

Metabolic water is the water produced during oxidation of the energy-containing nutrients in the body. Oxygen combines with the hydrogen atoms contained in carbohydrate, protein, and fat to produce water molecules. The metabolism of fat produces the greatest amount of metabolic water on a weight basis, and protein catabolism produces the smallest amount.[18] For every 100 g of fat, carbohydrate, and protein oxidized by the body, 107, 55, and 41 milliliters (ml) of metabolic water are produced, respectively. The rate of metabolic water production depends on an animal's metabolic rate and the type of diet. But regardless of these factors, metabolic water is fairly insignificant because it accounts for only 5% to 10% of the total daily water intake of most animals.

The last source of water intake is voluntary drinking. Factors affecting a pet's voluntary water consumption include the ambient temperature, type of diet, level of exercise, physiological state, and health. Water intake increases with both increasing environmental temperature and increasing exercise because more evaporative water is lost as a result of the body's cooling mechanisms. The amount of calories consumed also affects voluntary water consumption. As energy intake increases, more metabolic waste products are produced and the heat produced by nutrient metabolism increases. In these circumstances, the body requires more water to excrete waste products in the urine and to contribute to thermoregulation.

Diet type and composition can also dramatically affect voluntary water intake. A study on dogs found that when test animals were fed a diet containing 73% moisture, they obtained only 38% of their daily water needs from drinking water. When they were abruptly switched to a diet containing only 7% water, voluntary water intake immediately increased to 95% or more of the total daily intake.[19] For both dogs and cats, increasing the salt content of the diet caused an increased drinking response. When the level of salt in the diet of a group of cats was increased from 1.3% to 4.6%, voluntary water intake nearly doubled.[19] This effect may have practical significance given the high level of salt present in some commercial pet foods. Generally, if fresh, palatable water is available and proper amounts of a well-balanced diet are fed, most pets are able to accurately regulate water balance through voluntary intake of water.

C H A P T E R

2

Carbohydrates

 Carbohydrates are the major energy-containing constituents of plants, making up between 60% and 90% of dry-matter (DM) weight. This class of nutrients comprises the elements carbon, hydrogen, and oxygen. Carbohydrates can be classified as monosaccharides, disaccharides, or polysaccharides. *Monosaccharides,* often referred to as the *simple sugars,* are the simplest form of carbohydrate. A monosaccharide is comprised of a single unit containing between three and seven carbon atoms. The three hexoses (6-carbon monosaccharides) that are nutritionally and metabolically the most important are glucose, fructose, and galactose (Figure 2-1).

Glucose is a moderately sweet, simple sugar found in commercially-prepared corn syrup and sweet fruits such as grapes and berries. It is also the chief end product of starch digestion and glycogen hydrolysis in the body. Glucose is the form of carbohydrate found circulating in the bloodstream and is the primary form of carbohydrate used by the body's cells for energy. Fructose, commonly referred to as *fruit sugar,* is a very sweet sugar found in honey, ripe fruits, and some vegetables. It is also formed from the digestion or acid hydrolysis of the disaccharide sucrose. Galactose is not found in a free form in foods. However, it makes up 50% of the disaccharide lactose, which is present in the milk of all species. Like fructose, galactose is released during digestion. Within the body, galactose is converted to glucose by the liver and eventually enters the circulation in the form of glucose.

Disaccharides are made up of two monosaccharide units linked together. Lactose, the sugar found in the milk of all mammals, contains a molecule of glucose and a molecule of galactose. It is the only carbohydrate of animal origin that is of any significance in the diet. Sucrose, commonly recognized as table sugar, contains a molecule of glucose linked to a molecule of fructose. It is found in cane, beets, and maple syrup. Maltose is made up of two glucose molecules linked together. This disaccharide is not commonly found in most foods, but it is formed as an intermediate product in the body during the digestion of starch.

Polysaccharides are comprised of many single monosaccharide units linked together in long and complex chains. Starch, glycogen, dextrins, and dietary fiber are all polysaccharides. Starch is the chief carbohydrate source present in most

15

FIGURE 2-1

Basic carbohydrate structure.

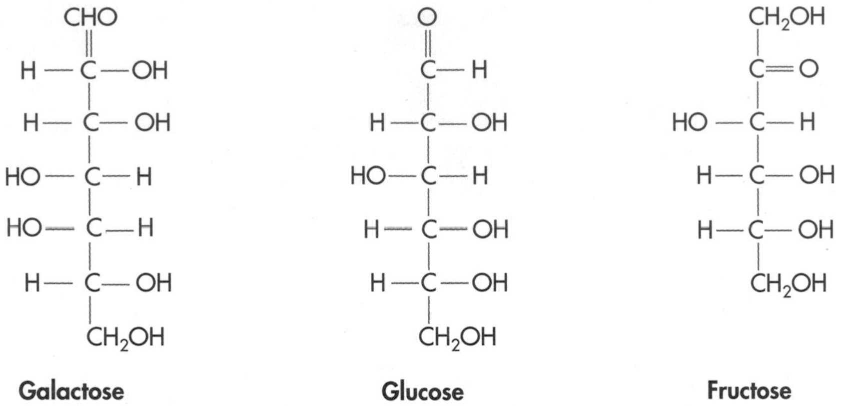

CHO
$\|$
H — C — OH
$|$
H — C — OH
$|$
HO — C — H
$|$
HO — C — H
$|$
H — C — OH
$|$
CH$_2$OH

Galactose

O
$\|$
C — H
$|$
H — C — OH
$|$
HO — C — H
$|$
H — C — OH
$|$
H — C — OH
$|$
CH$_2$OH

Glucose

CH$_2$OH
$|$
C = O
$|$
HO — C — H
$|$
H — C — OH
$|$
H — C — OH
$|$
CH$_2$OH

Fructose

commercial pet foods. Cereal grains such as corn, wheat, sorghum, barley, and rice are the major ingredients that provide this starch. Glycogen is the storage form of carbohydrate in the body. It is found in the liver and muscle, and it functions to help maintain normal glucose homeostasis in the body. Dextrins are polysaccharide compounds that are formed as intermediate products in the breakdown of starch. They are created during normal digestive processes in the body and through the commercial processing of some foods. The monosaccharide units found in starch, glycogen, and dextrin molecules have an alpha-configuration and are linked together by alpha-bonds. This type of bond can be readily hydrolyzed by the endogenous enzymes of the gastrointestinal tract and yields monosaccharide units upon either digestion or chemical hydrolysis.

Dietary fiber is plant material that consists primarily of several forms of carbohydrate. The major carbohydrate components of dietary fiber include cellulose, hemicellulose, pectin, and the plant gums and mucilages. Lignin, a large phenylpropane polymer, is the only noncarbohydrate component of fiber. Plant fiber differs from starch and glycogen in that its monosaccharide units have a beta-configuration and are linked together by beta-bonds. These bonds resist digestion by the endogenous enzymes of the gastrointestinal tract. As a result, dietary fiber cannot be broken down to monosaccharide units for absorption in the small intestine.

Although dogs and cats do not directly digest dietary fiber, certain microbes found in the large intestine (colon) are able to break down fiber to varying degrees. This bacterial fermentation produces short-chain fatty acids (SCFAs) and other end products. The SCFAs that are produced in greatest abundance are acetate, propionate, and butyrate. The magnitude of bacterial digestion depends on factors such as the type of fiber present in the diet, the gastrointestinal transit time, and the intake of other dietary constituents.[26] For example, in dogs and cats, pectin and other

TABLE 2-1

Dietary Fiber Fermentation in Dogs

Fiber Type	Solubility	Fermentability
Beet pulp	Low	Moderate
Cellulose	Low	Low
Rice bran	Low	Moderate
Gum arabic	High	Moderate
Pectin	Low	High
Carboxymethylcellulose	High	Low
Methylcellulose	High	Low
Cabbage fiber	Low	High
Guar gum	High	High
Locust bean gum	High	Low
Xanthan gum	High	Moderate

From Reinhart GA, Sunvold GD: In vitro fermentation as a predictor of fiber utilization. In *Recent advances in canine and feline nutritional research: proceedings of the 1996 Iams International Nutrition Symposium,* Wilmington, Ohio, 1996, Orange Frazer Press.

soluble fibers are highly fermentable, beet pulp is moderately fermentable, and cellulose is nonfermentable (Table 2-1). Ruminants and herbivorous animals are able to derive a significant amount of energy from the SCFAs produced by the bacterial fermentation of fiber. However, nonherbivores, such as the dog and the cat, cannot do this because of the relatively short and simple structure of their large intestine. Although SCFAs are produced in these species, there is no mechanism for the absorption of large amounts of SCFAs in the large intestine. Therefore the total energy balance of dogs and cats is not significantly affected by the production of SCFAs from dietary fiber.

However, the SCFAs that are produced from fiber are an important energy source for the epithelial cells lining the gastrointestinal tract in dogs and cats. The enterocytes and colonocytes of the large intestine are active cells that have a high turnover rate and rely on SCFAs as a significant energy source. Recent research has shown that dogs that are fed diets containing moderately fermentable fiber have increased colon weights, mucosal surface area, and mucosal hypertrophy when compared with dogs fed a diet containing a nonfermentable fiber source (Table 2-2).[27] These changes provide a measure of the absorptive capacity of the colon and indicate increased cellular activity and health. Although a highly fermentable fiber source has similar effects on colon weight and morphology, diets containing this type of fiber result in poor stool quality. It appears that the best fiber sources for companion animals are those that are moderately fermentable and provide adequate levels of SCFAs for the intestinal mucosa.[27,28,29] Fiber in the diets of dogs and cats also functions as an aid in the proper functioning of the gastrointestinal tract and as a dietary diluent that decreases the total energy density of the diet (see Section 2, p. 92, and also Section 5, pp. 324-326).

TABLE 2-2

Effects of Fiber Source on the Canine Colon

	Cellulose	Beet Pulp	Pectin/Gum Arabic	Interpretation
Colon weight (g/kg body weight)	6.09	6.52	6.62	More is better
Surface: area ratio	0.146	0.156	0.154	More is better
Cryptitis (number per five dogs)	4	1	3	Less is better
DNA content (microgram [μg]/mg)	47.4	40.4	38.4	Less is better

Data from Reinhart GA, Moxley RA, Clemens ET: Dietary fibre source and its effects on colonic microstructure and histopathology of Beagle dogs, *J Nutr* 124:2701S-2703S, 1994.

In the body, carbohydrate has several functions. The monosaccharide glucose is an important energy source for many tissues. A constant supply of glucose is necessary for the proper functioning of the central nervous system (CNS), and the glycogen present in the heart muscle is an important emergency source of energy for the heart. Glycogen in the liver and muscle can be hydrolyzed to supply additional carbohydrate fuel to cells when circulating glucose is low. Carbohydrate also supplies carbon skeletons for the formation of nonessential amino acids and is needed for the synthesis of other essential body compounds such as glucuronic acid, heparin, chondroitin sulfate, the immunopolysaccharides, deoxyribonucleic acid (DNA), and ribonucleic acid (RNA). When conjugated with proteins or lipids, some carbohydrates also become important structural components in the body's tissues.

Dietary carbohydrate provides animals with a source of energy and assists in proper gastrointestinal tract functioning. Only a limited amount of carbohydrate can be stored in the body as glycogen, so when dietary carbohydrate is consumed in excess of the body's energy needs, most is metabolized to body fat for energy storage. Therefore consumption of dietary carbohydrate in excess of an animal's energy needs can lead to increased body fat and obesity. In addition to its function in supplying energy to the body, digestible carbohydrate also has a protein-sparing effect. Just as animals eat to meet their energy needs, the body satisfies its energy requirement before using energy-containing nutrients in the diet for other purposes. If adequate carbohydrate is supplied in the diet, protein will be spared from being used for energy and can then be used for tissue repair and growth. Although dietary fiber does not contribute appreciably to energy balance in dogs and cats, a moderate level in the diet is beneficial. Plant fiber provides SCFAs to cells lining the intestine, helps to stimulate normal peristalsis, provides bulk to intestinal contents, and reduces gastrointestinal transit time (see Section 2, p. 92).

3

Fats

Dietary fat is part of a heterogeneous group of compounds known as the *lipids*. These compounds are classified together because of their solubility in organic solvents and their insolubility in water. They can be further categorized into simple lipids, compound lipids, and derived lipids. The simple lipids include the triglycerides, which are the most common form of fat present in the diet, and the waxes. Triglycerides are made up of three fatty acids linked to one molecule of glycerol (Figure 3-1), and waxes contain a greater number of fatty acids linked to a long-chain alcohol molecule. Compound lipids are composed of a lipid, such as a fatty acid, linked to a nonlipid molecule. Lipoproteins, which function to carry fat in the bloodstream, are a type of compound lipid. The derived lipids include sterol compounds, such as cholesterol, and the fat-soluble vitamins.

Triglyceride is the most important type of fat in the diet; it can be differentiated in foods according to the types of fatty acids that each triglyceride contains. Fatty acids vary in carbon-chain length and may be saturated, monounsaturated, or polyunsaturated. Most food triglycerides contain predominantly long-chain fatty acids (with an even number of carbon atoms ranging between 16 and 26). Two exceptions are butter and coconut oil, which contain appreciable amounts of short-chain fatty acids (SCFAs). Saturated fatty acids contain no double bonds between carbon atoms and thus are "saturated" with hydrogen atoms. Monounsaturated fatty acids have one double bond, and polyunsaturated fatty acids (PUFAs) contain two or more double bonds (Figure 3-2). In general, the triglycerides in animal fats contain a higher percentage of saturated fatty acids than do those in vegetable fats. Most plant oils, with the exception of palm, olive, and coconut oils, contain between 80% and 90% unsaturated fat; animal fats contain between 50% and 60% unsaturated fat.[7]

Fat has numerous functions within the body. Triglycerides are the body's primary form of stored energy. Major depots of fat accumulation are present under the skin (as subcutaneous fat), around the vital organs, and in the membranes surrounding the intestines. Some of these depots can be readily observed in obese dogs and cats. Fat depots have an extensive blood and nerve supply and are in a

FIGURE **3-1**

Triglyceride structure.

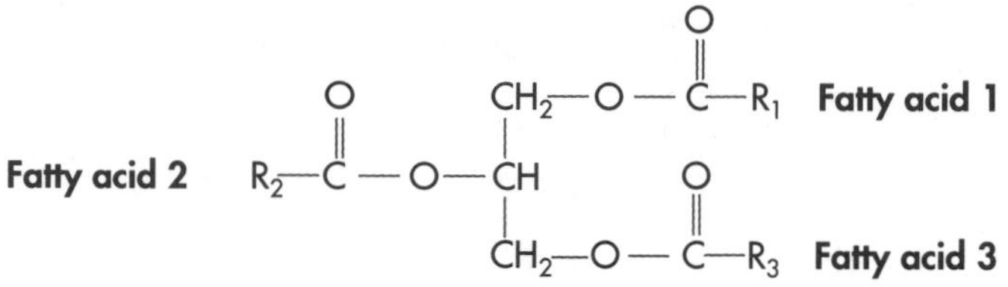

FIGURE **3-2**

Types of fatty acids.

Saturated

Lauric acid

CH_3—CH_2—CH_2—CH_2—CH_2—CH_2—CH_2—CH_2—CH_2—CH_2—CH_2—COOH

Monounsaturated

Palmitoleic acid

CH_3—CH_2—CH_2—CH_2—CH_2—CH_2—CH=CH—CH_2—CH_2—CH_2—CH_2—CH_2—CH_2—CH_2—COOH

Polyunsaturated

Linoleic acid

CH_3—CH_2—CH_2—CH_2—CH_2—CH=CH—CH_2—CH=CH—CH_2—CH_2—CH_2—CH_2—CH_2—CH_2—CH_2—COOH

Alpha-linolenic acid

CH_3—CH_2—CH=CH—CH_2—CH=CH—CH_2—CH=CH—CH_2—CH_2—CH_2—CH_2—CH_2—CH_2—CH_2—COOH

Arachidonic acid

CH_3—CH_2—CH_2—CH_2—CH_2—CH=CH—CH_2—CH=CH—CH_2—CH=CH—CH_2—CH=CH—CH_2—CH_2—CH_2—COOH

constant state of flux, providing energy in times of need and storage in times of energy surplus. They also serve as insulators, protecting the body from heat loss, and as a protective layer that guards against physical injury to the vital organs. Although animals have a very limited capacity to store carbohydrate in the form of glycogen, they have an almost limitless capacity to store surplus energy in the form of fat.

In addition to providing energy, fat has numerous metabolic and structural functions. Fat insulation surrounds myelinated nerve fibers and aids in the transmission of nerve impulses. Phospholipids and glycolipids serve as structural components for cell membranes and participate in the transport of nutrients and metabolites across these membranes. Lipoproteins provide for the transport of fats through the bloodstream. Cholesterol is used by the body to form the bile salts necessary for proper fat digestion and absorption, and it is also a precursor for the steroid hormones. Along with other lipids, cholesterol forms a protective layer in the skin that prevents excessive water loss and the invasion of foreign substances. The essential fatty acid (EFA) arachidonic acid is the precursor of a group of physiologically and pharmacologically active compounds called *prostacyclins, prostaglandins, leukotrienes,* and *thromboxanes.* These compounds perform extensive hormone-like actions in the body and are involved in processes such as vasodilation and vasoconstriction, muscle contraction, blood pressure homeostasis, gastric acid secretion, regulation of body temperature, regulation of blood clotting mechanisms, and control of inflammation.

In the diet, fat provides the most concentrated form of energy of all the nutrients. Although the gross energy (GE) of protein and carbohydrate is approximately 5.65 and 4.15 kilocalories per gram (kcal/g), the GE of fat is 9.4 kcal/g. In addition to containing more energy, the digestibility of fat is also usually higher than that of protein and carbohydrate. When mixtures of plant and animal fat were fed to adult dogs, estimates of apparent fat digestibility ranged between 80% and 95%.[30] A second study reported that the apparent digestibility of the fat in several commercially prepared dry-type dog foods varied between 70% and 90%.[31] Within each brand of food, the apparent fat digestibility was consistently higher than either protein or carbohydrate digestibility. Therefore increasing the percentage of fat in a pet's diet provides a very concentrated, readily digested source of energy that substantially increases the caloric density of the food.

Dietary fat also provides a source of EFAs and acts as a carrier that allows the absorption of the fat-soluble vitamins. The body has a physiological requirement for two distinct families of EFAs, the n-6 and the n-3 series.[32] This terminology denotes the position of the first double bond in the molecule, counting from the terminal (methyl) end of the chain. The most important fatty acid of the n-6 series is linoleic acid (see Figure 3-2). In most animals, gamma-linolenic acid and arachidonic acid can be synthesized from linoleic acid by alternating desaturation and elongation reactions. Therefore if adequate linoleic acid is provided in the diet, there is not a dietary requirement for gamma-linolenic acid or arachidonic acid. Although the dog is able to synthesize these fatty acids, the cat is one of the few species that requires a dietary source of arachidonic acid, even when adequate linoleic acid is present in the diet (see Section 2, pp. 94-95). In the n-3 family, alpha-linolenic acid also appears to have EFA properties.[33] Beneficial effects of n-3 fatty acids have been seen when these compounds are included in the diet at nutritional levels and balanced with n-6 fatty acid content. These effects relate to the fatty acid composition of cell membranes and the production of eicosanoids. When increased proportions of n-3 fatty acids are fed, proinflammatory compounds are minimized; feeding a high ratio of n-6 to n-3 fatty acids (a ratio of 25:1 or greater) causes increased production of proinflammatory eicosanoids (see Section 6, pp. 436-438).

All of the EFAs are polyunsaturated. Linoleic acid and the linolenic acids contain 18 carbon atoms and 2 and 3 double bonds, respectively. Arachidonic acid contains 20 carbon atoms and 4 double bonds (see Figure 3-2). In most animals the best sources of linoleic acid are vegetable oils such as corn, soybean, and safflower oils. Poultry fat and pork fat also contain appreciable amounts of linoleic acid, but beef tallow and butter fats contain very little. Arachidonic acid, on the other hand, is found only in animal fats. Some fish oils are rich in this EFA, and pork fat and poultry fat also supply a small amount.[7]

Fat in the diets of companion animals also plays a role in contributing to the palatability and texture of food. This is obviously a critical function because no pet food, regardless of how well-formulated it is, can be nutritious if it is not eaten. A study conducted with cats found that diets containing 25% to 40% fat were preferred to low-fat diets, but increasing the fat content further tended to decrease the diet's acceptability.[34] This effect of dietary fat is complicated by the fact that as the fat content in the diet increases, so does energy density. Animals require decreased quantities of calorie-dense foods to satisfy their energy requirements. However, the increased palatability of foods high in fat can encourage some pets to overconsume. Therefore, although fat does lend increased palatability to a diet, this effect can rapidly lead to overeating as the energy density of the diet rises. For this reason, well-balanced pet foods that are energy-dense and contain moderate to high levels of fat must often be fed on a portion-controlled basis.

4

Protein and Amino Acids

Proteins are complex molecules that, like carbohydrates and fats, contain carbon, hydrogen, and oxygen. In addition, all proteins contain the element nitrogen, and the majority contain sulfur. All proteins contain approximately 16% nitrogen. This consistency has resulted in the development of the nitrogen balance test, which is used to estimate an animal's body protein status. Nitrogen balance tests measure intake and excretion of nitrogen in animals that are fed a test diet. Net loss or gain of nitrogen then indicates increases or decreases in total body protein reserves (see Section 2, p. 99). Amino acids are the basic units of proteins and are held together by peptide linkages to form long protein chains (Figures 4-1 and 4-2). Proteins can range in size from several amino acids to large, complex molecules that consist of several intricately folded peptide chains, and they can be classified as either simple or complex forms. Once hydrolysis begins, simple proteins yield only amino acids or their derivatives. Examples include albumin in blood plasma, lactalbumin in milk, zein in corn, and the structural proteins keratin, collagen, and elastin. Complex or conjugated proteins are made up of a simple protein combined with a nonprotein molecule. Some types of complex proteins include the nucleoproteins, glycoproteins, and phosphoproteins.

Proteins in the body have numerous functions. They are the major structural components of hair, feathers, skin, nails, tendons, ligaments, and cartilage. The fibrous protein collagen is the basic material that forms most of the connective tissue throughout the body. Contractile proteins such as myosin and actin are involved in regulating muscle action. All of the enzymes that catalyze the body's essential metabolic reactions and are essential for nutrient digestion and assimilation are also protein molecules. Many hormones that control the homeostatic mechanisms of various systems in the body are composed of protein; for example, insulin and glucagon are two protein hormones involved in the control of normal blood glucose levels. Proteins found in the blood act as important carrier substances. These substances include hemoglobin, which carries oxygen to tissues; transferrin, which transports iron; and retinol-binding protein, which carries vitamin A. In addition to their transport functions, plasma proteins also contribute to the regulation of acid-

FIGURE 4-1

Peptide linkage.

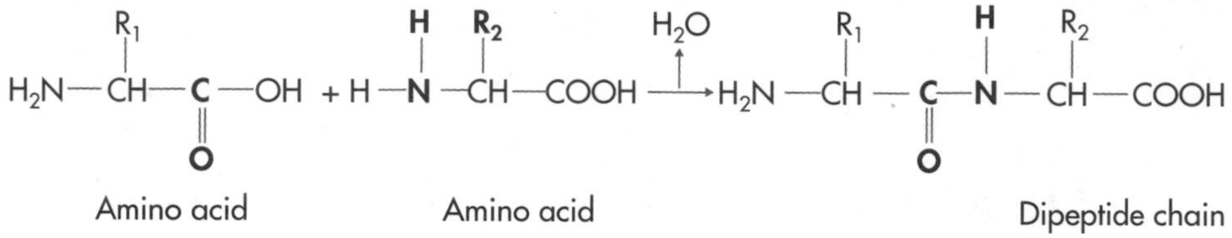

Amino acid — Amino acid — Dipeptide chain

FIGURE 4-2

Simple protein chain.

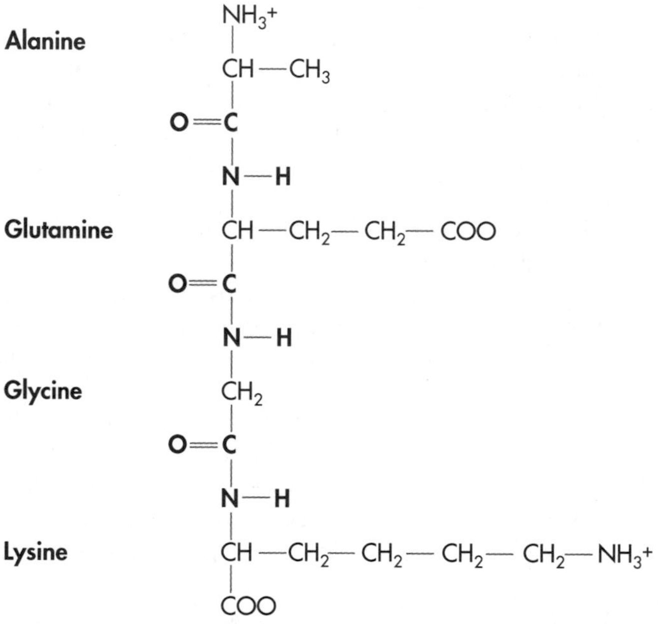

base balance. Finally, the body's immune system relies on protein substances; the antibodies that maintain the body's resistance to disease are all composed of large protein molecules.

Protein present in the body is not static; it is in a constant state of flux involving degradation and synthesis. Although tissues vary greatly in their rate of turnover, all protein molecules in the body are eventually catabolized and replaced. During growth and reproduction, additional protein is needed for the accretion of new tissue. A regular influx of protein and nitrogen, supplied by the diet, is necessary to maintain normal metabolic processes and provide for tissue maintenance and growth. The body has the ability to synthesize new proteins from amino acids, pro-

BOX 4-1

Essential and Nonessential Amino Acids for Dogs and Cats

Essential Amino Acids	Nonessential Amino Acids
Arginine	Alanine
Histidine	Asparagine
Isoleucine	Aspartate
Leucine	Cysteine
Lysine	Glutamate
Methionine	Glutamine
Phenylalanine	Glycine
Taurine (cats only)	Hydroxylysine
Tryptophan	Hydroxyproline
Threonine	Proline
Valine	Serine
	Tyrosine

vided that all of the necessary amino acids are available to the tissue cells. At the tissue and cellular level it is inconsequential whether the amino acids that are present were synthesized by the body, supplied from the diet as single amino acid units, or supplied from the diet in the form of intact protein. Therefore it is correct to state that the body does not really have a protein requirement per se but rather has a requirement for certain amino acids and a level of nitrogen. This requirement is still addressed as a protein requirement in the diet because most practical diets contain intact protein sources, not individual amino acids.

There are 22 alpha-amino acids found in protein chains. The term *alpha* denotes the attachment of the amino group (NH₂) to the first (alpha-) carbon in the molecule. Of these 22 alpha-amino acids, if an adequate source of nitrogen is supplied in the diet, dogs and cats are able to synthesize 12 at a sufficient rate to meet the body's needs for growth, performance, and maintenance. These are called the *nonessential,* or *dispensable, amino acids,* and they may be either supplied in the diet or synthesized by the body. The remaining 10 amino acids cannot be synthesized at a rate that is sufficient to meet the body's needs. These are the *essential amino acids,* and they must be supplied in the pet's diet. In addition to these 10, the cat has an additional requirement for taurine, a beta-sulfonic acid (see Section 2, pp. 108-111). The essential and nonessential amino acids are listed in Box 4-1.

Dietary protein serves several important functions. It provides the essential amino acids, which are used for protein synthesis in the growth and repair of tissue, and it is the body's principal source of nitrogen. Nitrogen is essential for the synthesis of the nonessential amino acids and of other nitrogen-containing molecules, such as nucleic acids, purines, pyrimidines, and certain neurotransmitter substances. Amino acids supplied by dietary protein can also be metabolized for energy. The gross energy (GE) of amino acids is 5.65 kilocalories per gram (kcal/g).

BOX 4-2

Methods to Determine Protein Quality

Chemical Score

$$\frac{\text{Limiting amino acid in the test protein (\%)}}{\text{Particular amino acid in the reference protein (\%)}}$$

Essential Amino Acid Index (EAAI)

$$\left.\frac{\text{Amino acid in the test protein (\%)}}{\text{Same amino acid in the reference protein (\%)}}\right\} \text{Summed for all essential amino acids}$$

Total Essential Amino Acid Content (E/T)

$$\frac{\text{Amount of nitrogen from essential amino acids in the protein source}}{\text{Amount of total nitrogen in the protein source}}$$

Protein Efficiency Ratio (PER)

$$\frac{\text{Weight gained by animals (g)}}{\text{Protein consumed by animals (total g)}}$$

Biological Value (BV)

$$\frac{\text{Food nitrogen} - (\text{fecal nitrogen} + \text{urinary nitrogen})}{\text{Food nitrogen} - \text{fecal nitrogen}}$$

Net Protein Utilization (NPU)

BV of protein × Digestibility of protein

When fecal and urinary losses are accounted for, the metabolizable energy (ME) of protein in dog and cat diets is approximately 3.5 kcal/g, approximately the same amount of energy that is supplied by dietary carbohydrate. Animals are unable to store excess amino acids. Surplus amino acids are used either directly for energy or are converted to glycogen or fat for energy storage. An ancillary function of the protein in dog and cat diets is to provide a source of flavor. Different flavors are created when food proteins are cooked in the presence of carbohydrate and fat.[35] In general, as the protein content of a diet increases, so does its palatability and acceptability.

The degree to which a dog or cat is able to use dietary protein as a source of amino acids and nitrogen is affected by both the digestibility and the quality of the protein included in the diet. Proteins that are highly digestible and contain all of the essential amino acids in their proper proportions relative to the animal's needs are considered high-quality proteins. In contrast, those that are either low in digestibility or limiting in one or more of the essential amino acids are of lower quality. The higher the quality of a protein in a diet, the less quantity will be needed by the animal to meet all of its essential amino acid needs. Various methods for evaluating the protein quality in foods have been developed (Box 4-2). Each of these methods has specific advantages and disadvantages with respect to efficacy of evaluating the overall quality of protein sources included in foods formulated for companion animals.

Several analytical tests predict protein quality based entirely on the protein's essential amino acid composition. *Chemical score* is an index that involves comparing the amino acid composition of a given protein source with the amino acid pattern of a reference protein of very high quality. Egg protein is typically used as the reference protein and is given a chemical score of 100. The essential amino acid that is in greatest deficit in the test protein is called the *limiting amino acid* because it will limit the body's ability to use that protein. The percentage of that amino acid present in the protein relative to the corresponding value in the reference protein determines the chemical score of the test protein. The three amino acids in food proteins that are most often limiting are methionine, tryptophan, and lysine. In some pet foods, arginine and isoleucine have also been reported to be limiting according to analysis by chemical score.[36] Although a chemical score provides useful information concerning the amino acid deficits of a protein source, its value is based entirely on the level of the most limiting amino acid in the protein and does not take into account the proportions of all of the remaining essential amino acids.

A modified version of chemical score, called the *essential amino acid index* (EAAI), measures the contribution that a protein makes to all of the essential amino acids, rather than only to the one in greatest deficit. A protein's EAAI is calculated as the geometric mean of the ratios of each of the essential amino acids in the test protein to their corresponding values in the reference protein.[37]

Finally, the *total essential amino acid content* (E/T) is calculated as the proportion of the total nitrogen in a protein source that is contributed by essential amino acids. Although chemical score and EAAI both indicate the quality of a protein's amino acid profile, the E/T measures the total quantity of essential amino acids within a particular protein source.

Estimations of protein quality from amino acid composition are helpful in assessing protein quality when combinations of different proteins are used in a food and for assessing protein sources that have been supplemented with purified amino acids. However, these tests are limited by the fact that they provide no information regarding the digestibility of a protein or the availability of its amino acids. For example, the heat used in processing can damage food protein, resulting in a decreased availability of certain amino acids. Simply using an analytical analysis based on amino acid composition would not reveal this change. Therefore a thorough assessment of a protein source ultimately requires that feeding trials be conducted in which the protein in question is fed to a predetermined number of test animals.

Protein efficiency ratio (PER) is one of the simplest and most commonly used feeding tests for measuring protein quality. Weanling male rats or growing chicks are fed an adequate diet containing the test protein for up to 28 days. Weight changes are measured and PER is calculated as the g in weight gained divided by the total g of protein consumed. The PER value indicates the ability of a protein source to be converted into tissue in a growing animal. One criticism of using PER as a measure of protein quality in dog and cat foods is that this test assumes that weight gain in growing animals is directly related to nitrogen retention. Although this has been proven to be true in rats, some investigators believe this may not be a consistent relationship in growing dogs.[34] In addition, any factor that influences the test animals' rate of growth during the study, regardless of whether it is related to protein quality, will affect the calculated PER value. One method of accounting for these problems is to include a positive and negative control group in the PER study. The positive control group is fed a diet containing a reference protein (egg), and the negative group is fed a protein-free diet. The effects of the non-protein group are subtracted from the effects in the test protein group when the study is completed.

Biological value (BV) and net protein utilization provide accurate measures of protein quality, but they are more time-consuming and labor intensive to conduct than are PER tests. BV is defined as the percentage of absorbed protein that is retained by the body. It is a measure of the ability of the body to convert absorbed amino acids into body tissue. Nitrogen balance studies must be conducted in which nitrogen from food, feces, and urine is collected and measured. Animals must be in a state of physiological maintenance, and the diet must contain adequate carbohydrate and fat to ensure that the protein in the diet is not metabolized for energy. True BV can be determined by first accounting for fecal and urinary losses of endogenous nitrogen when the animal is consuming a protein-free diet. One problem with using BV as a measurement of protein quality is that it does not account for protein digestibility. Theoretically, if the small portion of a very indigestible protein that is absorbed is used efficiently by the body, it could still have a very high BV value.

Net protein utilization (NPU) is calculated as the product of a protein's BV and its digestibility. NPU therefore measures the proportion of consumed protein that is retained by the body. A protein that is 100% digestible would have BV and NPU values that were the same. On the other hand, a poorly digested protein would have a much lower NPU value than BV value. Although BV and NPU are considered very important indicators of protein quality, data collected in nitrogen balance experiments can be affected by the level of protein in the diet, the energy intake, and the physiological state of the animal. Overall, in addition to one or more of the tests described earlier, the quality of protein in a pet food should always be assessed through trials in which the food is fed to the animals for which it was developed. Long-term effects on health and vitality must also be evaluated to fully determine the quality of a particular protein or mixture of proteins in a food.

CHAPTER

5

Vitamins

Vitamins are organic molecules that are needed in minute amounts to function as essential enzymes, enzyme precursors, or coenzymes in many of the body's metabolic processes. Although they are organic molecules, vitamins are not classified as carbohydrate, fat, or protein; they are not used as energy sources or structural compounds. With a few exceptions, most vitamins cannot be synthesized by the body and must be supplied in the food.

A general classification scheme for vitamins divides them into two groups: the fat-soluble vitamins and the water-soluble vitamins. The fat-soluble vitamins are A, D, E, and K; the water-soluble group includes vitamin C and members of the B-complex vitamin group. Fat-soluble vitamins are digested and absorbed using the same mechanisms as dietary fat, and their metabolites are excreted primarily in the feces through the bile. In contrast, most of the water-soluble vitamins are absorbed passively in the small intestine and are excreted in the urine. Excesses of fat-soluble vitamins are stored primarily in the liver. With the exception of cobalamin, the body is unable to store significant levels of the water-soluble vitamins. As a result, the fat-soluble vitamins, specifically vitamins A and D, have a much higher potential for toxicity than do the water-soluble vitamins. Similarly, because they can be stored, deficiencies of fat-soluble vitamins develop much more slowly in animals than do deficiencies of the water-soluble vitamins. A summary of food sources and signs of deficiency and excess for the vitamins is given in Table 5-1.

VITAMIN A

The general term *vitamin A* actually includes several related chemical compounds called *retinol, retinal,* and *retinoic acid.* Of these molecules, retinol is the most biologically active form. In the body, vitamin A has functions involving vision, bone growth, reproduction, and maintenance of epithelial tissue. This vitamin's role in vision is well established. In the rods of the retina, retinal combines with a protein called *opsin* to form *rhodopsin,* also known as *visual purple.* Rhodopsin is a light-sensitive pigment that enables the eye to adapt to changes in light intensity. When

TABLE 5-1

Vitamin Deficiencies, Excesses, and Major Dietary Sources

Vitamin	Deficiency	Excess	Sources
A	Impaired growth, reproductive failure, loss of epithelial integrity, dermatoses	Skeletal abnormalities, hyperesthesia	Fish liver oils, milk, liver, egg yolk
D	Rickets, osteomalacia, nutritional secondary hyperparathyroidism	Hypercalcemia, bone resorption, soft-tissue calcification	Liver, some fish, egg yolk, sunlight
E	Reproductive failure, pansteatitis in cats	Nontoxic; may increase vitamin A and D requirements	Wheat germ, corn and soybean oils
K	Increased clotting time, hemorrhage	None recorded	Green leafy plants, liver, some fish meals
Thiamin	CNS dysfunction, anorexia, weight loss	Nontoxic	Meat, wheat germ
Riboflavin	CNS dysfunction, dermatitis	Nontoxic	Milk, organ meats, vegetables
Niacin	Black tongue disease	Nontoxic	Meat, legumes, grains
Pyridoxine	Microcytic hypochromic anemia	None recorded	Organ meats, fish, wheat germ
Pantothenic acid	Anorexia, weight loss	None recorded	Liver, kidney, dairy products, legumes
Biotin	Dermatitis	Nontoxic	Eggs, liver, milk, legumes
Folic acid	Anemia, leukopenia	Nontoxic	Liver, kidney, green leafy vegetables
Cobalamin	Anemia	Nontoxic	Meat, fish, poultry
Choline	Neurological dysfunction, fatty liver	Diarrhea	Egg yolk, organ meats, legumes, dairy products
C	Not required by dogs and cats	Nontoxic	Citrus fruit, dark green vegetables

exposed to light, rhodopsin splits into retinal and opsin, and the energy that is released produces nerve transmissions to the optic nerve. In the dark, rhodopsin can then be regenerated by the combination of new retinal and opsin molecules. During periods of vitamin A deficiency, less retinal is available to regenerate rhodopsin; thus the rods of the eye become increasingly sensitive to light changes, which eventually results in night blindness.

Vitamin A is also essential for the formation and maintenance of healthy epithelial tissue. This tissue includes the skin and the mucous membranes lining the respiratory and gastrointestinal tracts. Vitamin A is believed to be necessary for both the proliferation and differentiation of cells and for the production of the mucoproteins found in the mucus produced by some types of epithelial cells.[38] Mucous secretions of epithelial tissue maintain the integrity of the epithelium and provide a barrier against bacterial invasion. In the absence of vitamin A, the differentiation of new epithelial cells beyond the squamous type to mature mucus-secreting cells fails to occur, and normal epithelial cells are replaced by dysfunctional, stratified, keratinized cells.[39] Epithelial tissue that does not function properly leads to lesions in the epithelium and increased susceptibility to infection.

Normal skeletal and tooth development and reproductive performance also depend on vitamin A. The vitamin's role in bone growth appears to involve the activity of the osteoclasts and osteoblasts of the epithelial cartilage and may be related to cellular division and the maintenance of cell membranes through glycoprotein synthesis. Experiments with laboratory animals have shown that vitamin A is also essential for spermatogenesis in males and normal estrous cycles in females.[38]

The origin of all vitamin A is the carotenoids, which are synthesized by plant cells. Carotenoids are dark red pigments that provide the deep yellow/orange color to many plants. Vegetables such as carrots and sweet potatoes contain high amounts of these compounds. Deep green vegetables also contain these pigments, but their color is masked by the deep green color of chlorophyll. When animals consume the carotenoids in plants, an enzyme located in the intestinal mucosa converts these compounds (which are commonly called *provitamin A*) to active vitamin A (Figure 5-1). The active vitamin is then absorbed and stored in the liver.

Although several different carotenoids are capable of providing vitamin A, beta-carotene is the most plentiful in foods and has the highest biological activity. Animal products do not contain carotenoids but can provide active vitamin A when included in the diet. Fish liver oils contain the highest amounts, and more common foods such as milk, liver, and egg yolk also contain vitamin A.

Like most animals, dogs are capable of converting carotenoids to active vitamin A; therefore they do not require an animal source of this vitamin in the diet. However, the enzyme that is essential for splitting the beta-carotene molecule is either absent or grossly deficient in the domestic cat. As a result, the cat is unable to convert carotenoid pigments to vitamin A and must receive a source of preformed vitamin A in the diet (see Section 2, pp. 117-119). In addition to providing a source of vitamin A, carotenoid pigments also have a role in modulating immune response. Recent studies have shown that both dogs and cats readily absorb beta-carotene and a related carotenoid called *lutein,* and that these pigments may have a function in cell-mediated and humoral immune response in these species.[39]

VITAMIN D

Vitamin D consists of a group of sterol compounds that regulate calcium and phosphorus metabolism in the body. As with vitamin A, there are provitamin forms of this vitamin. These are vitamin D_2 (ergocalciferol) and vitamin D_3 (cholecalciferol). Vitamin D_2 is formed when the compound ergosterol, which is found in many plants, is exposed to ultraviolet (UV) radiation. This conversion occurs only in harvested or injured plants, not in living plant tissue. Therefore this form of vitamin

FIGURE 5-1

Conversion of beta-carotene to vitamin A.

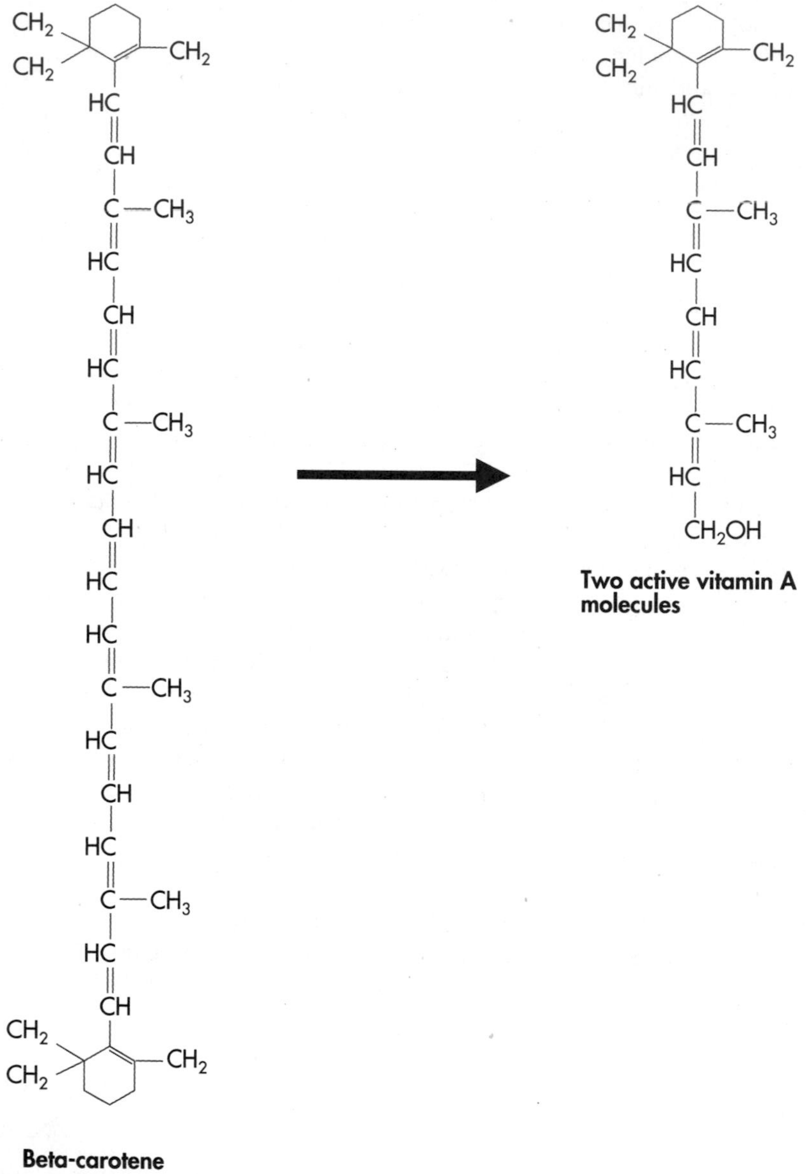

Beta-carotene

Two active vitamin A molecules

D is only of significance to ruminants and nonruminant herbivores that are consuming sun-dried or irradiated plant materials. The second form of provitamin D, vitamin D_3, is the form that is of greatest nutritional importance to omnivores and carnivores, such as the dog and cat. It is synthesized by the body when

7-dehydrocholesterol, a compound found in the skin of animals, is exposed to UV light from the sun. This form of vitamin D can be obtained either through synthesis in the skin or from the consumption of animal products that contain cholecalciferol. Because active vitamin D is synthesized by the body and because of the regulatory functions that it performs within the body, some controversy exists regarding its classification. Although some scientists believe that vitamin D should be considered a hormone, others continue to classify it as a vitamin. Regardless of its categorization, precursors of vitamin D are obtained through the diet, and vitamin D's functions are intricately involved with normal calcium and phosphorus homeostasis in the body.

Both ingested and endogenous vitamin D_3 (cholecalciferol) are stored in liver, muscle, and adipose tissue. Cholecalciferol is an inactive storage form of vitamin D. To become active, it must first be transported from the skin or intestines to the liver; there it is hydroxylated to 25-hydroxycholecalciferol. This compound is then transported through the bloodstream to the kidneys, where it is further converted to one of several possible metabolites. Metabolites include 1,25-dihydroxycholecalciferol, also called *calcitriol,* which is the most active form of vitamin D (Figure 5-2). The conversion of 25-hydroxycholecalciferol to calcitriol in the kidneys occurs in response to elevated parathyroid hormone (PTH), which is released from the parathyroid gland in response to decreasing serum calcium. A decrease in serum phosphorus also stimulates the formation of active vitamin D in the kidneys. Although inactive vitamin D is considered a vitamin, calcitriol is often classified as a hormone because it is produced in the body and because of its mechanism of action in the body.

Active vitamin D functions in normal bone tissue development and maintenance and is an important component in the homeostasis of the body's calcium and phosphorus pools. These effects are mediated through the influence of vitamin D on calcium and phosphorus absorption from the gastrointestinal tract and their deposition in bone tissue. At the site of the intestine, vitamin D stimulates the synthesis of calcium-binding protein, which is necessary for the efficient absorption of dietary calcium and phosphorus. Vitamin D also affects normal bone growth and calcification by acting with PTH to mobilize calcium from bone and by causing an increase in phosphate reabsorption in the kidneys. The net effect of vitamin D's actions in intestines, bones, and kidneys is an increase in plasma calcium and phosphorus to the level that is necessary to allow for the normal mineralization and remodeling of bone. A deficiency of vitamin D causes impaired bone mineralization and results in osteomalacia in adult animals and rickets in growing animals (see Section 2, pp. 119-121).

Sources of vitamin D for dogs and cats are varied. Endogenous vitamin D is produced when exposure to sunlight results in the conversion of the precursor 7-dehydrocholesterol in the skin to cholecalciferol. Irradiation is most effective in animals that have light-colored skin and sparse hair coats. Darkly pigmented skin and heavy coats can substantially decrease an animal's ability to produce endogenous vitamin D. The effectiveness of sunlight also depends on the intensity and wavelength of the light that is absorbed and the amount of time that the animal

FIGURE **5-2**

Conversion of 7-dehydrocholesterol to active vitamin D.

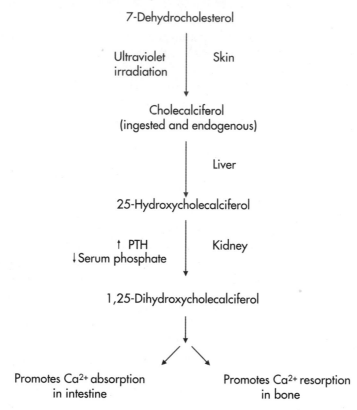

spends outside. Sunlight during the summer months and at high altitudes is most effective as a stimulus for vitamin D production. In general, most natural food substances contain very little vitamin D, although egg yolks, liver, and certain types of fish contain moderate amounts. Among the few concentrated food sources of vitamin D are the fish liver oils, particularly cod liver oil. Because natural foods are low in this vitamin, most commercially prepared pet foods are enriched with vitamin D to ensure that dogs and cats receive adequate amounts of this vitamin, regardless of the amount of daily sunlight that they receive.

VITAMIN E

Vitamin E is made up of a group of chemically related compounds called the *tocopherols* and *tocotrienols*. Alpha-tocopherol is the most active form of vitamin E and is the compound most commonly found in pet foods. Several active synthetic forms of vitamin E have also been produced and are commonly included in processed foods. Within the body, vitamin E is found in at least small amounts in almost all tissues; the liver is able to store appreciable amounts.

Vitamin E's chief function in the diet and in the body is as a potent antioxidant. Unsaturated fatty acids that are present in foods and in the lipid membranes of the body's cells are very vulnerable to oxidative damage. Vitamin E interrupts the oxidation of these fats by donating electrons to the free radicals that induce lipid peroxidation (see Section 3, Figure 16-2, p. 181). Peroxidation of the body's lipids can destroy the structural integrity of cell membranes, resulting in impairment of normal cellular functioning. Peroxidation of fats in foods causes rancidity and a loss of the nutritional value of the food's essential fatty acids (EFAs). In addition to its action on polyunsaturated fatty acids (PUFAs), vitamin E also protects vitamin A and the sulfur-containing amino acids from oxidative damage. As a direct result of these functions, an animal's requirement for dietary vitamin E depends on the level of PUFAs in its diet. Increasing PUFA levels in pet foods causes a concomitant increase in a dog's or cat's vitamin E requirement.

A second important interrelationship exists between the trace mineral selenium and vitamin E. Selenium is a cofactor for the enzyme glutathione peroxidase, which functions to reduce the peroxides that are formed during the process of fatty acid oxidation. The inactivation of these peroxides by glutathione peroxidase protects the cell membranes from further oxidative damage. By preventing the oxidation of cell-membrane fatty acids and the formation of peroxides, vitamin E spares selenium. Likewise, selenium creates a similar effect and is able to reduce an animal's vitamin E requirement.

In nature, vitamin E is synthesized by a variety of different plants. Food sources that are rich in the tocopherols include wheat germ and the oils of corn, cottonseed, soybean, and sunflower. In general, the vitamin E content of an oil increases along with its linoleic acid concentration. Most animal food sources supply only limited amounts of vitamin E. Egg yolk can contain a moderate amount of vitamin E depending on the diet of the hen, but milk and dairy products are very poor sources. The vitamin E in commercially prepared foods is susceptible to oxidation and destruction along with the fat in the diet. Therefore proper storage of foods is necessary both to prevent oxidative changes to fat and to maintain proper vitamin E levels.

VITAMIN K

Vitamin K comprises a group of compounds called the quinones. Vitamin K_1 (phylloquinone) occurs naturally in green plants, and vitamin K_2 (menaquinone) is synthesized by bacteria in the large intestine. Several synthetic analogues have also been prepared. Menadione (vitamin K_3), the most common form of synthetic vitamin K, has a vitamin activity two to three times higher than that of natural K_1. Like all animals, dogs and cats have a metabolic need for vitamin K. However, at least a proportion of this requirement can be obtained from bacterial synthesis of the vitamin in the intestine.

The best-known function of vitamin K is its role in the blood clotting mechanism. Specifically, it is required for the liver's synthesis of prothrombin (factor II) and three other clotting factors—factors VII, IX, and X—in the liver. Vitamin K acts as a cofactor for the enzyme that carboxylates glutamic acid residues in a prothrombin-precursor protein to form gamma-carboxyglutamic acid. The conversion of these amino acids facilitates the binding of prothrombin to calcium and phospholipids, a process necessary for the occurrence of normal blood clotting. It appears that vitamin K has a similar role in the activation of other proteins that contain glutamic acid residues in bone and kidney tissue.[40]

Vitamin K is found in green, leafy plants such as spinach, kale, cabbage, and cauliflower. In general, animal sources contain lower amounts of vitamin K; liver, egg, and certain fish meals are fairly good sources. The synthesis of vitamin K by bacteria in the large intestine of dogs and cats can contribute at least a portion, if not all, of the daily requirement in these species. Therefore a dietary supply of this vitamin only becomes significant when bacterial populations in the large intestine are reduced, such as during medical treatment with certain types of antibiotics, or when there is interference with the absorption or use of vitamin K from bacterial sources.

B-COMPLEX VITAMINS

The B-complex vitamins are water-soluble vitamins that were originally grouped together because of similar metabolic functions and occurrence in foods. These nine vitamins act as coenzymes for specific cellular enzymes that are involved in energy metabolism and tissue synthesis. Coenzymes are small organic molecules that must be present with an enzyme for a specific reaction to occur. The vitamins thiamin, riboflavin, niacin, pyridoxine, pantothenic acid, and biotin are all involved in the use of food energy. Folic acid, cobalamin, and choline are important for cell maintenance and growth and/or blood cell synthesis.

Thiamin

Thiamin, also referred to as vitamin B_1, is a component of the coenzyme thiamin pyrophosphate, which plays an important role in carbohydrate metabolism. Thiamin pyrophosphate is necessary for the decarboxylation and transketolation reactions that are involved in the use of carbohydrate for energy and conversion to fat and the metabolism of fatty acids, nucleic acids, steroids, and certain amino acids. Because of its importance in carbohydrate metabolism, an animal's thiamin requirement depends on the level of carbohydrate present in the diet. A deficiency of thiamin can significantly affect the functioning of the central nervous system (CNS) because of the system's dependency on a constant source of carbohydrate for energy. Natural food sources of thiamin include lean pork, beef, liver, wheat germ, whole grains, and legumes. Although it is present in a large variety of foods, thiamin is a heat-labile vitamin and thus readily destroyed by the high heat involved in the processing of many pet foods. To ensure adequate levels in pet foods, most companies supplement with an excess quantity of this vitamin before processing to ensure that the amount in the finished product is still sufficient. Naturally occurring thiamin deficiency is very rare in dogs and cats and is usually the result of the presence of antithiamin factors in the diet rather than an absolute vitamin deficiency (see Section 5, pp. 349-350).

Riboflavin

Riboflavin (vitamin B_2) is named for its yellow color (flavin) and because it contains the simple sugar D-ribose. It is relatively stable to heat-processing but is easily destroyed by exposure to light and irradiation. Riboflavin functions in the body as a component of two different coenzymes, flavin mononucleotide and flavin adenine dinucleotide. Both of these coenzymes are required in oxidative enzyme systems that function in the release of energy from carbohydrates, fats, and proteins, as well as in several biosynthetic pathways. Food sources of riboflavin include milk, organ meats, whole grains, and vegetables. In addition, microbial synthesis of riboflavin occurs in the large intestine of most species. The quantity that is synthesized appears to depend on both the species of animal and the level of carbohydrate that is fed.[7] However, the extent to which this source contributes to the daily riboflavin requirement of the dog and cat is unknown.

Niacin

Niacin (nicotinic acid), the third B vitamin, is closely associated with riboflavin in cellular oxidation-reduction enzyme systems. After absorption, niacin is rapidly converted by the body into nicotinamide, the metabolically active form of the vitamin. Nicotinamide is then incorporated into two different coenzymes, nicotinamide adenine dinucleotide and nicotinamide adenine dinucleotide phosphate. These coenzymes function as hydrogen-transfer agents in several enzymatic pathways involved in the use of fat, carbohydrate, and protein. Meat, legumes, and grains all contain high amounts of niacin. However, a large proportion of the niacin present in many plant sources is in a bound form and unavailable for absorption.[41] The niacin in animal sources is found primarily in an unbound, available form. In addition to consuming niacin in the diet, most animals also synthesize this vitamin as an end product of the metabolism of tryptophan, an essential amino acid. As a result, the level of tryptophan in the diet directly affects an animal's dietary requirement for niacin. Dogs are capable of synthesizing niacin from tryptophan. However, cats cannot synthesize niacin from tryptophan and must receive all of their niacin requirement from the diet.

Pyridoxine

Pyridoxine, vitamin B_6, comprises three different compounds: pyridoxine, pyridoxal, and pyridoxamine. Pyridoxal, which is a component of the coenzyme pyridoxal

5'-phosphate, is the biologically active form. This coenzyme is necessary for many of the transamination, deamination, and decarboxylation reactions of amino acid metabolism and is active to a lesser extent in the metabolism of glucose and fatty acids. Pyridoxal 5'-phosphate is also required for the synthesis of hemoglobin and the conversion of tryptophan to niacin. In the same manner that the thiamin requirement varies with the carbohydrate level in the diet, the pyridoxine requirement of an animal depends on the level of protein in the diet. Pyridoxine is widespread in foods, with organ meats, fish, wheat germ, and whole grains providing adequate amounts. Dietary deficiencies of this vitamin in dogs and cats have not been reported.

Pantothenic Acid

Pantothenic acid was named after the Greek term *pan*, meaning *all*, because this vitamin occurs in all body tissues and all forms of living tissue. Once absorbed, pantothenic acid is phosphorylated by adenosine triphosphate (ATP) to form coenzyme A. This coenzyme is essential to the process of acetylation, a universal reaction involved in many aspects of carbohydrate, fat, and protein metabolism within the citric acid cycle. Pantothenic acid is found in virtually all foods. As a result, deficiencies of this vitamin are extremely rare. Rich sources of pantothenic acid include organ meats, such as liver and kidney; egg yolk; dairy products; and legumes.

Biotin

The vitamin biotin is a coenzyme required in several carboxylation reactions. It acts as a carbon dioxide carrier in reactions in which carbon chains are lengthened; specifically, biotin is involved in certain steps of fatty acid, nonessential amino acid, and purine synthesis. Biotin is found in many different foods, but its bioavailability varies greatly. Eggs provide a very rich source of biotin, but egg white contains a compound called *avidin*, which binds biotin and makes it unavailable for absorption. Thoroughly cooking eggs destroys avidin and allows the biotin in the yolk to be used. Other food sources of biotin include liver, milk, legumes, and nuts. Intestinal bacteria also synthesize biotin; it is believed that a large proportion, if not all, of an animal's requirement can be met from this source.[7,11] Deficiencies are not generally a problem; however, the treatment of dogs and cats with antibiotics that decrease the bacterial population of the large intestine can cause an increase in the dietary requirement for biotin.

Folic Acid

Folic acid (folacin) is active in the body as tetrahydrofolic acid. This compound functions as a methyl-transfer agent, transporting single-carbon units in a number of metabolic reactions. An important role of folic acid is its involvement in the synthesis of thymidine, a component of deoxyribonucleic acid (DNA). When folic acid is deficient in the body, the inability to produce adequate DNA leads to decreased cellular growth and maturation. This is manifested clinically as anemia and leukopenia in deficient animals. Food sources of folic acid include green, leafy vegetables and organ meats such as liver and kidney. Like several of the other B vitamins, folic acid is synthesized by the bacteria of the large intestine in dogs and cats. It appears that most, if not all, of the daily requirement of dogs and cats can be met from this source.

Cobalamin

Cobalamin (vitamin B_{12}) contains the mineral cobalt and is unique in that it is the only vitamin that contains a trace element. Similar to folic acid, cobalamin is involved in the transfer of single-carbon units during various biochemical reactions. It is also involved in fat and carbohydrate metabolism and is necessary for the synthesis of myelin. As a result, a deficiency of vitamin B_{12} leads to both anemia and impairment of neurological functioning. In most animals, absorption of cobalamin from the diet is facilitated by a protein called *intrinsic factor,* which is produced in the intestine. The absence of this factor can lead to vitamin B_{12} deficiency. Although the presence of intrinsic factor has not been demonstrated in dogs or cats, it is likely that absorption occurs through the same mechanism in these species.

Cobalamin is only found in foods of animal origin. Rich sources of cobalamin include meat, poultry, fish, and dairy products. This vitamin is also unique for a B vitamin because, once absorbed from the diet, excesses can be stored by the body. The liver is the primary storage tissue; muscle, bone, and skin also contain small amounts of cobalamin. Deficiencies of cobalamin are extremely rare as a result of the very small amounts that are needed by the body and the body's ability to store appreciable amounts of the vitamin.

Choline

The last B vitamin, choline, acts as a donor of methyl units for various metabolic reactions in the body. Choline is a precursor for the neurotransmitter substance acetylcholine and is necessary for normal fatty-acid transport within cells. Unlike other vitamins, choline is also an integral part of cellular membranes. Choline is a component of two important phospholipids—phosphatidylcholine (lecithin) and sphingomyelin. Lecithin is essential for normal cell-membrane structure and function, and sphingomyelin is found in high concentrations in nervous tissue.

The body is capable of synthesizing choline from the amino acid serine. In this reaction, methionine acts as a methyl donor; folacin and vitamin B_{12} are also necessary. It is not known if sufficient choline is produced by dogs and cats to maintain health without a dietary source of this compound. Because choline and methionine both function as methyl donors in the body, diets that are high in methionine can replace some of an animal's choline requirement. Choline is also widespread in food sources. Egg yolk, organ meats, legumes, dairy products, and whole grains all supply high amounts of choline. Because of its synthesis in the body, its presence in many foods, and the ability of methionine to spare choline, dietary deficiencies of choline have not been reported in dogs and cats.

VITAMIN C (ASCORBIC ACID)

Ascorbic acid, commonly known as vitamin C, has a chemical structure that is closely related to the monosaccharide sugars. It is synthesized from glucose by plants and most animal species, including dogs and cats. When present in foods, ascorbic acid is easily destroyed by oxidative processes. Exposure to heat, light, alkalies, oxidative enzymes, and the minerals copper and iron all contribute to losses of vitamin C activity. Oxidative loss of vitamin C is inhibited to some extent by an acid environment and by the storage of foods at low temperatures.

The body requires ascorbic acid for the hydroxylation of the amino acids proline and lysine in the formation of collagen. Collagen is the primary constituent of osteoid, dentine, and connective tissue. It is produced in quantity by osteoblasts during skeletal growth; therefore it is important for normal bone formation. When ascorbic acid is not available, the synthesis of several types of connective tissue within the body is impaired. In animal species that have a dietary requirement for vitamin C, such as humans and guinea pigs, this results in a condition called scurvy. Clinical signs of scurvy include impaired wound healing, capillary bleeding, anemia, and faulty bone formation. Bone abnormalities that are associated with scurvy are the result of impaired cartilage synthesis.

With the exception of humans and a few other animal species, all animals are capable of producing adequate levels of endogenous vitamin C and therefore do not have a dietary requirement for this vitamin. Ascorbic acid is produced in the liver from either glucose or galactose through the glucuronate pathway. The adult dog produces approximately 40 milligrams per kilogram (mg/kg) body weight of ascorbate each day.[42] This is a relatively low amount compared to other mammalian species. However, controlled research studies in the dog have shown that this species does not require an exogenous source of vitamin C for normal development and maintenance.[43,44,45] Similarly, no requirement for dietary ascorbic acid has been demonstrated to exist in the cat.[11,46]

In recent years a number of breeders, dog show enthusiasts, and pet owners have been routinely administering high levels of supplemental vitamin C to their dogs' diets in the hopes of preventing or curing certain developmental skeletal disorders. To date, no controlled research studies have been published that show any efficacy of supplemental ascorbic acid in this role; on the other hand, a substantial amount of evidence exists that directly refutes this claim.[47,48] Currently the use of high amounts of supplemental vitamin C in the diets of healthy dogs and cats is not recommended and may even be contraindicated (see Section 5, pp. 343-344).

6

Minerals

Minerals are inorganic elements that are essential for the body's metabolic processes. Only about 4% of an animal's total body weight comprises mineral matter; however, like the vitamins, the presence of these elements is essential for life. A general classification scheme divides minerals into two groups, macrominerals and microminerals. *Macrominerals* are those minerals that occur in appreciable amounts in the body and account for most of the body's mineral content. They include calcium, phosphorus, magnesium, sulfur, iron, and the electrolytes sodium, potassium, and chloride. *Microminerals,* often referred to as the *trace elements,* include a larger number of minerals that are present in the body in very small amounts. These minerals are required in very small quantities in the diet.

Minerals have a variety of functions in the body. They activate enzymatically catalyzed reactions, provide skeletal support, aid in nerve transmission and muscle contractions, serve as components of certain transport proteins and hormones, and function in maintaining water and electrolyte balance. Significant interrelationships exist among many of the mineral elements that can affect mineral absorption, metabolism, and functioning. Specifically, excesses or deficiencies of some minerals can significantly affect the body's ability to use other minerals in the diet. As a result, the level of most minerals in the diet should be considered in relation to other components of the diet, with a goal of achieving an optimal overall dietary balance. Although most of the minerals are discussed separately in this section, the importance of these interrelationships is addressed when they are of practical significance to the nutrition of dogs and cats. A summary of food sources and signs of mineral deficiency and excess is shown in Table 6-1.

CALCIUM AND PHOSPHORUS

Calcium and phosphorus are usually discussed together because their metabolism and the homeostatic mechanisms that control their levels within the body are closely interrelated. Calcium is a principal inorganic component of bone. As much as 99% of the body's calcium is found in the skeleton; the remaining 1% is

TABLE 6-1

Mineral Deficiencies, Excesses, and Major Dietary Sources

Mineral	Deficiency	Excess	Sources
Calcium	Rickets, osteomalacia, nutritional secondary hyperparathyroidism	Impaired skeletal development; contributes to other mineral deficiencies	Dairy products, poultry and meat meals, bone
Phosphorus	Same as for calcium deficiency	Causes calcium deficiency	Meat, poultry, fish
Magnesium	Soft-tissue calcification, enlargement of long bone metaphysis, neuromuscular irritability	Dietary excess unlikely; absorption is regulated according to needs	Soybeans, corn, cereal grains, bone meals
Sulfur	Not reported	Not reported	Meat, poultry, fish
Iron	Hypochromic microcytic anemia	Dietary excess unlikely; absorption is regulated according to needs	Organ meats
Copper	Hypochromic microcytic anemia, impaired skeletal growth	Inherited disorder of copper metabolism causes liver disease	Organ meats
Zinc	Dermatoses, hair depigmentation, growth retardation, reproductive failure	Causes calcium and copper deficiency	Beef liver, dark poultry meat, milk, egg yolks, legumes
Manganese	Dietary deficiency unlikely; impaired skeletal growth, reproductive failure	Dietary excess unlikely	Meat, poultry, fish
Iodine	Dietary deficiency unlikely; goiter, growth retardation, reproductive failure	Dietary excess unlikely; goiter	Fish, beef, liver
Selenium	Dietary deficiency unlikely; skeletal and cardiac myopathies	Dietary excess unlikely; necrotizing myocarditis, toxic hepatitis and nephritis	Grains, meat, poultry
Cobalt	Dietary deficiency unlikely; vitamin B_{12} deficiency, anemia	Not reported	Fish, dairy products

distributed throughout the extracellular and intracellular fluids. Phosphorus is also an important component of bone. Approximately 85% of the body's phosphorus is found in inorganic combination with calcium as hydroxyapatite in bones and teeth. Most of the remaining portion of this mineral is found (in combination with organic substances) in the soft tissues.

The calcium in bone provides structural integrity to the skeleton and also contributes to the maintenance of proper blood calcium levels through ongoing resorption and deposition. The calcium in bone tissue is not in a static state but is constantly being mobilized and deposited as bone growth and maintenance take place and as the body's needs for plasma calcium fluctuate. The level of circulating plasma calcium is strictly controlled through homeostatic mechanisms and is independent of an animal's dietary intake of calcium. Circulating calcium has essential roles in nerve impulse transmission, muscle contraction, blood coagulation, the activation of certain enzyme systems, the maintenance of normal cell-membrane permeability and transport, and cardiac function.

Phosphorus that is present in bone is found primarily in combination with calcium in the compound called hydroxyapatite. Like calcium, this phosphorus lends structural support to the skeleton and is also released into the bloodstream in response to homeostatic mechanisms. The phosphorus that is found in the soft tissues of the body has a wide number of functions and is involved in almost all of the body's metabolic processes. It is a constituent of cellular deoxyribonucleic acid (DNA) and ribonucleic acid (RNA), several B-vitamin coenzymes, and the cell membrane's phospholipids, which are important for regulating the transport of solutes into and out of cells. Phosphorus is also necessary for the phosphorylation reactions that are part of many oxidative pathways for the metabolism of the energy-containing nutrients. Phosphorus is a component of the high-energy phosphate bonds of adenosine triphosphate (ATP), adenosine diphosphate, and cyclic adenosine monophosphate.

As mentioned previously, the body has several strictly controlled homeostatic mechanisms that are designed to maintain a constant level of circulating plasma calcium. These mechanisms involve parathyroid hormone (PTH), calcitonin, and active vitamin D (calcitriol). PTH is released into the bloodstream in response to a slight decrease in plasma calcium. This hormone stimulates the synthesis of active vitamin D in the kidneys and increases the resorption of calcium and phosphorus from bone. It also works on the kidney tubules to increase calcium reabsorption and decrease phosphorus reabsorption, resulting in increased retention of calcium in the body and increased losses of urinary phosphate. In turn, the active vitamin D produced by the kidneys in response to PTH acts at the site of the intestine to increase the absorption of dietary calcium and phosphorus. In conjunction with PTH, vitamin D also enhances the mobilization of calcium from bone by increasing the activity of osteoclasts. Overall, the net action of PTH is to increase the serum concentration of calcium and decrease the serum concentration of phosphorus. The net effect of active vitamin D is to increase levels of both serum calcium and phosphorus (Figure 6-1).

When the blood calcium level is normal, PTH secretion is inhibited through a negative feedback mechanism, and calcitonin, a hormone produced by the parafollicular cells (C cells) of the thyroid gland, is released. Calcitonin functions to reduce blood calcium levels by acting primarily to increase osteoblastic activity and decrease osteoclastic activity in bone tissue. The end result is a decrease in calcium mobilization from the skeleton. Calcitonin is also released in response to

FIGURE **6-1**

Regulation of calcium and phosphorus balance.

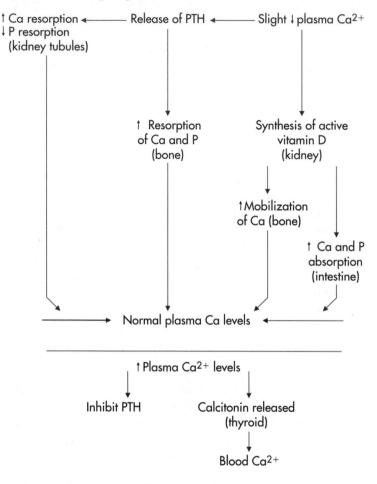

↑ Ca resorption ◄——— Release of PTH ◄——— Slight ↓ plasma Ca2+
↓ P resorption
(kidney tubules)

↑ Resorption   Synthesis of active
of Ca and P   vitamin D
(bone)   (kidney)

↑ Mobilization
of Ca (bone)

↑ Ca and P
absorption
(intestine)

Normal plasma Ca levels

↑ Plasma Ca2+ levels

Inhibit PTH   Calcitonin released
                        (thyroid)

Blood Ca2+

hypercalcemia and the release of certain hormones, such as gastrin. Under normal physiological circumstances, PTH and active vitamin D are the most important regulators of calcium homeostasis, with calcitonin playing a more minor role. However, calcitonin may be of increased importance in the normal homeostatic mechanisms of calcium regulation during growth, pregnancy, and lactation.

In addition to having common homeostatic mechanisms in the body, calcium and phosphorus also have an important relationship to each other within the diet. Once adequate levels of calcium and phosphorus have been included in the diet, it is important to consider the ratio of the amount of calcium to phosphorus. Excess dietary calcium forms an insoluble complex with phosphorus, resulting in decreased phosphorus absorption. Similarly, high levels of phosphorus or phytate in the diet can inhibit calcium absorption. Phytate is a phosphorus-containing compound found in the outer husks of cereal grains. Although this compound is high in phosphorus, the mineral is poorly available to the body. The recommended ratio of calcium to phosphorus in pet foods is between 1.2:1 to 1.4:1 in dogs and 0.9:1 to 1.1:1 in cats.[7,11,49] Feeding animals foods that have an improper calcium:phosphorus ratio or supplementing balanced foods with high amounts of either one of these minerals can lead to calcium or phosphorus imbalance. Such problems are usually manifested as skeletal disease in growing and adult animals (see Section 5, pp. 337-339).

Foods vary greatly in their calcium content. Dairy products and legumes contain high amounts, but cereal grains, meat, and organ tissues contain very little. Phosphorus, on the other hand, is widely distributed in foods. Foods that contain both phosphorus and calcium include dairy products and legumes. Fish, meats, poultry, and organ meats are also very rich sources of phosphorus. However, these foods are very deficient in calcium, and so their inclusion in the diets of dogs and cats must be balanced by a dietary source of calcium to ensure that an adequate calcium:phosphorus ratio is still maintained.

MAGNESIUM

Although magnesium is a macromineral, its amount in the body is much lower than that of calcium and phosphorus. Approximately 60% to 70% of the magnesium found in the body exists in the form of phosphates and carbonates in bone. Most of the remaining magnesium is found within cells, and a very small portion is present in the extracellular fluid. In addition to its role in providing structure to the skeleton, magnesium functions in a number of metabolic reactions; a magnesium-ATP complex is often the form of ATP that is used as a substrate in many of these processes. As a cation in the intracellular fluid, magnesium is essential for the cellular metabolism of both carbohydrate and protein. Protein synthesis also requires the presence of ionized magnesium. Balanced in the extracellular fluids with calcium, sodium, and potassium, magnesium allows muscle contraction and proper transmission of nerve impulses.

Magnesium is widespread in food sources and is abundant in whole grains, legumes, and dairy products. A deficiency of this mineral is not common in dogs and cats. However, excess magnesium in the diets of cats has been implicated as having a possible causal role in the occurrence of feline lower urinary tract disease (see Section 6, pp. 412-416).

SULFUR

Sulfur is required by the body for the synthesis of a number of sulfur-containing compounds. These include chondroitin sulfate, a mucopolysaccharide found in cartilage; the hormone insulin; and the anticoagulant heparin. As part of the amino acid cysteine, sulfur is found in the regulatory tripeptide glutathione. Glutathione is present in all cells and functions with the enzyme glutathione peroxidase to protect cells against the destructive effects of peroxides. It may also have a role in the transport of amino acids across cell membranes. In addition, sulfur is a constituent of the two B vitamins biotin and thiamin. Within the body, sulfur exists almost entirely as a component of organic compounds. The largest proportion of the body's sulfur is found within proteins as a component of the sulfur-containing amino acids cystine and methionine.

Most dietary sulfur is provided by methionine and cystine. Inorganic sulfates present in the diet are very poorly absorbed by the body and do not contribute an appreciable amount of sulfur. Sulfur deficiency has not been demonstrated in either dogs or cats, and it is believed that diets containing adequate amounts of the sulfur-containing amino acids do provide adequate amounts of sulfur.

IRON

Iron is present in all body cells, but the largest proportion of the body's iron is found as a component of the protein molecules hemoglobin and myoglobin. Hemoglobin is found in red blood cells and transports oxygen from the lungs to the tissues; myoglobin binds oxygen for immediate use by muscle cells. Iron is also a cofactor for several other enzymes and is a component of the cytochrome enzymes, which function in hydrogen ion transport during cellular respiration.

Dietary iron is poorly absorbed by most animals. Only about 5% to 10% of the iron present in the diet is absorbed by the body.[50,51] The amount of iron that is absorbed is affected by several factors, including the body's need for the mineral, the environment of the intestinal lumen, and the types of foods that are fed. Iron that is in the ferrous state (+2) is more readily absorbed than iron that is in the ferric state (+3). Therefore an acidic (reducing) environment in the intestine generally enhances iron absorption. Similarly, heme iron, which originates from the hemoglobin and myoglobin in animal food sources, is better absorbed than nonheme iron, which is found in plant sources and some animal foods. Low stores of iron in the body and increased metabolic need, such as during periods of growth and gestation, result in increased efficiency of iron absorption. Dietary factors that can inhibit iron absorption include the presence of phytate, phosphates, and oxalates in the diet and the intake of excess dietary zinc.[52,53]

Iron is transported in the bloodstream while bound to the transport protein transferrin, and it is stored in tissues while bound to two other proteins, ferritin and hemosiderin. Ferritin and transferrin are also involved in the regulation of iron absorption and transport. Chief storage sites for iron in the body are the liver, spleen, and bone marrow. Most animals are very efficient at conserving iron, so losses of this mineral from the body are minimal. The iron of hemoglobin is recycled and reused when red blood cells are catabolized, and only minute amounts are lost by renal excretion. As a result, the requirement for iron only increases drastically during periods of unusual blood loss, such as in cases of parturition, major surgery, injury, or severe parasitic infection or gastrointestinal disease. Iron deficiency results in a hypochromic, microcytic anemia, which is often manifested clinically by fatigue and depression. Conversely, iron, like most trace elements, is toxic if ingested in excessive amounts.

Organ meats such as liver and kidney are the richest sources of iron; meat, egg yolk, fish, legumes, and whole grains also provide adequate amounts. All of the iron in plants and approximately 60% of the iron in animal foods is in the form of non-heme iron, which is not absorbed as efficiently as heme iron. Anemia as a result of a dietary deficiency of iron is extremely rare in dogs and cats. A chronic blood loss that occurs during severe parasitic infections or hemorrhage is more likely to be the cause of iron deficiency in these species.

COPPER

The metabolism and functions of copper are closely tied to those of iron. Copper is necessary for normal absorption and transport of dietary iron. Along with iron, copper is essential for the normal formation of hemoglobin. Most of the copper found in blood is bound to the plasma protein ceruloplasmin. This protein is a copper-dependent ferroxidase that functions as a carrier of copper and also in the oxidation of plasma iron, which is necessary for binding to transferrin. Ceruloplasmin may also be involved in the mobilization of iron from storage sites in the liver. As a component of several different metalloenzymes, copper is required for the conversion of the amino acid tyrosine to the pigment melanin, for the synthesis of the connective tissues collagen and elastin, and for the production of ATP in the cytochrome oxidase system. Another copper metalloenzyme, superoxide dismutase, functions to protect cells from damage by superoxide radicals. Copper is also necessary for normal osteoblast activity during skeletal development.

The highest concentration of copper in the body is found in the liver. After absorption from the intestine, copper, complexed with the plasma protein albumin, is transported through the portal vein to the liver. Metallothioneins, small–molecular-weight cytoplasmic proteins, bind copper and are involved in regulating its transport into the liver. Copper is stored in the liver, where it is incorporated into ceruloplasmin and other proteins for use by the body. Excess copper is excreted in the bile.

Not surprisingly, copper deficiency results in a hypochromic, microcytic anemia similar to that seen with iron deficiency. Other signs of deficiency include depigmentation of colored hair coat and impaired skeletal growth in young animals. Although copper deficiency is not common in dogs and cats, an inherited disorder of copper metabolism that results in copper toxicosis occurs in several different breeds of dogs (see Section 6, pp. 387-388).

ZINC

The trace mineral zinc is widely distributed in many tissues of the body, and its actions influence carbohydrate, lipid, protein, and nucleic acid metabolism. Zinc is a component of many of the metalloenzymes, which include carbonic anhydrase, lactic dehydrogenase, alkaline phosphatase, carboxypeptidase, and aminopeptidase. Zinc also functions as a cofactor in the synthesis of DNA, RNA, and protein and is essential for normal cellular immunity and reproductive functioning. Like iron, the absorption of zinc from the diet is affected by several factors. The body's efficiency of zinc absorption increases with increasing need for this mineral. Animal sources of zinc, such as meat and eggs, are generally more readily absorbed than are plant sources. Dietary compounds that act to decrease zinc absorption include excess levels of calcium, iron, copper, and fiber, and the presence of phytates.[54] Metallothioneins have a high affinity for binding to zinc and are involved in the regulation of zinc absorption and metabolism.

Because of its role in protein synthesis, zinc deficiency is usually associated with growth retardation in young animals. Other clinical signs include anorexia, testicular atrophy, impaired reproductive performance, immune system dysfunction, conjunctivitis, and the development of skin lesions. In dogs and cats, skin and hair coat changes are usually the first clinical signs of zinc deficiency; these signs have been described as dull, coarse hair coat and skin lesions that show parakeratosis and hyperkeratinization.[55] Although not common, naturally occurring zinc-responsive dermatoses have been identified in companion animals.[56,57,58] In addition, a genetically influenced abnormality in zinc absorption and metabolism may exist in some breeds, resulting in an increased zinc requirement in affected animals (see Section 6, pp. 388-389).

MANGANESE

Like most of the other microminerals, manganese functions as a component of several cell enzymes that catalyze metabolic reactions. A large proportion of manganese is located in the mitochondrion of cells where it activates a number of metal-enzyme complexes that regulate nutrient metabolism. These complexes include pyruvate carboxylase and superoxide dismutase. Manganese is also necessary for normal bone development and reproduction. Foods that are good sources of manganese include legumes and whole-grain cereals. Animal-based ingredients are generally poor sources of manganese. Naturally occurring manganese deficiency has not been reported in either dogs or cats. However, manganese deficiency is characterized in other species by decreased growth, impaired reproduction, and disturbances in lipid metabolism.

IODINE

Iodine is required by the body for the synthesis of the hormones thyroxine and tri-iodothyronine by the thyroid gland. Thyroxine stimulates cellular oxidative processes and regulates basal metabolic rate. The principal sign of iodine deficiency is goiter, an enlargement of the thyroid gland. Cretinism, a syndrome characterized by failure to grow, skin lesions, central nervous system (CNS) dysfunction, and multiple skeletal deformities, can occur in young animals that are fed a severely deficient diet. However, naturally occurring iodine deficiency does not commonly occur in dogs or cats.

SELENIUM

As an essential component of the enzyme glutathione peroxidase, selenium protects cell membranes from oxidative damage. Glutathione peroxidase deactivates lipid peroxides that are formed during oxidation of cell-membrane lipids. In this role, selenium has a close relationship with vitamin E and the sulfur-containing amino acids methionine and cystine. Vitamin E protects the polyunsaturated fatty acids (PUFAs) in cell membranes from oxidative damage, and thus it prevents the release of lipid peroxides. By reducing the number of peroxides that are formed, vitamin E spares the cellular use of selenium. The sulfur-containing amino acids are important in selenium metabolism because they are necessary for the formation of glutathione peroxidase. Sources of selenium include cereal grains, meat, and fish. Because selenium is abundant in foods, naturally occurring deficiencies are not a problem in dogs and cats. However, like other trace elements, the ingestion of excess selenium is toxic.

COBALT

Cobalt is a constituent of vitamin B_{12}. Currently no function for cobalt in the body has been identified. Additional cobalt does not appear to be required by dogs and cats when their diet contains adequate amounts of vitamin B_{12}.

CHROMIUM

Chromium is a component of the organic complex known as *glucose tolerance factor*. This factor functions to enhance the action of the hormone insulin, which is necessary for the normal metabolism of glucose and other nutrients. In humans, chromium deficiency has been shown to be associated with abnormal glucose utilization and insulin resistance.[59] It has also been suggested that a low dietary intake of chromium or an impaired metabolism of chromium may be a factor associated with the development of diabetes (see Section 6, pp. 406-407). Recent studies with dogs have reported that supplementation with chromium affects glucose metabolism by enhancing glucose clearance from the blood following an intravenous glucose tolerance test, suggesting that chromium has a similar role in dogs as it does in humans.[60]

OTHER MICROMINERALS

There are several trace elements that have been shown to be required by other species of mammals, but they have not yet been demonstrated to be essential for dogs and cats. These include molybdenum, tin, fluorine, nickel, silicon, vanadium, and arsenic. It is highly likely that dogs and cats also require these elements, even though minimum requirements have not yet been established. These minerals are widespread in food ingredients and are required by the body in very minute amounts. Conversely, all have been shown to be highly toxic when fed in large doses.

ELECTROLYTES

Potassium

Potassium is the main cation in the intracellular fluid. Approximately one third of a cell's potassium is bound to protein; the rest is found in the ionized form. Ionized potassium within cells provides the osmotic force that maintains proper fluid volume. Cellular potassium is also required for numerous enzymatic reactions. The small concentration of potassium present in the extracellular fluid aids in the transmission of nerve impulses and the contraction of muscle fibers. The maintenance of potassium balance is especially important for the normal functioning of heart muscle. Many foods contain potassium. Meats, poultry, and fish are all rich sources, and whole-grain cereals and most vegetables also contain high amounts. Because of the abundance of potassium in most foods, potassium deficiency of a dietary origin is highly unusual in dogs and cats.

Sodium

Ionized sodium is the major cation found in the extracellular fluid. Sodium in this compartment provides the primary osmotic force that maintains the aqueous environment of the extracellular fluid. It functions in conjunction with other ions to maintain the normal irritability of nerve cells and the contractibility of muscle fibers. Sodium is also necessary for the maintenance of the permeability of cell membranes. The sodium "pump" controls the electrolyte balance between the intracellular and extracellular fluid compartments. The chief source of sodium in the diet is table salt (sodium chloride), which is used for food preservation in most commercially prepared foods. In addition to processed products, foods that have a naturally high sodium content include dairy products, meat, poultry, fish, and egg white. Because of this mineral's abundance in foods, sodium deficiency is not a problem in dogs and cats. Conversely, excess sodium intake has been implicated as a possible causal factor in hypertension in some human populations.[61,62] These observations, coupled with the high sodium content of some commercial pet foods, has led investigators to examine the effects of high sodium intake in dogs. Results indicate that hypertension is not a common problem in this species. Moreover, dogs appear to be physiologically resistant to excess salt intake.[63,64]

Chloride

Chloride ions account for about two thirds of the total anions present in the extracellular fluid. They are necessary for the regulation of normal osmotic pressure, water balance, and acid-base balance in the body. Chloride is also necessary for the formation of hydrochloric acid (HCl) in the stomach. HCl is required for the activation of several gastric enzymes and for the initiation of digestion in the stomach. Because most of the chloride that animals consume is associated with sodium, the daily amount consumed generally parallels sodium intake. Like potassium and sodium, dietary chloride deficiency has not been found to be a common problem in dogs and cats.

C H A P T E R

7

Digestion and Absorption

The process of digestion breaks down the large, complex molecules of many nutrients into their simplest, most soluble forms so that absorption and use by the body can take place (Table 7-1). The two basic types of action involved in this process are mechanical digestion and chemical (or enzymatic) digestion. Mechanical digestion involves the physical mastication (chewing), mixing, and movement of food through the gastrointestinal tract. Chemical digestion involves splitting the chemical bonds of the complex nutrients through enzymatically catalyzed hydrolysis. The three major types of foods that require digestion are fats, carbohydrates, and proteins. Before absorption takes place, most of the fat in food is hydrolyzed to glycerol, free fatty acids (FFAs), and some monoglycerides and diglycerides. Complex carbohydrates are broken down to the simple sugars—glucose, galactose, and fructose. Protein molecules are hydrolyzed to single amino acid units and some dipeptides. As dietary nutrients are digested, they are transported down the digestive tract by a series of contractions of the muscular walls of the gastrointestinal tract. The process of digestion and absorption begins when food first enters the mouth and ends with the excretion of waste products and undigested food particles in the feces.

MOUTH

In all species, the mouth functions to bring food into the body, initiate physical mastication, and mix the food with saliva. Saliva is secreted in response to the sight and smell of food. It acts as a lubricant to facilitate both chewing and swallowing and also serves to solubilize the dietary components that stimulate the taste buds and impart flavor to food. Compared to many ruminant and herbivorous species that thoroughly masticate their food, dogs and cats often swallow large boluses of food with little or no chewing. An examination of the teeth of dogs and cats presents important distinctions between these two species. Although domesticated dogs and cats have the same number of incisor and canine teeth (six incisors and two canines

TABLE 7-1

Digestive End Products of Carbohydrate, Protein, and Fat

Nutrient	Enzymes	End Products
Carbohydrate	Amylase	Glucose
	Lactase	Galactose
	Sucrase	Fructose
	Maltase	
Protein	Dipeptidase	Dipeptides
	Amino peptidase	Single amino acids
	Pepsinogen	
	Pepsin	
	Nucleotidase	
	Nucleosidase	
	Trypsin	
	Chymotrypsin	
	Carboxypeptidase	
	Nuclease	
Fat	Intestinal lipase	Glycerol
	Pancreatic lipase	FFAs
		Monoglycerides, diglycerides

on both the top and bottom jaws), the mouth of a dog contains more premolars and molars than does a cat's mouth. These teeth are associated with an increased capacity to chew and crush food, which is indicative of a diet containing a larger proportion of plant material. Thus the dentition of dogs is suggestive of a more omnivorous diet than is the dentition of cats, which is more typical of the pattern seen in most obligate carnivores.[65] Although both dogs and cats are "meat-eaters," the dog has evolved to consume a diet that is slightly more omnivorous in nature than that of the cat.

ESOPHAGUS

Food passes from the mouth to the stomach through the esophagus. The cells of the mucosal lining of the esophagus secrete mucus, which further aids in lubricating food as it passes to the stomach. As the food reaches the end of the esophagus, the cardiac sphincter, a ring of muscle at the junction between the esophagus and stomach, relaxes to allow food to enter the stomach. This ring relaxes in response to the peristaltic movements of the esophagus. It then immediately constricts after food has passed to prevent reflux of the stomach contents back into the lower esophagus.

STOMACH

The stomach acts as a reservoir for the body, allowing food to be ingested as a meal rather than continuously throughout the day. In addition to its storage function, the stomach also initiates the chemical digestion of protein, mixes food with gastric secretions, and regulates the entry of food into the small intestine. The gastric glands, which are located in the mucosal lining of the corpus portion of the stomach, secrete mucus, hydrochloric acid (HCl), and the proteolytic enzyme pepsinogen. Mucous secretions protect the gastric mucosa and also lubricate the ingested food. HCl is necessary to maintain a proper pH for the occurrence of enzymatic action. It functions to slightly alter the composition of ingested fat and protein in preparation for further action by digestive enzymes in the small intestine. Along with previously formed pepsin, HCl also converts pepsinogen to the enzyme pepsin. This enzyme initiates hydrolysis of protein molecules to smaller polypeptide units.

Both neurological and hormonal stimuli are important for the secretion of HCl and mucus by the stomach. Neurological stimuli are produced in response to the anticipation of eating, the sight and smell of food, and the presence of food in the stomach. In addition, psychological stimuli such as fear, stress, and anxiety can affect gastric secretions and gastrointestinal functioning in animals. The hormone gastrin is released in response to the presence of food and distention of the stomach. It is produced by mucosal glands in the antrum portion of the stomach. Gastrin stimulates the secretion of HCl and mucus and also increases gastric motility. Another local hormone, enterogastrone, is produced by glands located in the duodenal mucosa. Enterogastrone is secreted in response to the presence of fat entering the duodenum and counteracts gastrin's activity by inhibiting acid production and gastric motility.

Peristaltic movements of the stomach slowly mix the ingested food with gastric secretions, preparing it for entry into the small intestine. The mucosal cells located in the antral portion of the stomach secrete a mucus that has a more alkaline pH and is low in digestive enzymes. Thorough mixing in this portion results in the production of a semifluid mass of food called chyme. Chyme must pass through the pyloric sphincter to enter the small intestine for further digestion. Like the cardiac sphincter, the pyloric sphincter is a ring of muscle that is usually in a constricted state. This ring relaxes in response to the strong peristaltic contractions that originate in the stomach and travel toward the intestine. While open, this sphincter allows small amounts of chyme to enter the duodenum. The pyloric sphincter serves to control the rate of passage of food from the stomach into the small intestine. The rate of gastric emptying is affected by the osmotic pressure, particle size, and viscosity of the chyme, as well as the degree of gastric acidity and volume. In general, large meals have a slower rate of emptying than small meals, liquids leave the stomach faster than solids, and very high-fat meals may cause a decrease in stomach-emptying rate. Diets that contain soluble fiber as a fiber source cause a decreased rate of stomach emptying when compared with diets that contain insoluble dietary fiber.

SMALL INTESTINE

Before reaching the small intestine, most of the digestive processes that occur in dogs and cats are mechanical in nature. The chyme that is delivered through the pyloric sphincter to the duodenum is a semifluid mass made up of food particles mixed with gastric secretions. Carbohydrates and fats are almost unchanged in composition, but the protein in the food has been partially hydrolyzed to smaller polypeptides. Even this digestion is not crucial, however, because the enzymes of the small intestine are capable of completely digesting intact dietary protein. Therefore the major task of chemical digestion and the subsequent absorption of nutrients occurs in the small intestine.

Further mechanical digestion also occurs in the small intestine through the co-ordinated contractions of its muscle layers. These movements thoroughly mix the food mass with intestinal secretions, increase the exposure of digested food particles to the mucosal surface, and slowly propel the food mass through the intestinal tract. Constant sweeping motions of the intestinal villi that line the surface of the mucosa mix the chyme that is in contact with the intestinal wall and increase the efficiency of absorption of digested particles. After food has entered the small intestine, large quantities of mucus are secreted by the Brunner's glands, which are located immediately inside the duodenum. This mucus protects the intestinal mucosa from irritation and erosion by the gastric acids that are entering from the stomach and further lubricates the food mass.

Both the pancreas and the glands located in the duodenal mucosa secrete enzymes into the intestinal lumen that chemically digest fat, carbohydrate, and protein. Enzymes secreted by the intestinal cells include intestinal lipase, amino peptidase, dipeptidase, nucleotidase, nucleosidase, and enterokinase. Intestinal lipase converts fat to monoglycerides, diglycerides, glycerol, and FFAs. Amino peptidase breaks the peptide bond located at the N-terminal of the protein molecule, slowly releasing single amino acids from the protein chain. Dipeptidase breaks the peptide bond of dipeptides to release two single amino acid units. Both nucleosidase and nucleotidase hydrolyze nucleoproteins to their constituent bases and pentose sugars. Lastly, enterokinase converts inactive trypsinogen, a proenzyme secreted from the pancreas, to its active form. The final digestion of carbohydrate takes place at the brush border of the small intestine. The cells of the brush border secrete the enzymes maltase, lactase, and sucrase, which convert the disaccharides maltose, lactose, and sucrose to their constituent monosaccharides—glucose, fructose, and galactose.

Protease enzymes secreted by the pancreas include trypsin, chymotrypsin, carypeptidase, and nuclease. Several of these are secreted in an inactive form and are activated by other components in the small intestine after release. In addition, pancreatic lipase and amylase are released into the intestinal lumen and respectively function to hydrolyze dietary fat and starch into smaller units. Cholesterol esterase secreted by the pancreas catalyzes the formation of cholesterol esters. Free cholesterol must be esterified to fatty acids to facilitate its absorption into the body. The pancreas also secretes a large volume of bicarbonate salts into the small intestine.

These salts function to neutralize the acid chyme and provide the proper pH for the digestive enzymes to function.

Bile is another important component of nutrient digestion in the small intestine. It is produced by the liver and stored in the gallbladder. Bile's primary function in the small intestine is the emulsification of dietary fat and the activation of certain lipases. These two processes result in the formation of very small, water-soluble globules called *micelles*. The formation of micelles results in an increased surface area for the action of lipase and also arranges lipid molecules into water-miscible forms that are able to gain access to the aqueous layer covering the microvilli, ultimately facilitating absorption of fat into the body.

Hormonal control of digestion in the small intestine involves several components. Secretin is produced by the mucosa of the upper portion of the duodenum in response to the entry of acidic chyme into the duodenum. It stimulates the release of bicarbonate from the pancreas and controls the rate of bile flow from the gallbladder. Cholecystokinin is also released from this portion of the intestinal mucosa in response to the presence of fat in the food mass. This hormone stimulates contraction of the gallbladder, resulting in a release of bile into the intestinal lumen. Cholecystokinin (also referred to as *pancreozymin*) also stimulates secretion of the pancreatic enzymes.

In dogs and cats, the chemical digestion of food is completed in the small intestine. Digestible protein, carbohydrate, and fat are hydrolyzed to amino acids, dipeptides, monosaccharides, glycerol, FFAs, and monoglycerides and diglycerides. As these small units are produced, they are absorbed by the body along with dietary vitamins and minerals. Absorption involves the transfer of digested nutrients from the intestinal lumen into the blood or lymphatic system for delivery to tissues throughout the body. Like digestion, the greatest part of absorption takes place in the small intestine.

The structure of the inner wall of the small intestine is designed to provide a high amount of surface area for the absorption of nutrients. The mucosal folds, villi, and microvilli of the mucosa produce an absorptive inner surface area that is approximately 600 times that of the outer serosal layer of the intestine. Villi are fingerlike projections that cover the convoluted folds of the mucosa. Each individual villus contains a vascular network of venous and arterial capillaries and a lymph vessel called a *lacteal*. These function to transport absorbed nutrients to either the portal or lymphatic circulations. The surface of each villus is covered with numerous, minute projections called *microvilli*. These are often collectively referred to as the *brush border* of the small intestine. The cells lining the luminal surface of the villi are highly specialized absorptive cells called *enterocytes*. These cells have a lifespan of only 2 to 3 days, during which they absorb nutrients from the lumen of the small intestine. Old cells are continually sloughed off and excreted in the feces, giving these cells one of the highest turnover rates of any tissue in the body.

Nutrient absorption is accomplished in the small intestine through several processes. Some small molecules are absorbed by passive diffusion according to the osmotic gradient; for example, electrolytes and water molecules both flow across the mucosa in response to osmotic pressure. Facilitated diffusion involves the transport of large molecules across the cellular membrane in concurrence with the pressure gradient. Carrier proteins located in the membranes of the enterocytes facilitate transport of these nutrients into the cells. In contrast, active transport involves the transport of nutrient molecules across the intestinal epithelial membrane against a concentration gradient. This transport mechanism differs from passive diffusion in that more energy is required to transport materials against a concentration gradient. For example, the most common type of active transport mechanism involves a membrane protein carrier coupled with the active transport of sodium (the sodium pump).

Although some passive diffusion is believed to occur, most simple carbohydrates are absorbed by the body through an active process that is linked to sodium transport and uses a specific carrier protein. Single amino acids and some dipeptides and tripeptides are also absorbed in this manner. Small peptides that are absorbed into the cell are immediately hydrolyzed to single amino acid units before being released into the portal circulation. Sugars and amino acids are absorbed into the villus capillaries and from there enter the portal vein, which transports these nutrients to the liver. Absorption of fat involves the interaction of the fat-containing micelles with the aqueous layer surrounding the brush border. Micelles contain bile acids, monoglycerides, diglycerides, and long-chain fatty acids. Because they are water-miscible, the micelles are able to travel to the brush border, where they are disrupted and their component fat particles are absorbed into the cell. The bile remains in the lumen and eventually moves down the intestine to be reabsorbed and circulated back to the liver. Within the enterocyte, most of the fatty acids and glycerol are resynthesized into triglycerides, combined with cholesterol, phospholipid, and protein, and released into the central lacteal as either chylomicrons or very–low-density lipoprotein (VLDL) transport particles. The central lacteal drains into the major lymph vessels, and the particles eventually enter the blood circulation near the heart.

The liver functions to further process the absorbed monosaccharides and amino acids that arrive through the portal circulation. Some monosaccharides are converted to the storage carbohydrate form glycogen, and a certain quantity of glucose is secreted directly into the circulation. Some amino acids are released into the bloodstream, where they circulate to tissues for absorption into cells. Excess amino acids are either converted to other nonessential amino acids or metabolized by the liver for energy.

Most minerals are absorbed by the body in an ionized form. The water-soluble vitamins are transported by passive diffusion, but some may be absorbed by an active process when the diet contains low levels. Vitamin B_{12} is unique in its requirement for an intrinsic factor for proper absorption. Fat-soluble vitamins are made soluble by combination with bile salts and are then absorbed by passive diffusion through the lipid phase of the mucosal cell membrane. In general, when there is normal fat absorption, there is normal fat-soluble vitamin absorption.

LARGE INTESTINE (COLON)

The contents of the small intestine enter the large intestine through the ileocecal valve. The cecum is an intestinal pocket located next to the junction of the colon and the small intestine. This portion of the intestine varies in size and functional capacity among species of mammals. The cecum of nonruminant herbivores such as the horse and rabbit is relatively large and has a highly enhanced digestive capacity. Likewise, both the cecum and large intestine of the omnivorous pig are enlarged when compared with those of the carnivorous species. Microbial digestion of dietary fiber in the cecum and colon of nonruminant herbivores contributes significantly to the nutrient intake and balance of these animals. In comparison, carnivorous species such as the cat and mink have a vestigial cecum, and the length of their large intestine is relatively short. Relative to body size, the dog's cecum is not as large as the pig's, but it is somewhat larger than the cat's.[63] This observation is consistent with the fact that the dog has adapted to consuming a diet that is more omnivorous in nature than that of the cat. The extent to which bacterial digestion of dietary fiber in the cecum and colon contribute to energy balance in these species is small compared to the contribution for nonruminant herbivore species. However, recent research has shown that the short-chain fatty acids (SCFAs) produced by bacterial fermentation of fiber are an important energy source for colonocytes and may contribute to intestinal health in dogs (see Section 6, pp. 497-501).[27,28]

A chief function of the large intestine in dogs and cats is the absorption of water and certain electrolytes. Unlike the small intestine, the large intestine has no villi and therefore has a lower capacity for absorption. Although it is able to efficiently absorb water and electrolytes, it has no mechanisms for active transport. Along with a large volume of water, sodium is absorbed into the body from the large intestine. As mentioned previously, the bacterial colonies of the colon are capable of digesting some of the indigestible fiber and other nutrients in the diet that have escaped digestion in the small intestine. The products of this bacterial digestion give the feces of dogs and cats their characteristic smell and color. Undigested food residues, sloughed cells, bacteria, and unabsorbed endogenous secretions make up the fecal matter that eventually reaches the rectum and is excreted from the body.

Fecal characteristics in dogs and cats can be significantly affected by the quantity and type of indigestible matter that is present in the animal's diet. Bacterial digestion of these materials produce various gases, SCFAs, and other byproducts. When protein reaches the large intestine in an undigested state, bacterial degradation results in the production of the amines indole and skatole. In addition, hydrogen sulfide gas is produced from the sulfur-containing amino acids of undigested or poorly digested protein. Hydrogen sulfide gas, indole, and skatole impart strong odors to fecal matter and intestinal gas. Certain types of carbohydrates found in legumes such as soybeans are resistant to digestion by the endogenous enzymes of the small intestine. These carbohydrates reach the colon and are attacked by bacteria, with a resultant production of intestinal gas (flatulence). Hydrogen, carbon dioxide, and methane gases are produced from the bacterial digestion of carbohydrates. A similar effect occurs with certain types of fiber. While nonfermentable fibers resist digestion in the small intestine and fermentation in the large intestine, fermentable fibers are used as an energy source by intestinal bacteria, resulting in the production of gases and SCFAs. The degree to which flatulence and strong fecal odors occur in dogs and cats that are fed poorly digestible materials varies with the amounts and types of materials fed and the intestinal flora present in the colons of individual animals.

KEY POINTS

- Nutrition is the study of food, its nutrients, and other components, including an examination of the actions of specific nutrients, their interactions with each other, and their balance within a diet. The science of nutrition also studies ingestion, digestion, and absorption and use of nutrients. The six categories of nutrients—water, carbohydrates, proteins, fats, minerals, and vitamins—have specific functions and contribute to growth, body tissue maintenance, and optimal health.

- Energy is needed by the body to perform metabolic work, which includes maintaining and synthesizing body tissues, engaging in physical work, and regulating normal body temperature. Because of its critical importance, energy is always the first requirement met by an animal's diet.

- Although all companion animals have the ability to self-regulate their energy intake, some do not always do so, and obesity is the result. Free-choice feeding of highly palatable foods and a lack of appropriate exercise are frequently to blame. Portion-controlled feeding and appropriate levels of exercise are the best methods for controlling a pet's energy balance, growth rate, and weight.

- The metabolizable energy (ME) of a diet or feed ingredient for a given species can be determined by using one of three methods: (1) direct determination in feeding trials, (2) calculation method, and (3) extrapolation of data from other species. Although direct determination with feeding trials is the most accurate method, it is time-consuming and costly and requires large numbers of test animals. A quick and simple method of calculating the ME uses the minimum percentage of fat listed on the food's label in the following formula: $ME = 3.075 + 0.066 (fat)$

- Energy density (the number of calories provided by a food in a given weight or volume) is the most important factor in determining the quantity of food that a pet should eat each day. Energy density directly affects the amount of all other essential nutrients that an animal ingests. Expressing nutrient content on an energy density basis is the most accurate method. It puts the nutrients in a meaningful format.

- **Tip:** Reading food labels and comparing contents of foods in the store can be very confusing. For example, when the protein content is expressed as a percentage of weight, merely reading the protein content printed on the label of a canned dog food (7% protein) and a dry dog food (27% protein) does not tell the whole story. But when a simple formula is applied to determine the protein as a percentage of calories, one can see that the protein content of the dry and canned foods in this example is almost exactly the same (see Table 1-2).

- For an animal to survive, water is the single most important nutrient for the body. Water within the cells is necessary for most metabolic processes and chemical reactions, is important for temperature regulation, and is an essential component of normal digestion.

- Pets obtain water from food, metabolic water, and drinking water. If the water content of food is increased or decreased, most pets are naturally able to achieve water balance by increasing or decreasing their intake of drinking water.

- Moderately fermentable fiber sources (as opposed to highly fermentable and nonfermentable fiber sources) that are a source of bulk and provide adequate levels of short-chain fatty acids (SCFAs) in the large intestine are the best fiber sources for cats and dogs. These sources contribute to the health of the large intestine.

- Because carbohydrates are an excellent energy source for the body, they should be provided adequately in the diet so that protein will be not be used for energy and can instead be used for tissue repair and growth.

- Fat provides the most concentrated form of energy of all the nutrients, is a source of essential fatty acids (EFAs), and allows the absorption of fat-soluble vitamins. Fat also contributes to the palatability and texture of food. As the fat content increases, so does the energy density of the diet. Portion-controlled feeding is usually the best method when feeding a well-balanced, energy-dense pet food containing moderate to high levels of fat.

- Proteins are the major structural components of hair, feathers, skin, nails, tendons, ligaments, and cartilage. Enzymes essential for nutrient digestion are proteins, as are many hormones, such as insulin and glucagon. Blood proteins, such as hemoglobin, act as important carrier substances. The antibodies that enable the body to resist disease are composed of large protein molecules. Because the protein in the body is in a constant state of flux, a regular intake of dietary protein is necessary to maintain normal metabolic processes and provide for tissue maintenance and growth. Like fat, protein content contributes to the palatability and acceptability of food.

- **Tip:** Although there are several laboratory tests available for evaluating the quality of protein in food, all have their limitations. In addition to the tests available, the quality of pet food protein should always be assessed by trials in which the food is fed to the animals for which it was developed. The true quality of a protein or proteins in food must also be evaluated on a long-term basis by assessing the overall health and vitality of the pet.

- Most vitamins cannot be synthesized by the body and must be supplied in food. Well-balanced pet foods are formulated to provide the necessary supplementation. Vitamin C, however, is one vitamin that can be synthesized from glucose by dogs and cats; in contrast, humans must receive vitamin C from dietary sources.

- Minerals are inorganic elements that make up only about 4% of an animal's total body weight; nonetheless, the essential minerals must be present to sustain life.

- An electrolyte is a substance that dissociates into ions when in solution and thus becomes capable of conducting electricity; in other words, an ionic solute.

- Digestion and absorption actually begin in the mouth, with the mastication (chewing) of food and its mixture with saliva. Digestion continues throughout the gastrointestinal system and ends with the excretion of waste products and undigested food particles in the feces.

- Most of the important tasks of chemical digestion and the subsequent absorption of nutrients occur in the small intestine.

- In contrast to the small intestine, a primary function of the large intestine (colon) in dogs and cats is the absorption of water and certain electrolytes, especially sodium.

SECTION 1

REFERENCES

1. Cowgill GR: The energy factor in relation to food intake: experiments on the dog, *Am J Physiol* 85:45-64, 1928.
2. Durrer JL, Hannon JP: Seasonal variations in caloric intake of dogs living in an arctic environment, *Am J Physiol* 202:375-384, 1962.
3. Romsos DR, Hornshus MJ, Leveille GA: Influence of dietary fat and carbohydrate on food intake, body weight and body fat of adult dogs, *Pro Soc Exp Bio Med* 157:278-281, 1978.
4. Romsos DR, Belo PS, Bennink MR: Effects of dietary carbohydrate, fat and protein on growth, body composition and blood metabolite levels in the dog, *J Nutr* 106:1452-1464, 1976.
5. Romsos DR, Ferguson D: Regulation of protein intake in adult dogs, *J Am Vet Med Assoc* 182:41-43, 1983.
6. Armstrong J, Lund EM: Obesity: research update. In *Proceedings of the Petfood Forum*, Chicago, 1997, Watts Publishing.
7. National Research Council: *Nutrient requirements of dogs*, Washington, DC, 1985, National Academy of Sciences, National Academy Press.
8. Harris LE: *Biological energy interrelationships and glossary of energy terms*, Washington, DC, 1966, National Academy of Sciences, National Academy Press.
9. Kendall PT, Burger IH, Smith PM: Methods of estimation of the metabolizable energy content of cat foods, *Fel Pract* 15:38-44, 1985.
10. Kuhlman G, Laflamme DP, Ballam JM: A simple method for estimating the metabolizable energy content of dry cat foods, *Fel Pract* 21:16-20, 1993.
11. National Research Council: *Nutrient requirements of cats*, Washington, DC, 1986, National Academy of Sciences, National Academy Press.
12. Kealy RD, Olsson SE, Monti KL, and others: Effects of limited food consumption on the incidence of hip dysplasia in growing dogs, *J Am Vet Med Assoc* 201:857-863, 1992.
13. Hedhammer A, Wu FM, Krook L, and others: Overnutrition and skeletal disease: an experimental study in growing great Dane dogs, *Cornell Vet* 64(suppl 5):1-160, 1974.
14. Kasstrom H: Nutrition, weight gain and development of hip dysplasia, *Acta Radiol* 344(suppl):135-179, 1975.
15. Richardson DC: The role of nutrition in canine hip dysplasia, *Vet Clin North Am Small Anim Pract* 22:529-540, 1992.
16. Bjorntorp P: The role of adipose tissue in human obesity. In Greenwood MRC, editor: *Obesity: contemporary issues in clinical nutrition*, New York, 1983, Churchill Livingstone.
17. Bjorntorp P, Sjostrom L: Number and size of fat cells in relation to metabolism in human obesity, *Metabolism* 20:703-706, 1971.
18. Maynard LA, Loosli JK, Hintz HF, and others: *Animal nutrition*, ed 7, New York, 1979, McGraw-Hill.
19. Anderson RS: Water content in the diet of the dog, *Vet Ann* 21:171-178, 1981.
20. Burger IH, Blaza SE: Digestion, absorption, and dietary balance. In *Dog and cat nutrition*, ed 2, Oxford, England, 1988, Pergamon Press.
21. Caldwell GT: Studies in water metabolism of the cat, *Physiol Zool* 4:324-355, 1931.
22. Danowski TS, Elkinton JR, Winkler AW: The deleterious effect in dogs of a dry protein ration, *J Clin Invest* 23:816-823, 1944.
23. Prentiss PG, Wolf AV, Eddy HE: Hydropenia in cat and dog: ability of the cat to meet its water requirements solely from a diet of fish or meat, *Am J Physiol* 196:625-632, 1959.
24. Anderson RS: Water balance in the dog and cat, *J Small Anim Pract* 23:588-598, 1982.

25. Wilde RO, Jansen T: The use of different sources of raw and heated starch in the ration of weaned kittens. In Burger IH, Rivers JPW, editors: *Nutrition of the dog and cat*, Cambridge, England, 1989, Cambridge University Press.

26. van Soest PJ: The uniformity and nutritive availability of cellulose, *Fed Proc* 32:1804-1808, 1973.

27. Reinhart GA, Moxley RA, Clemens ET: Dietary fibre source and its effects on colonic microstructure, function and histopathology of Beagle dogs, *J Nutr* 124:2701S-2703S, 1994.

28. Sunvold GD, Fahey GC Jr, Merchen NR, and others: Fermentability of selected fibrous substrates by dog fecal microflora as influenced by diet, *J Nutr* 124:2719S-2720S, 1994.

29. Hallman JE, Moxley RA, Reinhart GA, and others: Cellulose, beet pulp, and pectin/gum arabic effects on canine colonic microstructure and histopathology, *Vet Clin Nutr* 2:137-142, 1995.

30. Orr NWM: The food requirements of Antarctic sledge dogs. In Graham-Jones O, editor: *Canine and feline nutritional requirements*, London, 1965, Pergamon Press.

31. Huber TL, Wilson RC, McGarity SA: Variations in digestibility of dry dog foods with identical label guaranteed analysis, *J Am Anim Hosp Assoc* 22:571-575, 1986.

32. Mead JF: Functions of the n-6 and n-3 polyunsaturated fatty acid acids. In Taylor TG, Jenkins NK, editors: *Proceedings of the XIII International Congress of Nutrition*, London, 1986, John Libbey.

33. Carlson SE: Are n-3 polyunsaturated fatty acids essential for growth and development? In Nelson GJ, editor: *Health effects of dietary fatty acids*, Champaign, Ill, 1990.

34. Kane E, Morris JG, Rogers QR: Acceptability and digestibility by adult cats of diets made with various sources and levels of fat, *J Anim Sci* 53:1516-1523, 1981.

35. Brown RG: Protein in dog foods, *Can Vet J* 30:528-531, 1989.

36. Kronfeld DS: Protein quality and amino acid profiles of commercial dog foods, *J Am Anim Hosp Assoc* 18:679-683, 1982.

37. Oser BL: An integrated essential amino acid index for predicting the biological value of proteins. In *Protein and amino acid nutrition*, New York, 1959, Academic Press.

38. Goodman DS: Vitamin A and retinoids in health and disease, *N Engl J Med* 310:1023-1031, 1984.

39. Chew BP, Park JS, Wong TS, and others: Importance of beta-carotene nutrition in the dog and cat: uptake and immunity. In Reinhart GA, Carey DP, editors: *Recent advances in canine and feline nutrition*, vol 2, Iams Nutrition Symposium Proceedings, Wilmington, Ohio, 1998, Orange Frazer.

40. Gallop PM: Carboxylated calcium–binding proteins and vitamin K, *N Engl J Med* 302:1460-1465, 1980.

41. Ghosh HP, Sarkar PK, Guha BC: Distribution of the bound form of nicotinic acid in natural materials, *J Nutr* 79:451-458, 1963.

42. Belfield WO, Stone I: Megascorbic prophylaxis and megascorbic therapy: a new orthomolecular modality in veterinary medicine, *J Int Acad Prev Med* 2:10-25, 1975.

43. Innes JRM: Vitamin C requirements in the dog: attempts to produce experimental scurvy. In *Report of the Cambridge Institute of Animal Pathology*, Cambridge, England, 1931.

44. Naismith DH: Ascorbic acid requirements of the dog, *Proc Nutr Soc* 17:21, 1958.

45. Naismith DH, Pellett PL: The water-soluble vitamin content of blood, serum and milk of the bitch, *Proc Nutr Soc* 19:15, 1960.

46. Carvalho da Silva A, Fajer AB, DeAngelis RC, and others: The domestic cat as a laboratory animal for experimental nutrition studies. II. Comparative growth and hematology on stock and purified rations, *Acta Physiol Latin Am* 1:26-43, 1950.

47. Grondalen J: Metaphyseal osteopathy (hypertrophic osteodystrophy) in growing dogs: a clinical study, *J Small Anim Prac* 17:721-735, 1976.

48. Teare JA, Krook L, Kallfelz FA, and others: Ascorbic acid deficiency and hypertrophic osteodystrophy in the dog: a rebuttal, *Cornell Vet* 69:384-401, 1979.

49. Association of American Feed Control Officials: *Official publication*, 1994, The Association.

50. Stewart WB, Bambino SR: Kinetics of iron absorption in normal dogs, *Am J Physiol* 201:67-77, 1961.

51. Pollack S, Balcerzak SP, Crosby WH: Transferrin and absorption of iron, *Blood* 21:33-39, 1963.

52. Erdman JW: Oilseed phytates: nutritional implications, *J Am Oil Chem Soc* 56:736, 1979.

53. Bafundo KW, Baker DH, Fitzgerald PR: The iron-zinc interrelationship in the chick as influenced by *Eimeria acervulina* infection, *J Nutr* 114:1306-1311, 1984.

54. Hunt JR, Johnson PE, Swan PB: Dietary conditions influencing relative zinc availability from foods to the rat and correlations with in vitro measurements, *J Nutr* 117:1913-1923, 1987.

55. Sanecki RK, Corbin JE, Forbes RM: Tissue changes in dogs fed a zinc-deficient ration, *Am J Vet Res* 43:1642-1646, 1983.

56. Sousa CA, Stannard AA, Ihrke PH: Dermatosis associated with feeding generic dog food: 13 cases (1981-1982), *J Am Vet Med Assoc* 192:767-680, 1988.

57. Wolf AM: Zinc-responsive dermatosis in a Rhodesian ridgeback, *Vet Med* 82:908-912, 1987.

58. Wright RP: Identification of zinc-responsive dermatoses, *Vet Med* 80:37-40, 1985.

59. Anderson RA: Chromium, glucose tolerance and diabetes, *Biol Trace Element Res* 32:19-24, 1992.

60. Keeling KL: Effect of chromium picolinate on glucose metabolism and immune response in dogs (master's thesis), Raleigh, NC, 1997, North Carolina State University.

61. Schribner BH: Salt and hypertension, *J Am Med Assoc* 250:388-389, 1983.

62. Houston MC: Sodium and hypertension, *Arch Intern Med* 146:179-185, 1986.

63. Swales JD: Blood pressure and the kidney, *J Clin Pathol* 34:1233-1240, 1981.

64. Wilhelmj CM, Waldmann EB, McGuire TF: Effect of prolonged high sodium chloride ingestion and withdrawal upon blood pressure of dogs, *Proc Soc Exp Bio Med* 77:379-382, 1951.

65. Morris JG, Rogers QR: Comparative dog and cat nutrition. In Burger IH, Rivers JPW, editors: *Nutrition of the dog and cat,* Cambridge, England, 1989, Cambridge University Press.

2

NUTRIENT REQUIREMENTS OF DOGS AND CATS

Pets must be fed a proper diet that supplies all of the essential nutrients in their correct quantities and proportions in order to maintain health throughout all stages of life. The primary goals of feeding companion animals include maintaining optimal health, promoting a normal (but not excessive) growth rate, supporting gestation and lactation, and, in some cases, contributing to high-quality performance. Proper feeding throughout the pet's life also contributes to long-term health, vitality, and longevity.

As a result of the advances that have been made in companion animal nutrition during the past 30 years, frank nutrient deficiencies are extremely rare in dogs and cats today. Rather, changes in nutrient status occur more often as a result of overfeeding, excessive supplementation, or exposure to inhibitory substances. It is important to recognize that individual nutrients do not function in isolation; interactions among essential nutrients are necessary for normal cellular metabolism. These relationships affect nutrient absorption, use, and excretion.

Pet food companies use this information to formulate balanced and complete pet foods for various stages of companion animals' lives. Because of the intricate interactions between dietary components, the balance of nutrients within the diet and the absolute quantity of each individual nutrient must always be considered.

All dogs and cats require an adequate intake of nutrients every day to maintain optimal health. Requirements for energy and certain nutrients can vary significantly during the lifetime of an individual pet. Increased demands occur during growth, reproduction, and physical work. A decreased requirement for energy and some nutrients occurs as animals attain adulthood and as they age. In addition to changing needs within the life cycle, the nutrient requirements of individual animals also vary considerably. For example, the energy needs for an adult Pug that spends a lot of time dozing on the couch will be significantly lower than the energy requirement of an adult Cairn Terrier that weighs the same amount but has an inherently higher activity level.

Standards of nutrient requirements for dogs and cats are necessary to provide general guidelines for commercial pet food companies to use when formulating diets. Ideally these standards should include current information concerning minimum and maximum levels of nutrients, nutrient requirements for different stages of life and activity levels, and estimates of the bioavailability of nutrients in commonly used pet food ingredients. Currently there are two sets of published standards that provide nutrient requirement information for dogs and cats. The National Research Council (NRC) compiles lists of minimum nutrient requirements of companion animals. A second group, the Association of American Feed Control Officials (AAFCO), has developed standards of practical *Nutrient Profiles* for dog and cat foods based on commonly used ingredients.

The recommendations of the NRC are compiled by committees of companion animal nutritionists. Two publications, the *Nutrient Requirements of Dogs* and the *Nutrient Requirements of Cats,* are issued by these committees. These publications are revised and updated as new knowledge becomes available. The nutrient recommendations for dogs were last updated in 1985, and the publication for cats was revised in 1986. These recommendations are lists of the minimum daily requirements (MDRs) of nutrients for dogs and cats. The MDRs denote the minimum quantity of available nutrients that must be supplied in the diet each day to allow normal body metabolism. It is important to realize that the MDR recommendations of the NRC do not include safety factors that account for variability within the pet population. In addition, most of the research on which these recommendations are based was conducted using purified or semipurified diets. Such diets contain nutrients that are generally more available than those found in normal pet food ingredients. As a result, if correction factors for differences in bioavailability are not included, the use of the NRC's recommendations to formulate commercial dog and cat foods can result in deficient levels of nutrients. However, no other comprehensive standard was available or acceptable to the AAFCO until late 1991, so almost all pet food companies in the United States used the NRC's guidelines for dogs and cats to formulate their pet foods. The NRC's recommendations were also the standard that companies were required to use to comply with regulations governing inclusion of the term "complete and balanced pet food" on their product labels (see Section 3, pp. 146-147).

The AAFCO's *Nutrient Profiles* were first published in 1992. These profiles provide recommendations for practical minimum and maximum levels of nutrients in commercial pet foods. The levels of nutrients listed in these reports are intended for processed foods at the time of feeding. Minimum nutrient levels are reported for two different categories. The first category is growth and reproduction; the second is adult maintenance. Maximum nutrient levels are reported for nutrients with a potential for overuse or toxicosis. The *Canine Nutrition Report* was adopted by the AAFCO in August 1991. All pet food companies are now required to use this profile rather than the NRC's recommendations when formulating dog foods to meet established nutrient levels. The *Feline Nutrition Report* was written in late 1991, and pet food manufacturers were required to use it starting in January 1993 (see Section 3, p. 146).

CHAPTER

8

Nutritional Idiosyncrasies
of the Cat

Although the dog and cat have about equal status as companion animals in our society, it is important to recognize that they belong to two separate species. This truth is evidenced by well-defined physiological, behavioral, and dietary differences. In the following chapters, differences between the cat's and the dog's requirements for a number of nutrients are discussed in detail. These differences include the cat's unique energy and glucose metabolism, higher protein requirement, requirement for dietary taurine, sensitivity to a deficiency of the amino acid arginine, inability to convert beta-carotene to active vitamin A, and inability to convert the amino acid tryptophan to niacin.

An examination of the phylogeny and evolutionary relationship of the domestic dog and cat offers some clues to their inherent dietary dissimilarities. Although both species are of the class Mammalia and the order Carnivora, the dog belongs to the modern day Canoidea superfamily and the cat belongs to the Feloidea superfamily.[1] Included with the dog in the Canoidea superfamily are several families with very diverse dietary habits. For example, the Ursid (bear) and the Procyonid (raccoon) families are both omnivorous, but species of the Alurid (panda) family are strictly herbivorous. The only carnivorous species included with dogs are the Musetilids (weasels). The Feloidea superfamily, on the other hand, includes three families: the Viverrids (genet), the Hyaenids (hyena), and the Felids (cat) (Figure 8-1). All of the species in these families, including the cat, have evolved as strict carnivores. The evolutionary history of the dog suggests a predilection for a diet that is more omnivorous in nature. The history of the cat indicates that this species has consumed a purely carnivorous diet throughout its evolutionary development.

The adherence of the cat to a highly specialized diet has resulted in specific metabolic adaptations that manifest themselves as peculiarities in nutritional requirements. The consequence of these changes is an animal that cannot obtain all necessary nutrients solely from plants and plant products and therefore requires the

FIGURE 8-1

Phylogenic tree of the dog and cat.

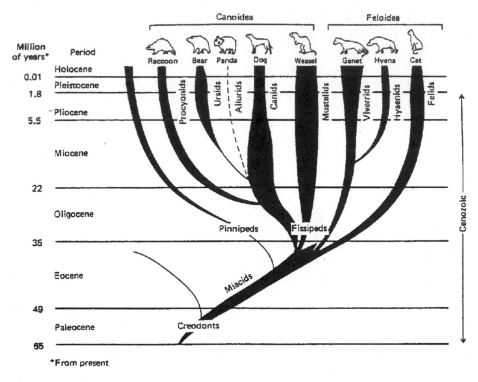

(From Morris J, Rogers Q. In Burger IH, Rivers JPW, editors: *Nutrition of cat and dog*, Cambridge, England, 1989, Cambridge University Press.)

BOX 8-1

Nutritional Idiosyncrasies of the Cat	
Idiosyncrasies of Practical Importance	**Idiosyncrasies of Academic Interest**
High protein requirement	Unique energy and glucose metabolism
Taurine requirement	Sensitivity to arginine deficiency
Arachidonic acid requirement	Inability to convert tryptophan to niacin
Preformed vitamin A requirement	

consumption of animal tissues to meet certain nutrient requirements. These specific nutritional idiosyncrasies are exhibited in the domestic cat *(Felis catus)* but not in its frequent housemate, the domestic dog *(Canis familiaris)*. This fact is of practical significance in light of the prevailing belief among some pet owners that cats may be fed as if they were small dogs.

The nutritional idiosyncrasies of the cat result in more stringent dietary requirements than those of a more omnivorous species, such as the dog. While all of these nutritional peculiarities are of metabolic significance, some are of greater practical importance than others when considering the optimal nutrition and proper feeding practices for pet cats (Box 8-1). The domestic cat's high protein requirement, along with its need for taurine, arachidonic acid, and preformed vitamin A, imposes a requirement for the inclusion of animal tissues in the diet of this species. Although it may be possible to develop a cereal-based ration for cats, such a formulation would require appropriate supplementation with purified forms of taurine, arachidonic acid, and preformed vitamin A.[2,3]

9

Energy Balance

All animals must meet their bodies' energy needs. Energy balance is achieved when energy expenditure is equal to energy intake, resulting in minimal changes in the body's store of energy. Positive energy balance occurs when caloric intake exceeds energy expenditure. In growing and pregnant animals, excess energy is converted predominately to lean body tissue. In adult, nonreproducing animals, positive energy balance results primarily in an increase in the quantity of fat stored by the body. Negative energy balance occurs when caloric intake is lower than energy expenditure. Weight loss and decreases in both fat and stores of lean body tissue occur during negative energy balance. The daily energy requirement for dogs and cats depends on the amount of energy that the body expends each day. Many factors can influence the energy requirement of a pet, and these factors must all be considered when determining the number of calories and the quantity of food required by a particular companion animal.

ENERGY EXPENDITURE

The body's energy expenditure can be partitioned into three major components: *resting metabolic rate* (RMR), *voluntary muscular activity, and meal-induced thermogenesis*.[4] A fourth component, called *adaptive* or *facultative thermogenesis,* represents energy that is expended in response to environmental conditions and yields heat but no useful work. Adaptive thermogenesis has been shown to exist in small, warm-blooded animals and is essential for cold adaptation.[5] It is theorized that this component may also function to increase thermogenesis during periods of overeating, thus protecting an animal from excessive weight gain. However, the importance of adaptive thermogenesis in the energy balance equation for species other than small rodents is not known.

Resting Metabolic Rate

The RMR contributes the greatest portion of an animal's total energy expenditure. The RMR is defined as the amount of energy expended while sitting quietly in a comfortable environment several hours after a meal or physical activity. It represents the energy cost of maintaining homeostasis in all of the integrated systems of the body during periods of rest.[4] Homeostasis refers to a state of internal stability within the body. The slightly lower value of the basal metabolic rate (BMR) is similar to the RMR, but it is measured shortly after waking and following an overnight fast. The RMR accounts for approximately 60% to 75% of an animal's total daily energy expenditure. Factors influencing RMR include sex and reproductive status, thyroid gland and autonomic nervous system function, body composition, body surface area, and nutritional state.[4] Research has shown that RMR is positively correlated with the total amount of respiring cell mass present in the body. Fat-free mass or lean body mass is the closest approximation available of the total respiring cell mass. Therefore the amount of fat-free mass or lean body tissue is the strongest predictor of an animal's metabolic rate, followed by body surface area and body weight.[6,7,8] Subsequently, as a pet's lean body mass and body surface area increase, RMR increases proportionately.

Voluntary Muscular Activity

Voluntary muscular activity is the most variable component of energy expenditure. Muscular activity contributes approximately 30% of the body's total energy expenditure in moderately active individuals.[9] The metabolic efficiency of performing physical work is invariable, but the total amount of energy expended is affected by both the duration and the intensity of the activity. In addition, the energy cost of any type of weight-bearing activity, such as walking or running, rises as body weight increases. This effect is a direct result of the added energy necessary to move a greater body mass. Therefore the energy expenditure of a pet with a high activity level depends on the duration and intensity of the exercise and the size and weight of the animal.

Meal-Induced Thermogenesis

Meal-induced thermogenesis refers to the heat produced following the consumption of a meal. The ingestion of nutrients causes an obligatory increase in heat production by the body. This increase is primarily the result of the metabolic cost of digestion, absorption, metabolism, and storage of nutrients. When a meal containing a mixture of carbohydrate, protein, and fat is consumed, meal-induced thermogenesis uses approximately 10% of the ingested calories. However, the magnitude of this heat production is influenced by the caloric and nutrient composition of the meal and the nutritional state of the individual.[9]

Adaptive Thermogenesis

Adaptive thermogenesis is an additional energy expenditure that is not accounted for by the obligatory and short-term thermogenesis of meal ingestion. Although this component is well documented in several species of small mammals, the signifi-

TABLE **9-1**

Factors Affecting Components of Energy Expenditure

Component	Factors
RMR	Gender, reproductive status, hormonal status, autonomic nervous system function, body composition, body surface area, nutritional stage, age
Voluntary muscular activity	Weight-bearing activity, duration of exercise, intensity of exercise, size and weight of animal
Meal-induced thermogenesis	Caloric and nutrient composition of meal, nutritional state
Adaptive thermogenesis	Ambient temperature, alterations in food intake, emotional stress

cance of adaptive thermogenesis to energy balance in larger mammals, such as dogs, cats, and humans, has not been conclusively established. Adaptive thermogenesis is manifested primarily as a change in the RMR in response to environmental stresses. These stresses include changes in ambient temperature, alterations in food intake, and emotional stress.[9] Cold adaptation in small mammals has been shown to rely on increased heat production that is disassociated from any productive work and separate from shivering thermogenesis.[5,10] Similarly, when energy intake increases, some animals are capable of increasing thermogenesis above the normal levels necessary for the metabolism of food and the maintenance of body temperature. This increased energy loss is a result of less efficient use of food calories. In the long term, the amount of weight gained during the period of overeating is significantly less than that normally expected from the increased caloric intake. This process may represent the body's tendency to protect the status quo of energy balance; thus adaptive thermogenesis regulates energy expenditure in an attempt to maintain body energy balance. Although this process has been shown to occur in laboratory animals and some human subjects, its significance in maintaining energy balance in companion animals is not yet known.[10,11]

Factors Affecting Energy Expenditure

Various factors influence a pet's total daily energy expenditure (Table 9-1). The RMR is affected by body composition, age, caloric intake, and hormonal status. The RMR component of energy expenditure naturally decreases as a pet ages, primarily as a result of a gradual loss of lean body tissue. Changes in RMR can also occur as a result of food restriction. When caloric intake is decreased, an initial decrease in RMR occurs because of hormonal influences. If caloric restriction continues, the loss of lean body tissue due to weight loss causes a persistent reduction in RMR. This decrease will not be corrected until normal levels of lean body tissue have been restored. Similarly, persistent overeating can lead to an increase in energy expenditure. Part of this increase results from the increase in lean body tissue with weight

BOX 9-1

Factors Affecting Energy Intake	
Internal Signals	**External Stimuli**
Gastric distention	Food availability
Physiological response to sight, sound, and smell of food	Timing and size of meals
	Food composition and texture
Changes in plasma concentrations of specific nutrients, hormones, and peptides	Diet palatability

gain and increased meal-induced thermogenesis. In addition, adaptive thermogenesis may increase energy expenditure as the body attempts to maintain energy balance in the face of increased energy intake. A pet's reproductive status also affects RMR. A recent study of the metabolic effects of neutering in cats found that gonadectomized (neutered) male and female cats had significantly lower estimated RMR values than those for intact cats of the same age.[12] These differences affected the cat's body composition and suggest that neutering alters a pet's daily energy needs (see Section 5, pp. 308-309).

Changes in voluntary activity and exercise level can significantly affect energy expenditure in dogs and cats. Just like people, companion animals tend to become more sedentary as they age. This change is usually first observed when the pet reaches maturity. In many breeds, play behaviors do not persist strongly into adulthood, and the onset of maturity is accompanied by a decline in physical activity. Later in life, voluntary activity may decline further because of chronic disease, the onset of arthritis, or a decreased tolerance for exercise. These changes will be reflected in a decline in the pet's total energy requirement. It follows that increasing a pet's daily exercise will increase the energy requirement. A portion of the higher energy expenditure occurs because of the direct calorie-consuming benefit of exercise. However, just as importantly, the long-term, cumulative effects of a regular exercise program will cause changes in body weight and composition. Regular exercise results in a higher proportion of lean tissue to fat tissue in the pet's body. The amount of exercise necessary to decrease body fat and maintain or increase lean body tissue is related to the duration and intensity of the physical activity. As discussed previously, an increase in lean body tissue increases RMR. Therefore voluntary activity not only directly burns energy, it also contributes to a higher percentage of lean body tissue and a higher RMR over a long-term period.

FOOD AND ENERGY INTAKE

The other half of the energy balance equation is energy intake. Food intake is regulated in all animals by a complex system involving both internal physiological controls and external cues. The internal signals and external stimuli that affect appetite, hunger, and satiety are presented in Box 9-1. Little research has been conducted on the internal signals that govern food intake in dogs and cats. Information involving these signals has been collected primarily in laboratory animals and can be used to provide insight into mechanisms that may be operating in other species.

Internal Controls of Food Intake

In all mammals the natural state for the body is one of hunger. This state is held in check by the presence of food in the gastrointestinal tract; the digestion, absorption, and metabolism of nutrients; and the amount of nutrients stored in the body at any one time. A small number of specific compounds appear to stimulate the appetite, and a much larger number of metabolic substrates satisfy the body.[13]

The hypothalamus is known to be involved in mediating both quantitative and qualitative changes in food intake. Several different neurotransmitter substances are believed to be involved in this process. Stimulatory neurotransmitters include catecholamine, norepinephrine, and three classes of neuropeptides (opioids, pancreatic polypeptides, and galanin).[13] Injections of these components directly into the hypothalamus of rats potentiates eating in both hungry and satiated animals. In addition, obesity as a result of overeating can be induced in laboratory animals by the chronic administration of norepinephrine.[13] The medial paraventricular nucleus is the area of the hypothalamus most sensitive to these neurotransmitters. Interestingly, there is evidence suggesting that these substances affect specific nutrient selection by animals, as opposed to simply increasing total caloric intake. Norepinephrine injection causes an increase in the consumption of carbohydrates, and the administration of opioids and galanin results in increased fat consumption.[13]

Substances that inhibit eating include the neurotransmitters dopamine and serotonin.[14] Synthesis of serotonin in the brain depends on the availability of the amino acid tryptophan, which is serotonin's precursor. In rats the specific action of serotonin appears to be the suppression of carbohydrate ingestion.[15] Other substances that inhibit food intake include the gut peptides cholecystokinin, glucagon, and bombesin.[16] Injections of glucagon in human subjects prior to eating cause a significant decrease in food intake.[17] The inhibitory effect of cholecystokinin (CCK) on food intake has been reported in several species, including humans.[16,18,19,20] In fact, the wolf appears to be one of the few species that does not alter food intake in response to CCK.[21] Bombesin is a peptide that has been investigated recently. The exogenous administration of this gut peptide to human subjects also results in decreased food intake.[22]

Insulin may be an important internal control signal for both appetite and satiety. The exogenous administration of this hormone stimulates hunger and increases food intake in human subjects. The mechanisms involved appear to be an insulin-induced decrease in the use of cellular glucose (glucoprivation) and severe hypoglycemia.[23] Insulin may also act directly on the hypothalamus to mediate this effect. Studies with rats have shown that both insulin and the adrenal glucocorticoid corticosterone function synergistically with central neurotransmitter substances to stimulate eating.[13] In human subjects, feelings of hunger are positively correlated with low levels of blood glucose.[24] Excess plasma glucose, however, does not depress food intake.[25]

Insulin may also be involved in signaling satiety and the cessation of eating. It has been theorized that the size of the fat deposit in an animal's body may be regulated by the concentration of insulin in the cerebrospinal fluid.[26] The insulin level in the cerebrospinal fluid increases and decreases proportionately as fat cells increase and decrease in size. These changes happen without the daily fluctuations that occur in plasma insulin levels. The insulin receptors of the cerebrospinal fluid, which are not accessible to the plasma insulin pool, appear to be involved in the regulation of food intake and total body adiposity. A study with rats demonstrated that when insulin was infused into the cerebrospinal fluid over a period of several weeks, food intake and body weight decreased significantly.[27] On the other hand, when the spinal pool of insulin was experimentally decreased by the injection of insulin antibodies, food intake and body weight both increased. These changes occurred independently of changes in plasma insulin concentration. Insulin levels in cerebrospinal fluid may modulate the brain's response to other internal satiety signals, such as the release of gut peptides, and may be important in the long-term control of body fat stores.

A final internal control mechanism for food intake is the gastric distention that occurs following meal ingestion. Physical distention of the stomach and the distal small intestine stimulates the vagus nerve and relays satiety information to the brain. However, the presence of food in the stomach alone will not inhibit food intake until gastric distention reaches pathological proportions. This is most likely a result of the stomach's natural ability to expand greatly in size. Other internal mechanisms are probably more important in signaling postprandial satiety than are stomach fullness or gastric distention.[25]

Aberrations in any of the internal control systems for appetite, hunger, and satiety can result in pathological changes in food intake. For example, lesions involving the ventromedial center of the hypothalamus lead to overeating, but lesions of the lateral nucleus result in an inhibition of food intake. Endocrine imbalances such as insulinoma, hypopituitarism, hyperadrenocorticism, and possibly hypothyroidism may affect food intake. Any metabolic dysfunction that affects neurotransmitter substances or the gut peptides could also potentially result in changes in food intake. Little research has been conducted in dogs and cats concerning internal satiety signals. It can be speculated that such mechanisms are operating in these species, but the degree of their importance in controlling food intake in domestic pets is not known.

External Controls of Food Intake

External controls of food intake include stimuli such as diet palatability, food composition and texture, and the timing and environment of meals. Exposure to highly palatable foods is considered a primary environmental factor contributing to food overconsumption in humans, laboratory animals, and companion animals.[28,29] Studies with human subjects have demonstrated that the quantity of food consumed varies directly with its palatability, and palatability does not appear to increase with levels of food deprivation. In other words, if food is perceived to be very appealing, an individual tends to consume more of it, regardless of the initial level of hunger.[4,30] Similarly, when rats are offered a highly palatable diet, they overeat and become obese.[31] This effect has been observed with high-fat diets, calorically dense diets, and "cafeteria" diets that provide a large variety of palatable food items.[32]

Dogs and cats have definite preferences for certain flavors and types of pet foods. A flavor preference test for dogs showed that the majority of those studied preferred canned and semimoist pet food over dry food.[33] Beef appears to be the most preferred type of meat, and cooked meat is overwhelmingly preferred to uncooked meat.[34] It is theorized that early experience with cooked meat, such as that present in commercial pet foods, is the cause of the development of this strong preference for cooked products compared with fresh products. Dogs also have a strong preference for sucrose, while cats do not seem to enjoy the taste of sugar.[35,36] In both species, warm food is preferred to cold food, and palatability generally increases along with the fat content of the diet.[36,37] Many of the taste preferences of dogs and cats can be explained by the type of taste buds or "units" found on their tongues.[38] For example, both dogs and cats have a high proportion of taste buds that are sensitive to amino acid flavors. It is postulated that these provide them with the ability to distinguish between the different types of meats that may be found in a carnivorous diet.

Palatability is an important diet characteristic that is heavily promoted in the marketing of commercial pet foods (see Section 3, pp. 200-202). Many pet owners select a pet food based on their own perceptions of the food's appeal and their pet's acceptance of the diet, rather than on indicators of nutritional adequacy. Semimoist foods contain high amounts of simple sugars, a taste that is preferred by many dogs. Canned pet foods, on the other hand, are often very high in fat. Fat contributes both to the palatability and the caloric density of the food. Feeding pets highly palatable foods on an ad libitum basis may encourage overeating in some pets and ultimately lead to weight gain and obesity.

The timing and social setting of meals also influence eating behavior. Dogs and cats rapidly become conditioned to receiving their meals at a particular time of day. This conditioning manifests itself both behaviorally and physiologically. Pets generally show increased activity levels at mealtime, and gastric secretions and gastric motility increase in anticipation of eating. In addition, dogs tend to increase food intake when consuming food in the presence of others.[25] This process is called *social facilitation*. It is not uncommon for pet owners to report that their dog was quite finicky before the introduction of a second pet. In most pets, social facilitation causes a moderately increased interest in food and an increased rate of eating. In some pets, the increase in food intake that occurs in response to another animal's presence can be extreme enough to singularly cause excessive food intake.[25] In some situations, however, the development of social hierarchies between dogs has the opposite effect on food consumption. Subordinate pets may be intimidated enough by dominant animals to inhibit eating during mealtimes.

The frequency with which meals are provided affects both food intake and metabolic efficiency. Increasing meal frequency may have opposing effects on weight gain. An increase in the number of meals per day results in an increased energy loss as a result of meal-induced thermogenesis. In a study with adult dogs, a group that was fed four times per day increased oxygen consumption 30%, but a second group that was fed the same amount of food in one meal daily exhibited only a 15% increase in oxygen consumption.[39] There is also evidence indicating that a decrease in lipogenesis occurs when multiple meals are fed as compared with the consumption of the same number of calories in only one or two meals.[40] In contrast, it is known that the presence of food, particularly palatable food, is a potent external cue for meal ingestion. An increased number of meal offerings each day may lead to excess consumption in individuals that are highly sensitive to external cues.[41] A study was conducted to compare the effects of free-choice feeding with portion-controlled feeding on the growth and development of growing puppies.[42] Puppies that had access to food throughout the day gained weight more rapidly and were heavier than puppies fed using the portion-controlled regimen. However, the two groups exhibited similar amounts of skeletal growth as measured by forelimb and body length. These results indicate that both groups were developing maximally, but the free-choice fed group was depositing more body fat than was the portion-controlled group. Continual exposure to a highly palatable food throughout the day may lead to overconsumption and excess weight gain in some dogs and cats. This tendency to overconsume may more than compensate for the increased energy loss that results from meal-induced thermogenesis.

A final external factor that may contribute to food intake is the nutrient composition of the diet. Nutrient composition affects both the efficiency of nutrient metabolism and the amount of food that is voluntarily consumed. Dietary fat and simple sugar appear to be the nutrients of greatest concern. Although most animals decrease their intake of a high-fat diet in an attempt to balance energy needs, the greater caloric density of the diet and its increased palatability can still cause increased energy consumption in some individuals. Additionally, the metabolic efficiency of converting dietary fat to body fat for storage is higher than the efficiency of converting dietary carbohydrate or protein to body fat. Only 3% of the energy content of fat is lost when it is stored as body fat. This loss can be compared with a loss of 23% of the energy content of dietary carbohydrate and protein when these nutrients are converted to body fat.[9,43] Therefore, if an animal is consuming more than its caloric requirement of a particular diet and if the excess calories are provided by fat, more weight will be gained than if the excess calories are coming from either carbohydrate or protein. This effect has been demonstrated in companion animals; puppies that consume a high-fat diet show similar growth in lean body mass when compared with puppies fed diets lower in fat, but the former accumulate more body fat.[44] When adult dogs were fed either a high-fat or a high-carbohydrate diet, the dogs fed the high-fat diet consumed only 13% more energy than those fed the high-carbohydrate diet, but they retained 117% more energy.[45] Even though a portion of this increased weight gain was attributed to the small difference in energy intake, there appeared to be increased efficiency of fat deposition in the dogs consuming the high-fat diet.

The amount of simple sugar in a diet may also affect energy balance in some animals. Rats will increase their caloric consumption of standard rat food when they are provided with a water/sucrose solution to drink along with the food. Prolonged feeding of the solution results in increased fat deposition and weight gain.[46] The mechanism responsible for this effect may be an insulin-induced hypoglycemia that occurs after sucrose consumption, resulting in increased feelings of hunger.[24] Increasing the simple sugar content of a diet increases its palatability in most species, with the exception of the cat.

A diet that is highly varied and contains calorically dense, palatable food items can also cause changes in food intake. This type of feeding regimen is commonly referred to as a "cafeteria" diet and has been shown to cause dramatic increases in total food intake, meal size, meal frequency, and body weight in normal adult rats.[47] It appears that the novelty of being presented with several different types of palatable foods can override normal satiety signals.[48] A practice that is similar to the "cafeteria" diet and is occasionally observed in companion animals is the feeding of a variety of table scraps and calorically dense treats or the constant offering of new types of foods. The persistent feeding of highly desirable and appealing treats to some dogs and cats may override the body's natural tendency to balance energy intake and lead to the overconsumption of energy (see Section 5, pp. 310-311).

DETERMINATION OF ENERGY REQUIREMENT OF DOGS AND CATS

The total daily energy requirement of an animal is the sum of the energy that is needed for the RMR, meal-induced thermogenesis, voluntary muscular activity, and maintenance of normal body temperature when exposed to adverse weather conditions. Adult animals in a state of maintenance only require enough energy to support activity and maintain the body's normal metabolic processes and tissue stores. On the other hand, dogs and cats that are growing, reproducing, or working have increased energy requirements.

Dogs

Formulating an exact equation for the estimate of energy requirements for dogs is a difficult task because of the wide variety of body sizes and weights seen in this species. The amount of energy that is used by the body is correlated with total body surface area. Body surface area per unit of weight decreases as animals increase in size. As a result, the energy requirements of animals with widely differing weights are not well correlated with body weight; they are more closely related to body weight raised to a specified power, which is called *metabolic body weight*. Metabolic body weight accounts for differences in body surface area between animals of varying sizes. Although several different values have been suggested, compilation of the data that is available on energy requirements for dogs indicates that

BOX 9-2

Calculation of Energy Requirements of Adult Dogs at Maintenance

Formula 1 (recommended)

ME requirement = $K \times W_{kg}^{0.67}$

K = 99 Inactive
132 Active
160 Very active

Examples: ME requirement of a 10 kg (22 lb) dog = $132 \times (10 \text{ kg})^{0.67}$ = 617.4 kcal of ME/day
ME requirement of a 40 kg (88 lb) dog = $132 \times (40 \text{ kg})^{0.67}$ = 1562.9 kcal of ME/day

Formula 2

ME requirement = $100 \times W_{kg}^{0.88}$

Examples: ME requirement of a 10 kg (22 lb) dog = $100 \times (10 \text{ kg})^{0.88}$ = 758.5 kcal of ME/day
ME requirement of a 40 kg (88 lb) dog = $100 \times (40 \text{ kg})^{0.88}$ = 2569.3 kcal of ME/day

Formula 3

ME requirement = $132 \times W_{kg}^{0.75}$

Examples: ME requirement of a 10 kg (22 lb) dog = $132 \times (10 \text{ kg})^{0.75}$ = 742.3 kcal of ME/day
ME requirement of a 40 kg (88 lb) dog = $132 \times (40 \text{ kg})^{0.75}$ = 2099.5 kcal of ME/day

the best power function to use is 0.67.[49] The allometric equation for the metabolizable energy (ME) requirement, represented as ME = K (representing a constant) $\times$ weight $(W)_{kilograms\ (kg)}^{0.67}$ provides an accurate estimate of daily energy requirements for different sizes of adult dogs experiencing different activity levels. Values for K range between 99 and 160 (Box 9-2). Two other equations can also be used to estimate ME for adult dogs. The first uses the power 0.88 in the equation ME = $100 \times W_{kg}^{0.88}$. This equation provides a reasonable estimate of the daily energy requirements of active dogs weighing between 1 and 60 kg. However, studies have shown that this equation may overestimate the energy requirements of adult dogs that have low to normal activity levels. The third equation, ME = $132 \times W_{kg}^{0.75}$, provides a good estimate for small and medium size breeds during maintenance.[50] However, this equation may underestimate the energy needs of some of the larger breeds of dogs. Regardless which of the three equations is used to predict energy needs, the resulting number should be used only as a starting point to determine the daily energy requirement of a particular animal. Variability among individual dogs and the environmental conditions under which dogs are kept can result in a requirement that is up to 25% greater or less than the predicted amount.

The estimates provided by these equations can be adjusted according to the dog's long-term response to feeding. For example, using the first equation, an active adult dog weighing 10 kg (22 pounds [lbs]) would require approximately 617 kilocalories (kcal) of ME per day. If a food containing 3800 kcal/kg (1727 kcal/lb) was fed, the dog would require 0.16 kg (160 grams [g]) of food. This is equal to 5.6 ounces (oz). One 8-oz cup of dry dog food contains 3 to 4 oz of food. Therefore the initial feeding level of this dog should be a little more than 1½ cups of food per day (Table 9-2).

TABLE **9-2**

Calculation of the Amount of Food to Feed Dogs and Cats

	Energy Requirement (kcal of ME/kg)		Energy Density (kcal/kg)		Quantity (kg)				Pounds		Ounces		Cups Per Day
Dog (10 kg)	617	÷	3800	=	0.16	×	2.2	=	0.352	=	5.6	=	1.6
Cat (4 kg)	240	÷	4200	=	0.057	×	2.2	=	0.125	=	2.0	=	0.57
Puppy (10 kg)	1234	÷	3800	=	0.325	×	2.2	=	0.715	=	11.4	=	3.26
Kitten (1 kg)	250	÷	4200	=	0.059	×	2.2	=	0.129	=	2.06	=	0.58

TABLE **9-3**

Energy Requirements for Different Stages of Life

Stage	Energy Requirement
Dogs	
Post weaned	2 × adult maintenance ME*
40% adult body weight	1.6 × adult maintenance ME
80% adult body weight	1.2 × adult maintenance ME
Late gestation	1.25 to 1.5 × adult maintenance ME
Lactation	3 × adult maintenance ME
Prolonged physical work	2 to 4 × adult maintenance ME
Decreased environmental temperature	1.2 to 1.8 × adult maintenance ME
Cats	
Post weaned	250 kcal ME/kg body weight
20 weeks	130 kcal ME/kg body weight
30 weeks	100 kcal ME/kg body weight
Late gestation	1.25 × adult maintenance ME
Lactation	3 to 4 × adult maintenance ME

*Adult maintenance for a dog of comparable weight.

The energy requirements predicted by these three equations are specific for adult maintenance. Stages of life that result in increased energy needs include growth, gestation, lactation, periods of strenuous physical work, and exposure to extreme environmental conditions (Table 9-3). After weaning, growing puppies require approximately twice the energy intake per unit of body weight as adult dogs of the same weight. An active puppy that weighs 10 kg would require 2 × 617 kcal, or 1234 kcal, per day. This would correspond to approximately 3¼ cups of food per day (see

Table 9-2). When puppies reach about 40% of their adult weight, this level of food should be reduced to 1.6 times maintenance levels; it should be further reduced to 1.2 times maintenance levels when 80% of adult weight is achieved.[49] The age at which a puppy will attain these proportions of adult weight will vary with the adult size of the dog. In general, large breeds of dogs mature more slowly than do small breeds. Most puppies achieve 40% of their adult weight between 3 and 4 months of age and 80% between 4½ and 8 months, depending on the breed. Although large breeds of dogs do not attain full adult size until they are more than 10 months of age, small breeds reach adult size at a slightly earlier age.[51]

Energy needs increase substantially for bitches during gestation and lactation. During the first 3 to 4 weeks of the 9-week gestation, energy needs remain the same as for maintenance. After the fourth week of pregnancy, energy requirements increase gradually to provide for rapid fetal growth. The energy needs of a pregnant bitch will increase to approximately 1.25 to 1.5 times the normal maintenance requirement by the end of the gestation period.[52] Lactation is one of the most energy-demanding stages of life for an animal. Depending on the size of the litter, the energy needs of a bitch during lactation can increase to as much as three times the normal maintenance requirement. Using the previous example, a bitch with a normal weight of 10 kg and maintenance energy needs of 617 kcal will require 3 × 617 kcal, or 1851 kcal, during peak lactation. This is equal to about 5 cups of food per day. The ability of a bitch to consume this amount of food may be limited by the size of her stomach. Therefore it is important to feed a food that is highly digestible and nutrient dense during this stage of life (see Section 4, pp. 230-231).

Both physical work and environmental stresses can cause increased energy needs in dogs. Short bouts of intense physical exercise may cause only a small increase in energy needs, but a regular program of prolonged exercise may cause increased needs of up to 2 to 4 times maintenance levels.[49] In addition, cold and hot weather conditions can also increase the energy requirement. Dogs must expend additional energy to support normal body temperature in cold conditions and to enhance body cooling mechanisms in warm conditions. Depending on the severity, living in cold conditions can increase energy requirements by 1.2 to 1.8 times the normal maintenance needs in dogs.[53]

Recent data from feeding studies with dogs suggest that the body type and conformation of particular breeds affect daily energy requirements.[54] For example, adult Newfoundland dogs have lower energy requirements than adult Great Danes of similar weight. This difference may be a reflection of variation in proportions of lean body tissue in the two breeds. More research into energy differences in different breeds is necessary because such information may be helpful in explaining the predisposition to obesity seen in certain breeds and breed-types.

Cats

The mature body weight of most domestic cats varies between about 2 and 6 kg (4 and 13 lbs). Because cats do not show the extreme variability in body size and weight that dogs do, it is possible to express their energy requirement on a body

BOX 9-3

Calculation of Energy Requirements of Adult Cats at Maintenance

Formula 1

Sedentary house cats: 50 kcal/kg × W_{kg}
Examples: ME requirement of a 4 kg cat = 50 kcal × 4 kg = 200 kcal of ME/day
  ME requirement of a 6 kg cat = 50 kcal × 6 kg = 300 kcal of ME/day

Formula 2

Moderately active cats: 60 kcal/kg × W_{kg}
Examples: ME requirement of a 4 kg cat = 60 kcal × 4 kg = 240 kcal of ME/day
  ME requirement of a 6 kg cat = 60 kcal × 6 kg = 360 kcal of ME/day

Formula 3

Very active cats: 70 kcal/kg × W_{kg}
Examples: ME requirement of a 4 kg cat = 70 kcal × 4 kg = 280 kcal of ME/day
  ME requirement of a 6 kg cat = 70 kcal × 6 kg = 420 kcal of ME/day

weight basis. Thus it is not as important to account for differences in body surface area in this species. Various estimates for the ME requirement for adult maintenance in cats have been published.[55,56,57] An estimate of 60 kcal/kg of body weight for moderately active adult cats and 70 kcal/kg of body weight for very active adult cats provides a reasonable starting point when determining the energy needs of an individual.[58,59] Although few studies have been conducted with purebred cats, available results indicate that breed differences in energy requirements are probably minor in the domestic cat.[60]

Sedentary house cats receiving little or no daily exercise require as little as 50 kcal/kg (Box 9-3). For example, an active adult cat weighing 4 kg (8.8 lbs) would require approximately 240 kcal of ME per day. If a dry food containing 4200 kcal/kg is fed, 0.057 kg or 57 g of food should be fed. This amount is equal to about 2 oz of food. If a cup of this food weighs 3.5 oz, the cat should be given approximately ½ cup of food per day (see Table 9-2).

Like dogs, the energy requirements of cats increase during growth, reproduction, physical activity, and extreme environmental conditions (see Table 9-3). The energy and nutrient requirements of growing kittens are highest per unit of body weight at about 5 weeks of age.[59] Young, rapidly growing kittens require approximately 250 kcal of ME per kg of body weight. This requirement declines to 130 kcal/kg by 20 weeks of age and to 100 kcal/kg by 30 weeks of age. A 3-month-old kitten weighing 1 kg (2.2 lbs) would require approximately 250 kcal/day. If a dry kitten food containing 4300 kcal/kg is fed, the kitten should be given 58 g or 2 oz of food. This is equal to a little more than ½ cup of food per day.

Studies with reproducing queens have indicated that energy requirements of cats increase throughout gestation, rather than only during the last 4 to 5 weeks.[61] By the end of the 9-week gestation, an increase of about 25% above normal maintenance energy needs is usually required. It appears that the accretion of excess maternal body tissues during gestation allows the queen to prepare adequately for the intense energy demands of lactation. The queen then uses these maternal stores and additional dietary energy to meet her energy requirements during lactation. In practical situations, queens often gain too much weight if allowed excess food intake during the first few weeks of gestation. As with dogs, intake should still be strictly monitored to ensure only a moderate increase in weight during the first 4 to 5 weeks of gestation. Depending on the size of the litter, a queen's dietary energy requirement may be as high as 250 kcal/kg body weight during peak lactation.[61] Increases of approximately 120 to 180 kcal/kg body weight are typical for queens that are in good physical condition at the time of parturition.[59] Using the same adult cat as an example, this would be equal to 720 kcal/day, or about 1¾ cups of food containing 4200 kcal/kg. During all physiological stages, the energy requirement of a particular cat vary with age, activity level, environmental temperature, body condition, and length and thickness of the cat's coat. Therefore these estimates should be used only as a starting point when determining the exact needs of an individual animal. Evaluation of the cat's body weight and condition can then be used to adjust the initial energy requirement estimate.

WATER

The daily drinking water requirement of a dog or cat depends on several factors. Voluntary water intake will increase in response to any change that causes an increase in water losses from the body, such as increased physical activity, increased body or environmental temperature, changes in the kidneys' ability to concentrate urine, or the onset of lactation. In addition, the amount of water present in the pet's food can significantly affect voluntary water intake. If the water content of the food is very high, both dogs and cats are able to maintain normal water balance with no additional drinking water.[62,63]

Generally, a pet's total exogenous water requirement, expressed in milliliters (ml), for maintenance in a thermoneutral environment is equal to two to three times the dry-matter (DM) intake of food, expressed in grams.[49,58] For example, if an adult dog requires 1000 kcal/day and is given a dry food that has an energy density of 3500 kcal/kg, the dog should receive 285 g of food per day. Dry pet foods contain approximately 8% moisture. Therefore the dog will be consuming 262 g of dry matter (DM). Multiplying this number by 3 gives an estimated water requirement of 785 ml of water per day. Other recommendations suggest that pets require an amount of drinking water that is roughly equal to the number of kcal that are consumed per day.[64] In this case, the requirement would then be equal to 1000 ml/day. The best method of ensuring adequate water intake in both dogs and cats is to provide fresh, clean water at all times, regardless of the animal's physiological state, caloric needs, or DM intake.

10

Carbohydrate Metabolism

All animals have a metabolic requirement for glucose. This requirement can be supplied either through endogenous synthesis or from dietary sources of carbohydrate. Gluconeogenic pathways in the liver and kidneys use propionic acid, lactic acid, glycerol, and certain amino acids to produce glucose, which is then released into the bloodstream to be carried to the body's tissues. Some data suggest that gluconeogenic pathways are active at all times in carnivorous species.[65,66] For example, the cat has been shown to be able to maintain normal blood glucose levels even during prolonged periods of fasting.[65]

The dog is capable of meeting its metabolic requirement for glucose from gluconeogenic pathways throughout growth and adult maintenance, provided that sufficient fat and protein are included in the diet.[44,67] However, the need for an exogenous source of carbohydrate during the metabolically stressful periods of gestation and lactation has been debated. During gestation the bitch's needs increase because glucose provides a major energy source for fetal development. Similarly, during lactation, additional glucose is needed for the synthesis of lactose, the disaccharide present in milk. It is assumed that the queen's glucose requirement also increases.

An early study with dogs examined the degree of reproductive success in bitches that were fed diets with varying levels of carbohydrates. The data indicated that bitches did require a source of carbohydrate to whelp and rear healthy puppies. Females who had been fed a carbohydrate-free diet throughout gestation became hypoglycemic, hypoalanemic, and ketotic near the end of their pregnancies. Only 63% of their puppies were alive at birth, and puppy mortality was high shortly after birth.[52] However, these results were subsequently refuted by data from a second experiment that also examined the effects of feeding a carbohydrate-free diet to bitches throughout gestation and lactation.[68] The latter group of researchers found that a carbohydrate-free diet did not affect duration of gestation, litter size, litter weight, or puppy viability. The difference in the results of the two experiments were attributed to differences in the protein levels of the diets that were fed. The diet in the first study contained only 26% protein, compared with 51% and 45% protein diets in the second set of experiments. It appears that the higher protein diets supplied the bitches with sufficient amounts of gluconeogenic amino acids to allow the maintenance of plasma glucose levels despite the heavy demands of gestation and lactation. Alanine, glycine, and serine appear to be the principle gluconeogenic amino acids in dogs.[69] The fact that the dogs in the first study exhibited hypoalanemia suggests that insufficient alanine was available to allow adequate gluconeogenesis. The hypoglycemia observed in these bitches was probably a result of the lack of gluconeogenic precursors rather than an innate inability to synthesize sufficient glucose during gestation and lactation.

These results were further supported by a study that examined the ability of varying levels of dietary protein to ameliorate the effects of carbohydrate-free diets on gestation and lactation.[70] The data confirm that feeding carbohydrate-free diets to pregnant and lactating bitches can cause adverse effects. However, performance was not impaired when the protein level in the diet was sufficiently high. The investigators estimated that if carbohydrate is provided in the diet, bitches require about 7 grams (g) of digestible crude protein per unit of metabolic body weight. However, if no carbohydrate is supplied in the diet, this protein requirement must be increased to approximately 12 g of protein. Lactating bitches appear to require between 13 and 18 g of protein per unit of metabolic weight when fed a diet containing carbohydrate and 30 g when fed a carbohydrate-free diet. This information indicates that although carbohydrate is physiologically essential for the dog, it is not an indispensable component of the diet, even during the metabolically demanding stages of gestation and lactation. Although specific studies have not been conducted during pregnancy and lactation in the cat, this species' unique pattern of gluconeogenesis, coupled with its carnivorous nature, suggests that it too can survive all stages of life while consuming a carbohydrate-free diet.

Compared with the dog and other omnivorous species, the cat has several unique mechanisms for metabolizing dietary carbohydrate. The cat's ability to maintain normal blood glucose levels and health when fed a carbohydrate-free diet is probably at least partly related to its different pattern of gluconeogenesis. In most animals, maximal gluconeogenesis for the maintenance of blood glucose levels occurs during the postabsorptive state, when dietary soluble carbohydrate is no longer available. However, carnivorous species are similar to ruminant species in that they maintain a constant state of gluconeogenesis with a slightly increased rate immediately after feeding.[71] Because the body is limited in its ability to conserve amino acids, and a carnivorous diet contains little soluble carbohydrate, this immediate use of gluconeogenic amino acids for the maintenance of blood glucose levels is a distinct advantage.

The enzyme activity values in the cat's liver indicate that gluconeogenic amino acids in the diet are deaminated and converted to glucose, rather than being directly oxidized for energy.[72] Liver phosphoenolpyruvate carboxykinase (PEPCK), a major gluconeogenic enzyme, does not change in activity level when cats that were previously fed high-protein diets are subjected to fasting.[65] In addition, no significant changes in hepatic PEPCK activity occurs when cats are switched from a low-protein diet (17.5%) to a high-protein diet (70%).[73] These data support the supposition that the hepatic gluconeogenic enzymes in cats always have a high rate of activity, necessitating the rapid conversion of excess dietary amino acids to glucose.

There also may be differences between cats and omnivores in the relative importance of various gluconeogenic and carbohydrate-metabolizing pathways. Compared with omnivorous species, the cat has a high hepatic activity of the enzyme serine-pyruvate aminotransferase and low activity of the enzyme serine dehydratase.[73,74] It appears that the cat is able to convert the amino acid serine to glucose by a route that does not involve either pyruvate or serine dehydratase. An alternate pathway has been proposed for the conversion of serine to glucose.[75] It has been observed that a high activity of the first enzyme in this alternate pathway, serine-pyruvate aminotransferase, appears to be associated with carnivorous dietary habits in mammals.[73]

After glucose is absorbed into the body, it must be phosphorylated to glucose-6-phosphate before it can be metabolized. The liver of most omnivorous animals, including the domestic dog, has two enzymes that catalyze this reaction, glucokinase and hexokinase. Hexokinase is active when low levels of glucose are delivered to the liver, and glucokinase operates whenever the liver receives a large load of glucose from the portal vein. The feline liver has active hexokinase but does not have active glucokinase.[76] Consequently, the rate of glucose metabolism in the liver of the cat cannot increase in response to high levels of soluble carbohydrate in the diet to the same degree as the rate in the liver of a species possessing both enzymes. It can be postulated that species having both enzymes have a greater capacity to handle high-glucose diets than do those that possess only hexokinase.

The fact that dogs and cats do not require carbohydrate in their diets is usually immaterial because most commercial foods include at least a moderate level of this nutrient. In general, dry pet foods contain the highest amount of carbohydrate. Commercial dry foods may include between 30% and 60% carbohydrate, and canned foods contain anywhere between 0% and 30%.[77] The largest proportion of carbohydrate in pet foods is provided by starch. Cooked starch is well digested by both dogs and cats.[44,78,79] It provides an economical and digestible energy source, and it is also essential for the extrusion process used in the preparation of most dry pet foods. The digestibility of dietary starch by dogs and cats is affected by the heat treatment and size of the starch granules. Heating greatly increases digestibility, and finely ground starch is more digestible than coarsely ground granules.[77,80]

Although cooked starch provides an excellent energy source, certain individual disaccharides, such as sucrose and lactose, are not well tolerated by pets.[81] An animal's ability to digest and use these sugars is governed by the levels of sucrase (beta-fructofuranosidase) and lactase (beta-galactosidase) found in the cells of the intestinal lumen. As in most species, the activity of lactase in dogs and cats tends to decrease with age. Queen's milk contains approximately 3% to 5% lactose, which provides about 20% of its metabolizable energy (ME).[82] Although kittens can digest this high level of lactose, some adult cats may exhibit diarrhea when consuming high levels of lactose. As a result of a loss of lactase activity with age, feeding adult companion animals large amounts of milk or other dairy products often results in maldigestion.[83] Small quantities of these foods can be digested by most pets, but large quantities cause diarrhea because of the osmotic effect of the sugar that escapes digestion and the volatile fatty acids that are produced by bacterial fermentation of the sugar in the large intestine. Although it has not been demonstrated in dogs or cats, data from other species indicate that very young animals have low levels of sucrase activity during the first few weeks of life. For this reason, sucrose solutions should not be used as energy sources for very young or orphaned puppies and kittens.[49]

Fiber is the other carbohydrate component commonly present in pet foods. Although dietary fiber is not a required nutrient per se, the inclusion of optimal amounts of fiber in the diets of companion animals is necessary for normal functioning of the gastrointestinal tract. Insoluble fiber functions to increase the bulk of the diet, contributes to satiety, and maintains normal intestinal transit time and gastrointestinal tract motility. Soluble fiber delays gastric emptying and, when fermented by colonic bacteria, produces short-chain fatty acids (SCFAs) that are important energy sources for colonocytes, the mucosal cells of the colon (see Section 6, pp. 499-501). Common sources of dietary fiber in pet foods include wheat middlings; tomato, citrus, and grape pomace; beet pulp; and the hulls of soybeans and peanuts. Corn, rice, wheat, and barley all contribute digestible carbohydrates and supply small amounts of fiber. In addition, protein sources in cereal-based pet foods add varying amounts of dietary fiber to the ration. The amount of fiber in pet foods varies with the type of food and the ingredients that are included. In general, the guaranteed maximum crude fiber content of most commercial pet foods ranges between 3% and 6% of the dry matter (DM) of the diet.[84] However, pet foods that contain higher quantities (5% to 25% crude fiber) are also available.[85]

11

Fats

FAT AS AN ENERGY SOURCE

The fat requirement of dogs and cats depends on the animal's need for essential fatty acids (EFAs) and a calorically dense diet. In pet foods, dietary fat contributes approximately 8.5 kilocalories (kcal) of metabolizable energy (ME) per gram (g), and protein and carbohydrate provide about 3.5 kcal/g. In addition to its high energy content, fat is also a highly digestible nutrient. The apparent digestibility of the fats found in high-quality pet foods is usually greater than 90%.[37,80] Because of its digestibility and higher energy content, increasing the level of fat in a pet's diet appreciably increases energy density. Both dogs and cats are able to maintain health when consuming diets that contain wide ranges of fat content, provided that other nutrients are adjusted to account for the changes in energy density.[44,49,58] Because animals normally eat or are fed to meet their energy needs, consumption of a more energy-dense ration will result in decreased consumption of the total volume of food. Therefore, if nutrients are not adjusted in relation to fat, multiple nutrient deficiencies can result.

Periods of high energy demand occur during growth, gestation, lactation, and prolonged periods of physical exercise. Feeding an energy-dense, high-fat diet during these periods allows an animal to consume adequate calories without having to ingest excessive amounts of dry matter (DM). In addition, feeding a high-fat diet during strenuous physical work may have metabolic benefits. Fatty acids are the primary source of energy used by the body during prolonged physical exertion. Consumption of a high-fat diet by dogs appears to result in an enhanced ability to use fatty acids for energy, ultimately contributing to improved endurance.[86,87] Most dry dog foods that are marketed for adult maintenance contain between 5% and 13% fat.[49] In comparison, the fat content of dry dog foods that are formulated for gestation, lactation, or performance may be 20% or greater.[88] In general, cat foods contain slightly higher amounts of dietary fat than do most dog foods. High levels of dietary fat can be fed to both dogs and cats with no detrimental results, provided that all nutrients are balanced and that the animals are fed to meet, and not exceed, their energy requirements.

Most adult pets that live relatively sedentary lifestyles do not need foods containing high levels of fat. Although high-fat pet foods are capable of providing good nutrition and supporting optimal health, sedentary animals may be inclined to overconsume these diets because of their high palatability and energy density. If adult pets are fed performance diets, strict portion-controlled feeding should be used to prevent excessive energy consumption and weight gain. Likewise, feeding high-fat, energy-dense foods during periods of rapid growth should be strictly monitored. Careful monitoring is especially important for large breeds of dog. High-fat foods that are balanced for all essential nutrients are capable of supporting a high rate of growth in dogs and cats if they are fed ad libitum. However, maximal growth rate has been shown to be incompatible with proper skeletal development in dogs.[89,90,91] Portion-controlled feeding should therefore be used to control a growing pet's weight gain, rate of growth, and body condition (see Section 4, pp. 251-254, and Section 5, pp. 333-337).

FAT AS A SOURCE OF ESSENTIAL FATTY ACIDS

In addition to providing energy, fat is necessary in the diet of dogs and cats as a source of EFAs. The fatty acids necessary for normal metabolism are linoleic acid and arachidonic acid of the n-6 series and, possibly, alpha-linolenic acid of the n-3 series (see Section 1, p. 21). All of these necessary fatty acids are long-chain, polyunsaturated fatty acids (PUFAs). Like most animals, dogs are able to meet their requirements for the n-6 fatty acids from an adequate dietary source of linoleic acid. Two key enzymes in the pathway for the synthesis of gamma-linolenic and arachidonic acid from linoleic acid are delta-6-desaturase and delta-5-desaturase. Unlike the dog, the cat is unable to synthesize adequate amounts of arachidonic acid because of low activity of delta-6-desaturase and delta-5-desaturase in the liver.[92,93,94,95] The cat also has low levels of delta-8-desaturase and delta-4-desaturase enzymes.[96,97]

When linoleic acid but not arachidonic acid is included in the diet, cats develop impaired platelet aggregation and thrombocytopenia, and queens fail to deliver viable kittens.[98,99] Interestingly, the male cat's reproductive performance is not impaired by arachidonic acid deficiency, which appears to be because of the teste's ability to produce adequate arachidonic acid from linoleate for its own use. In addition, cats that are deficient in arachidonic acid exhibit slight increases in hepatic neutral fat content and mild mineralization of the kidneys. Other clinical signs may include poor coat condition, retarded growth, impaired wound healing, and the development of skin lesions.[93] The addition of arachidonic acid at a level of 0.04% of ME to purified diets containing adequate linoleic acid results in normal reproductive performance in female cats.[100]

Only linoleic acid is required in the diet of dogs, but a cat's diet must contain both linoleic acid and arachidonic acid. The parent fatty acid linoleate is essential for the maintenance of normal skin functions, such as the regulation of water permeability.101 Linoleic acid also functions as the precursor for several derived fatty acids that are essential to the body for proper membrane structure, normal growth, maintenance of skin and coat condition, and lipid transport in the blood. Dietary arachidonic acid is required by the cat for functions that depend primarily on the formation of eicosanoids from arachidonic acid, such as reproduction and platelet aggregation.[99]

DIETARY FAT AND ESSENTIAL FATTY ACID REQUIREMENTS

Dogs

The EFA requirement of the dog is usually expressed in terms of linoleic acid content because the dog's physiological requirement for EFAs can be met by sufficient dietary linoleic acid. In addition, it is of practical value to denote the requirement in this way because linoleic acid is the most prevalent EFA in most foods.[49] The National Research Council (NRC) and the Association of American Feed Control Officials' (AAFCO's) *Nutrient Profile* for dogs both recommend that the canine diet for adult maintenance provide a minimum of 1% of the dry weight as linoleic acid and 5% total fat.[49,102] The AAFCO's recommendations further suggest that this level be increased to 8% total fat during periods of growth and reproduction.[102]

Cats

Reliable estimates for EFA requirements in cats are difficult to make because adequate levels of linoleic acid in the diet decrease the requirement for arachidonic acid, and high levels of arachidonic acid can meet some of the needs for linoleic acid.[100] One study demonstrated that dietary linoleic acid at a level of 6.7% of dietary calories is more than adequate to prevent signs of deficiency in the cat.[101] Extrapolation of data on the unsaturation index of liver lipids and comparisons with data reported for the rat were used to determine a linoleic acid requirement estimate of 2.5% of the calories in the diet.[103,104,105] Other data demonstrated that 0.04% of the energy supplied as arachidonic acid would support adequate reproduction in queens, provided that other interfering PUFAs were not present in the diet.[99] Many fish oils contain n-3 fatty acids that can interfere with the body's ability to use arachidonic acid. The NRC recommends that arachidonic acid supply 0.02% of the dry weight in a diet with an energy density of 5000 kcal of ME/kilogram (kg).[58] This recommended amount is equivalent to 0.04% of the metabolizable calories. The same group recommends that linoleic acid should supply a minimum of 1% of the metabolizable calories in the dry diet to meet the needs for all stages of the cat's life.[58] The AAFCO's *Nutrient Profiles* for cat foods recommends 0.5% linoleic acid and 0.02% arachidonic acid in diets containing 4000 kcal of ME/kg.[102]

DEFICIENCIES AND EXCESSES

Low amounts of fat in the diet can lead to deficiencies in both total energy and EFAs. The palatability of dog and cat diets is strongly affected by fat content. To a limit, increasing fat results in enhanced palatability. Similarly, decreasing fat below a certain level causes decreased acceptability of the diet. This effect is believed to be the result of both the consistency and the flavor that fat contributes to a pet food. Because low-fat diets may not be readily accepted by pets, their potential for causing an energy or EFA deficiency is exacerbated by their causing a decrease in food intake.

In dogs, an EFA deficiency results in a dry, dull coat; hair loss; and the eventual development of skin lesions. Over time, the skin becomes pruritic, greasy, and susceptible to infection. A change in the surface lipids in the skin alters the normal bacterial flora and can predispose the animal to secondary bacterial infections.[106] Epidermal peeling, interdigital exudation, and otitis externa have also been reported in EFA-deficient dogs.[107] Because EFAs are important for the maintenance of the epidermal barrier, and because skin cells have a high rate of turnover, the skin is particularly vulnerable to EFA deficiencies. Linoleic acid deficiency in cats results in similar dermatological signs. In addition, kittens will fail to grow normally, and they may develop fatty degeneration of the liver and fat deposition in the kidneys.[100,108,109]

EFA deficiencies are not common in dogs and cats. These deficiencies develop only over a long period. When they do occur, deficiencies are usually associated with the consumption of diets that are either poorly formulated or have been stored improperly. Most well-formulated diets contain sufficient amounts of EFAs, but exposure to high environmental temperatures and humidity for long periods can promote oxidation of the unsaturated fatty acids in the food. This process is commonly referred to as *rancidity*. If insufficient antioxidants are present, EFA activity is destroyed. As the unsaturated fats are destroyed by oxidation, not only is EFA activity lost, but so are the vitamins D, E, and biotin. EFA deficiency in dogs and cats can also occur as a complication of other diseases, such as pancreatitis, biliary disease, hepatic disease, and malabsorption.[106]

Although commercially prepared foods will not normally cause fat or EFA deficiency, many pet owners believe that supplementing their pet's diet with corn oil or some other type of fat will improve coat quality. This supplement is only effective if the pet is truly suffering from an EFA or fat deficiency. If that is the case, completely changing the diet to a well-formulated pet food that supplies all of the essential nutrients in their correct proportions, including fat and EFAs, is recommended. Simply adding a source of fat or EFAs to a deficient diet may or may not solve the EFA deficit and has the potential to further imbalance a diet that is already inadequate. In some cases, fatty-acid supplementation may be effective in treating certain inflammatory and hyperproliferative skin diseases in companion animals. Recent research indicates that providing certain types of PUFAs promotes the formation of fewer inflammatory agents, resulting in a lessening of clinical signs (see Section 6, pp. 435-443).

Excess fat intake can also be detrimental to a pet's health. Both dogs and cats are able to digest and assimilate diets containing high levels of fat.[45,110] However, providing more fat than the gastrointestinal tract can effectively digest and absorb results in fatty stools (steatorrhea) and diarrhea. This problem is most commonly observed when pet owners provide their dog or cat with table scraps composed predominantly of fatty foods. In addition, the long-term consumption of diets that are very high in fat may lead to weight gain and obesity because of the high palatability and energy density of the diet. Feeding diets that are very high in fat and do not have all other nutrients balanced relative to energy density may result in the development of deficiencies in other essential nutrients. Lastly, excessive levels of PUFAs in the diet cause an increase in an animal's vitamin E requirement. Vitamin E functions as an antioxidant in the body, protecting cellular membrane lipids from peroxidation. The vitamin is preferentially oxidized before the unsaturated fatty acids, thus protecting the fatty acids from rancidity; however, vitamin E is destroyed in this process. Therefore as the level of unsaturated fatty acids in the diet of an animal increases, so does its requirement for vitamin E. If a pet food contains very high levels of PUFAs or if an owner is supplementing a balanced diet with high amounts of corn or vegetable oil, vitamin E in the diet must concomitantly be increased. A condition called *pansteatitis,* or "yellow fat disease," occurs in cats when their diets are high in unsaturated fatty acids and marginal or low in vitamin E (see Section 5, pp. 345-346).

C H A P T E R

12

Protein and Amino Acids

Protein is required by the body for two major purposes: to provide the essential amino acids that may be used for protein synthesis and to supply nitrogen for the synthesis of dispensable amino acids and other essential nitrogen-containing compounds (see Section 1, p. 23). Animals do not have a dietary requirement for protein per se, but they require the essential amino acids and a certain level of nitrogen. This requirement is commonly expressed as a protein requirement because amino acids and nitrogen are most typically supplied in the diet in the form of intact protein. Adult animals require dietary protein to replace protein losses in skin, hair, digestive enzymes, and mucosal cells; protein also replaces amino acid losses from normal cellular protein catabolism. Young animals have these same maintenance requirements plus an added requirement for the growth of new tissue. If protein is deficient in the diet, adult animals will experience negative nitrogen balance and the loss of lean body tissue, and immature animals will exhibit decreased weight gain or weight loss and impaired growth and development.

An animal's *protein requirement* is defined as the minimum intake of dietary protein that promotes optimal performance.[111] The criteria that have been used most often to evaluate performance when determining protein requirements in dogs and cats are nitrogen balance and growth rate. Nitrogen balance studies are based upon the fact that protein, on the average, contains 16% nitrogen. The nitrogen content of food and excreted matter is commonly measured using an analytical test called the *Kjeldahl method*.[112] A measurement of nitrogen intake and excretion by the body provides a rough estimate of the body's protein status. Nitrogen balance is calculated as Nitrogen balance = nitrogen intake − nitrogen excretion through urine and feces. The nitrogen in the feces is made up of unabsorbed dietary protein and nitrogen from endogenous sources. Urinary nitrogen is composed primarily of urea, which is the end product of protein catabolism. Further nitrogen losses occur from desquamated cells of the skin surface, hair, and nails. However, these losses are very difficult to measure and are usually not considered when measuring nitrogen balance in experimental studies.

Requirement studies with growing animals use maximum positive nitrogen balance or maximum growth rate to indicate an adequate level of protein in the diet;

TABLE 12-1

States of Nitrogen Balance

State	Balance	Physiological Stage
Zero	N intake = N excretion	Maintenance
Positive	N intake > N excretion	Growth, gestation, recovery from illness
Negative	N intake < N excretion	Inadequate nutrition, severe illness or injury, urinary N loss during renal failure, gastrointestinal tract loss during certain diseases

N, Nitrogen.

studies for adult companion animals use zero nitrogen balance to indicate dietary protein adequacy. *Zero nitrogen balance* means that the body's daily loss of protein is replaced by intake, without a net gain or loss in total body protein. Although the vast majority of requirement studies have used zero nitrogen balance to assess the protein requirement of adult animals, it is important to recognize that diets containing this level of protein may not be adequate to promote optimal performance and health. For example, adult dogs that were fed diets containing just enough protein to attain zero nitrogen balance were found to be more susceptible to the toxicity of certain drugs.[113] In addition, higher levels of protein in the diet may be needed to maintain optimal protein reserves.[114] Although protein is not stored in the body as is fat and, to a lesser degree, carbohydrate, the term *reserves* refers to the ability of the body to mobilize protein from prioritized body tissues during periods of stress. It is possible that the requirements obtained using zero nitrogen balance may represent a minimum protein requirement for adult animals. If this is the case, it would be prudent to feed slightly higher levels of protein than this minimum amount to healthy adults, especially during periods of stress.[111]

Nitrogen equilibrium (zero balance) is the normal state for healthy adult animals during maintenance. An animal is described as being in a state of positive nitrogen balance when protein intake exceeds excretion. Positive nitrogen balance occurs when new tissue is being synthesized by the body, such as during the physiological stages of growth and gestation or the recovery phase after prolonged illness or injury. Negative nitrogen balance results when protein excretion exceeds intake. An animal that exhibits negative balance is losing nitrogen from tissues more rapidly than it is being replaced. This loss of nitrogen may occur for several reasons. If the animal is consuming an insufficient amount of energy, body tissues must be catabolized to provide energy to the body. If inadequate levels of available protein and/or amino acids are fed, tissue replacement cannot occur. Severe or prolonged illness or injury results in a catabolic state in animals that is evidenced by excessive breakdown of the body's tissues and negative nitrogen balance. Excess losses of nitrogen from the urine during renal failure or from the gastrointestinal tract during some types of gastrointestinal disease can also cause negative nitrogen balance to occur (Table 12-1).

BOX 12-1

Factors Affecting Protein Requirement

Protein quality: As protein quality increases, protein requirement decreases.
Amino acid composition: As amino acid composition improves, protein requirement decreases.
Protein digestibility: As protein digestibility increases, protein requirement decreases.
Energy density: As energy density increases, protein requirement as a percentage of the diet, increases.

FACTORS AFFECTING PROTEIN REQUIREMENTS

The determination of the exact protein requirements for dogs and cats is a difficult task because many factors can affect an individual animal's need for this nutrient. Dietary factors that affect nitrogen balance include protein quality and amino acid composition, protein digestibility, and the energy density of the diet. In addition, an animal's activity level, physiological state, and prior nutritional status can all influence the protein requirement as determined by nitrogen balance or growth rate (Box 12-1).

An animal's protein requirement varies inversely with the protein source's digestibility and with its ability to provide all of the essential amino acids in their correct quantities and ratios. As protein digestibility and quality increase, the level of protein that must be included in the diet to meet the animal's needs decreases. Most of the protein requirement studies that have been conducted with dogs and cats have used either purified or semipurified diets; the protein and amino acids in these diets are highly digestible and available. However, most of the protein sources used in today's commercial pet foods have comparatively low digestibility coefficients. For example, protein digestibility in a semipurified diet approaches 95%, but that of high-quality, commercial diets ranges between 80% and 90%. On the other hand, low-quality, commercial pet foods can have protein digestibilities of less than 75%.[59] As a result of these differences, requirement studies with purified or semipurified diets tend to underestimate the protein requirements of animals that are consuming mixed protein diets that contain less available nutrients.

Protein quality also influences an animal's protein requirement. The higher the biological value of a protein, the less the amount that is needed to meet all of an animal's essential amino acid needs (see Section 1, pp. 26-28). Therefore, as the quality of the protein in the test diet increases, the estimated requirement decreases. Again, the diets that were used in most amino acid and protein requirement studies had amino acid contents that were adjusted to carefully fit the needs of the experiment. Few, if any, naturally occurring protein sources have amino acid compositions that specifically fit the requirements of companion animals. Most practical sources of protein contain excesses of some amino acids and slight or severe deficiencies of others relative to an animal's requirement. Commercial pet foods correct for these inadequacies by using mixtures of protein sources that have complimentary profiles of essential amino acids.

Correction factors can be applied to requirement estimates that were determined using purified or high-quality protein sources. These factors account for differences in protein digestibility and quality in the sources included in commercially prepared pet foods.[49,58] However, the ingredients that are used in the formulation of commercial rations can vary greatly in protein digestibility and quality.[115,116] Therefore much care must be taken when interpreting and using requirement data that have been derived from studies using purified diets. In the end, the only totally effective means of evaluating the amino acid or protein content of a particular diet is to feed the diet and thoroughly evaluate the results.

The caloric density of the diet used in the requirement study significantly affects the estimated protein requirement. The presence of nonprotein calories has a protein-sparing effect. A diet must first meet an animal's energy needs before the energy-containing nutrients can be used for other purposes. Therefore adequate nonprotein calories in the form of carbohydrate or fat spare the protein in the diet from being metabolized for energy. If sufficient nonprotein calories are not provided, at least a portion of the dietary protein will be metabolized as an energy source. At caloric intakes that are less than the animal's energy requirement, protein will not be available for the building or replacing of body tissues because it will all be used for energy. Therefore, when a diet is limiting in both energy and protein, weight loss and a loss of lean body tissue result. Nitrogen balance studies have shown that when the dietary protein level is held constant, nitrogen retention increases as caloric intake increases and approaches the animal's energy requirement.[117]

A second aspect of the relationship between protein and energy must also be examined. Assuming that adequate nonprotein energy is present in the diet, as the energy density of the diet increases, a higher total concentration of protein is required for maximal nitrogen retention. The most important factors that affect the energy density of commercial pet foods are dietary fat concentration and diet digestibility. The relationship between energy density and protein content is illustrated by the results of a study with growing dogs.[118] When a diet containing 25% crude protein and 20% fat was fed, maximal growth rate resulted. However, when the fat content of the diet was increased to 30%, 29% crude protein was necessary to support maximal growth. The reason for this change relates to an animal's tendency to eat to satisfy its energy needs. Provided that these controls are in place, an animal will naturally consume less of a more energy-dense ration. Pet owners who use portion-controlled feeding regimens usually adjust quantity according to their pet's body weight and/or growth rate. Therefore portion-controlled feeding schedules are still regulated according to the pet's energy requirements. When lower quantities of food are fed, protein must contribute a higher proportion of the diet so that the animal is still able to meet its total protein needs. Although protein is the most commonly used example, this relationship with energy also applies to all other essential nutrients.[119]

Protein requirement studies must also take into account an animal's prior nutritional status and physiological state. The amount of absorbed protein needed to produce nitrogen equilibrium depends on the degree of protein depletion. Dogs with depleted body protein reserves require lower levels of nitrogen to achieve nitrogen balance than do dogs with normal reserves.[120] This effect may be the result of an increased efficiency of absorption and use of dietary protein when in a depleted state or due to a decreased rate of protein catabolism. Ensuring that all dogs are in positive nitrogen balance and have adequate body protein reserves by feeding a high-protein diet before the onset of a requirement study has been used to eliminate this discrepancy. Physiological state also directly affects nitrogen balance and will therefore affect the outcome of requirement studies that use nitrogen balance. In growing puppies and kittens, the rate of growth and, subsequently, the protein requirement decrease slightly with age.[115,121,122,123,124]

PROTEIN REQUIREMENTS

Dog

Numerous studies have been conducted on the minimum protein requirement of the adult dog. However, differences in the protein sources, energy densities, and amino acid balance of the experimental diets have led to a great deal of confusion regarding this requirement. Generally when diets containing very high-quality protein sources are fed, adult dogs require between 4% and 7% of their metabolizable energy (ME) calories to be supplied as protein.[125,126,127] However, when lower-quality protein sources are included in the diet, the requirement increases to more than 20% of the ME calories.[57,111,128] This value is equivalent to 21% protein in a typical dry dog food containing 3.5 kilocalories (kcal) of ME/gram (g). The protein requirement of growing puppies is significantly higher than that of adult dogs. Early studies using mixed protein sources reported minimum protein requirements of between 17% and 22% of ME for growing dogs. These experiments used maximum weight gain as an indicator of minimum protein needs.[118,129,130] A more recent study, which also used weight gain as the criterion, reported a slightly lower requirement.[131] However, the protein source used in this experiment was of high quality when compared with that used in the earlier studies. Nitrogen balance data in this study provided a protein requirement estimate of 20% of ME or greater.[131] It appears that weight gain in growing dogs is maximized at lower protein intakes than is nitrogen retention. It has been estimated that a minimum of 19.5% of a diet's calories should be supplied as high-quality protein to maximize nitrogen retention in puppies between the ages of 8 and 17 weeks.[111] Another recent study suggested a value of 16% of ME calories as a minimum for growth in dogs.[132] However, the diets used in this study were composed of purified amino acids, not intact protein, so they were almost 100% available. The investigators found that a level of 16% of ME supported greater T-cell responses and resulted in greater nitrogen retention in growing puppies than did a

TABLE **12-2**

Suggested Minimum Levels of Protein in the Diets of Dogs and Cats
as a Percentage of Metabolizable Energy

	NRC*	AAFCO
Dogs		
Adult maintenance	—[†]	18% ME
Growth and reproduction	11.4% ME	22% ME
Cats		
Adult maintenance	10% ME	23% ME
Growth and reproduction	17% ME	26% ME

*NRC 1985, 1986.
[†]Estimate not provided.

diet containing 12% protein. It was emphasized that this value should be taken as a minimum, because all of the amino acids in the diets were highly available, there were no amino acid excesses or imbalances, and no allowances had to be made for losses due to processing or storage.[132]

The importance of considering protein digestibility and amino acid content when determining an animal's protein requirement is well illustrated by a comparison of the protein requirement estimates provided by the 1974 and 1985 National Research Council's (NRC's) *Nutrient Requirements for Dogs*.[49,50] The 1985 NRC recommendations suggest a minimum protein requirement for growing dogs of 11.4% of ME calories.[49] This amount is approximately half the value that was proposed in their 1974 publication. The change in 1985 was a direct result of the publication of a number of studies that determined the dog's requirement for most of the essential amino acids. Although these studies provided valuable information concerning the minimum amino acid requirements of the dog, they all included diets containing carefully controlled levels of purified amino acids. The use of these studies to derive recommendations for protein levels in practical dog foods resulted in estimates that were much lower than those based on mixed protein diets. As a result, difficulty in the interpretation and use of the 1985 recommendations led some pet food companies to return to the 1974 requirement recommendations for formulation of their pet foods. When the Canine Nutrition Expert Committee of the Association of American Feed Control Officials (AAFCO) published the *Nutrient Profiles* for dog foods in 1992, they reinstated the original protein requirements for growth and reproduction that were published in the 1974 NRC report. The committee recommended a minimum level of 18% protein on a dry-matter basis (DMB) for adult maintenance and 22% protein for growth and reproduction (Table 12-2).[102] These values are equivalent to 18% and 22% of ME in a food containing 3.5 kcal/g. If the energy density of the diet is higher, appropriate adjustments in protein content must be made.

Cat

Early studies of the cat's nutrient requirements showed that it has a protein requirement substantially higher than that of other mammals, including the dog.[59,122,133] When growing kittens were fed varying levels of dietary protein, supplied as minced herring and minced liver, growth was reported to be satisfactory only when protein exceeded 30% of the dry weight of the diet.[122] In comparison, growing puppies fed mixed diets required only 20% protein for adequate growth and development.[124] One of the first studies of the protein requirement of the adult cat reported that 21% dietary protein was necessary to maintain nitrogen balance when cats were fed a mixed diet containing liver and whitefish as the primary protein sources.[128]

More recently, experimentation using crystalline amino acids and protein isolates has allowed more precise definition of the minimum protein requirements of growing kittens and adult cats. One study reported a protein requirement of 18% to 20% (by weight) in growing kittens fed either crystalline amino acid diets or casein diets supplemented with methionine.[134] A second study reported requirements as low as 16% of ME calories when growing kittens were fed a purified diet containing all of the essential amino acids in their correct concentrations and ratios.[123] Using a similar semipurified diet, the protein requirement of adult cats was determined to be 12.5% of ME.[135] The profound effect that protein digestibility, amino acid balance, and amino acid availability have on determining an animal's dietary protein requirement is illustrated by the substantially lower values that were obtained when semipurified and purified diets were used to determine requirements. However, the comparison of these current figures with ideal minimum protein requirements of other mammals still demonstrates that the cat, together with other obligate carnivores such as the fox and the mink, has a higher requirement for dietary protein. For example, although the cat requires 20% of a 100%-available, well-balanced ideal protein for growth and 12% for maintenance, the dog requires only 12% and 4% respectively.[121] It should be noted that these values are substantially lower than the protein requirement of a cat fed a practical diet containing protein sources that are not perfectly balanced or 100% available.

The 1986 NRC recommendations for cats suggest a minimum of 240 g of protein/kilogram (kg) in the diets of growing kittens and 140 g/kg in the diets of adult cats. These values are calculated on the assumption that diet energy densities are 5 kcal/g. This amount is equivalent to 24% protein or only 17% of ME calories for growing kittens and 14% protein or 10% of ME calories for adults (see Table 12-2). These values assume highly available and well-balanced protein sources. The NRC recommendations note that a variable proportion of the protein included in commercially prepared cat foods is indigestible and that processing methods may result in changes in the availability of certain amino acids. Therefore it is suggested that pet food companies make allowances for the amino acid composition of the proteins included in their foods and for the digestibility and availability of the protein. A range of 80% to 90% availability is suggested for high-quality ingredients and 60% to 70% for lower-quality ingredients (see Section 3, pp. 202-205).[58]

The NRC provides recommendations for minimum nutrient requirements for dogs and cats, not recommended allowances for inclusion in pet foods. The AAFCO profiles that were established by the Feline and Canine Nutrition Expert Committees provide nutrient estimates for use in the actual formulation of pet foods. Therefore, it is not surprising that the AAFCO's *Nutrient Profiles* for cat foods suggest a substantially higher level of protein for inclusion in commercially prepared cat foods.[102] A level of 30% of the diet (on a DMB) is suggested for growth and reproduction in diets containing 4 kcal of ME/g of food. This value is equivalent to 26% of ME calories. A level of 26% of the diet is suggested for adult maintenance. This level is equivalent to about 23% of ME calories (see Table 12-2). Other investigators have suggested a minimum level of 15% of ME calories provided by a high-quality protein for adult maintenance in cats. This level corresponds to 17% (by weight) of a diet containing 4 kcal/kg.[111]

The cat's comparatively high dietary requirement for protein is the result of increased needs for the maintenance of normal body tissue, rather than increased needs for growth. Approximately 60% of the growing kitten's protein requirement is used for the maintenance of body tissues; only 40% is used for growth.[124] The opposite is true in most of the other species that have been studied. For example, the growing rat requires only 35% of its dietary protein for maintenance and 65% for growth;[50] similarly, the growing dog uses only 33% of its protein requirement for maintenance and 66% for growth.[121]

The elevated protein requirement for maintenance in the cat results from the inability of the nitrogen catabolic enzymes in the cat's liver to adapt to changes in dietary protein intake.[73] When most mammals are fed diets high in protein, the enzymes involved in amino acid catabolism, nitrogen disposal, and gluconeogenesis increase in activity to use surplus amino acids and convert excess nitrogen to urea. Conversely, when low-protein diets are fed, the activity of these enzymes declines, resulting in conservation of nitrogen.[136,137,138] This adaptive mechanism is a distinct advantage because it allows animals to conserve amino acids while consuming low-protein diets; it also provides a mechanism to catabolize excess amino acids when consuming high-protein diets. One study involved feeding two groups of adult cats either high-protein (70%) or low-protein (17.5%) diets for 1 month.[73] The activities of three urea cycle enzymes and seven nitrogen catabolic enzymes in the liver were then measured. With the exception of one transaminase enzyme, no significant differences in enzyme activity were found between the cats fed the low-protein diet and the cats fed the high-protein diet. Several gluconeogenic and lipogenic enzymes were also measured, none of which exhibited any change in activity in response to the changes in dietary protein level. On the other hand, similar rat hepatic enzymes increase in activity from 2.75-fold to 13-fold after rats are changed from a low-protein diet to a high-protein diet.[139]

In addition to the inability of the cat's protein-catabolizing enzymes to adapt to changes in dietary protein levels, the enzymes involved in nitrogen catabolism function at relatively high rates of activity.[73] This metabolic state causes the cat to catabolize a substantial amount of protein after each meal, regardless of its protein content. Thus the cat does not have the capability to conserve nitrogen from the body's general nitrogen pool. The only alternative that ensures adequate conservation of body protein stores is the consistent consumption of a diet containing high levels of protein.[124] It can be theorized that because of the cat's strict adherence to a carnivorous diet, it experienced little selective pressure throughout its evolutionary history to develop metabolic adaptations to low-protein diets. As a result, the cat is now obliged to always consume meals that contain high levels of dietary protein.

Another factor that contributes to an animal's dietary protein requirement is its need for essential amino acids. When the protein nutrition of the cat was first studied, it was postulated that its high dietary requirement might be the result of an unusually high requirement for one or more of the essential amino acids. The results of several experimental studies showed that with the exception of slightly higher requirements for leucine, threonine, methionine, and arginine, as well as a unique dietary requirement for taurine, the requirements for specific essential amino acids are not significantly greater in the cat than in the rat, dog, or pig.[105,124] Therefore elevated essential amino acid requirements are not the cause of the cat's high protein requirement. The domestic cat does have two unique amino acid requirements, however. The first involves the cat's inability to synthesize adequate arginine for normal functioning of the urea cycle and protein synthesis; the second concerns the cat's dietary requirement for taurine, an amino sulfonic acid.

Arginine Requirement The amino acid arginine is not considered a dietary essential in most adult animals because most species can synthesize adequate amounts to meet their metabolic needs. However, arginine has been shown to be indispensable for both dogs and cats throughout life.[140,141] Arginine is needed by the body for normal protein synthesis and as an essential component of the urea cycle. Arginine functions in the urea cycle as an ornithine precursor and urea cycle intermediate. In this capacity arginine allows the large amounts of ammonia generated after the consumption of a high-protein meal to be converted to urea for excretion from the body.

A lack of arginine in the diet causes an immediate and severe deficiency response in the cat. Cats will develop severe hyperammonemia within several hours of consuming a single arginine-free meal.[142] Clinical signs include emesis (vomiting), muscle spasms, ataxia, hyperesthesia (sensitivity to touch), and tetanic spasms. These signs can eventually lead to coma and death. Dogs show similar, but less severe, clinical signs of arginine deficiency following consumption of an arginine-free meal.[140,143]

There appear to be two basic reasons for the cat's extreme sensitivity to arginine deficiency. First of all, the cat is unable to synthesize de novo ornithine. Ornithine is an arginine precursor within the urea cycle. In most animals, the amino acids glutamate and proline act as precursors for ornithine synthesis in the intestinal mucosa. However, the cat's intestinal mucosal cells have extremely low levels of active pyrroline-5-carboxylate synthase, an essential enzyme in this pathway. The cat also has low activity of a second essential enzyme, ornithine aminotransferase.[144]

In addition to being unable to synthesize ornithine, the cat is also unable to synthesize arginine from ornithine for use by extrahepatic tissues, even if dietary

TABLE 12-3

Arginine Synthesis

Reaction	Most Mammals	Cats
Glutamate + Proline → Ornithine (intestine)	Normal	Low
Ornithine → Citrulline (intestine)	Normal	Little activity
Citrulline travels to the kidney	Does occur	Does not occur
Citrulline → Arginine (kidney)	Does occur	Does not occur

ornithine is provided. Studies in the rat demonstrated that the normal route of arginine synthesis for use by extrahepatic tissues involves both the liver and the kidneys.[145] Arginine cannot leave the liver to provide for extrahepatic tissues because high activity of liver arginase prevents its accumulation to a concentration above that of the bloodstream. However, citrulline, which is produced from ornithine either in the intestinal mucosa or in a urea cycle intermediate in the liver, can travel to the kidneys where it is then converted to arginine. This arginine provides the kidneys and other tissues of the body with their needs for normal growth and tissue maintenance. In the cat, citrulline is not produced in the intestinal mucosa (because of the inability to produce ornithine), and the citrulline produced in the liver appears to be unable to leave the hepatocyte to be converted to arginine by the kidneys.[55,124]

As a direct result of these two metabolic deficiencies, arginine becomes an essential amino acid for both urea cycle function and for normal growth and maintenance in the cat (Table 12-3). The importance of arginine for normal functioning of the urea cycle, coupled with the cat's high and inflexible rate of protein catabolism, causes the cat to be extremely sensitive to arginine deficiency. Like the cat, the growing dog also has a dietary requirement for arginine. However, the response of the growing dog to an arginine-deficient diet is not as severe as that observed in the immature cat.[140,143]

The growing kitten's requirement for arginine is estimated to be approximately 1.1% of a dry diet containing an ME of approximately 4.7 kcal/g.[105,140] Because arginine is found in adequate amounts in most protein sources, an arginine deficiency is generally not a practical problem in cats, provided they are fed a diet containing adequate levels of protein.

Taurine Requirement Taurine is a unique beta–amino-sulfonic acid that is not incorporated into large proteins but is found as a free amino acid in tissues or as a constituent of small peptides. It is synthesized by most mammals from methionine and cysteine during normal sulfur amino acid metabolism (Figure 12-1). The myocardium and retina contain high concentrations of free taurine, and these two tissues are able to concentrate taurine to levels that are 100-fold to 400-fold greater

FIGURE **12-1**

Taurine synthesis and metabolism in the cat.

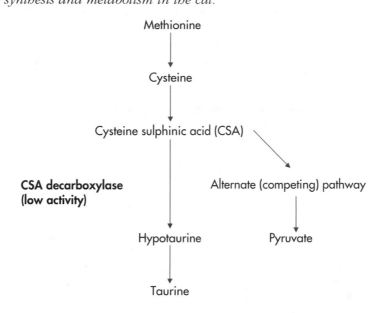

than those found in plasma.[146] Although taurine may be involved in many aspects of metabolism, it is known to have important roles in bile acid conjugation, retinal function, and normal functioning of the myocardium.[146,147,148] Taurine is also necessary for normal reproductive performance in queens.[149]

Cats are able to synthesize only small amounts of taurine.[150] This inability is partially the result of the cat's low activity of two enzymes that are essential for taurine synthesis, cysteine dioxygenase and cysteine sulfinic acid decarboxylase. In addition, a competing pathway of cysteine metabolism exists in the cat and results in the production of pyruvate rather than taurine from methionine and cysteine (see Figure 12-1).[151] The cat is not unique in its limited capacity for taurine synthesis. Low levels of de novo synthesis have been reported in humans, Old World monkeys, rabbits, and guinea pigs.[152] However, the cat is the only species in which taurine deficiency occurs. This is the result of this species' unusually high metabolic demand for taurine. The domestic cat uses only taurine for bile-salt formation and, in contrast to other animals, cannot convert to conjugation of bile acids with glycine when the taurine supply is limited.[147] As a result, the cat has a continual requirement for taurine to replace fecal losses that occur from incomplete recovery of bile salts by the enterohepatic circulation. The dog also uses only taurine to conjugate bile acids, but it appears to be able to synthesize enough taurine to meet its metabolic needs.[153] Although humans and Old World monkeys also have only a limited capacity for taurine synthesis and prefer to conjugate bile acids with taurine, they will switch to glycine conjugation when dietary taurine is low.

Feline central retinal degeneration (FCRD) was the first clinical deficiency syndrome caused by taurine deficiency in the cat to be recognized. Taurine's primary role in the proper functioning of the retina involves the photoreceptor cells, where it regulates the flux of calcium and potassium ions across the photoreceptor pigment–epithelial cell barrier.[148] When taurine is absent, the photoreceptor cell membranes become disrupted and dysfunctional, which eventually leads to cellular death and the loss of cells. A concomitant degeneration of the underlying tapetum lucidum can also occur.[154] Although abnormalities in electroretinograms can be observed within 5 to 6 months of consuming taurine-deficient diets, visual impairment is only observed clinically when cats are in the later stages of retinal degeneration.[155,156] At this point, irreversible blindness occurs in most cats.

Taurine is also necessary for normal functioning of the myocardium. Although it is not the only underlying cause in cats, a deficiency of taurine results in the development of dilated cardiomyopathy (DCM).[146] This degenerative disease has been reported in several species and causes decreased myocardial contractility, which eventually leads to cardiac failure. Along with the retina, the myocardium is one of the tissues in the body that is able to concentrate taurine to levels much greater than those found in the plasma.[157] Heart studies indicate that taurine may confer a calcium- and potassium-stabilizing effect on heart tissue and may thereby ensure cationic stability and membrane integrity.[158]

One study reported data from 21 clinical cases of DCM in pet cats.[146] All of the cats were found to have significantly lower plasma taurine concentrations when compared with clinically normal cats. When the affected cats were supplemented with taurine (0.5 g twice daily), all the cats clinically improved within 2 weeks. At 3 to 4 weeks, the cats showed improved echocardiographs that eventually resulted in complete normalization of left ventricular function. When the study was published, all surviving cats were clinically and echocardiographically normal. In addition, two experimental cats that had been fed a purified diet containing marginally low levels of taurine for 4 years developed DCM. These cats also exhibited full recovery as a result of taurine supplementation. The authors of the study proposed that low levels of taurine in plasma and myocardial tissue are a major cause of the development of DCM in cats.

The dietary requirement for taurine in the cat somewhat depends on the level of sulfur amino acids (SAAs) in the diet. Research studies have shown that the cat's taurine requirement increases when the SAA content of the diet is less than 1.55%.[159] Additional studies found that when weanling kittens were fed a taurine-deficient diet containing a level of SAAs near the requirement, all of the kittens developed FCRD. However, when the level of SAAs was doubled in the diet, none of the kittens developed FCRD during the 12-month study period.[55] These results are relevant to the reported occurrence of FCRD in cats that have been fed only commercial dog food.[160] In general, dog foods have lower protein levels and lower SAA contents than commercial rations that have been formulated for cats.

In 1986, the NRC recommended a taurine level of 500 to 750 parts per million in the dry diet of cats to prevent taurine deficiency and maximize tissue stores.[58] However, some diets formulated at these levels were found to be inadequate.[151]

Subsequent studies showed that the amount of dietary taurine required to maintain normal whole blood and plasma taurine levels in cats is dependent upon the type of diet.[161,162,163] For expanded dry diets, a concentration of 1000 milligrams (mg)/kg of diet is adequate. However, concentrations as high as 2500 mg/kg are required for canned cat foods. This is necessary because the taurine requirement of cats consuming canned foods is substantially higher than that of cats consuming dry foods.[164,165]

A series of studies was conducted to determine the underlying cause for this difference. The effects of heat processing and of the level and source of protein on taurine status in adult cats were examined.[153] Results suggest that thermal processing that results in the production of Maillard products increases microbial degradation of taurine in the intestine and subsequently increases fecal losses of taurine. A substantial proportion of the taurine requirement of adult cats is required to replace taurine lost in the feces as a result of the microbial degradation of taurine-containing bile acids. Therefore, any factor that increases microbial degradation of taurine will lead to an increased dietary requirement. *Maillard products* are complexes of reducing sugars and proteins that are formed during heat treatment. Because these products are less digestible than untreated protein, they may provide an intestinal environment that favors increased numbers of taurine-degrading bacteria or facilitates taurine's exposure to bacteria. Maillard products may also affect taurine status by indirectly influencing the release of the hormone cholecystokinin (CCK). One of the effects of CCK is to stimulate the release of bile acids into the intestinal lumen during digestion. By binding certain proteolytic enzymes in the small intestine, Maillard products facilitate CCK release, causing increased amounts of bile acids to be released into the intestine and enhancing fecal losses through microbial degradation.[153,165] Because of the observed effects of heat processing upon taurine status, the AAFCO's *Nutrient Profiles* for cat foods require that canned cat foods contain a minimum of 2000 mg of taurine/kg and that dry foods contain a minimum of 1000 mg/kg.[102]

Taurine is present only in animal tissues. High concentrations (200 to 400 mg/kg of wet weight) are found in meat, poultry, and fish. Shellfish are extremely rich sources of taurine, containing up to 2500 mg/kg.[105] Although a carnivorous diet ensures the cat an adequate taurine intake, the consumption of a diet containing high amounts of plant products and cereal grains may not provide sufficient taurine. Of special concern are cereal-based dog foods that contain lower levels of protein and taurine. As previously mentioned, unlike the cat, the dog does not require dietary taurine.[75] Therefore, while these diets are adequate for dogs, the practice of feeding dog foods to cats may result in taurine deficiency and the development of FCRD.[160]

ESSENTIAL AMINO ACIDS OF SPECIAL CONCERN

The following amino acids have been identified as being essential for growing puppies and kittens: arginine, histidine, isoleucine, leucine, lysine, methionine, phenylalanine, threonine, tryptophan, and valine. Although both the dog and the cat have a dietary requirement for arginine, the cat is unusual in its immediate and severe reaction to the consumption of an arginine-free meal. The other amino acids that are of special concern in the feeding of dogs and cats are lysine and the SAAs methionine and cysteine. Of less practical concern, but of academic interest, is the cat's inability to convert the amino acid tryptophan to the B vitamin niacin.

Lysine

The growing dog's dietary requirement for lysine appears to increase as the level of total protein in the diet increases.[166] This effect has been demonstrated in other species and may be the result of amino acid imbalances and antagonisms with lysine at higher levels of protein intake.[111] This effect may be especially important because lysine is often the first limiting amino acid in cereal-based dog foods.[167] In addition, the lysine that is present in the diet is susceptible to certain types of processing damage that can occur in commercially prepared pet foods. The exposure of protein to excessive heat induces cross-linking between amino acids, resulting in decreased digestibility of the ration's total protein. Even mild heat treatment can result in a reaction between the epsilon-amino group of lysine and the amino groups of free amino acids with reducing sugars. The resultant Maillard products are resistant to digestion and result in a reduction in the amount of available lysine that can be supplied by the food. Therefore the lysine content of commercial pet foods must be closely monitored.

The limiting amino acids in cereal proteins are lysine and tryptophan. However, meat products contain adequate amounts of these amino acids. The inclusion of meat proteins with cereal proteins in a pet food, coupled with properly controlled processing methods, ensures that the ration contains an adequate level of available lysine. In a completely cereal-based dog food, either supplemental lysine or a meat source of lysine must be added (see Section 3, pp. 176-177).

Methionine and Cysteine

The SAA methionine is essential for dogs and cats, but cysteine is dispensable. However, because methionine is used by the body to synthesize cysteine, approximately half of an animal's methionine requirement can be met by adequate levels of cysteine.[168,169] Therefore it is preferable to address a total SAA requirement rather than a specific methionine requirement for animals. The SAA requirement is substantially higher in the cat than it is in other mammals. Although growing dogs require a minimum of 1.06 g/1000 kcal of ME, the minimum requirement of growing cats is approximately 1.5 times this amount.[49,58] This high requirement may be a result of several factors. First, the cat is unique in its production of a compound called *felinine*. Felinine is synthesized from cysteine and is excreted in the urine of all cats. It is found in its highest concentration in the urine of adult, intact males.[170] Although its exact role is unknown, it has been suggested that felinine may be a urinary component involved in territorial marking or in the regulation of sterol metabolism in the feline species.[171] Other possible reasons for the cat's high SAA requirement are its needs for the maintenance of a thick hair coat and for the increased methylation reactions necessary for the synthesis of phospholipids. Increased phospholipid synthesis is believed to be necessary for the absorption and transport of the high level of fat that is normally included in a cat's diet. Lastly, the cat's requirement for dietary taurine further adds to the cat's total requirement for SAAs in the diet.

In addition to the difference in SAA requirements between dogs and cats, there is some evidence that there may be differences in methionine requirements among breeds of dogs. One study showed that growing Labrador Retrievers required higher levels of total SAAs to maximize growth and nitrogen retention than did growing Beagles.[131] Methionine is usually the first limiting amino acid in most commercial pet foods that contain animal tissues and plant protein sources.[172] This fact, coupled with the high SAA requirement for cats, results in methionine being an important consideration for pet food companies during the formulation of nutritionally balanced pet foods.

Cat's Inability to Convert Tryptophan to Niacin

The requirement for the B vitamin niacin is met in most animals through both the consumption of dietary nicotinamide and through the conversion of the essential amino acid tryptophan to nicotinic acid (Figure 12-2). The efficiency of conversion of tryptophan to niacin varies among species but is generally quite low (3%).[173] This is a result of the existence of more dominant competing pathways of tryptophan metabolism. A branch point in the pathway involved in tryptophan catabolism results in the synthesis of either quinolinic acid or picolinic acid. Quinolinic acid is further metabolized to form niacin; picolinic acid is converted to glutarate. Although most species have high levels of picolinate carboxylase activity that result in a higher production of picolinic acid, a substantial amount of niacin is still produced from the quinolinic acid branch. The activity of picolinate carboxylase in cats is 30 to 50 times higher than its activity in rats, resulting in negligible niacin synthesis from tryptophan in the cat.[173]

Animal tissues are well supplied with nicotinamide. The regular consumption of a carnivorous diet throughout evolutionary history would probably not result in selective pressure for the cat to synthesize niacin from precursor substances. However, it has been postulated that the high-protein diet of the cat would exert pressure toward a high rate of tryptophan catabolism (i.e., the picolinic acid branch of the pathway). The rapid metabolism of tryptophan would prevent the accumulation of the amino acid and its intermediates, such as serotonin, to toxic levels. Animal proteins contain significantly higher levels of tryptophan than do plant proteins. Thus the high activity of picolinic carboxylase in the cat may prevent the accumulation of tryptophan and its byproducts in the bloodstream following the consumption of a meal containing high amounts of animal protein.[75]

The inability of the cat to convert tryptophan to niacin is of little practical significance to the feeding management of pet cats because nicotinamide is widely distributed in feed ingredients. Sources of this vitamin in commercial pet foods include

FIGURE **12-2**
Niacin synthesis.

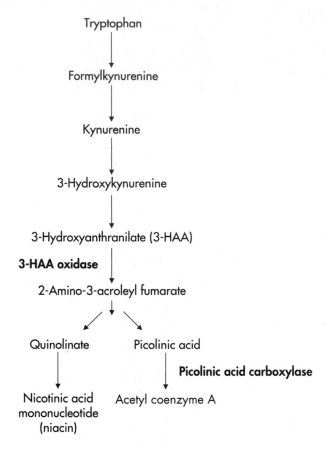

Tryptophan

↓

Formylkynurenine

↓

Kynurenine

↓

3-Hydroxykynurenine

↓

3-Hydroxyanthranilate (3-HAA)

3-HAA oxidase

↓

2-Amino-3-acroleyl fumarate

Quinolinate   Picolinic acid

Picolinic acid carboxylase

Nicotinic acid   Acetyl coenzyme A
mononucleotide
(niacin)

animal and fish byproducts, distillers' grains and yeast, and certain oil meals. Therefore the chance of inducing a niacin deficiency through improper feeding practices is slim, regardless of the cat's inability to convert tryptophan to niacin for use by the body.

PROTEIN DEFICIENCY IN DOGS AND CATS

Signs of protein deficiency include retarded growth in young animals and weight loss and impaired reproductive and work performance in adults. A deficiency of protein commonly occurs with energy deficiency; this state is referred to as *protein/calorie malnutrition* (PCM). When PCM occurs, the animal exhibits lethargy, reduced digestive efficiency, and reduced resistance to infectious disease.[174] Lowered plasma protein levels occur after prolonged protein deficiency and can eventually lead to edema or ascites. There is also some evidence in other species that general undernutrition and protein deficiency during development can affect brain development and learning capabilities later in life.[175,176]

Protein deficiency is uncommon in companion animals that are fed balanced commercial pet foods. This is probably because the majority of commercial foods contain more protein than is needed to meet the minimum requirement.[84] When protein deficiency does occur, it is usually because owners are attempting to economize by feeding low-quality, poorly formulated rations during periods of high nutrient need, such as pregnancy or lactation. Additionally, cats that are fed cereal-based dog foods that contain marginally adequate levels of protein are at risk for the development of protein and/or taurine deficiency.

PROTEIN EXCESS IN DOGS AND CATS

As mentioned previously, there is some evidence suggesting that it may be beneficial to feed animals levels of protein that are higher than the minimum level necessary to maintain nitrogen equilibrium.[113,114] The additional protein may be used to provide protein reserves that contribute to the body's ability to withstand stress and infectious disease challenges. There are two possible uses for dietary protein that exceeds the body's total needs. If the animal is in zero energy balance, the excess protein will be used as an energy source. If the animal is in positive energy balance (i.e., consuming more energy than it is expending), then the excess protein will be metabolized to fat for energy storage in the body. Unlike fat and small amounts of carbohydrate, excess amino acids are not stored by the body for future use.

All companion animals have the ability to metabolize excess protein. This process results in the production of urea and its excretion in the urine. In recent years, the potential detrimental effects of excess protein intake in companion animals have interested a number of investigators. As a result of studies that were conducted with rats, it was theorized that feeding high levels of dietary protein over long periods to dogs and cats may contribute to the development of chronic kidney disease.[177,178,179] Some researchers also believe that protein excess can lead to nephropathy in animals that are already in renal compromise.[177,180] Protein restriction is often used in the dietary management of companion animals with uremia caused by chronic kidney disease. In these cases, restriction of dietary protein to levels that meet, but do not exceed, the animal's requirement minimizes urea production and reduces some of the clinical signs associated with uremia.[181] However, there is no conclusive evidence showing that protein intake actually contributes to the development of kidney dysfunction in healthy animals (see Section 6, pp. 455-458).[88]

Reduced renal weight and a gradual decline in kidney function are normal occurrences of aging and have been extensively studied in humans and rats.[182,183,184] A study with dogs evaluated clinical changes in renal function in a colony of Beagles for a period of 13 years. The data from this study indicate that normal kidney aging can lead to a nephron loss of up to 75% before clinical or biochemical signs occur.[185] Pets with less than a 75% loss are usually clinically normal, but they may be more susceptible to renal insult than are younger animals still possessing renal reserve capacity.[185] This knowledge has led to the practice of systematically reducing the protein content in the diets of elderly animals in an attempt to prevent or minimize the progression of kidney dysfunction.[186] However, it is also important that normal geriatric dogs and cats receive adequate amounts of high-quality protein to minimize losses of body protein reserves and satisfy maintenance protein needs. Although there is evidence that a reduction in protein intake has a significant effect on clinical signs once a high level of kidney dysfunction is observed, there is no evidence indicating a need to systematically reduce protein levels in the diets of healthy older pets. It is recommended that protein in the diets of geriatric dogs should not be restricted simply because of old age. Rather, elderly pets should receive diets containing adequate, but not excessive, levels of high-quality protein. If a pet is diagnosed with chronic renal disease, moderate protein restriction can then be implemented to minimize extrarenal effects.[185] The primary function of this restriction is to improve the blood chemistry aberrations and some of the clinical signs associated with chronic renal disease (see Section 6, pp. 462-465).[187,188]

13

Vitamins and Minerals

FAT-SOLUBLE VITAMINS

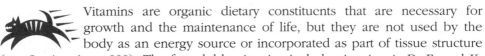 Vitamins are organic dietary constituents that are necessary for growth and the maintenance of life, but they are not used by the body as an energy source or incorporated as part of tissue structure (see Section 1, p. 000). The fat-soluble vitamins include vitamins A, D, E, and K. These vitamins are absorbed from the small intestine in much the same way as dietary fat and are stored primarily in the liver.

Vitamin A

All animals have a physiological requirement for active vitamin A, or retinol. However, most mammals, including the dog but with the exception of the cat, have the ability to convert vitamin A precursors to active vitamin A (see Section 1, pp. 29-31). Carotenoid pigments, of which beta-carotene is the most important, are cleaved by a dioxygenase enzyme in the intestinal mucosa to yield vitamin A aldehyde (retinal). Retinal is then reduced by a second enzyme to form active vitamin A (retinol). Retinol is esterified to fatty acids and absorbed into the body along with dietary fat.[189,190,191] The dioxygenase enzyme that is essential for the splitting of the beta-carotene molecule is either absent or grossly deficient in the domestic cat. Studies have shown that neither dietary nor intravenous beta-carotene can prevent the development of vitamin A deficiency in this species.[192] As a result, the cat must have preformed vitamin A present in the diet. The most common forms of preformed vitamin A in foods are derivatives of retinol, such as retinyl palmitate and retinyl acetate. These compounds are found in the largest quantities in fish liver oils and animal livers.

Nutrient requirements for vitamin A and its content in pet foods are expressed either as international units (IUs) or retinol equivalents. One IU of vitamin A is equal to 0.3 micrograms (μg) of retinol or 0.6 μg of beta-carotene. The 1985 National Research Council (NRC) recommendations report a minimum requirement in

TABLE **13-1**

*Recommended Minimum Fat-Soluble Vitamin Requirements**

	Vitamin A	Vitamin D	Vitamin E	Vitamin K
Dog				
NRC	3710 IU	404 IU	22 IU	—[†]
AAFCO	5000 IU	500 IU	50 IU	—
Cat				
NRC	3333 IU	500 IU	30 IU	0.1 mg
AAFCO	5000 IU	500 IU	30 IU	0.1 mg[††]

*Per kg of diet.
[†]No requirement established.
[††]For cats consuming diets containing greater than 25% fish (on a DMB).

the growing dog of 3710 IU/kilogram (kg) of diet in a diet containing 3.67 kilo-calories of metabolizable energy per kg (kcal of ME/kg).[49] However, the Association of American Feed Control Officials (AAFCO) *Nutrient Profiles* for dog foods recommend that dog foods containing an energy density of 3.5 kcal/kg should include a minimum of 5000 IU/kg for growth, reproduction, and maintenance.[102] The NRC's 1986 *Nutrient Requirements of Cats* reports a vitamin A minimum requirement of 3333 IU/kg of dry diet for growing kittens and 6000 IU/kg of dry diet during pregnancy and lactation.[58] This requirement is based on a diet with a ME of 5 kcal/gram (g) of dry matter (DM) (Table 13-1). Although adequate research on the minimum daily vitamin A requirement for maintenance in mature cats has not been conducted, it is presumed that the levels provided for the growing kitten are adequate for adults during maintenance.[58] The AAFCO's *Nutrient Profiles* suggest a level of 5000 IU/kg of diet on a dry-matter basis (DMB) to be included in all commercially prepared cat foods, as compared with the minimum requirements for cats recommended by the NRC.[102]

Vitamin A deficiency is rarely observed in dogs and cats because commercial pet foods contain adequate amounts and because dogs are able to convert the carotenoids found in plant matter into active vitamin A. In young, growing animals, vitamin A deficiency results in abnormal bone growth and neurological disorders. Stenosis of the neural foramina causes pinching of cranial and spinal nerves as they pass through the abnormally shaped bone. If the deficiency persists, shortening and thickening of the long bones occur, along with abnormal development of the bones of the skull.[193,194] Vitamin A deficiency in adult animals affects reproduction, vision, and functioning of the epithelium. Clinical signs include anorexia, xerophthalmia and conjunctivitis, corneal opacity and ulceration, skin lesions, and multiple disorders of the epithelial layers in the body.[49,58]

Vitamin A toxicity is not common in the animal kingdom because the precursor for vitamin A, beta-carotene, is not a toxic substance. The intestinal mucosa regulates the hydrolysis of beta-carotene and the subsequent absorption of retinol into the body. However, the cat cannot use carotenoids and must consume all of its vitamin A as preformed retinyl palmitate or free retinol from animal tissues. The absorption of preformed vitamin A is not regulated by the intestinal mucosa, and a toxic level of this vitamin is readily absorbed by the body. The domestic cat is more likely to be fed excessive levels of vitamin A than are other species of domesticated pet. If cats are fed foods that contain excessively high levels of vitamin A, they are unable to protect themselves from absorbing toxic levels. These foods include organ meats, such as liver and kidney, and various fish oils. Vitamin A toxicosis in cats results in a disorder called deforming cervical spondylosis. The effects of excess vitamin A on bone growth and remodeling cause the development of bony exostoses (outgrowths) on the cervical vertebrae. These changes eventually cause pain, difficult movement, lameness, and crippling in severe cases (see Section 5, pp. 346-349).

Vitamin D

Vitamin D is essential for normal calcium and phosphorus metabolism and homeostasis. The actions of vitamin D on the intestine, skeleton, and kidneys result in increased plasma levels of calcium and phosphorus. These increased levels allow normal mineralization and remodeling of bone and cartilage and maintain the concentration of calcium in the extracellular fluid that is necessary for normal muscle contraction and nervous tissue excitability. Many animals have the ability to synthesize vitamin D_3 from 7-dehydrocholesterol when the skin is exposed to ultraviolet (UV) radiation. The inactive form of the vitamin is then stored in the liver. Biochemical conversions, first in the liver and then in the kidneys, convert vitamin D_3 to its active form when necessary (see Section 1, pp. 31-34).

Dietary requirements for vitamin D depend on calcium and phosphorus levels in the diet, the ratio of these two minerals, and the age of the animal. Because of the skin's ability to produce vitamin D, adult animals that are consuming diets with adequate levels of calcium and phosphorus have very low requirements for cholecalciferol. During growth, vitamin D is important for the normal development and mineralization of bone. Still, even with this added need, very low levels of dietary vitamin D appear to be necessary for companion animals, provided that adequate calcium and phosphorus are present (see Table 13-1).

There are conflicting data from studies that have measured the ability of companion animals to produce adequate levels of vitamin D in the skin to meet their daily needs. When a group of growing kittens were fed a diet containing adequate levels of calcium and phosphorus, normal bone growth occurred in the absence of dietary vitamin D and exposure to UV light.[195] It was speculated that the kittens in this study were able to use body stores of vitamin D that had been acquired during suckling. Another study reported that when a group of weanling English Pointer and German Shepherd dogs were fed a diet containing no supplemental cholecalciferol, no signs of vitamin D deficiency developed.[196] The dogs were fed the diet for 2 years and were housed in indoor/outdoor runs. A second group was fed the same ration and supplemented with 60.5 mg of cholecalciferol/kg of diet. During the treatment period there were no significant differences in growth rate, body length, or serum calcium and phosphorus levels between the two groups of dogs. Periodic radiographic examinations revealed no differences in skeletal development. The authors of the study concluded that dogs that are fed practical diets and exposed to adequate sunlight do not require supplemental cholecalciferol during the first 2 years of life. It is important to note that vitamin D levels of the diets in this study were not analyzed. Therefore it is possible that adequate levels of vitamin D were present in one or more of the ingredients included in the basal diet.

Other data have shown that dogs and cats do not synthesize sufficient amounts of vitamin D in the skin to meet their daily requirements, even when daily irradiation with UV light is provided.[195,197,198] When dogs were fed a dry food to which no supplemental vitamin D had been added, both the radiated and nonradiated groups developed biochemical, radiological, and histological signs of rickets.[197] Clinical signs included broadened growth plates and bowed legs. When the vitamin D-deficient diet was replaced with a commercial dog food containing 1800 IU of vitamin D/kg, the signs resolved, normal bone mineralization was observed, and circulating levels of vitamin D metabolites increased to normal values. Vitamin D deficiency was also produced in kittens that were fed a diet containing no vitamin D and 1% calcium and phosphorus.[195] Deficiency signs were exacerbated when the diet's phosphorus level was decreased to 0.65% and calcium was increased to 2%. More recently, studies of growing kittens showed that kittens fed purified diets devoid of vitamin D and containing moderately low levels of calcium and phosphorus had declining plasma levels of 25-hydroxycholecalciferol and eventually developed clinical signs of vitamin D deficiency.[198] Kittens that were provided daily exposure to sunlight or UV light in the spectral range for vitamin D synthesis were affected to the same degree as kittens with no exposure to radiation. Further studies by the same group showed that the concentration of vitamin D's precursor, 7-dehydrocholesterol, is very low in the skin of cats when compared with the concentration seen in other mammals. This is caused by high activity of the enzyme 7-dehydrocholesterol-delta-7-reductase, which catalyzes the conversion of 7-dehydrocholesterol to cholesterol. Because cats rapidly convert 7-dehydrocholesterol to cholesterol, they have limited capacity for synthesizing cholecalciferol and, ultimately, active vitamin D (see Section 1, pp. 31-34).

The interrelationship between vitamin D, calcium, and phosphorus in the diet has been demonstrated by studies that have produced experimental vitamin D deficiencies in dogs and cats by limiting or imbalancing calcium and phosphorus levels in the diet.[195,199,200,201] Recent studies with kittens showed that clinical signs of vitamin D deficiency did not occur when the level of calcium in a vitamin D–deficient diet was increased from 7 g/kg to 12 g/kg.[202] However, plasma levels of 25-hydroxycholecalciferol were less than normal in these kittens and increased significantly when the kittens were switched to a diet containing 124 IUs of vitamin D/kg. Normal plasma levels of 25-hydroxycholecalciferol were maintained when the diet's vitamin D content was further increased to 250 IU/kg. The authors concluded that commercial diets formulated for growing kittens should contain a minimum concentration of 250 IUs of vitamin D/kg.

Vitamin D deficiency results in rickets in growing animals and osteomalacia in adults. Rickets is characterized by bone malformation caused by insufficient deposition of calcium and phosphorus. The long bones are affected, resulting in bowing of the legs and thickening of the joints. Osteomalacia is caused by decalcification of bone and an increased tendency of the long bones to fracture. Cats with vitamin D deficiency become reluctant to move and show decreased inclination to groom themselves. A progressive posterior paralysis develops, eventually leading to quadriparesis in advanced cases. These neurological changes are associated with degeneration of the spinal cord caused by abnormal growth and remodeling of cervical vertebrae.[198] In most animals, vitamin D deficiency develops concomitantly with deficiencies or imbalances in dietary calcium and phosphorus. Low levels of these minerals exacerbate vitamin D deficiency and may precipitate the signs of rickets in growing animals.

Excess levels of vitamin D can be toxic to dogs and cats and result in excessive calcification of soft tissues in the body. Chronic ingestion of high levels of vitamin D may eventually lead to skeletal abnormalities and deformations of the teeth and jaws in growing companion animals. Oversupplementation with vitamin D is the most common cause of vitamin D toxicity in dogs and cats. A survey of commercial cat foods marketed in the United States found that none of the foods was deficient in vitamin D content, based upon a requirement of 250 IU/kg, but some did contain less than the AAFCO minimum of 500 IU/kg.[198] In addition, 20 of the 49 foods sampled had more than 7500 IU/kg and 15 had greater than 10,000 IU/kg. The AAFCO's maximum allowance for vitamin D is 5000 IU/kg. The effects of long-term ingestion of vitamin D levels this high are not known. While no reports of clinical vitamin D toxicity in cats have been reported in the United States, there have been clinical cases among cats in Japan that were fed a commercial pet food containing fish products with high vitamin D concentrations.[203]

Vitamin E

Vitamin E functions as a biological, chain-breaking antioxidant that neutralizes free radicals and prevents the peroxidation of lipids within cellular membranes. An animal's requirement for vitamin E depends on dietary levels of polyunsaturated fatty acids (PUFAs) and selenium, a trace mineral. Vitamin E and selenium function synergistically. Although vitamin E protects cell membrane fatty acids by quenching the free radicals formed during oxidation, selenium (as a component of the enzyme glutathione peroxidase) reduces peroxide formation. This process further protects membrane fatty acids from oxidative damage (see Section 1, pp. 34-35).

Increasing the level of unsaturated fat in the diet causes an increase in an animal's vitamin E requirement. In commercial pet foods, vitamin E also protects unsaturated fats from destructive oxidation. The vitamin is preferentially oxidized before the unsaturated fatty acids, thus protecting them from rancidity. However, in this process, vitamin E is destroyed. Therefore, as the level of unsaturated fatty acids in pet foods increases, the amount of vitamin E should increase.

A naturally occurring deficiency of vitamin E is not common in dogs and cats. However, the ingestion of poorly prepared or poorly stored foods or supplementation with large amounts of PUFAs can precipitate a deficiency of this vitamin. Vitamin E deficiency in dogs has been associated with skeletal muscle degeneration, decreased reproductive performance, retinal degeneration, and impaired immunological response.[204] A deficiency of this nutrient has also been implicated in the development of certain dermatological disorders in dogs. The occurrence of demodicosis has been associated with decreased blood levels of vitamin E.[205] It has also been postulated that a subclinical vitamin E deficiency causes suppression of the immune system, which in turn increases a dog's susceptibility to demodectic mange infestation. When dogs with demodicosis were treated with supplemental vitamin E, significant levels of improvement were reported. However, other researchers have been unable to reproduce these results.[206] More controlled research is necessary before definitive conclusions can be made concerning the role of vitamin E in the control of demodectic mange. Supplementation with large amounts of vitamin E has also been shown to have antiinflammatory effects on some dogs with skin disorders.[207,208] This treatment has been used with varying levels of success in dogs with discoid lupus erythematosus, dermatomyositis, and acanthosis nigricans (see Section 6, pp. 432-433).

There is recent evidence that dogs engaging in prolonged strenuous activity may have increased vitamin E needs.[208] Racing Alaskan sled dogs demonstrated increased lipid peroxidation and metabolic signs of skeletal muscle damage following a 3-day period of strenuous work. These changes were associated with a concurrent decline in serum vitamin E concentration. It is possible that alterations in antioxidant capacity associated with exercise may be prevented or ameliorated through vitamin E supplementation. However, studies that examine the effects of vitamin E supplementation during strenuous activity in dogs are needed before recommendations can be made.

A condition called *pansteatitis,* or "yellow fat disease," occurs in cats that are fed diets containing marginal or low levels of alpha-tocopherol and high amounts of unsaturated fatty acids. Signs of pansteatitis include anorexia, depression, pyrexia (fever), hyperesthesia of the thorax and abdomen, a reluctance to move, and the presence of "swollen fat."[209,210] A diet that contains high levels of fish oil may cause a three-fold to four-fold increase in a cat's daily requirement for alpha-tocopherol.[58] Early cases of pansteatitis occurred almost exclusively in cats that were fed a canned, commercial, fish-based cat food, of which red tuna was the principal type of fish. Later cases of the disease occurred in cats that were fed diets consisting wholly or largely of canned red tuna or fish scraps. Red tuna packed in oil contains high levels of PUFAs and low levels of vitamin E. The addition of large amounts of fish products to a cat's diet appears to be the primary cause of this disease in pet cats (see Section 5, pp. 345-346).

Vitamin K

Vitamin K includes a class of compounds known as the *quinones.* This vitamin is necessary for normal blood coagulation because of its role in the synthesis of prothrombin (factor II) and several other clotting factors (see Section 1, pp. 35-36). Evidence in both dogs and cats indicates very low dietary requirements for vitamin K, probably due to the ability of bacterial synthesis in the intestine to fully meet the animal's need for this nutrient. However, interference with vitamin K synthesis or absorption can cause a deficiency, with signs of hemorrhage and decreased levels of prothrombin in the blood.

Vitamin K deficiency is extremely rare in dogs and has only recently been reported in cats. In two separate situations, cats fed canned commercial cat foods containing either salmon or tuna developed signs of vitamin K deficiency.[211] Signs included the development of gastric ulcers, increased coagulation times, and decreased serum concentrations of vitamin K-dependent clotting factors. Surprisingly, the vitamin K concentration in the diets was 60 mg/kg diet, a level considered to be adequate for companion animals. Surviving animals responded positively to vitamin K supplementation and demonstrated normalized clotting times within 24 hours of vitamin K therapy. A subsequent series of studies by the same laboratory failed to induce vitamin K deficiency in cats fed various types of purified diets. The experimental diets contained low levels of vitamin K (4 to 30 mg/kg of diet) and various factors with the potential to interfere with vitamin K synthesis or absorption. These results suggest that kittens fed purified diets have very low dietary vitamin K requirements and that there may be a factor present in canned cat foods containing fish products that interferes with vitamin K synthesis or absorption. Although this factor has not been identified, it is recommended that canned fish-based cat diets contain more than 60 mg of vitamin K/kg and a supplemental source of vitamin K.

WATER-SOLUBLE VITAMINS

The water-soluble vitamins that are of importance to the dog and cat are all B-complex vitamins. Most of these vitamins are involved in the use of food and the production of energy in the body (see Section 1, pp. 36-39). Because of the availability of well-formulated and well-balanced pet foods today, simple deficiencies of the B-complex vitamins are extremely rare in companion animals. However, there are several situations in which B-vitamin nutrition may be of concern in the nutritional management of dogs or cats. Thiamin deficiency can occur when dogs or cats are fed certain types of raw fish containing an enzyme that destroys this vitamin, while biotin deficiency can be induced by feeding animals large amounts of raw egg whites (see Section 5, p. 350).[212,213,214,215] Genetics can also play a role in B-vitamin metabolism. An inherited disorder in Giant Schnauzers causes malabsorption of vitamin B_{12} (see Section 6, pp. 000-000). The requirement for vitamin B_6 (pyridoxine) is directly affected by the level of protein in the diet. As the protein level in the diet increases, so does a dog's or cat's requirement for vitamin B_6.[216,217,218,219]

MINERALS

As with most other nutrients, problems with mineral nutrition in dogs and cats are often a result of excesses or imbalances from interactions with other nutrients rather than a result of frank deficiencies in the diet. This section focuses on those minerals that are of most practical significance in the nutrition and feeding management of dogs and cats today.

Calcium and Phosphorus

Calcium and phosphorus are macrominerals necessary for the formation and maintenance of the skeleton. These nutrients are involved in a wide range of metabolic reactions (see Section 1, pp. 41-45). When considering canine and feline requirements for these nutrients, the availability of the calcium and phosphorus that is present in the diet must be taken into account. Studies have shown that requirements for available calcium are quite low. Levels of 0.37% available calcium or 0.5% to 0.65% total calcium have been shown to be adequate for growing puppies.[49,220] The NRC's 1985 report recommends a level of 0.59% calcium on a DMB for growing dogs.[49] However, other data indicate that 0.55% total calcium may be inadequate for normal growth in large breeds of dogs.[221] Calcium requirement estimates for growth in cats are reported to vary between 200 and 400 milligrams (mg)/day. This amount is equivalent to approximately 0.6% to 0.8% of the diet.[58,222] However, when cats are fed purified diets, normal growth can be supported by as little as 150 to 200 mg of calcium/day.[222]

Both the NRC's recommendations and the AAFCO's *Nutrient Profiles* have established requirement estimates for calcium and phosphorus in the diets of dogs and cats.[49,58,102] The NRC's recommendations set minimum requirements for available nutrients; these reports do not contain safety margins to allow for processing losses of nutrients or variability in nutrient availability. On the other hand, the AAFCO's standards provide estimates for minimum amounts of nutrients to be included in commercially prepared pet foods; safety margins are included in all requirement estimates to account for differences in availability among ingredients. Accounting for varying levels of availability is especially important with respect to most minerals, including calcium and phosphorus. The AAFCO's *Nutrient Profiles* for dogs recommend a minimum level of 1.0% calcium and 0.8% phosphorus for growth and 0.6% and 0.5% for adult maintenance. Recommendations for cats are 1.0% calcium and 0.8% phosphorus for growth and reproduction and 0.6% calcium and 0.5% phosphorus for adult maintenance.[102] Although there is evidence that adult cats can consume diets with a ratio as low as 0.6:1 with no adverse effects, calcium/phosphorus ratios between 1.2:1 to 1.4:1 are considered optimal by most nutritionists.[102,223]

When formulating rations, pet food manufacturers must account for differences in calcium and phosphorus availability in the various ingredients that are used. Absorption coefficients for calcium have been reported to vary between 0% and 90%, depending on the composition of the diet, the age of the animal, and the total calcium content of the diet.[220,224] Within limits, as the calcium content of a diet decreases, the dog's efficiency of absorption tends to increase.[221] Increasing the amount of vitamin D in the diet also increases the body's ability to absorb dietary calcium and phosphorus.

Pet food ingredients vary in their ability to provide available calcium and phosphorus. In general, the calcium and phosphorus in plant products are less available than the minerals found in animal products. Cereal grains contain phytate, a phosphorus-containing compound that can bind other minerals, including calcium, and make them unavailable for absorption. Although phytate is very high in phosphorus, the availability of phytate phosphorus is only about 30%.[58] On the other hand, many of the animal products included in pet foods are very high in phosphorus but low in calcium; these products include fresh meat or poultry, meat or fish meals, and organ meats. As a result, pet foods must be carefully formulated to ensure that both adequate levels and a proper ratio of calcium to phosphorus are maintained.

Deficiencies of calcium and phosphorus are unusual today because of the production of well-formulated pet foods. Because phosphorus is present in so many foods, a dietary deficiency of this mineral is extremely rare. However, calcium imbalance in growing dogs or cats still occurs as a result of improper feeding practices. A calcium deficiency develops most commonly when puppies or kittens are fed a "table scrap" diet consisting primarily of muscle or organ meats. This type of diet results in a syndrome called *nutritional secondary hyperparathyroidism*. The low calcium and extremely high phosphorus content of an all-meat diet leads to inadequate absorption of calcium and a transient hypocalcemia. The lowered blood levels of calcium stimulate the release of parathyroid hormone (PTH). PTH increases bone resorption of calcium, resulting in a restoration of normal blood calcium. When calcium is deficient in the diet, chronically elevated levels of PTH maintain blood calcium levels within a normal range. However, these elevated PTH levels lead to bone demineralization and a loss of bone mass.[225,226] In dogs the mandibles (jaw bones) show the earliest signs of bone demineralization; this leads to periodontal disease and loss of teeth. Over time, severe bone loss leads to compression of the spinal vertebrae and spontaneous fractures of the long bones. Affected dogs and cats exhibit joint pain and swelling, lameness, and a reluctance to move. Splaying of the toes, excessive sloping of the metatarsal and metacarpal bones, and lateral deviation of the carpus are also observed. Treatment involves correction of the diet through provision of a nutritionally complete and balanced ration. It is advisable to completely replace the deficient diet with a commercially prepared pet food rather than attempt to balance the current diet through the addition of calcium supplements (see Section 5, p. 353).

A second problem that involves calcium homeostasis in the body is the occurrence of puerperal tetany or eclampsia in lactating bitches and queens. Eclampsia is a disease that is seen most commonly in small breeds of dogs and, less frequently, in cats. Eclampsia usually occurs immediately before or 2 to 3 weeks after parturition and is caused by the failure of the dam's calcium regulatory mechanisms to maintain serum calcium levels when there is a loss of calcium to the milk. One of the roles of ionized calcium in the body is to stabilize electrical charges across nerve and muscle cell membranes. In the absence of normal serum calcium levels, cell membranes become hyperexcitable, leading to convulsive seizures and tetany. In the case of eclampsia, serum calcium levels may decrease to less than 7 mg/deciliter (dl). Normally, serum calcium is strictly maintained at a level of 9.5 to 10.5 mg/dl.

Prompt medical care is necessary and consists of intravenous administration of calcium borogluconate.[227,228] Prognosis is very good if the disorder is treated at an early stage.

Although controlled research has not been conducted with companion animals, research with dairy cattle has demonstrated that the consumption of a diet high in calcium during pregnancy actually increases the incidence of this disorder, but moderately low intakes of calcium can prevent its occurrence.[229,230] It is believed that a relative hypercalcemia, caused by a high-calcium diet or calcium supplementation during pregnancy, exerts negative feedback on PTH synthesis and secretion by the parathyroid gland. This effect causes a decrease in both the body's capability to mobilize calcium stores from bone and its ability to increase calcium absorption in the intestine. When calcium is suddenly needed for lactation, the body's regulatory mechanisms are unable to adapt quickly enough to the sudden calcium loss. Calcium is diverted preferentially to milk production, and the animal's serum calcium decreases. Although a correlation between excess calcium during pregnancy and eclampsia has not been proven in dogs or cats, it is prudent to avoid calcium supplements during pregnancy in these species. If a bitch or queen is being fed a high-quality commercial food that has been formulated for feeding through gestation and lactation, calcium supplementation is not necessary and is probably contraindicated.

Just as too little calcium during growth can be detrimental to dogs and cats, so can excessive amounts. The most common cause of excess calcium in a pet's diet is supplementation of an already complete and balanced pet food with high-calcium foods or mineral supplements. Although adequate calcium is essential for normal bone growth and skeletal development, several health risks are taken when excessively high levels of calcium are added to an adequate diet. Excess calcium can produce deficits in other nutrients and has the potential for causing several serious health disorders (see Section 5, pp. 337-343).

Magnesium

Magnesium is present in both soft tissues and bone. It is essential for normal muscle and nervous tissue functioning and plays a key role in a number of enzymatic reactions (see Section 1, p. 45). A deficiency of magnesium in the diet results in muscle weakness, ataxia, and, eventually, convulsive seizures. However, naturally occurring magnesium deficiency is not normally seen in dogs and cats. Excess magnesium has been implicated as a risk factor in the development of feline lower urinary tract disease (see Section 6, pp. 412-416).

Copper

Copper is needed by the body for iron absorption and transport, hemoglobin formation, and normal functioning of the cytochrome oxidase enzyme system (see Section 1, p. 47). The normal metabolism of copper in the body involves the passage of excess copper through the liver and its excretion in bile. Disorders that affect bile excretion often result in an accumulation of copper in the liver, sometimes to toxic levels. In these cases, liver copper toxicosis is a secondary disorder that develops as an effect of the primary liver disease. However, a primary hepatic copper-storage disease exists in certain breeds of dogs. In these cases, the underlying cause of the disease is an accumulation of copper in the liver that eventually results in degenerative liver disease (see Section 6, pp. 387-388).

Zinc

With the exception of iron, zinc is the most abundant micromineral present in the body's tissues. It is important for normal carbohydrate, lipid, protein, and nucleic acid metabolism, and it is necessary for the maintenance of normal epidermal integrity, taste acuity, and immunological functioning.[231,232] The problem of zinc deficiency has been reported in a variety of animal species, including dogs and cats.[233,234,235,236] Clinical signs of deficiency that are common to most species include growth retardation, abnormalities in hair and skin condition, gastrointestinal disturbances, and impaired reproductive performance.[237] The disruption of normal cellular division and maturation processes is believed to be the underlying cause of many of these signs.

Experimental studies of zinc deficiency in dogs and cats have found that skin and coat changes are usually the first clinical signs to develop in these species. Within 2 weeks of consuming a zinc-deficient ration, dogs develop desquamating skin lesions on the foot pads, extremities, joints, and groin. Lesions first appear as small, erythematous areas that eventually enlarge and merge into dry, crusty, brown lesions. Microscopically, the lesions show parakeratosis, hyperkeratinization, and an inflammatory infiltration of neutrophils, lymphocytes, and macrophages.[236,237] Coat changes have also been reported to occur with zinc deficiency. Affected dogs develop a dry, harsh hair coat with fading coat color.[237] When a diet containing adequate zinc is provided, these clinical signs rapidly resolve.

There are several underlying causes of naturally occurring zinc deficiency in dogs and cats. A syndrome called "generic dry dog food disease" has been described that involves the development of zinc deficiency in dogs that are fed poorly formulated, inexpensive, dry dog foods.[235,238] Young, rapidly growing dogs of the large and giant breeds seem to be most susceptible, but several cases have also been reported in adult animals (Figure 13-1) (see Section 3, pp. 195-196).[234,235,238,239] Another dietary cause of zinc deficiency is feeding a diet excessively high in calcium or providing calcium supplements (see Section 5, p. 339). An inherited disorder of zinc metabolism occurs in certain breeds of dogs and also causes clinical signs of zinc deficiency (see Section 6, pp. 388-389).

Sodium

The concern over the connection between sodium intake and essential hypertension in humans has resulted in interest in the sodium content of pet foods and its

FIGURE **13-1**

Zinc deficiency in a young, rapidly growing Bernese Mountain Dog due to in-creased requirements during growth.

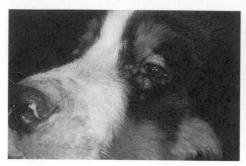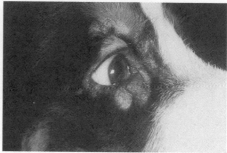

(Reprinted with permission from Candace Sousa, DVM, Animal Dermatology Clinic, Sacramento, California.)

implications for companion animal health. An animal's requirement for sodium is primarily influenced by the unavoidable daily loss of this mineral from the body.[240] In adults during maintenance, these losses are usually quite low. The body's ability to conserve sodium results in a very low dietary sodium requirement in dogs and cats. Maintenance requirements of adults are estimated to range between 0.03% to 0.09% sodium in DM, with slight increases required during pregnancy and lactation.[102,240] Most commercial pet foods contain well above these amounts of sodium.[88]

In all animals the immediate effect of increased salt intake is increased water consumption. Sodium balance in dogs is maintained primarily through changes in urinary excretion of the mineral.[241] An increase in intake above the body's requirement is accompanied by increases in urinary water and sodium excretion. The most important risk attributed to long-term salt excess is its effect on blood pressure. Although this association has been shown to be a causal factor in the development of essential hypertension in certain human subpopulations, there are no data supporting the existence of such a relationship in dogs and cats. Essential hypertension is very rare in companion animals. Data from studies that examined the effect of salt intake on canine blood pressure indicate that this species is resistant to salt retention and hypertension.[242,243,244] Adult dogs that were fed high-sodium diets were able to resist very high levels of salt intake without weight gain or edema, and their renal systems adjusted quickly to changes in dietary sodium.[243,244] When hypertension does occur in dogs and cats, it is usually a secondary disorder occurring as a result of renal disease.[242,245]

Although additional controlled research needs to be conducted, the dog appears to be resistant to the development of salt-induced hypertension. Companion animals readily adapt to the sodium levels in pet foods by altering urinary excretion of sodium. It is probable that these levels are of no harm when fed to animals that are healthy and have free access to fresh water.[240]

KEY POINTS

- Although equally popular as pets, dogs and cats have diverse nutritional needs. Dogs are omnivores, while cats have remained carnivores throughout their evolution. Cats cannot obtain all necessary nutrients from plants and plant products and must consume some animal tissues in order to meet their needs for high protein levels, taurine, arachidonic acid, and preformed vitamin A.

- There are three major components of energy expenditure: (1) the energy expended during rest (resting metabolic rate [RMR]), (2) the energy expended during voluntary muscle activity, and (3) the energy/heat produced by thermogenesis.

- As pets age, regular exercise is important to maintain adequate energy expenditure. Voluntary activity burns energy, increases lean body tissue, and results in a higher RMR.

- Not surprisingly, most dogs prefer canned and semimoist pet food rather than dry; cooked rather than uncooked meat; beef over other meats; and warm food rather than cold. To a degree, palatability increases along with the fat content of the diet.

- More energy is required to convert dietary carbohydrate and protein to body fat, as compared to dietary fat. Thus if an animal consumes more than its caloric requirement and the excess calories are provided by fat, the animal will gain more weight than if the excess calories come from carbohydrate or protein sources.

- "Cafeteria" feeding, or giving a varied diet of high-calorie, palatable foods such as table scraps, may override the body's natural tendency to balance intake and lead to overconsumption.

- The energy requirements of cats and dogs are higher during growth, reproduction, physical activity, and exposure to cold environmental conditions. During lactation, the energy needs of dogs and cats can increase as much as three times normal, depending on litter size. Table 9-3 provides methods of calculating energy requirements and the amounts to feed.

- As dogs and cats reach maturity, their ability to digest milk and other dairy products decreases as a result of decreased activity of lactase in the intestinal mucosa. Similarly, it is thought that very young animals have low levels of sucrase, which indicates that sucrose solutions are not recommendable for very young or orphaned puppies and kittens.

- Although deficiencies of essential fatty acids (EFAs) in dogs and cats are uncommon, dermatological changes are usually the first indication of a problem. EFA deficiency usually results from poorly formulated or rancid foods, but it can occur as a complication of pancreatitis, biliary disease, hepatic disease, or malabsorption. Close attention should be paid to the pet's coat and skin.

- Protein in the diets of adult dogs, adult cats, puppies, and kittens is necessary for the replacement of protein losses in the skin, hair, digestive enzymes, and mucosal cells, as well as amino acid losses from normal cellular protein catabolism. Puppies and kittens also require protein for growth. Protein-deficient adults have a negative nitrogen balance and begin to lose lean muscle mass; puppies and kittens experience impaired growth and development.

- The protein requirement of the cat is higher than that of the dog as a result of the cat's greater needs for the maintenance of normal body tissues rather than from increased needs for growth. This is because of the inability of certain catabolic enzymes in the cat's liver to adapt to changes in dietary protein intake.

- Arginine deficiency in the cat has immediate and devastating effects. Severe hyperammonemia, emesis, muscle spasms, ataxia, hyperesthesia, and tetanic spasms can lead to coma and death. Taurine deficiency can lead to retinal degeneration and dilated cardiomyopathy (DCM).

- Feeding cereal-based dog foods to cats can be harmful; such foods have lower protein and taurine levels and can cause protein and taurine deficiency.

- Contrary to popular belief, there is no research-based, conclusive evidence that protein ingestion contributes to the development of kidney dysfunction in healthy dogs and cats. Moreover, there is no evidence that the protein intake of geriatric dogs should be restricted just because of old age.

- Vitamin A toxicity is uncommon but possible in cats. Because cats must consume preformed vitamin A, and because the absorption is not regulated by the intestinal mucosa, a toxic level can be absorbed. Foods with high levels of vitamin A, such as organ meats (liver and kidney) and various fish oils, should be fed sparingly. Vitamin A toxicosis causes the growth of bony protuberances on the cervical vertebrae that eventually cause pain, lameness, and even crippling in severe cases.

SECTION 2

REFERENCES

1. Colbert EH: *Evolution of the vertebrates,* ed 3, New York, 1980, John Wiley & Sons.
2. Czarnecki-Maulden GL: Nutritional idiosyncrasies of the cat. In *Proceedings of the annual meeting of the American Association of Zoo Veterinarians,* November 2-6, Chicago, 1986 (abstract).
3. Burger I, Edney A, Horrocks D: Basics of feline nutrition, *Practice* 9:143-150, 1987.
4. Danforth E, Landsberg L: Energy expenditure and its regulation. In Greenwood MRC, editor: *Obesity—contemporary issues in clinical nutrition,* New York, 1983, Churchill Livingstone.
5. Sellers EA, Reichman S, Thomas N, and others: Acclimatization to cold in rats: metabolic rates, *Am J Physiol* 167:651-655, 1951.
6. Ravussin E, Burnand B, Schutz Y, and others: Twenty-four hour energy expenditure and resting metabolic rate in obese, moderately obese and control subjects, *Am J Clin Nutr* 35:566-573, 1982.
7. Halliday D, Hesp R, Stalley SF, and others: Resting metabolic rate, weight, surface area and body composition in obese women, *Int J Obes* 3:1-6, 1979.
8. Forbes GB, Welle SL: Lean body mass in obesity, *Int J Obes* 7:99-107, 1983.
9. Horton ES: An overview of the assessment and regulation of energy balance in humans, *Am J Clin Nutr* 38:972-977, 1983.
10. Rothwell N, Stock MJ: Luxuskonsumption, diet-induced thermogenesis and brown fat: the case in favor, *Clin Sci* 64:19-23, 1983.
11. Sims EAH: Experimental obesity, dietary-induced thermogenesis, and their clinical implications, *Clin Endocrinol Metabol* 5:377-395, 1976.
12. Root MV: Early spay-neuter in the cat: effect on development of obesity and metabolic rate, *Vet Clin Nutr* 2:132-134, 1995.
13. Leibowitz SF: Hypothalamic neurotransmitters in relation to normal and disturbed eating patterns. In Wurtman RJ, Wurtman JJ, editors: *Human obesity,* New York, 1987, New York Academy of Sciences.
14. Leibowitz SF, Shor-Posner G: Brain serotonin and eating behavior, *Appetite* 7(suppl):1-14, 1986.
15. Caballero B, Finer N, Wurtman RL: Plasma amino acids and insulin levels in obesity: response to carbohydrate intake and tryptophan supplements, *Metabolism* 37:672-676, 1988.
16. Smith GP, Gibbs J: The effect of gut peptides on hunger, satiety and food intake in humans. In Wurtman RJ, Wurtman JJ, editors: *Human obesity,* New York, 1987, New York Academy of Sciences.
17. Penick SB, Hinkle LE Jr: Depression of food intake in healthy subjects by glucagon, *N Eng J Med* 264:893-897, 1961.
18. Smith GP, Jerome C, Norgren R: Afferent axons in abdominal vagus mediate satiety effect of cholecystokinin in rats, *Am J Physiol* 249:R638-R641, 1985.
19. Kissileff HR, Pi-Sunyer FX, Thornton J, and others: Cholecystokinin octapeptide (CCK-8) decreases food intake in man, *Am J Clin Nutr* 34:154-160, 1981.
20. Shaw MJ, Hughes JJ, Morley JE, and others: Cholecystokinin octapeptide action on gastric emptying and food intake in normal and vagotomized man. In Vanderhaeghen JJ, Crawley JN, editors: Neuronal cholecystokinin, *Ann NY Acad Sci* 448:640-641, 1985.
21. Morley JE, Levine AS, Plotka ED, and others: The effect of naloxone on feeding and spontaneous eating locomotion in the wolf, *Physiol Behav* 30:331-334, 1983.
22. Murrahainen NE, Kissileff HR, Thornton J, and others: Bombesin: another peptide that inhibits feeding in man, *Soc Neurosci* 9:183, 1983 (abstract).
23. Silverstone T, Besser M: Insulin, blood sugar and hunger, *Postgrad Med J* 47:427-429, 1971.
24. Geiselman PJ, Novin D: The role of carbohydrates in appetite, hunger and obesity, *Appetite* 3:203-223, 1982.

25. Houpt KA, Hintz HF: Obesity in dogs, *Canine Pract* 5:54-57, 1978.

26. Itallie TB, van Kissileff HR: The physiologic control of energy intake: an econometric perspective, *Am J Clin Nutr* 38:978-988, 1983.

27. Woods SC, Porte D Jr, Bobbioni E: Insulin: its relationship to the central nervous system and to the control of food intake and body weight, *Am J Clin Nutr* 42:1063-1071, 1985.

28. Vasselli JR, Cleary MP, van Itallie TB: Modern concepts of obesity, *Nutr Rev* 41:361-373, 1983.

29. Houpt KA: Ingestive behavior problems of dogs and cats, *Vet Clin North Am Small Anim Pract* 12:683-690, 1982.

30. Hill SW: Eating responses of humans during meals, *J Comp Physiol Psychol* 86:652-657, 1974.

31. Scalafani A, Springer O: Dietary obesity in adult rats: similarities to hypothalamic and human obesity syndromes, *Physiol Behav* 17:461-471, 1976.

32. Slattery JM, Potter RM: Hyperphagia: a necessary precondition to obesity?, *Appetite* 6:133-142, 1985.

33. Kitchell RL, Baker GG: Taste preference studies in domestic animals. In Swan H, Lewis D, editors: *Proceedings of the Sixth Nutritional Conference,* Nottingham, England, 1972, Churchill Livingstone.

34. Lohse CL: Preferences of dogs for various meats, *J Am Anim Hosp Assoc* 10:187-192, 1974.

35. Bartoshuk LM, Harned MA, Parks LTD: Taste of water in the cat: effect of sucrose preference, *Science* 171:699-701, 1971.

36. Houpt KA, Smith SL: Taste preferences and their relation to obesity in dogs and cats, *Can Vet J* 22:77-81, 1981.

37. Kane E, Morris JG, Rogers QR: Acceptability and digestibility by adult cats of diets made with various sources and levels of fat, *J Anim Sci* 53:1516-1523, 1981.

38. Thorne CJ: Understanding pet response: behavioral aspects of palatability. In *Proceedings of the Petfood Forum,* Chicago, 1997, Watts Publishing.

39. Leblanc J, Diamond P: The effect of meal frequency on postprandial thermogenesis in the dog, *Fed Proc* 44:1678, 1985 (abstract).

40. Fabry P, Tepperman J: Meal frequency—a possible factor in human pathology, *Am J Clin Nutr* 23:1059, 1970.

41. Rodin J: The externality theory today. In Stunkard AJ, editor: *Obesity,* Philadelphia, 1980, WB Saunders.

42. Alexander JE, Wood LLH: Growth studies in Labrador retrievers fed a calorie-dense diet: time-restricted versus free choice feeding, *Can Pract* 14:41-47, 1987.

43. Danforth E Jr: Diet and obesity, *Am J Clin Nutr* 41:1132-1145, 1985.

44. Romsos DR, Belo PS, Bennink MR, and others: Effects of dietary carbohydrate, fat and protein on growth, body composition and blood metabolite levels in the dog, *J Nutr* 106:1452-1464, 1976.

45. Romsos DR, Hornshus MJ, Leveille GA: Influence of dietary fat and carbohydrate on food intake, body weight and body fat of adult dogs, *Proc Soc Exp Biol Med* 157:278-281, 1978.

46. Kanarek RB, Marks-Kaufmann R: Developmental aspects of sucrose-induced obesity in rats, *Physiol Behav* 23:881-885, 1979.

47. Rogers PJ, Blundell JE: Meal patterns and food selection during the development of obesity in rats fed a cafeteria diet, *Neurosci Biobehav Rev* 8:441-453, 1984.

48. Rolls BJ, Rowe EA, Turner RC: Persistent obesity in rats following a period of consumption of a mixed energy diet, *J Physiol (Lond)* 298:415-427, 1980.

49. National Research Council: *Nutrient requirements of dogs,* Washington, DC, 1985, National Academy of Sciences, National Academy Press.

50. National Research Council: *Nutrient requirements of dogs,* Washington, DC, 1974, National Academy of Sciences, National Academy Press.

51. Allard RL, Douglass GM, Kerr WW: The effects of breed and sex on dog growth, *Compan Anim Pract* 2:15-19, 1988.

52. Romsos DR, Palmer HJ, Muiruri KL, and others: Influence of a low carbohydrate diet on performance of pregnant and lactating dogs, *J Nutr* 111:678-689, 1981.

53. Blaza SE: Energy requirements of dogs in cold conditions, *Canine Pract* 9:10-15, 1982.

54. Earle KE: Calculations of energy requirements of dogs, cats and small psittacine birds, *J Small Anim Pract* 34:163-173, 1993.

55. Goggin JM, Schryver HF, Hintz HF: The effects of ad libitum feeding and caloric dilution on the domestic cat's ability to maintain energy balance, *Feline Pract* 21:7-11, 1993.

56. Kendall PT, Blaza SE, Smith PM: Comparative digestible energy requirements of adult Beagles and domestic cats for body weight maintenance, *J Nutr* 113:1946-1955, 1983.

57. Earle KE, Smith PM: Digestible energy requirements of adult cats at maintenance, *J Nutr* 121:S45-S46, 1991.

58. National Research Council: *Nutrient requirements of cats,* Washington, DC, 1986, National Academy of Sciences, National Academy Press.

59. Carey D: *Iams Technical Center data,* Lewisburg, Ohio, 1993, The Iams Company.

60. Finke MD, Lutschaunig MT: Energy requirements of adult Abyssinian cats, *Vet Clin Nutr* 2:64-67, 1995.

61. Loveridge GG, Rivers JPW: Body weight changes and energy intakes of cats during pregnancy and lactation. In Burger IH, Rivers JPW, editors: *Nutrition of the dog and cat,* New York, 1989, Cambridge University Press.

62. Danowski TS, Elkinton JR, Winkler AW: The deleterious effect in dogs of a dry protein ration, *J Clin Invest* 23:816-823, 1944.

63. Prentiss PG, Wolf AV, Eddy HE: Hydropenia in the cat and dog: ability of the cat to meet its water requirements solely from a diet of fish or meat, *Am J Physiol* 196:625-632, 1959.

64. Lewis LD, Morris ML, Hand MS: Nutrients. In Lewis LD, Morris ML, Hand MS, editors: *Small animal clinical nutrition,* ed 3, Topeka, Kan, 1987, Mark Morris Associates.

65. Kettlehut IC, Foss MC, Migliorini RH: Glucose homeostasis in a carnivorous animal (cat) and in rats fed a high-protein diet, *Am J Physiol* 239:R115-R121, 1978.

66. Migliorini RH, Linder C, Moura JL, and others: Gluconeogenesis in a carnivorous bird (black vulture), *Am J Physiol* 225:1389-1392, 1973.

67. Belo PS, Romsos DR, Leveille GA: Influence of diet on glucose tolerance, on the rate of glucose utilization and on gluconeogenic enzyme activities in the dog, *J Nutr* 106:1465-1472, 1976.

68. Blaza SE, Booles D, Burger IH: Is carbohydrate essential for pregnancy and lactation in dogs? In Burger IH, Rivers JPW, editors: *Nutrition of the cat and dog,* New York, 1989, Cambridge University Press.

69. Brady LJ, Armstrong MK, Muriuri KL, and others: Influence of prolonged fasting in the dog on glucose turnover and blood metabolites, *J Nutr* 107:1053-1061, 1977.

70. Kienzle E, Meyer H: The effects of carbohydrate-free diets containing different levels of protein on reproduction in the bitch. In Burger IH, Rivers JPW, editors: *Nutrition of the dog and cat,* New York, 1989, Cambridge University Press.

71. Morris JG, Rogers QR: *Nutritionally related metabolic adaptations of carnivores and ruminants,* Halkidiki, Greece, 1982, International Symposium on Plant, Animal and Microbial Adaptations to Terrestrial Environments, Man and the Biosphere.

72. Beliveau GP, Freedland RA: Metabolism of serine, glycine and threonine in isolated cat hepatocytes *(Felis domestica), Comp Biochem Physiol* 71B:13-18, 1982.

73. Rogers QR, Morris JG, Freedland RA: Lack of hepatic enzymatic adaptation to low and high levels of dietary protein in the adult cat, *Enzyme* 22:348-356, 1977.

74. Rowsell EV, Carnie JA, Wahbi SD, and others: L-serine dehydratase and L-serine-pyruvate aminotransferase activities in different animal species, *Comp Biochem Physiol* 63:543-555, 1979.

75. Morris JG, Rogers QR: Metabolic basis for some of the nutritional peculiarities of the cat, *J Small Anim Pract* 23:599-613, 1982.

76. Ballard FJ: Glucose utilization in mammalian liver, *Comp Biochem Physiol* 14:437-443, 1965.

77. De Wilde RO, Jansen T: The use of different sources of raw and heated starch in the ration of weaned kittens. In Burger IH, Rivers JPW, editors: *Nutrition of the cat and dog,* New York, 1989, Cambridge University Press.

78. Trudell JI, Morris JG: Carbohydrate digestion in the cat, *J Anim Sci* 41:329, 1975.

79. Pencovic TA, Morris JG: Corn and wheat starch utilization by the cat, *J Anim Sci* 41:325, 1975.

80. Morris JG, Trudell J, Pencovic T: Carbohydrate digestion by the domestic cat *(Felis catus), Br J Nutr* 37:365-373, 1977.

81. Burger IH: A basic guide to nutrient requirements. In Edney ATB, editor: *Dog and cat nutrition,* ed 2, Oxford, England, 1988, Pergamon Press.

82. Keen CL, Lonnerdal B, Clegg MS, and others: Developmental changes in composition of cats' milk: trace elements, minerals, protein, carbohydrate and fat, *J Nutr* 112:1763-1769, 1982.

83. Mundt HC, Meyer H: Pathogenesis of lactose-induced diarrhea and its prevention by enzymatic splitting of lactose. In Burger IH, Rivers JPW, editors: *Nutrition of the cat and dog,* New York, 1989, Cambridge University Press.

84. Kallfelz FA: Evaluation and use of pet foods: general considerations in using pet foods for adult maintenance, *Vet Clin North Am Small Anim Pract* 19:387-403, 1989.

85. Bartges J, Anderson WH: Dietary fiber, *Vet Clin Nutr* 4:25-28, 1997.

86. Downey RL, Kronfeld DS, Banta CA: Diet of Beagles affects stamina, *J Am Anim Hosp Assoc* 16:273-277, 1980.

87. Reynolds AJ, Fuhrer HL, Dunlap MD, and others: Lipid metabolite responses to diet and training in sled dogs, *J Nutr* 124:2754S-2759S, 1994.

88. Kallfelz FA, Dzanis DA: Overnutrition: an epidemic problem in pet animal practice?, *Vet Clin North Am Small Anim Pract* 19:433-446, 1989.

89. Dammrich K: Relationship between nutrition and bone growth in large and giant dogs, *J Nutr* 121:114S-121S, 1991.

90. Nap RC, Hazewinkel HAW: Growth and skeletal development in the dog in relation to nutrition: a review, *Vet Q* 1:50-59, 1994.

91. Hedhammer A, Wu F, Krook L, and others: Overnutrition and skeletal disease: an experimental study in growing Great Dane dogs, *Cornell Vet* 5 (suppl 64):1-159, 1974.

92. Rivers JPW, Sinclair AJ, Crawford MA: Inability of the cat to desaturate essential fatty acids, *Nature (Lond)* 258:171-173, 1975.

93. Rivers JPW, Sinclair AJ, Moore DP, and others: The abnormal metabolism of essential fatty acids in the cat, *Proc Nutr Soc* 35:66a-67a, 1976.

94. Hassam AG, Rivers JPW, Crawford MA: The failure of the cat to desaturate linoleic acid: its nutritional implications, *Nutr Metabol* 21:321-328, 1977.

95. Pawlowsky R, Barnes A, Salem N: Essential fatty acid metabolism in the feline: relationship between liver and brain production of long-chain polyunsaturated fatty acids, *J Lipid Res* 35:2032-2040, 1994.

96. Sinclair AJ, Slattery W, McLean JG, and others: Essential fatty acid deficiency and evidence for arachidonate synthesis in the cat, *Br J Nutr* 46:93-96, 1981.

97. Davidson BC, Traher CS: The importance of essential fatty acid evaluation and supplementation in feline diets, *J South Afric Vet Assoc* 58:39-41, 1987.

98. MacDonald ML, Anderson BC, Rogers QR, and others: Essential fatty acid requirements of cats: pathology of essential fatty acid deficiency, *Am J Vet Res* 45:1310-1317, 1984.

99. MacDonald ML, Rogers QR, Morris JG: Effects of linoleate and arachidonate deficiencies on reproduction and spermatogenesis in the cat, *J Nutr* 114:719-726, 1984.

100. MacDonald ML, Rogers QR, Morris JG: Nutrition of the domestic cat, a mammalian carnivore, *Ann Rev Nutr* 4:521-562, 1984.

101. MacDonald, ML, Rogers QR, Morris JG: Role of linoleate as an essential fatty acid for the cat, independent of arachidonate synthesis, *J Nutr* 113:1422-1433, 1983.

102. Association of American Feed Control Officials: *Official publication*, 1997, Association of American Feed Control Officials.

103. Rivers JPW, Frankel TL: Fat in the diet of cats and dogs. In Anderson RS, editor: *Nutrition of the dog and cat*, Oxford, England, 1980, Pergamon Press.

104. Mohrhauer H, Holman RT: The effect of dose level of essential fatty acids upon fatty acid composition of the rat liver, *J Lipid Res* 4:151-159, 1963.

105. O'Donnell JA III, Hayes KC: Nutrition and nutritional disorders. In Holzworth J, editor: *Diseases of the cat: medicine and surgery*, Philadelphia, 1987, WB Saunders.

106. Codner EC, Thatcher CD: The role of nutrition in the management of dermatoses, *Semin Vet Med Surg (Small Anim)* 5:167-177, 1990.

107. Hansen AE, Wiese HF: Fat in the diet in relation to nutrition of the dog. I. Characteristic appearance and changes of animals fed diets with and without fat, *Tex Rep Biol Med* 9:491-515, 1951.

108. Sinclair AJ, McLean JG, Monger EA: Metabolism of linoleic acid in the cat, *Lipids* 14:932-936, 1979.

109. Rivers JPW: Essential fatty acids in cats, *J Small Anim Pract* 23:563-576, 1982.

110. Humphreys ER, Scott PP: The addition of herring and vegetable oils to the diets of cats, *Proc Nutr Soc* 21:XVIII, 1962.

111. Schaeffer MC, Rogers QR, Morris JG: Protein in the nutrition of dogs and cats. In Burger IH, Rivers JPW, editors: *Nutrition of the dog and cat*, New York, 1989, Cambridge University Press.

112. Bradstreet RB: *The Kjeldahl method for organic nitrogen*, New York, 1965, Academic Press.

113. Allison JB, Wannemacher RW, Migliarese JF: Diet and the metabolism of 2-aminofluorene, *J Nutr* 52:415-425, 1954.

114. Wannemacher RE, McCoy JR: Determination of optimal dietary protein requirements of young and old dogs, *J Nutr* 88:66-74, 1966.

115. Case LP, Czarnecki-Maulden GL: Protein requirements of growing pups fed practical dry-type diets containing mixed-protein sources, *Am J Vet Res* 51:808-812,1990.

116. Maybee DM, Morgan AF: Evaluation by dog growth of egg yolk protein and six other partially purified proteins, some after heat-treatment, *J Nutr* 43:261-279, 1951.

117. Allison JB: Optimal nutrition correlated with nitrogen retention, *Am J Clin Nutr* 4:662-672, 1956.

118. Ontko, JA, Wuthier RE, Phillips PH: The effect of increased dietary fat upon the protein requirement of the growing dog, *J Nutr* 62:163-169, 1957.

119. Hilton JW, Atkinson JL: High lipid and high protein dog foods, *Can Vet J* 29:76-78, 1988.

120. Allison JB, Seeley RD, Brown JH, and others: The evaluation of proteins in hypoproteinemic dogs, *J Nutr* 31:237-242, 1946.

121. Payne PR: Assessment of the protein values of diets in relation to the requirements of the growing dog. In Graham-Jones O, editor: *Canine and feline nutritional requirements*, 1965, London, Pergamon Press.

122. Dickinson CD, Scott PP: Nutrition of the cat. II. Protein requirements for growth of weanling kittens and young cats maintained on a mixed diet, *Br J Nutr* 10:311-316, 1956.

123. Anderson PA, Baker DH, Sherry PA, and others: Nitrogen requirement of the kitten, *Am J Vet Res* 41:1646-1649, 1980.

124. Rogers QR, Morris JG: Why does the cat require a high protein diet? In Anderson RS, editor: *Nutrition of the dog and cat*, New York, 1980, Pergamon Press.

125. Arnold A, Schad JS: Nitrogen balance studies with dogs on casein or methionine-supplemented casein, *J Nutr* 53:265-273, 1954.

126. Kade CF Jr, Phillips JH, Phillips WA: The determination of the minimum requirement of the adult dog for maintenance of nitrogen balance, *J Nutr* 36:109-121, 1948.

127. Melnick D, Cowgill GR: The protein minima for nitrogen equilibrium with different proteins, *J Nutr* 13:401-424, 1937.

128. Greaves JP, Scott PP: Nutrition of the cat. III. Protein requirements for nitrogen equilibrium in adult cats maintained on a mixed diet, *Br J Nutr* 14:361-369, 1960.

129. Heiman V: The protein requirements of growing puppies, *J Am Anim Hosp Assoc* 111: 304-308, 1947.

130. Gessert CG, Phillips PH: Protein in the nutrition of the growing dog, *J Nutr* 58:415-421, 1956.

131. Burns RA, LaFaivre MH, Milner JA: Effects of dietary protein quantity and quality on the growth of dogs and rats, *J Nutr* 112:1843-1853, 1982.

132. Sheffy BE: The 1985 revision of the National Research Council nutrient requirements of dogs and its impact on the pet food industry. In Burger IH, Rivers JPW, editors: *Nutrition of the dog and cat,* New York, 1989, Cambridge University Press.

133. Jansen GR, Deuth MA, Ward GM, and others: Protein quality studies in growing kittens, *Nutr Rep Int* 11:525-536, 1975.

134. Smalley KA, Rogers QR, Morris JG: The nitrogen requirement of the kitten using crystalline amino acid diets or casein diets. In *Proceedings of the Twelfth International Congress on Nutrition,* San Diego, 96:538, Aug 16-21,1981 (abstract).

135. Burger IH, Blaza SE, Kendall PT: The protein requirement of adult cats, *Proc Nutr Soc* 40:102a, 1981.

136. Harper AE: Effect of variations in protein intake on enzymes of amino acid metabolism, *Can J Biochem* 43:1589-1597, 1965.

137. Kaplan JH, Pitot HC: The regulation of intermediary amino acid metabolism in animal tissues. In Munro HN, editor: *Mammalian protein metabolism,* vol 4, New York, 1970, Academic Press.

138. Schimke RT: Adaptive characteristics of urea cycle enzymes in the rat, *J Biol Chem* 237:459-467, 1962.

139. Szepesi B, Freedland RA: Alterations in the activities of several rat liver enzymes at various times after initiation of a high protein regimen, *J Nutr* 93:301-310, 1967.

140. Burns RA, Milner JA, Corbin JE: Arginine: an indispensable amino acid for mature dogs, *J Nutr* 111:1020-1024, 1981.

141. Anderson PA, Baker DH, Corbin JE: Lysine and arginine requirements of the domestic cat, *J Nutr* 109:1368-1372, 1979.

142. Morris JG, Rogers QR: Ammonia intoxication in the near-adult cat as a result of a dietary deficiency of arginine, *Science* 199(4327):431-432, 1978.

143. Czarnecki GL, Baker DH: Urea-cycle metabolism in the dog with emphasis on the role of arginine, *J Nutr* 114:581-586, 1984.

144. Costello MJ, Morris JG, Rogers QR: The role of intestinal mucosa in endogenous arginine biosynthesis in ureotelic mammals. In *Proceedings of the Twelfth International Congress on Nutrition, San Diego,* 96:538, Aug 16-21, 1981 (abstract).

145. Featherston WR, Rogers QR, Freedland RA: Relative importance of kidney and liver in synthesis of arginine by the rat, *Am J Physiol* 224:127-129, 1973.

146. Pion PD, Kittleson MD, Rogers, QR, and others: Myocardial failure in cats associated with low plasma taurine: a reversible cardiomyopathy, *Science* 237:764-768, 1987.

147. Rabin AR, Nicolosi RJ, Hayes KC: Dietary influence of bile acid conjugation in the cat, *J Nutr* 106:1241-1246, 1976.

148. Hayes KC, Sturman JA: Taurine in metabolism, *Ann Rev Nutr* 1:401-420, 1981.

149. Sturman JA, Gargano AD, Messing JM, and others: Feline maternal taurine deficiency: effect on mother and offspring, *J Nutr* 116:655-657, 1986.

150. Morris JG, Rogers QR: The metabolic basis for the taurine requirement of cats. In Lombardine JB, Schaffer SW, Azuma J, editors: Taurine: nutritional value and mechanisms of action, *Adv Exp Med Bio* 315:33-44, 1992.

151. Morris JG, Rogers QR: Why is the nutrition of cats different from that of dogs?, *Tijdschr Diergeneesk* 1:64S-67S, 1991.

152. Hayes KC: Nutritional problems in cats: taurine deficiency and vitamin A excess, *Can Vet J* 23:2-5, 1982.

153. Morris JG, Rogers QR, Seungwook WK, and others: Dietary taurine requirement of cats is determined by microbial degradation of taurine in the gut, *Vet Clin Nutr* 1:118-127, 1994.

154. Wen GY, Sturman JA, Wisniewski HM, and others: Tapetum disorganization in taurine-depleted cats, *Invest Ophthalmol Vis Sci* 18:1201-1206, 1979.

155. Sturman JA, Rassin DK, Hayes KC, and others: Taurine deficiency in the kitten: exchange and turnover of [^{35}S] taurine in brain, retina and other tissues, *J Nutr* 108:1462-1476, 1978.

156. Barnett KC, Burger IH: Taurine deficiency retinopathy in the cat, *J Small Anim Pract* 21: 521-526, 1980.

157. Hayes KC: A review of the biological role of taurine, *Nutr Rev* 34:161-165, 1976.

158. Huxtable R, Barbeau A: *Taurine*, New York, 1976, Raven Press.

159. O'Donnell JA III, Rogers QR, Morris JG: Effect of diet on plasma taurine in the cat, *J Nutr* 111:1111-1116, 1981.

160. Aguirre GD: Retinal degeneration associated with the feeding of dog food to cats, *J Am Vet Med Assoc* 172:791-796, 1978.

161. Earl KE, Smith PM: The effect of dietary taurine content on the plasma taurine concentration of the cat, *Brit J Nutr* 66:227-235, 1991.

162. Morris JG, Rogers R, Pacioretty LM: Taurine: an essential nutrient for cats, *J Small Anim Pract* 31:502-509, 1990.

163. Carey DP, Strieker MJ: Taurine essentials and clinical management. In *Iams Technical Report,* Lewisburg, Ohio, 1993, The Iams Company.

164. Hickman MA, Rogers QR, Morris JG: Effect of processing on the fate of dietary [14C] taurine in cats, *J Nutr* 120:995-1000, 1990.

165. Hickman MA, Morris JG, Rogers QR: Intestinal taurine and the enterohepatic circulation of taurocholic acid in the cat, *Adv Exp Med Biol* 315:45-54, 1992.

166. Milner JA: Lysine requirements of the immature dog, *J Nutr* 111:40-45, 1981.

167. Brown RG: Protein in dog foods, *Can Vet J* 30:528-531, 1989.

168. Teeter RG, Baker DH, Corbin JE: Methionine and cystine requirements of the cat, *J Nutr* 108:291-297, 1978.

169. Burns RA, Milner JA: Sulfur amino acid requirements of the immature Beagle dog, *J Nutr* 111:2117-2122, 1981.

170. Roberts RN: *A study of felinine and its excretion by the cat* (doctoral dissertation), Buffalo, 1963, State University of New York.

171. Shapiro IL: *In vivo studies on the metabolic relationship between felinine and serum cholesterol in the domestic cat* (doctoral dissertation), Newark, Del, 1962, University of Delaware.

172. Rogers QR, Morris, JG: Protein and amino acid nutrition of the cat. In *American Animal Hospital Association Proceedings,* 1983.

173. Ikeda M, Tsuji H, Nakamura S, and others: Studies on the biosynthesis of nicotinamide adenine dinucleotide. II. A role of picolinic carboxylase in the biosynthesis of nicotinamide adenine dinucleotide from tryptophan in mammals, *J Biol Chem* 240:1395-1401, 1965.

174. Maynard LA, Loosli JK, Hintz HF, and others: The proteins and their metabolism, In *Animal nutrition,* ed 7, New York, 1979, McGraw-Hill.

175. Levitsky DA, Massaro TF, Barnes RH: Maternal malnutrition and the neonatal environment, *Fed Proc* 32:1709-1719, 1973.

176. Barnes RH: Effect of postnatal dietary protein and energy restriction on exploratory behavior in young pigs, *Dev Psychobiol* 9:425-435, 1976.

177. Brenner BM, Meyer TW, Hostetter TH: Dietary protein intake and the progressive nature of renal disease: the role of hemodynamically mediated glomerular injury in the pathogenesis of progressive glomerular sclerosis in aging, renal ablation, and intrinsic renal disease, *N Eng J Med* 307:652-657, 1982.

178. Murphy DH: Too much of a good thing: protein and a dog's diet, *Int J Study Anim Prob* 4:101-107, 1983.

179. Saxton JA, Kimball GC: Relation of nephrosis and other diseases of albino rats to age and to modifications of diet, *Arch Pathol* 32:951-965, 1941.

180. Lalick JJ, Allen JR: Protein overload nephropathy in rats with unilateral nephrectomy, *Arch Pathol* 91:373-382, 1971.

181. Polzin DJ, Osborne CA: Conservative medical management of canine chronic renal failure: concepts and controversies, *Proc Am Coll Vet Int Med* 1:4-55 to 4-58, 1986.

182. Lowenstein LM: The rat as a model for aging in the kidney. In Gibson DC, Adelman RC, Finch C, editors: *Development of the rodent as a model system of aging,* Washington, DC, 1978, US Department of Health, Education, and Welfare.

183. Goldman R: Aging of the excretory system: kidney and bladder. In Finch EE, Hayflick L, editors: *Handbook of the biology of aging,* New York, 1977, Van Nostrand Reinhold.

184. Kaufman GM: Renal function in the geriatric dog, *Compend Cont Ed Pract Vet* 6:108-109, 1984.

185. Cowgill LD, Spangler WL: Renal insufficiency in geriatric dogs, *Vet Clin North Am Small Anim Pract* 11:727-749, 1981.

186. Branam JE: Dietary management of geriatric dogs and cats, *Vet Tech* 8:501-503, 1987.

187. Leibetseder JL, Neufeld KW: Effects of medium protein diets in dogs with chronic renal failure, *J Nutr* 121:S145-S149, 1991.

188. Polzin DJ, Osborne CA, Hayden DW, and others: Influence of reduced protein diets on morbidity, mortality and renal function in dogs with induced chronic renal failure, *Am J Vet Res* 45:506-517, 1984.

189. Glover J, Goodwin TW, Morton RA: Conversion of beta-carotene into vitamin A in the intestine of the rat, *Biochem J* 41:XLV, 1947.

190. Goodman DS, Huang HS, Kanai M, and others: The enzymatic conversion of all-trans beta-carotene into retinal, *J Biol Chem* 242:3543-3554, 1967.

191. Thompson SY, Braude R, Coates ME, and others: Further studies on the conversion of beta-carotene to vitamin A, *Br J Nutr* 4:398-420, 1960.

192. Gershoff SN, Andrus SB, Hegsted DM, and others: Vitamin A deficiency in cats, *Lab Invest* 6:227-239, 1957.

193. Mellanby E: The experimental production of deafness in young animals by diet, *J Physiol* 94:316-321, 1938.

194. Hayes KC: On the pathophysiology of vitamin A deficiency, *Nutr Rev* 29:3-6, 1971.

195. How KL, Hazewinkel HA, Mol JA: Dietary vitamin D dependence of cat and dog due to inadequate cutaneous synthesis of vitamin D, *Gen Comp Endocrinol* 96:12-18, 1994.

196. Kealy RD, Lawler DF, Monti KL: Some observations on the dietary vitamin D requirement of weanling pups. In Morris JG, Finley D, Rogers Q, editors: *Proceedings of the Waltham International Symposium on the Nutrition of Small Companion Animals,* Sept 4-8, University of California, Davis, Calif, 1990.

197. Hazewinkel HAW: Nutrition in relation to skeletal growth deformities, *J Small Anim Pract* 30:625-630, 1989.

198. Morris JF: Vitamin D synthesis by kittens, *Vet Clin Nutr* 3:88-92, 1996.

199. Campbell JR, Douglas TA: The effect of low calcium intake and vitamin D supplements on bone structure in young growing dogs, *Br J Nutr* 19:339-347, 1965.

200. Brickman AS, Chilumula RR, Coburn JW, and others: Biologic action of 1,25-dihydroxy-vitamin D_3 in the rachitic dog, *Endocrinology* 92:728-734, 1973.

201. Kelly PJ: Bone remodeling in puppies with experimental rickets. *J Lab Clin Med* 70:94-105, 1967.

202. Morris JG, Earle KE: Vitamin D and calcium requirements of kittens, *Vet Clin Nutr* 3:93-96, 1996.

203. Haruna A, Kawai K, Takaba T, and others: Dietary calcinosis in a cat, *J Anim Clin Found* 1:9-16, 1992.

204. Scott DW, Sheffy BE: Dermatosis in dogs caused by vitamin E deficiency, *Comp Anim Pract* 1: 42-46, 1987.

205. Figueriredo C: Vitamin E serum contents, erythrocyte and lymphocyte count, PCV, and hemoglobin determinations in normal dogs, dogs with scabies, and dogs with demodicosis. In *Proceedings of the Annual American Academy of Veterinary Dermatologists and the American College of Veterinary Dermatology,* 1985.

206. Miller WH: Nutritional considerations in small animal dermatology, *Vet Clin North Am Small Anim Pract* 19:497-511, 1989.

207. Scott DW, Walton DK: Clinical evaluation of oral vitamin E for the treatment of primary canine acanthosis nigricans, *J Am Anim Hosp Assoc* 21:345-350, 1985.

208. Hinchcliff KW, Reinhart GA, Reynolds AJ, and others: Exercise and oxidant stress. In Reinhart GA, Carey DP, editors: *Recent advances in canine and feline nutrition,* vol 2, 1998 Iams Nutrition Symposium Proceedings, Wilmington, Ohio, 1998, Orange Frazer Press.

209. Cordy DR: Experimental production of steatitis (yellow fat disease) in kittens fed a commercial canned cat food and prevention of the condition by vitamin E, *Cornell Vet* 44:310-318, 1954.

210. Gaskell, CJ, Leedale AH, Douglas SW: Pansteatitis in the cat: a report of five cases, *J Small Anim Pract* 16:117-121, 1975.

211. Strieker MJ, Morris JG, Feldman BF, and others: Vitamin K deficiency in cats fed commercial fish-based diets, *J Small Anim Pract* 37:322-326, 1996.

212. Smith DC, Proutt LM: Development of thiamine deficiency in the cat on a diet of raw fish, *Proc Soc Exp Biol Med* 56:1-5, 1944.

213. Houston D, Hulland TJ: Thiamine deficiency in a team of sled dogs, *Can Vet J* 29:383-385, 1988.

214. Pastoor FJH, Herck H, van Klooster A, and others: Biotin deficiency in cats as induced by feeding a purified diet containing egg white, *J Nutr* 121:S73-S74, 1991.

215. Shen CS, Overfield L, Murthy PNA, and others: Effect of feeding raw egg white on pyruvate and propionyl CoA carboxylase activities on tissues of the dog, *Fed Proc* 36:1169, 1977.

216. Miller EE, Baumann CA: Relative effects of casein and tryptophan on the health and xanthurenic acid excretion of pyridoxine deficient mice, *J Biol Chem* 157:551-562, 1945.

217. Gries CL, Scott ML: The pathology of pyridoxine deficiency in chicks, *J Nutr* 102:1259-1268, 1972.

218. Linkswiler HM: Vitamin B-6 requirements of men. In *Human vitamin B-6 requirements,* Washington, DC, 1978, National Academy of Science.

219. Bai SC, Sampwon DA, Morris JG, and others: The level of dietary protein affects the vitamin B-6 requirement of cats, *J Nutr* 121:1054-1061, 1991.

220. Jenkins KJ, Phillips PH: The mineral requirements of the dog. II. The relation of calcium, phosphorus and fat levels to minimal calcium and phosphorus requirements, *J Nutr* 70:241-246, 1960.

221. Hazewinkel HAW, Van Der Brom WE, van Klooster AT, and others: Calcium metabolism in Great Dane dogs fed diets with various calcium and phosphorus levels, *J Nutr* 121:S99-S106, 1991.

222. Scott PP: Minerals and vitamins in feline nutrition. In Graham-Jones O, editor: *Canine and feline nutrition requirements,* London, 1965, Pergamon Press.

223. Kealy RD, Lawler DF, Ballam JM: Dietary calcium:phosphorus ratio for adult cats, *Vet Clin Nutr* 3:28, 1996.

224. Hedhammer A: Nutrition as it relates to skeletal disease. In *Proceedings of the Kal Kan Symposium,* Columbus, Ohio, 1980, Kal Kan.

225. Bennett D: Nutrition and bone disease in the dog and cat, *Vet Rec* 98:313-320, 1976.

226. Hintz HF, Schryver HF: Nutrition and bone development in dogs, *Comp Anim Pract* 1:44-47, 1987.

227. Austad R, Bjerkas E: Eclampsia in the bitch, *J Small Anim Pract* 17:793-798, 1976.

228. Bjerkas E: Eclampsia in the cat, *J Small Anim Pract* 15:411-414, 1974.

229. Boda JM, Cole HH: The influence of dietary calcium and phosphorus on the influence of milk fever in dairy cattle, *J Dairy Sci* 37:360-372, 1954.

230. Wiggers KD, Nelson DK, Jacobson NL: Prevention of parturient paresis by a low-calcium diet prepartum: a field study, *J Dairy Sci* 58:430-431, 1975.

231. Catalanotto FA: The trace metal zinc and taste, *Am J Clin Nutr* 31:1098-1103, 1978.

232. Miller WH, Griffin CE, Scott DW, and others: Clinical trial of DVM Derm Caps in the treatment of allergic disease in dogs: a nonblinded study, *J Am Anim Hosp Assoc* 25:163-168, 1989.

233. Kane E, Morris JG, Rogers QR, and others: Zinc deficiency in the cat, *J Nutr* 111:488-495, 1981.

234. Wolf AM: Zinc-responsive dermatosis in a Rhodesian Ridgeback, *Vet Med* 82:908-912, 1987.

235. Van den Broek AHM, Thoday KL: Skin disease in dogs associated with zinc deficiency: a report of five cases, *J Small Anim Pract* 27:313-323, 1986.

236. Sanecki RK, Corbin JE, Forbes RM: Tissue changes in dogs fed a zinc-deficient ration, *Am J Vet Res* 43:1642-1646, 1982.

237. Banta CA: The role of zinc in canine and feline nutrition. In Burger IH, Rivers JPW, editors: *Nutrition of the dog and cat,* New York, 1989, Cambridge University Press.

238. Sousa CA, Stannard AA, Ihrke PJ: Dermatosis associated with feeding generic dog food: 13 cases (1981-1982), *J Am Vet Med Assoc* 192:676-680, 1988.

239. Fadok VA: Zinc responsive dermatosis in a Great Dane: a case report, *J Am Anim Hosp Assoc* 18:409-414, 1982.

240. Mitchell AR: Salt intake, animal health and hypertension: should sleeping dogs lie? In Burger IH, Rivers JPW, editors: *Nutrition of the dog and cat,* New York, 1989, Cambridge University Press.

241. Smith RC, Haschem T, Hamlin RL, and others: Water and electrolyte intake and output and quantity of faeces in the healthy dog, *Vet Med Sm Anim Clin* 59:743-748, 1964.

242. Spangler WL, Gribble DH, Weiser MG: Canine hypertension: a review, *J Am Vet Med Assoc* 170:995-998, 1977.

243. Ladd M, Raisz LG: Response of the normal dog to dietary sodium chloride, *Am J Physiol* 159:149-152, 1949.

244. Wilhelmj CM, Waldmann EB, McGuire TF: Effect of prolonged high sodium chloride ingestion and withdrawal upon blood pressure of dogs, *Proc Soc Exp Biol Med* 77:379-382, 1951.

245. Anderson IJ, Fisher EW: The blood pressure in canine interstitial nephritis, *Res Vet Sci* 9:304-313, 1968.

3

PET FOODS

The previous sections examined basic principles of nutrition and the specific nutrient requirements of dogs and cats. The practical application of this information is the provision of optimal nutrition to companion animals throughout life. This section provides information that enables pet owners and professionals to thoroughly evaluate and select appropriate foods for dogs or cats. The history and current regulation of commercial pet foods is examined, with special attention paid to current labeling requirements and measurements of nutritional adequacy. A study of the nutrient content of pet foods provides an overview of ingredients included in commercial pet foods and of methods used to measure nutrient content. Chapter 17, which examines the various types of available pet foods, facilitates easy categorization of foods for comparison purposes. Also, detailed information regarding the evaluation of pet foods allows owners and professionals to efficiently assess commercial products and select appropriate foods for individual animals.

14

History and Regulation
of Pet Foods

Pet owners generally have two options available when choosing the type of diet to feed their companion animals. They may either prepare a homemade diet or purchase a commercially prepared dog or cat food. Today the majority of pet owners in the United States feed their companion animals commercially prepared foods. The popularity of commercial products is evidenced by the growth of the pet food industry over the past 40 years. In 1958 total pet food sales in the United States were estimated to be $350 million. This amount increased to $1.43 billion in 1972 and to $5.1 billion in 1986.[1] In 1996, the U.S. market for pet foods and supplies sold through grocery stores and mass merchandise outlets was more than $11.5 billion.[2] More than 74% of these sales were for pet food. The Pet Food Institute's (PFI's) directory of pet food manufacturers lists more than 300 companies, and it is estimated that there are more than 3000 different brands of pet food products.[3]

HISTORY

Before the middle of the nineteenth century, diets for dogs and cats were not commercially prepared. Owners fed their pets table scraps or homemade formulas made from human foods and leftovers. The first commercial dog food to be marketed was in the form of a biscuit. It was produced and sold in 1860 by James Spratt, an American living in London.[4] Following success in England, Spratt began selling his product in the United States. In the early 1900s several other groups observed Spratt's success and began to develop and sell pet foods. The Chappel brothers of Rockford, Illinois were responsible for producing the first batches of canned food. The Chappels named their product Ken-L-Ration and followed it with the introduction of a dry product in the 1930s. Around the same time, Samuel Gaines broke into the market with a new type of dog food called a "meal." The meal consisted of a number of dried, ground ingredients that were mixed together and sold in 100 pound (lb) bags. Pet owners enjoyed the convenience of this new product because they were able to buy fairly large quantities at one time. In addition, very little preparation of the food was necessary before feeding.

In the early 1900s, pet foods were marketed only through feed stores. The National Biscuit Company (Nabisco), which purchased Milk Bone in 1931, was the first group to attempt to sell its product in grocery stores. Selling pet food in human food markets initially met with much resistance. Because most pet foods were made from byproducts of human foods, customers and store owners considered it unsanitary to sell such products next to foods that were meant for human consumption. However, Nabisco persisted, and Milk Bones finally made it into the supermarket. The convenience and economy of purchasing pet foods at grocery stores rapidly overcame customer concerns. Improved distribution and availability resulted in increased sales and popularity of commercial pet foods. By the mid 1930s many brands were sold in grocery stores. At this time, although some dry biscuits and meal products were available, canned pet foods were still the most popular type of pet food product sold in the United States.

With the onset of World War II, a shortage of metal resulted in fewer cans being available for the processing of pet food. The pet food industry responded by producing and selling a larger proportion of dry foods. However, once the war was over, canned foods again became more popular with pet owners. It was not until the development of the extrusion process that dry pet foods began to increase in popularity. The extrusion process and expanded pet foods (foods produced through the extrusion process) were first developed by researchers at Purina laboratories in the 1950s. *Extrusion* involves first mixing all of the pet food ingredients together and then rapidly cooking the mixture and forcing it through an extruder (specialized pressure-cooker). This process causes a rapid expansion of the bite-sized food particles, resulting in increased digestibility and palatability of the food. After extrusion and drying, a coating of fat or some other palatability enhancer is usually sprayed onto the outside of the food pieces. In 1957 Purina Dog Chow, an expanded product, was first introduced to grocery stores. A year later, this new product had become the bestselling dog food in the United States. Today the majority of dry pet foods sold in the United States are extruded products, and dry dog food makes up the largest proportion of the pet food market.

Because little was known about the nutrient requirements of dogs and cats when pet foods were first manufactured, the same food was commonly marketed for both species. Manufacturers merely labeled the cans or bags differently. However, as more knowledge was acquired about the different nutrient needs of dogs and cats, separate pet foods were formulated for each. In 1996 dry dog food made up the highest proportion of pet food retail sales, while dry cat food showed a substantial increase in sales.[2] As more knowledge becomes available about canine and feline nutrition, companies are developing diets that are designed for specific stages of life, physiological states, and health problems.[4] Although not all of these products are beneficial or necessary, they represent a response to the pet-owning pub-

TABLE 14-1

Governing Agencies of Commercial Pet Foods

Agency	Function
Association of American Feed Control Officials (AAFCO)	Sets standards for substantiation claims and provides an advisory committee for state legislation
National Research Council (NRC)	Collects and evaluates research and makes nutrient recommendations
Food and Drug Administration (FDA)	Specifies permitted ingredients and manufacturing procedures
United States Department of Agriculture (USDA)	Regulates pet food labels and research facilities
Pet Food Institute (PFI)	Trade organization that represents pet food manufacturers
Canadian Veterinary Medical Association (CVMA)	Administers voluntary product certification
State Feed Control Offices	Enforces the Commercial Feed Law within states
Environmental Protection Agency (EPA)	Regulates the use of pesticides in raw material and feeds; regulates processing plant discharges
Federal Trade Commission (FTC)	Regulates trade and advertising
Pet Food Association of Canada	Trade organization that represents pet food manufacturers

lic's desire to supply their companion animals with the best nutrition possible during all stages of life. The public's increased interest in nutrition and health, coupled with the large number of commercial products available, has led many pet owners, hobbyists, and professionals to critically evaluate the types of foods they select for their animals. An increasing number of pet owners are now interested in learning more about the regulation of the foods they buy and the formulation and nutrient content of these foods.

GOVERNING AGENCIES

A number of agencies and organizations regulate the production, marketing, and sales of commercial pet foods in the United States. Each agency has different and sometimes overlapping responsibilities and varying degrees of authority. Although some regulations are mandatory, others are optional suggestions. The following discussion identifies the major agencies and their roles in pet food regulation and provides an overview of the current regulations that govern the production and sale of pet foods in the United States (Table 14-1).

Association of American Feed Control Officials

The Association of American Feed Control Officials (AAFCO) is the most instrumental agency in the regulation of commercial pet foods. AAFCO was first formed in 1909 and is an association of state and federal feed control officials that acts in an advisory capacity to provide models for state legislation. For example, AAFCO's *Model Feed Bill* specifies labeling procedures and ingredient nomenclature for all animal feeds. Because AAFCO is an association and not an official regulatory body, its policies must be voluntarily accepted by state feed control officials for actual implementation. Pet food regulations can vary somewhat between states, and AAFCO's policy statements and regulations promote uniformity in feed regulations throughout the United States.

AAFCO's involvement in the pet food industry began in the 1960s. The PFI, a trade organization, worked with AAFCO to develop a set of policy statements and, eventually, regulations. Today AAFCO ensures that nationally marketed pet foods are uniformly labeled and nutritionally adequate.[5] These services include providing interpretations of AAFCO's pet food regulations and suggestions for uniform enforcement. A large proportion of AAFCO's regulations specify the type of information that companies are allowed to include on their pet food labels. The Pet Food Committee of AAFCO acts as the liaison between the pet food industry and AAFCO. Although a majority of the states follow AAFCO regulations for pet foods, not all states have a mechanism for inspection and enforcement of the regulations.

An important accomplishment of AAFCO during the 1990s has been the development of practical *Nutrient Profiles* to be used as standards for the formulation of dog and cat foods. Committees consisting of canine and feline nutritionists from universities, government, and the pet food industry worked together to establish two sets of standard nutrient profiles: one for dogs and one for cats. The profiles are based on ingredients commonly included in commercial foods, and nutrient levels are expressed for processed foods at the time of feeding. Minimum nutrient levels to be included in the pet food are provided for two categories: (1) growth and reproduction and (2) adult maintenance. Maximum levels are suggested for nutrients that have been shown to have the potential for toxicity or for when overuse is a concern. The AAFCO's *Nutrient Profiles* have replaced the previously used National Research Council (NRC) recommendations as the recognized authority for the substantiation of nutritional adequacy claims on labels (see Appendix 4, pp. 553-554). Although the goal of the NRC is to compile information concerning the basic nutrient requirements of dogs and cats, the AAFCO's *Nutrient Profiles* provide practical minimum and maximum levels of nutrients for inclusion in commercial pet foods. Therefore the *Nutrient Profiles* are more functional for the commercial pet food industry than were the NRC recommendations.

National Research Council

The NRC is a private, nonprofit organization that collects and evaluates research that has been conducted by others. The NRC functions as the working arm of the National Academy of Sciences, National Academy of Engineering, and Institutes of

Medicine, and it conducts services for the federal government, the scientific community, and the general public.[6] The NRC includes a standing committee on animal nutrition that identifies problems and needs in animal nutrition, recommends appointments of scientists to subcommittees, and reviews reports. Two NRC subcommittees were established for dog and cat nutrition. These groups developed reports that provided recommendations for the nutrient requirements of dogs and cats throughout various stages of life. Signs of nutrient deficiency and excess in these species were also included in these reports. The current NRC recommendations for dogs and cats, published in 1985 and 1986 respectively, are based primarily on research using purified or semipurified diets that contained nutrients in highly available forms. Although these studies provide valuable information about the minimum requirements of available nutrients for dogs and cats, they cannot be used as guidelines for the formulation of commercial pet foods without the inclusion of safety margins. Safety margins are needed to account for the decreased availability of nutrients in practical ingredients, variability of nutrient availability between ingredients, and loss of nutrients during processing.

Before the development and acceptance of the AAFCO's *Nutrient Profiles*, the NRC's reports on nutrient requirements for dogs and cats were the recognized authorities for pet food formulation and substantiation of nutritional adequacy claims on the labels of commercial pet foods. Because the 1985 and 1986 editions of the NRC requirements provided estimates only for available nutrients and did not include safety margins, pet food manufacturers were using the 1974 and 1978 NRC publications as their standards for pet food formulation. In the early 1990s, AAFCO's *Nutrient Profiles* replaced the NRC recommendations as the standard to be used by pet food manufacturers. In addition to providing suggested levels of nutrients to be included in foods, rather than the minimum nutrient requirements of the animals, AAFCO's *Nutrient Profiles* also include maximum levels for selected nutrients.

Currently the NRC has no regulatory responsibilities to the pet food industry. In 1991 the agency requested that their recommendations not be used to substantiate nutritional adequacy in dog and cat foods. However, the periodic revisions of the NRC's *Nutrient Requirements for Dogs* and *Nutrient Requirements for Cats* are a valuable resource for information for all groups involved in pet nutrition. These reports review current research concerning essential nutrient requirements of companion animals, signs of toxicity and deficiency, and interactions that can occur between nutrients within diets. Although these standards are not of practical use for the formulation of commercial pet foods, they do provide a compilation of pertinent research on the topic of companion animal nutrition.

Food and Drug Administration

All pet food manufacturers must follow the Food and Drug Administration (FDA) rules that specify proper identification of pet foods, a net quantity statement on the label, proper listing of ingredients and the manufacturer's name and address, and acceptable manufacturing procedures. Feed control officials within each state are usually relied upon to inspect facilities and enforce these regulations, although the FDA is authorized to take direct action if necessary. The FDA also regulates the inclusion of health claims on pet food labels. One type of health claim, a *drug claim,* is defined as the assertion or implication that the consumption of a food may help in the treatment, prevention, or reduction of a particular disease or diseases. The Center for Veterinary Medicine (CVM), a department of the FDA, has primary regulatory authority over health claims on pet food labels.

If a health claim is considered a drug claim, the CVM will not allow its use on the label. All new drugs are subjected to an FDA approval process before being marketed. New foods, on the other hand, are not required to undergo similar pre-market testing. Therefore, the inclusion of any health claims on a pet food that indicate that the consumption of the product will treat or prevent a specific disease constitutes a drug claim, and such a product would be subject to the same series of tests required of all new drugs. For example, the FDA has decreed that the word *hypoallergenic* cannot be used on pet food labels because this term may misrepresent the product. Similarly, the FDA's influence has led AAFCO to disallow inclusion of the term *low ash* on cat food labels because the statement may imply that the product has an effect on feline lower urinary tract disease.

United States Department of Agriculture

The United States Department of Agriculture (USDA) is responsible for ensuring that pet foods are clearly labeled to prevent human consumers from mistaking these products for human foods. This role includes the inspection of the meat ingredients used in pets foods to ensure proper handling and guarantee that such ingredients are not included in the human food supply. A second important role that the USDA plays in the pet food industry is to inspect and regulate research facilities. All kennels and catteries that are operated by pet food companies, private groups, or universities must fulfill USDA requirements for physical structure, housing and care of animals, and sanitation. Once these facilities have passed initial certification, they are regularly inspected by USDA officials. Although some pet food companies maintain their own kennels, others contract their feeding trials out to private research kennels or universities. Long-term feeding trials make up a large component of the testing conducted on quality, commercial pet foods. It is important that the facilities in which these tests are conducted maintain proper care of their animals and conform to sound sanitation practices.

Pet Food Institute

The PFI is a trade organization that represents manufacturers of commercially prepared dog and cat foods. The PFI works closely with the Pet Food Committee of the AAFCO to evaluate current regulations and make recommendations for changes. However, as a group, PFI does not have any direct regulatory powers over the production of pet foods, pet food testing, or statements included on labels.

Canadian Veterinary Medical Association Pet Food Certification Program

Like the PFI, the Canadian Veterinary Medical Association (CVMA) is not a regulatory agency. However, it administers a voluntary product certification program for pet food manufacturers in Canada. This program has been in operation since 1977 and involves two phases—an initial certification followed by an ongoing monitoring program. To achieve initial certification, a manufacturer must prove that the pet food is capable of meeting the nutritional needs of dogs or cats throughout all stages of life. The product must be tested using both feeding trials and laboratory analyses of nutrient levels. After a product has passed initial certification, its production is monitored every 2 months, and digestibility trials are conducted every 6 months. Involvement in the CVMA certification program is not mandatory. Rather, it provides a method of voluntary enforcement of certain standards for pet foods and is considered to be the CVMA's "seal of approval" for certified pet food products in Canada. Currently AAFCO does not allow the CVMA seal on Canadian pet foods shipped to the United States for sale.

CURRENT PET FOOD REGULATIONS

Most of the control over the nutrient content of pet foods, ingredient nomenclature, and label claims is relegated to AAFCO. As stated previously, AAFCO is not a regulatory agency per se; rather, it acts in an advisory capacity to state feed control officials. The Model Feed Bill that the AAFCO has developed and implemented is a template for state legislation; it specifies labeling procedures and ingredient nomenclature. Pet food regulations still vary somewhat from state to state, but adherence to AAFCO's regulations minimizes these differences. Each year the AAFCO publishes an official document that includes a section containing the current regulations for pet foods. These regulations govern the definitions and terms, label formats, brand and product names, nutrient guarantee claims, types of ingredients, drug and food additives, statements of calorie content, and descriptive terms that are to be used with or included in commercial pet foods. In addition, the AAFCO-sanctioned feeding protocols for proving nutritional adequacy and metabolizable energy (ME) are included.

Definitions, Terms, and Label Format

The definitions and terms section of the AAFCO's pet food regulations identify the Principal Display Panel (PDP) as the part of a container's label that is intended to be displayed to the customer for retail sales. This is followed by a section that defines the format to be used in the PDP and sets rules for ingredient and guaranteed analysis statements to be included on labels. Statements that are allowed on labels are described and strictly regulated; these are called *statements of nutritional adequacy* or *purpose of the product*. For example, the commonly used "complete and balanced nutrition for all stages of life" claim must be substantiated through one of two possible methods. The first method (option one) involves demonstrating through a series of feeding trials that the pet food satisfactorily supports health in a group of dogs or cats throughout gestation, lactation, and growth. The tests that the manufacturer uses must follow a set of feeding trial protocols that have been established and sanctioned by the AAFCO. The second method (option two) requires that the food be formulated to contain ingredients in quantities that are sufficient to provide the estimated nutrient requirements for all stages of life for the dog or cat. This can be achieved either through simple calculation using standard ingredient tables or through laboratory analysis of nutrients. If the second option is used, the AAFCO's *Nutrient Profiles* for dog and cat foods are used as the standard against which to measure nutrient content.

Limited label claims must be substantiated for the particular stage of life for which they are formulated. Most commonly, limited claims signify feeding for adult maintenance only. In these cases, the food must either be shown to meet the AAFCO's *Nutrient Profiles* for adult maintenance or have passed AAFCO's feeding trials for maintenance. Foods that contain the statement "intended for intermittent or supplemental use" do not meet requirements for either "complete and balanced" or for a limited claim and are therefore not expected to provide complete nutrition. The AAFCO also requires that all products labeled with the "complete and balanced" claim include specific feeding directions on the product label. If a secondary life stage is mentioned outside of the nutritional adequacy statement on the label, instructions for feeding pets in that life stage must also be included.

Brand and Product Names

Brand name refers to the name by which a pet food manufacturer's products are identified and distinguished from the pet foods of other companies.[5] The AAFCO regulates both brand and product names. For example, if a pet food product name includes a flavor designation, the flavor must be shown to be detectable by a recognized testing method, and the source of the flavor must be designated in the ingredient list. Similarly, the use of the term "all" or "100%" must mean that only the designated ingredient, an amount of water necessary for processing, and trace amounts of preservatives and condiments are present in the product. The inclusion of one or more ingredient names in a descriptive product name is allowed if the ingredients constitute a minimum of 25% of the pet food, singularly or in combination. If in combination, none of the named ingredients can be less than 3% of the formula. For example, the use of the name "lamb and rice dinner" requires that 25% or greater of the formula is lamb meat and rice, with rice making up the lesser of the two ingredients while still providing at least 3% of the formula. Any product claims of "new and improved" are only allowed to be stated on the PDP and can be used for a maximum period of 6 months after the introduction of the changes.

Nutrient Guarantees and Types of Ingredients

The AAFCO identifies acceptable terms for designating the guaranteed analysis for prescribed nutrients. Comparisons that are made between nutrient levels in the pet food and the AAFCO's *Nutrient Profiles* must be listed in the same units as those used in the published profile. When such comparisons are made, it is also required that the product must meet the *Nutrient Profiles* to which the comparison is made. Foods that are formulated as vitamin or mineral supplements are regulated separately and must state nutrient levels in the units designated by the AAFCO. All ingredients must be listed in the ingredient statement and shown in letters of the same font and size. The AAFCO also requires that no pet food, with the exception of those labeled as sauces, gravies, juices, or milk replacers, contain a moisture level greater than 78%.

Drug and Food Additives

Artificial color may be added to pet foods only if it has been shown to be harmless to pets. Such additives are approved and listed by the FDA. Health claims, including the inclusion of drugs or the pharmacologic use of nutrients, are regulated by the AAFCO through FDA state officials or through the FDA directly.

Statement of Caloric Content

In 1994, AAFCO accepted the inclusion of an optional caloric content statement on pet food labels. This statement must be presented separately from the guaranteed analysis table, and energy must be expressed as ME, in units of kilocalories (kcal) per kilogram (kg). The caloric content may also be expressed as kcal per lb, cup, or other commonly used household measuring unit. The calorie claim must be substantiated either by calculation using modified Atwater factors or through feeding trials specified by the AAFCO. The method that is used must be stated on the label.

Descriptive Terms

The AAFCO regulation "PF8" is the newest addition to the pet food regulations. First implemented in 1998, this regulation specifies the acceptable use of the terms "light" (or "lite"), "less or reduced calories," "lean," "low-fat," and "less or reduced fat."[7,8] This regulation reflects the current concern of consumers with the fat and energy content of pet foods and the formulation and marketing of pet foods for weight control and weight reduction. Specific maximum energy contents are designated for all pet foods marketed using the term "light" (or "lite"). For example, a "light" dry dog food can contain no greater than 3100 kcal of ME/kg. A dry dog food containing the designation of "less or reduced calories" must include the percentage of reduction from the product of comparison and a caloric content statement. The terms "lean" and "less fat" are similarly regulated by designating the maximum percentages of fat within categories of dog and cat food. For example, a dry dog food that is labeled "lean" can contain no greater than 9% crude fat. As with the "reduced calories" term, the term "less or reduced fat" must include the percentage of reduction from the product of comparison.

C H A P T E R

15

Pet Food Labels

The pet food label is an important component of commercial pet foods because many consumers rely primarily on the label for information about the product's nutritional adequacy and palatability. Current regulations require that all labels of pet foods manufactured and sold in the United States contain the following items: product name; net weight; name and address of the manufacturer; guaranteed analysis for crude protein, crude fat, crude fiber, and moisture; list of ingredients in descending order of predominance by weight; the words "dog food" or "cat food"; and a statement of nutritional adequacy or purpose of the product. Pet food manufacturers must also include a statement that indicates the method that was used to substantiate the nutritional adequacy claim, either through the Association of American Feed Control Officials' (AAFCO's) feeding trials or by formulating the food to meet the AAFCO's *Nutrient Profiles* (Box 15-1). An expiration date indicating the timespan from the date of production to the date of expiration of the product is optional, as is a "best if used by" date.

WHAT CONSUMERS CAN LEARN FROM THE PET FOOD LABEL

Guaranteed Analysis Panel

Most pet owners first look at the guaranteed analysis panel of the pet food because this gives them information regarding the amount of protein and fat contained in the product. Manufacturers are required to include minimum percentages for crude protein and crude fat and maximum percentages for moisture and crude fiber for both dog and cat foods. Optional guarantees that may be listed include, but are not limited to, magnesium (minimum percentage), taurine (minimum percentage), linoleic acid (minimum percentage), and ash (maximum percentage). It is important to recognize that these numbers represent only minimums and maximums and do not reflect the exact amounts of these nutrients in the product. For example, a pet

BOX **15-1**

Typical Commercial Pet Food Label

Wuf-Wuf Dog Food
Net weight 8 pounds (lbs)

Feeding Instructions	Cups per Day
Toy breeds (5-10 lbs)	0.5-1 cup
Small breeds (10-30 lbs)	1-2 cups
Medium breeds (30-50 lbs)	2-4 cups
Large breeds (50-80 lbs)	4-5 cups
Giant breeds (80-120 lbs)	5-7 cups

Guaranteed Analysis

Crude protein	Not less than 30%
Crude fat	Not less than 20%
Crude fiber	Not more than 4%
Moisture	Not more than 10%

Manufactured by Wuf-Wuf Inc., Bowserville, Ohio

Wuf-Wuf provides complete and balanced nutrition for all stages of a dog's life, as determined through AAFCO feeding studies.

Ingredients: Chicken, chicken byproduct meal, ground corn, rice flour, fish meal, chicken fat (preserved with mixed tocopherols and citric acid), ground grain sorghum, dried beet pulp, chicken digest, dried egg product, brewer's dried yeast, flax, dicalcium phosphate, calcium carbonate, DL-methionine, potassium chloride, mineral supplement, vitamin supplement.

food that has a label claim of "minimum crude fat: 11%" cannot have less than 11% fat, but may have more. Although one product with this claim may contain 13% fat, another carrying the same claim may have 11.5% fat. Assuming all other nutrients are comparable, the 1.5% difference in fat content can make a significant difference in the product's caloric density and palatability.

The terms *crude protein*, *crude fat*, and *crude fiber* all refer to specific analytical procedures used to estimate these nutrients in foodstuffs. On the average, protein contains 16% nitrogen. *Crude protein* is the estimate of total protein in a foodstuff that is obtained by multiplying analyzed levels of nitrogen by a constant. Slight inaccuracies in this estimate are caused by variations in nitrogen content between proteins and by the presence of nonprotein nitrogen compounds in the foodstuff. *Crude fat* is an estimate of the lipid content of a food that is obtained through extraction of the food with ether. In addition to lipids, this procedure also isolates certain organic acids, oils, pigments, alcohols, and fat-soluble vitamins. On the other hand, some complex lipids, such as phospholipids, may not be isolated with this method. *Crude fiber* represents the organic residue that remains after plant material has been treated with dilute acid and alkali solvents and after the mineral component has been extracted. Although crude fiber is used to report the fiber content of many commercial products, it usually underestimates the level of true dietary fiber in a product. It has been determined that the crude fiber method recovers only 50%

to 80% of the cellulose, 10% to 50% of the lignin, and less than 20% of the hemi-cellulose in a given sample.[9] Consequently, crude fiber may be a measurement of most of the cellulose in a sample, but it underestimates all of the other dietary fiber components. Consumers can use the guaranteed analysis panel to provide a rough estimate of protein, fat, and fiber content in a particular pet food. However, these numbers should only be considered as a starting point when comparing different products or brands, and they should not be assumed to represent the actual levels of these nutrients in the food.

When examining the guaranteed analysis panel of a pet food, consumers must always take into account the moisture (water) content of the product. The amount of water in a food significantly affects the values listed in the guaranteed analysis table because most pet foods display nutrient levels on an "as-fed" (AF) basis, rather than a dry-matter basis (DMB). AF means that the percentages of nutrients were calculated directly, without accounting for the proportion of water in the product. Pet foods can vary greatly in the amount of water they contain. For example, dry cat and dog foods usually contain between 6% and 10% water, but canned foods contain up to 78% water.[10] In order to make valid comparisons of nutrients in foods with different amounts of moisture, it is necessary to first convert nutrients to a DMB. Similarly, the caloric content of a pet food also affects the interpretation of the guaranteed analysis panel. Caloric density must always be considered when comparing levels of protein, fat, carbohydrate, and other nutrients in different pet foods (see pp. 205-206).

Ingredient List

The ingredient list is often the second place on the label that consumers look for information about the food they are buying. The list of ingredients must be arranged in decreasing order by predominance by weight. The terms used must be names assigned by the AAFCO when applicable, or they must be names that are commonly accepted as the standard by the feed industry. In no case can any single ingredient be given undue emphasis, nor can designations of the quality of ingredients be included. The ingredient list indicates where the principal components of a pet food come from—animal products or plant products. In general, if an ingredient from an animal source is listed first or second in a canned pet food or within the first three ingredients of a dry pet food, the food can be assumed to contain animal products as its principal protein source.

Most popular and generic brands of pet food are formulated as "variable-formula diets." This means that the ingredients used in the food will vary from batch to batch, depending on the availability and market prices of ingredients. In contrast, most of the premium foods sold at feed stores, pet stores, and through veterinarians are produced using fixed formulas. In this case, the company will not change the formulation in response to changes in market prices. Checking the ingredient list of several bags of a particular pet food over a period of time can indicate whether the company is using fixed or variable formulation. Although the pet owner may pay slightly more for a fixed formulation diet, the consistency between batches of food is a distinct advantage to the dog or cat that is consuming the food (see pp. 194-195).

Although the ingredient list can provide general information about the type of ingredients included in a food, it does not provide information about the quality of its components. Ingredients used in pet foods vary significantly in digestibility, amino acid content and availability, mineral availability, and the amount of indigestible material they contain. Unfortunately, there is usually no way of determining the quality of the ingredients by using the ingredient list. In fact, some premium foods with high-quality, highly available ingredients may have an ingredient list that is almost identical to that of a generic food that contains poor-quality ingredients with low digestibility and nutrient availability. Therefore the ingredient list alone should never be used to compare two pet foods because the differences in the qualities of ingredients are impossible to know from this information.

Like the guaranteed analysis, the list of ingredients can be deceptive in some cases because manufacturers are not required to list the ingredients on a DMB. This is usually not a problem in dry pet foods because most of the ingredients included in these diets have a relatively low moisture content. However, canned products may contain ingredients with vastly different amounts of moisture. As a result, an ingredient that actually contributes a low proportion of nutrients to the food may be listed first if it has a high water content, but an ingredient that contributes a large proportion of the nutrients to the food may be lower on the ingredient list if it has a low moisture content. A common example involves the use of texturized vegetable protein (TVP) in canned pet foods. TVP is composed of extruded soy flour that is dyed and shaped to resemble meat products. The actual meat ingredients in a product that contains TVP can be listed high on the ingredient list because they are added in a wet form; however, TVP is added to the formulation in a dry form and therefore appears to contribute very little on an AF basis. In reality, most of the protein in such a food is coming from the TVP and not from the animal-source ingredients listed first.

A second way that the ingredient list can be misleading is the manner in which certain ingredients are presented. Manufacturers may separate different forms of similar ingredients so that they can be listed separately on the label and appear further down the list. For example, an ingredient list may include kibbled wheat, ground wheat, wheat flour, flaked wheat, wheat middlings, and wheat bran. These ingredients are called "split ingredients" and may in some cases represent two or more forms of the same product. Examples of split ingredients are ground wheat and wheat flour, which differ only in the fineness of the grind used during processing. Individually, these ingredients make up only a small fraction of the diet and therefore can be listed low on the ingredient list. As a whole, wheat actually constitutes a large proportion of this diet. Consumers should be aware that listing different forms of the same ingredient suggests a legal but purposeful misrepresentation of the product's ingredient content on the part of the manufacturer.

Nutritional Adequacy

A final item that consumers may read on the pet food label is the claim of nutritional adequacy. With the exception of treats and snacks, the label of all pet foods

BOX 15-2

Label Claims of Nutritional Adequacy and How to Interpret Them

Claim 1: "Wuf-Wuf is formulated to meet the nutrient levels established by the AAFCO's *Nutrient Profiles* for dog foods for all life stages."

Interpretation: This dog food has not been subjected to AAFCO feeding tests. Although the food has been formulated to meet the AAFCO's *Nutrient Profiles*, there is no way of knowing from this substantiation claim whether or not feeding studies have been conducted on this food.

Claim 2: "Animal feeding tests using AAFCO procedures substantiate that Wuf-Wuf provides complete and balanced nutrition for all life stages."

Interpretation: This dog food has been subjected to the complete series of AAFCO feeding studies, including those for gestation, lactation, and growth. This substantiation method shows that the food is complete for all life stages.

Claim 3: "Animal feeding tests using AAFCO procedures substantiate that Wuf-Wuf provides complete and balanced nutrition for adult maintenance."

Interpretation: This food has undergone AAFCO feeding protocol studies for maintenance only and has not been tested for gestation, lactation, or growth. Feeding studies have been conducted, but the food has not been shown to be nutritionally complete for life stages other than maintenance.

Claim 4: "Wuf-Wuf Veterinary Diet (Gastrointestinal Formula) is intended for intermittent or supplemental feeding only. Use as directed by your veterinarian."

Interpretation: This food is intended for special nutritional or dietary needs that require the involvement of a veterinarian for diagnosis, management, and follow-up.

that are in interstate commerce must contain a statement and validation of nutritional adequacy. Current AAFCO regulations allow four primary types of nutritional adequacy statements. A common claim is "complete and balanced for all life stages." This statement signifies that the food has been formulated to provide complete and balanced nutrition for gestation, lactation, growth, and maintenance. A limited claim states that the food provides complete and balanced nutrition for a particular stage of life, such as adult maintenance. A third claim is found on products that are intended for intermittent or supplemental feeding only. Last, products that are intended for therapeutic feeding under the supervision of a veterinarian bear the statement "use only as directed by your veterinarian" (Box 15-2).

When the "complete and balanced nutrition" claim is used for any or all life stages, manufacturers must indicate the method that was employed to substantiate this claim. Currently, AAFCO regulations require that the manufacturer either performs AAFCO-sanctioned feeding trials on the food (option one) or formulates the diet to meet the AAFCO's *Nutrient Profiles* for dog and cat foods (option two). The first option, testing the food through a series of feeding trials, is the most thorough and reliable evaluation method. The terminology for labels of pet foods that have passed these tests is as follows: "Animal feeding tests using AAFCO procedures substantiate that (brand) provides complete and balanced nutrition for (life stages)."[7,11] The inclusion of the terms "feeding tests," "AAFCO feeding test protocols," or

BOX 15-3

Information Provided by the Pet Food Label

The pet food label *does* provide information about:	The pet food label *does not* provide information about:
Net weight of product	Exact levels of nutrients
Name and location of manufacturer or distributor	Digestibility and nutrient availability
Minimum crude protein and crude fat content	Quality of the ingredients
Maximum moisture and crude fiber content	
List of ingredients	
Nutritional adequacy statement	
Method of substantiation of adequacy claim	
Feeding instructions	
Caloric density (optional)	

"AAFCO feeding studies" in the statement all validate that the product has undergone feeding tests with dogs or cats. However, if the substantiation claim states only that the food has met the AAFCO's *Nutrient Profiles* (option 2), this indicates that AAFCO feeding trials were not conducted on the food. Although some companies that use option 2 measure the level of certain nutrients in the food through laboratory analysis, the best way to test the nutritional adequacy of a pet food is still through actual feeding trials.

Consumers should be aware that the use of feeding trials is not required if manufacturers use the second method of substantiation. This method is commonly referred to as the "calculation method" because it allows manufacturers to substantiate the "complete and balanced" claim by merely calculating the nutrient content of the formulation of the diet using standard tables of ingredients or analyzing the product through laboratory analyses without actually feeding the food to any animals. Although some manufacturers using this method of substantiation may still conduct some of their own feeding trials, there is no way of knowing this from the label unless they have used the AAFCO feeding trial protocols (Box 15-3).

THE CHANGING PET FOOD LABEL

Recent changes in the labeling of human food and an increased awareness on the part of the general public about the importance of proper nutrition has resulted in increased concern of pet owners about their pets' diets. Consumers are now demanding to know more about the foods they are feeding to their companion animals. One of the ways in which this information can be provided is through the pet food label.

The AAFCO has made some recent labeling changes and is continuing to study ways in which to improve the current pet food label so that it more adequately represents the food contained in the package. For example, in 1992 a new regulation was passed that required all dog and cat foods labeled "complete and balanced for any or all stages of life" to include feeding directions on the product label. At a minimum, these instructions must state "Feed (weight unit) of product per (weight unit) of dog or cat."[12] Before 1994 the inclusion of a caloric density statement on pet food labels was prohibited. In 1993 recommendations were made to the AAFCO for the measurement of metabolizable energy (ME) and the inclusion of ME values on pet food labels. This new provision was accepted in 1994, making the inclusion of a caloric density statement on the label optional for pet food manufacturers. The inclusion of such a statement, along with a breakdown of the percentage of calories that are contributed by fat, carbohydrate, and protein, provides information about the suitability of the food for different stages of a pet's life. For example, hard-working dogs may benefit from a diet with an increased proportion of ME calories supplied by fat. In addition, it is much more accurate to compare foods according to the percentage of calories that are contributed by carbohydrate, protein, and fat than to compare them by the percentage of these nutrients by weight (see pp. 205-206).

Information about additional nutrients on the guaranteed analysis panel is also beneficial to consumers. As discussed previously, current regulations require inclusion of only crude protein, crude fat, fiber, and moisture on this panel. Optional guarantees for ash, taurine, linoleic acid, omega-6 and omega-3 fatty acids, and magnesium are now allowed. The inclusion of guarantees for other essential nutrients such as calcium; phosphorus; sodium; vitamins A, E, and D; and certain trace minerals would give consumers more information to use when selecting a food. In the future, changing this panel to include actual amounts of these nutrients (i.e., proximate analysis) rather than the minimums and maximums that are currently required would be advantageous.

The AAFCO continues to consider and evaluate the use of descriptive terms on pet food labels. The challenge lies in providing consumers with factual information and claims that can be reliably substantiated by manufacturers. Two terms that had been under scrutiny were "natural" and "tartar control". Because the term "natural" has been overused in the marketing of human foods and pet foods and because the meaning of the term can be vague or misleading, the AAFCO established guidelines for inclusion of the word "natural" on the pet food label. These include stipulations that all ingredients and components of ingredients other than the vitamins and minerals in products labeled "natural" must not be chemically synthesized. If chemically synthesized vitamins or minerals are included, the product is labeled "natural with added vitamins and minerals". Guidelines for the use of "tartar control" claims have been recommended to the AAFCO by its Pet Food Committee. These indicate that pet foods and treats that claim to clean teeth, freshen breath, or whiten teeth by virtue of their mechanical (abrasive) action during chewing are acceptable. In contrast, claims of tartar reduction or prevention may be misleading and should not be used. Likewise, foods that imply pharmacological effects that prevent or control tartar are not permitted unless approved through established protocols as new animal drugs or pharmaceuticals.

The AAFCO's Pet Food Committee and the Pet Food Institute (PFI) are working together to develop more effective and efficient testing methods of label claim substantiation. One concept that is receiving attention is the use of product families. This idea originated with the PFI, who adopted a policy describing the families and made recommendations to the AAFCO. The AAFCO Pet Food Committee is currently finalizing guidelines for this concept. A *family* consists of pet food products that contain similar ingredients, use the same processing method, are within the same moisture control and energy category (these categories are designated as less than 20%, 20% to 65%, or greater than 65% moisture), and are intended to have the same label claim. One product within a family will be required to pass complete feeding trial protocols. This product is called the "lead product." If this product passes, it is assumed that the other products within the family will also pass because they are nutritionally similar to the lead product and contain similar ingredients. Once a particular nutritional claim is established for the lead product, pet foods within the same family are entitled to make the same nutritional claim. For the remaining products, only laboratory analyses of a select number of nutrients must be conducted. Although the family grouping concept is still not finalized, this new regulation would ensure that consumers would be able to distinguish between products that have actually been fed to cats or dogs and those that have just been analyzed.

As the AAFCO continues to review, evaluate, and revise its current regulations, it is probable that many of these changes will occur, resulting in a pet food label that can provide consumers with a greater amount of helpful information (see Box 15-3).

PET FOOD ADVERTISING

Pet food manufacturers are in a unique situation when they consider the marketing techniques used to sell their products. Although it is the dog or the cat that is consuming the food and the animal's health that is directly affected by the product's quality, it is the pet owner who is making the decision to buy the product. Therefore manufacturers must not only consider what is the most nutritious food to feed to dogs and cats, they must also consider the pet owner's perception of the best food to feed his or her companion animal. Most of today's marketing strategies are aimed toward convincing pet owners that a particular food offers some benefit to the pet that is above and beyond that of all other products. Because most foods carry the "complete and balanced" label claim, offering complete nutrition is not perceived by many owners to be a unique selling point. Rather, acceptability and palatability, cost, feeding convenience, digestibility, and suitability of the food for the pet's lifestyle, age, or physiological state are all important considerations for today's owner. In recent years, as knowledge about canine and feline nutrition has progressed, pet food companies have started to produce foods that specifically meet the needs of companion animals during different stages of life and for pets that live different lifestyles. Examples of these foods include high-performance diets for working dogs, growth diets for young dogs and cats, and maintenance diets for adult pets. The sale of these foods is accompanied by educational programs for pet owners about the nutrient needs of their companion animals.

The needs and perceptions of the pet owner are of primary concern when marketing a pet food. Identifying these needs is often the first task for pet food manufacturers. Although some pet owners are concerned primarily with providing the best nutrition for their companion animals, others are more interested in the cost of the food, its availability in stores, or the convenience of feeding it. In today's market there are products that appeal to all of these needs and to the many different types of pet owners.

Because there is no way to determine whether a food contains superior nutrition by examining it or by feeding it a few times, many pet owners rely on a product's palatability and acceptability as their chief selection criteria. Palatability is a subjective measure of how well an animal likes a particular food, and acceptability is an indication of whether the amount of food eaten is enough to meet the animal's caloric requirements.[13] These are both important considerations because regardless of a food's nutritional value, it cannot nourish an animal if it is not eaten. Palatability and acceptability are also very powerful marketing tools. Most pet owners enjoy giving their companion animal a food that is eagerly accepted and eaten, and they will be inclined to buy a food that they know their pet relishes. However, many highly palatable foods are high in fat and as a result are energy dense. This increased palatability, coupled with a high energy density, can lead to overeating and obesity if the food is fed on a free-choice basis. In recent years the prevalent use of palatability as a marketing tool for pet foods has probably contributed to the increasing problem of obesity in dogs and cats in the United States. Owners should certainly pick a food that their pet enjoys, but they should be aware that extremely palatable foods can induce overeating.

In today's busy society, convenience and ease of preparation are also important to many pet owners. The convenience of feeding dry pet foods and the availability of these foods in supermarkets contributed greatly to their initial success. Dry foods keep well after opening, do not require refrigeration, and require little if any preparation before feeding. Packaging foods in portion-sized bags is another technique that attracts pet owners who desire convenience. Many canned cat foods and semimoist pet foods are marketed to provide one meal per package, therefore eliminating even the need to measure out a portion of food before feeding.

Although it is not the chief consideration for some pet owners, for others the cost of the food is very important. There are a number of commercial foods available today that are advertised as being more economical to feed while still providing superior nutrition. However, it is important for pet owners to know that to produce a low-cost product, ingredients that are of lower quality, and thus lower cost, must be used. Therefore a cheaper product is probably going to be a lower quality food, even though the guaranteed analysis panel may not reflect this. In addition, when considering the price of a pet food, the actual cost of feeding the animal must be calculated, not the cost per unit weight of the food. Most low-quality, cheap ingredients have significantly lower digestibilities than the ingredients that are used in premium foods. A greater quantity of a food with low digestibility must be fed to an animal to provide the same amount of nutrition as that in a food with higher digestibility and nutrient availability. As a result, owners may find that they have to feed significantly larger portions of the cheaper food to their pet. Also, companies that produce inexpensive dog and cat foods may not have the funds or capability to conduct thorough testing of their products. In most cases, these foods are not tested using AAFCO feeding protocols because this testing will cost extra money. In general, when pricing dog and cat foods, it is safe to assume that buyers usually "get what they pay for." Premium products cost more primarily because they contain high-quality ingredients and because they have been subjected to more rigorous testing than inexpensive generic and name-brand products. Marketing techniques that promote low-priced foods as being equivalent in value to more costly products usually mislead the consumer into believing that the food offers the same benefits as a premium food but at a substantially lower cost.

In recent years a new technique that has been used to increase the sales of pet foods is "niche marketing."[4] This concept involves developing, marketing, and selling products that are designed for specific age groups, physiological states, activity levels, and health problems. As more knowledge has become available, nutritionists and pet food manufacturers have realized that optimum nutrition is often best provided through specialized products formulated for different stages of life or even for certain disease states. In general, more consumer education is necessary with these products, and most are sold only through feed stores, veterinarians, and pet supply stores. These products can be contrasted to the "all-purpose" pet foods that are developed and marketed for sale in grocery stores. Although specialized foods are marketed to appeal to involved pet owners who are interested in providing the best nutrition to their pets, the "all-purpose" foods are attractive to the pet owner who wishes to have a food that is balanced, fairly economical to feed, and convenient to buy.

Other commonly used marketing tools for pet foods include the development of products that resemble foods consumed by humans. This obviously appeals to the sense of taste of the pet owner, more so than that of the animal that will be eating the food. These products are varied and creative. Some foods have the appearance of chunks of meat, and others look like stews, containing a variety of meat and vegetables. The actual content of these foods is usually not the ingredient that they are made to resemble. For example, TVP can be shaped and dyed to resemble chunks of meat. Flavor varieties are also a strong selling tool. Because owners enjoy variety in their diets, they believe that this is also important for their pets. Almost all of the pet foods and treats that are sold in grocery stores come in a variety of flavors. Although these differences may appeal to owners, it is unknown whether individual pets have strong preferences between flavors. Nonetheless, it is the owner who buys the food, and some will be induced to buy a food that looks like ground steak or pronounces itself to be "liver-flavored."

Promoting the addition or deletion of a particular ingredient in a pet food is another tactic used to increase sales. Whether this information is grounded in fact is a moot point because there is always a segment of the pet-owning population that is willing to believe in the value or hazard of a given ingredient. For example, some owners believe that soy is a poor-quality ingredient. Pet foods that are marketed as containing no soy capitalize on this belief, whether or not it is founded in fact. Similarly, the pet-owning public can be convinced that the presence of a particular ingredient may contribute to a superior product. The use of fish and fish meal in cat foods is an example. Cats are actually desert animals by ancestry and probably had very little access to fish in their original diets. However, the use of clever and cute advertisements has convinced pet owners that all cats inherently love the taste of fish. The presence of fish in certain cat foods is then promoted as a distinct benefit. Although it is true that cats enjoy the taste of fish, this ingredient is no more palatable to most cats than are several other high-protein ingredients included in cat foods.

16

Nutrient Content of Pet Foods

The most important consideration in choosing a commercial pet food for a companion animal is its nutrient content. *Nutrient content* refers not only to the exact levels of nutrients in the food but also to the digestibility and availability of all the essential nutrients. Nutrients can be supplied in commercial pet food through a large number of different ingredients. Commonly used pet food ingredients vary greatly in form and quality, and it is this diversity that can make the selection of a suitable dog or cat food a difficult task. This chapter discusses the methods used to determine and express nutrient content in pet foods and reviews commonly used pet food ingredients and additives.

METHODS FOR DETERMINING NUTRIENT CONTENT

Laboratory Analysis

When pet food manufacturers formulate and produce pet foods, there are two ways they can determine the level of nutrients present in the product. The first and most accurate way is to conduct a laboratory analysis of the finished product. *Proximate analysis* is a commonly used panel of tests that provides information about a select group of nutrients. The laboratory procedures involved in proximate analysis provide the percentages of moisture, crude protein, crude fat, ash (minerals), and fiber that are contained in the food. Nitrogen-free extract (NFE), which represents a rough estimate of the soluble carbohydrate fraction of the food, can be calculated by subtraction (see Section 1, pp. 6-8). The guaranteed analysis panel of the pet food label is generated from the proximate analysis results and reports only maximum or minimum levels of a very limited number of nutrients.

Pet food companies that are producing high-quality products and are interested in the education of pet owners will provide consumers with information about the exact nutrient content of their foods. Because regulations do not allow the inclusion of these details on the pet food container itself, they are usually supplied to pet owners in the form of informational brochures and pamphlets. These publications can be obtained through the feed store, pet supply store, or veterinarian's office where the food is purchased or by contacting the pet food company directly. In addition to the proximate analysis of the food, the essential vitamin and mineral content and the energy density of the food are also usually included in these reports.

Calculation

The second method that manufacturers may use to determine nutrient content is calculation of the average nutrient content of the food's ingredients using values reported in standard tables. The amount of essential nutrients contributed by each ingredient in the food are then summed. Standard tables contain average levels of essential nutrients in common feed ingredients. Although this method of nutrient determination is certainly less costly and time-consuming than laboratory analysis, there are several significant problems with using calculation alone to determine the nutrient content of pet foods.

First, there is a lack of complete and accurate data for the nutrient content of many ingredients included in commercial pet foods. As a result, manufacturers must rely upon tables that contain approximations of the types of ingredients they are using. These tables may contain information that is outdated or misleading. For example, as grain yields have increased in recent years, the average percentage of protein in corn and soybeans has decreased.[14] Standard tables do not always reflect these changes. A study conducted by the Office of the Texas State Chemist recently measured the protein content of corn, oats, and grain sorghum samples taken from different locations within the state.[15] The average protein content in 200 samples of yellow corn was 7.87%, with a range of 5.97% to 10.25%. Protein values were less than 8% in 62% of the samples, and 31.5% of the samples had protein contents below 7.5%. The National Research Council's (NRC's) 1985 standard value for corn used in the formulation of dog foods is 9.4%. If this value is used when formulating a pet food using the calculation method, the pet food would most likely contain less corn protein than predicted. A similar trend of decreasing protein content was observed in oats and grain sorghum, which could lead to miscalculations with these grains. These discrepancies illustrate the need for pet food companies to directly analyze the nutrient content of their pet foods after formulation and not rely exclusively upon table values for the nutrient content of ingredients.

A second problem with the calculation method is that the quality of ingredients cannot be determined. Ingredient quality affects the level and availability of nutrients in finished pet foods. Standard tables represent averages and cannot reflect differences in ingredient quality among raw ingredients. The processing of a pet food further affects ingredient quality. Nutrient losses can occur during processing or storage, and studies have shown that the digestibility and nutrient availability of plant-based and animal-based ingredients are significantly affected by processing methods.[16,17,18] For example, dogs digest soybean flour more efficiently than soybean grits when incorporated into a canned diet.[16] This difference is probably related to the smaller particle size of the flour. Subsequent work showed that dogs fed different forms of rice assimilate blended rice more efficiently than whole rice.[17] This difference was attributed to reduced food particle size and possibly to increased damage to starch granules in the blended product. In either case, it is apparent that the processing method used for plant ingredients significantly affects digestion and nutrient availability. Differences in the type of processing system and the cooking temperature for animal-based ingredients are also important. When the effects of cooking temperatures and processing systems on 46 sources of meat and bone meal or poultry byproduct meal were examined, it was found that higher processing temperatures caused decreases in the true digestibility values of amino acids in the finished product.[18] Again, if table values alone are used to predict protein content, these effects cannot be predicted. Laboratory analysis of finished products and feeding trials with animals are the only methods for obtaining reliable information about nutrient availability after pet food processing.

Determination of Digestibility

Current Association of American Feed Control Officials (AAFCO) regulations do not require that companies determine the digestibility of their foods (see pp. 155-156). However, the digestibility of a pet food must always be considered. Digestibility provides a measure of the diet's quality because it directly determines the proportion of nutrients in the food that are available for absorption into the body. Pet food companies evaluate the digestibility of their products through feeding studies. The disappearance of nutrients as they pass through the gastrointestinal tract and are absorbed into the body is measured. The test diet is fed to the animals for a pretest period of 5 to 7 days to allow acclimation to the diet. Following this period, the amount of food consumed and the amount of fecal matter excreted are recorded for 3 to 5 days. The fecal matter that is collected represents the undigested residue of the food that was consumed. Laboratory analyses of both feed and fecal matter are conducted to provide the levels of nutrients in each, and amounts of digested nutrients are calculated by subtraction. These figures, expressed as percentages, are called *digestion coefficients*. In this type of study, the figures that are derived are called "apparent" digestibility coefficients because the fecal matter also contains metabolic waste products that originated from the animal and not from the food (Table 16-1).

True digestibility can be determined by deducting the normal metabolic loss of the nutrient from the amount of the nutrient measured in the fecal matter. True digestibility trials are most commonly conducted for protein. The animals are fed a protein-free or very-low-protein diet for a short period, and a baseline level of protein excretion is measured. This figure can then be used to account for the endogenous metabolic loss of protein in the feces when the digestibility trial is conducted. It can be argued that apparent digestibility is actually a better indication of a diet's ability to supply nutrients than is true digestibility. The endogenous losses that occur in the fecal matter represent cellular and enzymatic losses that are the

TABLE **16-1**

Variability in Pet Food Digestibility

	Diet		
	A	**B**	**C**
Protein digestibility (%)	70.25	80.99	85.86
Fat digestibility (%)	82.70	90.42	90.72
Fiber digestibility (%)	17.44	48.53	61.48
Fecal score*	3.95	4.47	4.48
Fecal volume	162.38	89.18	46.48

Data provided by Iams Technical Center, Lewisburg, Ohio, 1993.

*Based on a 1 to 5 rating: 1 = loose and watery; 5 = firm. Scores of 4 to 5 are considered normal.

BOX **16-1**

Effect of Different Digestibilities on the Amount of Protein Available to the Dog

Diet A

28% protein

70.25% of the protein is digestible

Therefore 70.25% of 28% protein = 0.7025 × 28 = **19.67%** digestible protein

Diet B

28% protein

85.9% of the protein is digestible

Therefore 85.9% of 28% protein = 0.859 × 28 = **24.05%** digestible protein

result of the cost of digesting and absorbing food. Therefore apparent digestibility represents the actual net gain to the animal from the digestion of the food.

Information about the nutrient content of a diet means little if the product's digestibility is not known. For example, laboratory analyses of two different dry dog foods reveal that they each contain 28% protein. If the protein digestibility of diet A is 70.25%, this means that the food actually provides less than 20% digestible protein. On the other hand, if the digestibility of diet B is 85.8%, it provides about 24% digestible protein (see Table 16-1 and also Box 16-1). The amount of protein available to the animal is higher in diet B than in diet A, even though laboratory analyses indicate that they have similar total protein contents. Digestibility also affects fecal volume and form and defecation frequency (see Table 16-1). As a diet's digestibility increases, fecal volume decreases significantly. In addition, a highly digestible pet food produces firm and well-formed feces. Although manufacturers are not required to conduct digestibility trials on their feeds, reputable companies that produce quality products always conduct these trials to ensure that their foods contain levels of nutrients that will meet animals' daily requirements for absorption into the body.

Determination of Metabolizable Energy

The metabolizable energy (ME) of a pet food is another important consideration when selecting a diet (see Section 1, p. 5). ME indicates the amount of energy in a pet food that is available to the animal for use. Although digestible energy (DE) measures the amount of energy that is absorbed across the intestinal wall, ME accounts for digestibility and for losses of energy in the urine and through expired gases (flatus). Although expired gases account for a significant proportion of energy in most farm animals, it is an insignificant energy loss in dogs and cats. Therefore the analysis of the ME of foods for dogs and cats includes only urinary losses of energy.

ME is the preferred unit for analyzing the energy content of pet foods because unlike gross energy (GE), which is a measure of the total energy in the diet, ME provides an accurate representation of the amount of energy that is actually available to the animal. ME can be determined either through feeding trials or, less accurately, by calculation using standard energy values for protein, carbohydrate, and fat. A rough estimate of the ME of a pet food can also be calculated using the values that are provided in the guaranteed analysis panel on the label (see Section 1, pp. 10-11).

The AAFCO allows, but does not require, the inclusion of caloric claims on pet food labels. If an ME statement is included, it must be separate and distinct from the guaranteed analysis panel and must be identified as "calorie content". A pet food's ME must be expressed as kilocalories (kcal) per kilogram (kg) of product. Additional units such as kcal per measuring cup or pound (lb) may also be listed on the label. Like the "complete and balanced" statement on the pet food label, the ME statement must be accompanied by a substantiation claim. AAFCO regulations allow manufacturers to determine ME content in one of three possible ways:

1. Calculation using modified Atwater factors and values for crude protein, crude fat, and NFE obtained from proximate analysis. (Samples must be taken from at least four production batches of the product.)
2. Calculation from digestible nutrients or DE. (Data are obtained from digestibility trials without urine collection.)
3. Direct determination from digestibility trials (including urine collection).

Although the inclusion of ME values on pet food labels will help pet owners select appropriate products for their pets, there is still some controversy regarding the methods of substantiation required.[19] The use of modified Atwater factors for the calculation of ME in commercial pet foods has been shown to overestimate the ME content for some foods. In contrast, calculation from DE using a correction factor for urine energy losses closely approximates ME values obtained through direct measurement. This discrepancy means that companies using either direct measurement of ME or calculation of ME from digestibility trial data will accurately represent the product's ME on the label. However, as with the "complete and balanced" claim, when the calculation method is used, the stated ME value may be less accurate. Ironically, the standard that is currently used to verify direct measurement and digestibility trial calculation methods for ME determination is the calculation method. The AAFCO requires that if digestibility trials are used to obtain ME values, the value on the label must not exceed or understate the value determined using the calculation method by more than 15%.[12] Therefore, as with the "complete and balanced" claim, pet food consumers should always make note of the method that was used to determine the ME value when selecting a pet food.

EXPRESSION OF NUTRIENT CONTENT

The guaranteed analysis panel of a pet food usually reports nutrient levels on an "as fed" (AF) basis. This means that the nutrient content in the diet is measured directly, without accounting for the amount of water in the product. This type of measurement is considered AF because it represents the level of nutrients in the food as they are consumed by the animal. For example, if 10 ounces (oz) of a semimoist cat food contains 2.5 oz of protein, it contains 25% ([2.5 ÷ 10] × 100) protein on an AF basis. Similarly, if 10 oz of a dry cat food also contains 2.5 oz of protein, it too has a protein content of 25% on an AF basis. Comparing these two foods on an AF basis would indicate that they contribute similar levels of protein to the cat. However, because of the large range in moisture content between different types of pet foods, the diluting effect of water makes comparisons between pet foods on an AF basis difficult to interpret.

Animals eat and are fed to meet their caloric needs. Therefore a food with a high water content has its nutrients essentially "diluted" when compared with a food containing less water. Regardless of the amount of moisture in the diet, an animal still needs to eat a certain amount of dry matter (DM) to meet its daily caloric requirement. Conversion of nutrient data to a dry-matter basis (DMB) allows more accurate comparisons to be made between different types of pet foods. For example, the semimoist cat food discussed earlier contains 25% water and 75% DM; the dry food contains 10% water and 90% DM. The percentage of protein on a DMB can be calculated by dividing the percentage of the nutrient on an AF basis by the proportion of DM in the diet. The protein content of the semimoist food on a DMB is approximately 33%, but the protein content of the dry diet is 28% (Box 16-2). Therefore, although their label guarantees indicate similar protein contents, the semimoist food actually contains a higher level of protein than does the dry food on a DMB.

One of the most accurate ways to compare foods is by calculating the levels of nutrients as a proportion of ME. This is called *nutrient density* and is the most accurate way to express a food's nutrient content because it allows an accurate comparison of nutrient content between all types of pet foods. Although the DM method eliminates differences in nutrient expression due to differences in water content, it does not account for differences in energy content. Nutrient density accounts for differences in both water content and caloric content, and it expresses nutrient levels in pet foods based upon the energy that is available for the animal to use (the ME). Because all animals eat or are fed to meet their energy needs, the amount of food consumed and thus the amount of nutrients taken in depends directly on the caloric content of the food. Nutrient density expresses the energy-

BOX 16-2

Converting Nutrients from an As-Fed to a Dry-Matter Basis

Formula

Percentage of nutrient on an AF basis ÷ proportion of DM in the diet

Example

Semimoist food contains: 25% protein
75% DM
Dry food contains: 25% protein
90% DM
For semimoist food: (25 ÷ 75) × 100 = **33%** protein on a DMB
For dry food: (25 ÷ 90) × 100 = **28%** protein on a DMB

TABLE 16-2

Protein Intake Relative to Dietary Metabolizable Energy

	Energy Requirement (Kcal)		Diet Energy Density (Kcal/g)		Food Intake (g)		Protein in Diet (%)				Protein Consumed (g)
Diet A	2000	÷	4.0	=	500	×	26	÷	100	=	130.0
Diet B	2000	÷	3.5	=	571	×	26	÷	100	=	148.5

containing nutrients such as protein, fat, and carbohydrate as a percentage of ME or as grams (g) per 1000 kcal of ME. The nutritional standard for nutrients that do not contain energy (vitamins and minerals) is units per 1000 kcal of ME.

For example, diets A and B contain the same amount of protein (26%) on a DMB. However, the two foods have different energy densities. Diet A contains 4000 kcal/kg and diet B contains 3500 kcal/kg. Because diet B is lower in calories, a greater quantity (volume of food) needs to be consumed to meet a particular animal's caloric needs. A dog that requires 2000 kcal/day would consume 500 g of diet A or approximately 570 g of diet B. If the two diets contain the same percentage of protein on a weight basis, the dog would consume more total protein when he was fed diet B as compared with diet A (Table 16-2). If the protein level is sufficiently high, excess protein will be consumed when the dog is fed diet B. Excess protein is invariably used directly for energy or converted to fat for the storage of energy. On the other hand, if the diets contain marginal levels of protein, the dog may be deficient in protein when consuming diet A, which had a higher caloric density. This example illustrates the need to increase nutrient density as the caloric density of a diet increases. Although protein is a commonly used example, this concept applies to all of the essential nutrients. Because an animal will be fed less of a calorically dense food, the percentage of nutrients by weight in these foods must be higher so that the animal can still meet its needs for all essential nutrients while

171

eating a lower quantity of food. The nutrient level in pet foods must be carefully balanced so that when caloric requirements are satisfied, the requirements for all other nutrients are met at the same time.

The simplest way to solve the confusion of differences in caloric densities is to express nutrients as a percentage of ME or as units per 1000 kcal of ME, rather than as a percentage of weight. This is certainly the most accurate way to present nutrient content data and compare different foods. Nutrient densities of foods with different moisture contents can be compared because water does not contribute any calories to the distribution. In addition, foods with differing caloric contents are equalized using this method, allowing for accurate representation of nutrient levels. Although using DM calculations eliminates distortions that are the result of differences in moisture content, such comparisons do not take into consideration the calories of the foods or the amounts that must be consumed by the animal to meet energy needs. Comparisons using nutrient densities calculated on a caloric basis can be used with foods of different DM and energy content and with different weights or volumes.

Comparisons of caloric distribution are also important. The three nutrient groups that contribute energy to the diet are protein, carbohydrate, and fat. The relative contributions that each of these groups make to a diet's energy content is an important consideration in choosing a suitable pet food for a particular animal. For example, a hard-working dog requires sufficient protein to supply needs for muscle development and maintenance and increased calories to supply the necessary energy for work. Diets for hard-working dogs should contain adequate protein and a fairly high proportion of fat. A suggested caloric distribution expressed as a percentage of ME calories for protein, fat, and carbohydrate is 32%, 56%, and 12%, respectively. In contrast, a diet formulated for less active adult animals during maintenance should have a lower proportion of fat and an increased proportion of soluble carbohydrates. A suggested distribution is 26%, 38%, and 36% of ME calories from protein, fat, and carbohydrate, respectively. A maintenance diet with this caloric distribution has an energy balance that is shifted from fat to carbohydrate. This profile better meets the reduced energy needs of a sedentary dog and makes weight gain less likely. A typical profile of ME distribution for growing dogs is 27% protein, 41% fat, and 32% carbohydrate, and a profile for growing cats is 30% protein, 48% fat, and 22% carbohydrate (Figure 16-1).

Pet food companies that provide nutritional information about their products to consumers in the form of brochures often include caloric distribution and nutrient density information in these materials. If the information is not available, pet owners can calculate a rough estimate of the food's ME and caloric distribution of protein, fat, and carbohydrate from the food's proximate analysis. If the proximate analysis is not known, the guaranteed analysis panel on the label can be used, although it is much less accurate. Calculations that can be used to estimate total ME per kg are provided in Section 1, pp. 4-8. The example used is a dry dog food that contains the following guaranteed analysis:

FIGURE **16-1**

Recommended caloric distribution of pet foods.

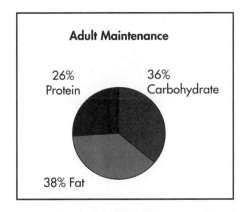

Adult Maintenance

26%
Protein

36%
Carbohydrate

38% Fat

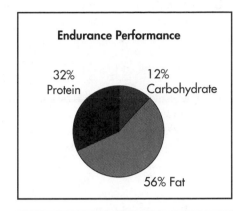

Endurance Performance

32%
Protein

12%
Carbohydrate

56% Fat

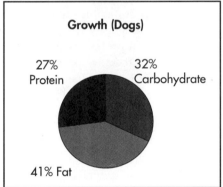

Growth (Dogs)

27%
Protein

32%
Carbohydrate

41% Fat

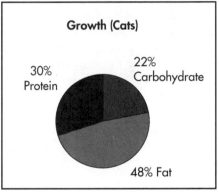

Growth (Cats)

30%
Protein

22%
Carbohydrate

48% Fat

- Crude protein: not less than 26%
- Crude fat: not less than 15%
- Crude fiber: not more than 5%

Mineral content is estimated to be about 7%, and carbohydrate content is determined by subtraction: 100% − 26% − 15% − 5% − 7% = 47%. Modified Atwater factors can be used to calculate the number of calories contributed by each nutrient in 100 g of food (see Table 1-3, p. 000). The total calories in 100 g of food equals 383. The total calories of ME per kg of this food is 3830, or 1741 kcal/lb of food. The percentage of ME calories contributed by protein is approximately 24%. The proportions of calories contributed by fat and carbohydrate are 33% and 43%, respectively (Box 16-3). This pet food has a distribution that would be appropriate for an adult dog during maintenance if it is not working hard.

BOX 16-3

Expression of Nutrients as a Percentage of Metabolizable Energy

Total calories in 100 g of food:
Protein = 3.5 kcal/g × 26 g = 91 kcal
Fat = 8.5 kcal/g × 15 g = 127.5 kcal
Carbohydrate = 3.5 kcal/g × 47g = 164.5 kcal
Total kilocalories = 91 + 127 + 164 = 383 kcal/100 g of food
Percentage of ME contributed by each nutrient (caloric distribution):
Protein = (91 kcal + 383 kcal) × 100 = **24%**
Fat = (127.5 kcal + 383 kcal) × 100 = **33%**
Carbohydrate = (164.5 kcal + 383 kcal) × 100 = **43%**

If a pet food's caloric distribution is calculated from the guaranteed analysis panel, it is important to recognize that the calculated numbers represent only a rough estimate and not the actual caloric distribution of the food. Companies that produce quality products and are aware of the importance of nutrient density will publish the ME and caloric distribution information for companion animal professionals and consumers. Because the calculation method can misrepresent a food by up to 15%, determination of these data is best accomplished through actual animal feeding studies.

COMMON PET FOOD INGREDIENTS

The ingredient list on a pet food label contains all of the food sources included in the formulation of the diet. Pet food regulations require the actual ingredients in each food to conform to the label, and the ingredient list cannot contain any reference to the quality of the ingredients that were used. Every ingredient that is part of a commercial pet food is included for a specific purpose. A few of the major ingredients may contain only one major nutrient or nutrient group, and others may contribute several essential nutrients to the diet. For example, corn is an excellent source of starch and is the principal source of digestible carbohydrate in many dry pet foods. Although corn contains a small percentage of protein, the amount of protein that is contributed to the total diet is small. Therefore corn is considered to be primarily a source of digestible carbohydrate when included in pet foods. Chicken contains high levels of protein and fat and is considered to be a source of both of these nutrients. A good rule for determining whether or not an ingredient in a pet food is a protein source is to compare the level of protein in the ingredient with the level of the ingredient in the food. Anything that has a protein content that is greater than its percentage in the diet is considered to be a source of protein for that ration. For example, if a pet food contains 20% chicken byproduct meal that has a protein content of 65%, chicken byproduct meal constitutes a protein source for that food.

When the ingredient list of a pet food is examined, the nutrient or nutrients contributed by each ingredient should be a primary concern. Both the amount and

BOX 16-4

Common Pet Food Ingredients

Primary Nutrient Contribution

Protein	Carbohydrate	Fat	Dietary Fiber
Beef	Alfalfa meal	Animal fat	Apple pomace
Brewer's dried yeast	Barley	Borage oil	Barley
Chicken meal	Brewer's rice	Chicken fat	Beet pulp
Chicken liver meal	Brown rice	Corn oil	Cellulose
Chicken byproduct meal	Dried kelp	Fish oil	Citrus pulp
Chicken	Dried whey	Flax seed (full fat form)	Oat bran
Chicken byproducts	Flax seed	Poultry fat	Peanut hulls
Corn gluten meal	Flax seed meal	Safflower oil	Pearled barley
Dried egg product	Grain sorghum	Soybean oil	Rice bran
Fish	Ground corn	Sunflower oil	Soybean hulls
Fish meal	Ground rice	Vegetable oil	Soybean mill run
Lamb	Ground wheat		Tomato pomace
Lamb meal	Molasses		
Meat byproducts	Oat meal		
Meat meal	Pearled barley		
Meat and bone meal	Rice flour		
Poultry byproduct meal	Wheat		
Soy flour	Wheat flour		
Soybean meal			

quality of the ingredient in the product determine how efficiently the ingredient can provide nutrition to animals consuming the complete diet. It is also important to consider that a pet food is made up of a number of ingredients, not just the first three or four provided at the start of the list. Nutrients that are contributed by all ingredients must be considered when evaluating a pet food. The following discussion reviews common pet food ingredients and the major nutrients that they contribute to commercial pet foods (Box 16-4).

Protein Sources

The protein in dog and cat foods can be supplied by animal sources, plant sources (grains), or a combination of the two. In general, high-quality animal source proteins provide superior amino acid balances for companion animals when compared with the amino acid balances supplied by grain proteins. However, animal protein sources can range from excellent quality to poor quality.[20] Characteristics of an ingredient, such as digestibility and amino acid availability, can only be determined through feeding trials. This information cannot be conveyed through the information presented on the pet food label. In contrast, grain protein sources are comparatively consistent in their quality and ability to supply amino acids. The protein in grains is not as balanced or available as the protein in high-quality animal sources, but it is higher in these characteristics than are poor-quality animal protein sources.

Animal protein sources that are commonly included in commercial pet foods include beef, chicken, chicken byproduct meal, chicken meal, dried egg, fish, fish meal, meat and bone meal, meat byproducts, and meat meal. In recent years lamb, lamb meal, and rabbit have also been included in some dog and cat foods. The term *meat,* as defined by the AAFCO, can represent any species of slaughtered mammal. Most commonly, this includes the striated muscle of pork, beef, sheep, or horse meat. When the term *byproduct* is included in the ingredient name, this means that secondary products are included with the ingredient in addition to the principal product. For example, when an ingredient is listed as "poultry," this means that it includes a clean combination of flesh and skin with or without bone derived from part or whole carcasses of poultry, exclusive of feathers, heads, feet, and entrails.[12] On the other hand, "poultry byproduct" refers to the clean parts of carcasses of slaughtered poultry, which may contain bone, heads, feet, and viscera, but no feathers. Because of the inclusion of heads and feet, poultry byproduct meal may be lower in nutritional value than fresh poultry or poultry meal. Depending on the supplier and the type of refining process that the pet food manufacturer uses, byproducts can vary greatly in the amount of indigestible material they contain. This is one of the factors contributing to the variability seen among animal protein sources. Another common term that is often part of an ingredient's name is *meal.* This term simply refers to any ingredient that has been ground or otherwise reduced in particle size. For example, "chicken meal" is the dry, ground, whole chicken, exclusive of heads, feet, viscera, or feathers.

Some animal protein sources contain varying amounts of bone. If meat and bone meal is included as an ingredient, the amount of bone contained in the product can affect its quality as a protein source as well as the mineral balance of the entire diet. The matrix of bone is composed of the protein collagen. Collagen is very poorly digested by dogs and cats, yet it will be analyzed as protein in the pet food. All muscle meats are very low in calcium content and have calcium/phosphorus ratios between 1:15 and 1:26. When bone is included with a meat ingredient, the calcium level of the product is increased, and the calcium/phosphorus ratio may be normalized. However, inexpensive meat and bone meals often contain excess levels of minerals. In this case, the problem becomes one of supplying too much calcium, phosphorus, and magnesium in the diet, rather than an insufficient amount of these nutrients. An excessively high calcium level in a pet food that contains meat and bone meal, poultry meal, or fish meal is an indication that the meal included in the product may be of poor quality and contains excessively high amounts of bone.

Grain protein sources that are used in pet foods include corn gluten meal, soy flour, soy grits, soybean meal, alfalfa meal, flax seed meal, and wheat germ. Pet foods that contain grain products as the major source of protein usually include a combination of soy products and corn gluten meal. Corn gluten meal is the dried residue that remains after most of the starch and germ-containing portions of the grain have been removed, and the bran has been separated and removed. As a protein source, corn gluten meal is relatively consistent in quality. This protein source is not as digestible as high-quality animal protein ingredients, but its protein is often more available than some of the poorer quality animal products.[21] On a DM basis, corn gluten meal contains a high proportion of protein, but its protein is deficient in the essential amino acids lysine and tryptophan.

Soybean products have been included in pet foods for a number of years. Defatted soybean meal, flour, and grits are the forms that are usually included in dry pet foods. Texturized vegetable protein (TVP) is the form that is often found in semimoist and canned foods. TVP is produced by the extrusion of defatted soy flour and has the advantage of retaining its meatlike texture and appearance through the high temperatures of the canning process.[22] The digestibility of soy protein by dogs varies between 71% and 87%, which is a slightly lower percentage than that for animal proteins.[23,24] Soy protein can complement corn gluten meal in a plant-based pet food because it is limiting in the sulfur amino acid methionine but is rich in lysine. When fed to cats, soy protein has been shown to affect taurine loss and bile acid kinetics. As a result, taurine supplementation may be necessary when soy is included as a protein source in cat foods.[25]

Although soy protein is well digested by dogs, soy carbohydrate is poorly digested in the canine small intestine. Undigested carbohydrate travels to the large intestine, where it is fermented by colon bacteria, resulting in the production of short-chain fatty acids (SCFAs) and gas. The osmotic action of the SCFAs and possible increased electrolyte concentrations in the colon cause increased fecal water content. This effect is pronounced in diets in which more than 50% of the protein is supplied by soy, and it can result in loose stools and flatulence.[22] These undesirable effects have been attributed to the oligosaccharides present in soy, specifically stachyose and raffinose. Investigations of the ability of dogs to digest and ferment soy carbohydrate found that when dogs were fed diets containing either conventional soybean meal or a low-oligosaccharide soybean meal, they digested the low-oligosaccharide meal as extensively as the conventional soybean meal.[26] Moreover, the total tract digestion of soy oligosaccharides was nearly 100% for both types of soy product. These results indicate that the canine colon is capable of fully fermenting the portion of soy carbohydrate that is indigestible in the small intestine. This information is significant when considering the proportion of soy included in a pet food because fecal consistency, defecation frequency, and colon health may be affected.

Raw soy contains phytate and several metabolic inhibitors that affect an animal's ability to digest and absorb other nutrients.[22] Soy trypsin inhibitors function to reduce the digestibility of protein in the diet. However, trypsin inhibitors, like many other antinutritional factors, are heat-labile and are largely destroyed by heating during the processing of pet foods. Hemagglutinins in soy are lectins that are capable of binding carbohydrate and agglutinating red blood cells. However, these have not been shown to be toxic, and like trypsin inhibitors, they are heat-labile. In contrast, phytate is not significantly affected by heat and is capable of interfering with the absorption of certain minerals even after processing. Therefore pet food manufacturers must account for the effects of phytate when balancing the mineral component of soy-containing foods.

Carbohydrate Sources

Ingredients that contribute digestible carbohydrates to commercial pet foods include various forms of corn, rice, grain sorghum, wheat, and oats. Barley, carrots, flax seed, molasses, peas, and potatoes may also be included, but usually in lesser amounts. With the exception of molasses, all of these ingredients contribute complex carbohydrates in the form of starch.

The cooking of starch greatly enhances its digestibility. Therefore heat treatment of these ingredients is necessary during the processing of the food to ensure maximal use by companion animals. In dry pet foods, a certain proportion of the diet must be made up of starch to allow for proper expansion of the food pellets. During expansion, temperatures within the extruder come close to 150° C. This temperature increases the size of the starch granules and improves digestibility and palatability.

Although it is not a digestible nutrient, dietary fiber is categorized with carbohydrates. Dietary fiber is not digested by intestinal enzymes, but it is required in the diet to promote normal gastrointestinal tract functioning (see Section 1, pp. 16-17). Sources of indigestible fiber in commercial pet foods include beet pulp; rice bran; apple and tomato pomace; peanut hulls; citrus pulp; the bran of oats, rice, and wheat; and cellulose. Bran is a milling byproduct that consists of the outer coarse coat (pericarp) of the cereal grain. During the production of flour, this portion is removed from the grain and separated. Pulp is the solid residue that remains after juices are extracted from fruits or vegetables; pomace specifically refers to the pulp of fruit. The beet pulp that is included in pet foods is derived from sugar beets (not red beets) and is considered to be a high-quality fiber source because it is moderately fermentable. Moderately fermentable fiber sources provide adequate bulk for gastrointestinal tract functioning and stool production while also promoting gastrointestinal cell health through the production of SCFAs (see Section 1 pp. 16-17, and Section 6, pp. 497-501).

Fat Sources

The fat in a pet food contributes calories and essential fatty acids (EFAs) and enhances palatability. Commonly used sources of fat in commercial pet foods include various types of animal fats and vegetable oils. The general term *animal fat* refers to fat that comes from the tissues of mammals and/or poultry. Animal fat must contain a minimum of 90% total fatty acids, not more than 2.5% unsaponifiable matter (the unsaponifiable portion of a fat contains lipid compounds other than triglycerides and fatty acids, such as sterols, pigments, and fatty alcohols), and not more than 1% insoluble impurities.[12] If the product is completely made up of a single type of fat, such as poultry or beef fat, a descriptive term denoting the species of the animal source must be used. Chicken fat and poultry fat are the two most common types of animal fat included in dog and cat foods. Therefore, if the ingredient list uses the term *animal fat,* the consumer must assume that the fat contains fats from several different types of mammals and/or poultry. Similarly, the terms *vegetable fat* or *vegetable oil* refer to the product obtained from the extraction of the oil from seeds. If a specific plant source is the exclusive source of the oil, this must be indicated on the label. Most commonly, corn, safflower, and soybean oils are used in commercial pet foods. Flax is an important plant source of fat because ground whole flaxseed is an excellent source of the omega-3 fatty acid alpha-linolenic acid. Borage oil, a source of alpha-linolenic acid and of the omega-6 fatty acid gamma-linolenic acid, may also be included in pet foods that contain adjusted ratios of omega-6 to omega-3 fatty acids.

In addition to specific fat sources, ingredients such as chicken, poultry, and various meat products also contribute a significant amount of fat to pet foods. Fish meal is an excellent protein source and also supplies fish oil, which contains long-chain omega-3 fatty acids. If an antioxidant has been added to the fat source as a preservative, this must be indicated following the listing of the product on the ingredient list.

Vitamin and Mineral Sources

Almost all of the major ingredients discussed earlier also contribute vitamins and minerals to the diet. When a balanced ration is formulated, vitamin and mineral levels are made adequate through the addition of purified or semipurified forms of these nutrients. Because only small amounts of vitamins and minerals are required by animals and because other ingredients also supply these nutrients, purified forms of vitamins and minerals are present in small amounts in pet foods and are listed low on the ingredient list of the label.

Minerals vary greatly in their bioavailability, and many factors can affect the mineral availability within a diet. It is important not only to have adequate amounts of each mineral relative to the animal's requirement but also to consider the relationship between minerals and the overall balance of the ration. Excess levels of any mineral may adversely affect the ability of the body to absorb other minerals in the diet. For example, excess levels of calcium, copper, and possibly vitamin D can all inhibit the absorption of zinc in dogs.[27] Manufacturers must always consider these relationships when balancing the mineral component of their pet foods.

One of the biggest concerns about vitamins in commercial pet foods is their loss during processing and storage. Adequate quantities of vitamins that account for losses during processing and storage must be added to pet foods to ensure that sufficient levels are present at the time of feeding. The high heat and pressure used in the canning process result in losses of the B vitamins thiamin and folic acid. Compensatory levels of these vitamins must be added to maintain adequate postprocessing levels. In dry, extruded pet foods, there are considerable losses of vitamin A, riboflavin, folic acid, niacin, and biotin. However, if vitamin A is added as part of the fat coating that is sprayed onto the food after extrusion, there is little to no loss of the vitamin during storage. In semimoist foods, slight losses of vitamin A and riboflavin have been observed.[28] Studies have provided recommendations for levels of vitamins to add to preprocessed pet food to ensure that levels after processing and storage are still sufficient to meet an animal's nutrient needs.[28] In addition, manufacturers who ensure thorough testing of their products conduct nutrient analyses of their finished products; this testing may not be done by manufacturers who use the calculation method for nutritional adequacy substantiation.

Ingredients that contribute vitamins and minerals to pet foods must be balanced in terms of their overall quantities, their bioavailability, and their relationships to each other. Commonly included sources of minerals in commercial pet foods include potassium chloride, calcium carbonate, dicalcium phosphate, monosodium phosphate, manganese sulfate or manganese oxide, copper sulfate, zinc oxide, sodium selenite, potassium iodide, ferrous sulfate, and cobalt carbonate. Examples of sources of vitamins include choline chloride, D-activated animal sterol (a source of vitamin D), alpha-tocopherol, thiamin or thiamin mononitrate, niacin, calcium pantothenate, pyridoxine hydrochloride, riboflavin, folic acid, biotin, menadione dimethylpyrimidinol (a source of vitamin K), vitamin A acetate, and vitamin B_{12}.

Additives and Preservatives

Additives are ingredients that are included in pet foods to enhance or preserve the product's color, flavor, texture, stability, or nutrient content. Preservatives are additives that are included with the express purpose of protecting nutrients in the food from oxidative or microbial damage. All preservatives are classified as additives, but not all additives have a function in food preservation.

One of the chief concerns in the production of commercial pet foods is safety. A product must be proven to be both nutritious and safe for consumption by companion animals throughout its designated shelf-life. The manufacturer must ensure that the food remains free of bacterial contamination and harmful toxins and is protected from degradation and the loss of nutrients during storage. The method of preservation that is used for a pet food depends to some degree on the type of food. The low moisture content of dry pet foods inhibits the growth of most organisms. The heat sterilization and anaerobic environment of canned foods kills all microbes. Semimoist pet foods often have a low pH and contain humectants that bind water within the product, making it unavailable for use by invading bacteria or fungi. Frozen pet foods, although less common, are protected by storage at extremely low temperatures. Many commercial foods also contain added compounds that aid in the preservation process. For example, potassium sorbate prevents the formation of mold and yeasts; glycerol and certain sugars act as humectants.

A primary nutrient in pet foods that requires protection during storage is dietary fat. In recent years the inclusion of high levels of fat in dry pet foods has resulted in the need for methods of protecting these fats from oxidative destruction during storage. Foods that are formulated for dogs and cats contain vegetable oils, animal fats, and the fat-soluble vitamins A, D, E, and K. These nutrients all have the potential to undergo oxidative destruction during storage. This oxidative degradation, called *lipid peroxidation,* occurs as a three-stage process.[29] *Initiation* occurs when a free radical, usually oxygen, attacks a polyunsaturated fatty acid (PUFA) and results in the formation of a fatty-acid radical. Exposure of the fat to heat, ultraviolet radiation, or certain metal ions such as iron and copper accelerate this process. The fatty acid radical continues to react with oxygen, resulting in the formation of peroxides. Peroxides react with other fatty acids to form more fatty-acid radicals and hydroperoxides (Figure 16-2). This second phase is called *propagation* because the reaction is autocatalyzed and increases geometrically in rate. The reaction is only terminated when all of the available fatty acids and vitamins have been oxidized. The subsequent *decomposition* of the hydroperoxides produces offensive odors, tastes, and changes in the texture of the food. In addition, oxidation of lipids in pet foods results in a loss of caloric content and the formation of toxic forms of peroxides that can be harmful to the health of companion animals.[30]

Pet food manufacturers include antioxidants in commercial pet foods to prevent the autooxidation process. The Food and Drug Administration (FDA) defines *antioxidants* as substances that aid in the preservation of foods by retarding deterioration, rancidity, or discoloration as the result of oxidative processes.[31] Various types of antioxidants have been accepted for use in human and animal foods since 1947.[32] These compounds do not reverse the effects of oxidation once it has started; rather, they retard the oxidative process and prevent destruction of the fat in the food. Therefore, to be effective, antioxidants must be included in the diet when it is initially mixed and processed. The inclusion of antioxidant compounds in commercial pet foods prevents rancidity; maintains the food's flavor, odor, and texture; and prevents the accumulation of the toxic end products of lipid degradation.

FIGURE **16-2**

Antioxidant action.

No Antioxidant

$$
\begin{array}{ccccc}
& & & O_2 & & & R\text{—}H \\
& & & \downarrow & & & \downarrow \\
R\text{—}H & \longrightarrow & R^* & \longrightarrow & R\text{—}O\text{—}O^* & \longrightarrow & R\text{—}O\text{—}O\text{—}H + R^* \\
\text{Fatty acid} & & \text{Free radical} & & \text{Peroxide} & & \text{Hydroperoxide}
\end{array}
$$

Antioxidant Added

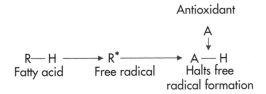

$$
\begin{array}{ccc}
& & \text{Antioxidant} \\
& & A \\
& & \downarrow \\
R\text{—}H & \longrightarrow R^* \longrightarrow & A\text{—}H \\
\text{Fatty acid} & \text{Free radical} & \text{Halts free} \\
& & \text{radical formation}
\end{array}
$$

Antioxidants can be categorized into two basic types—natural-derived products and synthetic products. Natural-derived antioxidants are commonly found in certain grains, vegetable oils, and some herbs and spices. While these compounds exist in nature, the term "natural" can be misleading to consumers because all of these compounds are processed in some way to make them available for use in commercial foods.[33] Vitamin E is probably the most widely distributed natural-derived antioxidant. Physiologically, vitamin E functions as an antioxidant in body tissues and will also function to protect fats in the diet from oxidative destruction. There are several forms in which vitamin E, or the tocopherols, exist in nature. Alpha-tocopherol has the strongest biological function in tissues of the body. In contrast, gamma-tocopherol and delta-tocopherol both have low biological activity, but they are more effective than alpha-tocopherol as feed antioxidants. Tocopherols for use in foods are obtained primarily from the distillation of soybean oil residue. Further processing of this byproduct separates gamma-tocopherols and delta-tocopherols from alpha-tocopherol. Because of the high market demand for physiologically active vitamin E, most commercial preparations contain primarily alpha-tocopherol. This form has lower value as a feed antioxidant, and commercial preparations are often modified to improve their delivery to the body. These changes may render the compound even less effective as a protector of fat within a pet food.[31] Mixed tocopherols, containing both delta-tocopherol and gamma-tocopherol, are the most effective natural-derived antioxidants and show the greatest efficacy in the protection of animal fats in pet foods. However, because the tocopherols are rapidly decomposed as they protect fat from oxidation, the shelf-life of pet foods stabilized with tocopherols alone is shorter than that of foods preserved with a mixture of several different antioxidants.[30,33,34]

Other natural-derived antioxidants that may be included in pet foods include ascorbic acid (vitamin C), rosemary extract, and citric acid. Ascorbic acid functions naturally as an antioxidant by scavenging oxygen. However, it is a water-soluble compound and is not easily solubilized with the lipid fraction of foods, which affects its function as an antioxidant for the fat in commercial pet foods. Vitamin C has been shown to work synergistically with other antioxidants, such as vitamin E and butylated hydroxytoluene, and it is often included in pet foods for this reason.[35] Ascorbyl palmitate is a compound that is similar in structure to ascorbic acid. Although ascorbyl palmitate is not normally found in nature, its hydrolysis yields ascorbic acid and the free fatty acid (FFA) palmitic acid, both of which are natural compounds. The antioxidant function of ascorbyl palmitate is the result of the ascorbic acid portion of the molecule.

Rosemary extract is obtained from the dried leaves of an evergreen shrub, *Rosemarinus officinalis*. It is effective as a natural-derived preservative in high-fat diets and has been shown to enhance antioxidant efficiency when included in combination with tocopherols, ascorbic acid and citric acid.[34] Citric acid is found in citrus fruits, such as oranges and lemons, and is often included in combination with other natural-derived antioxidants in pet foods. Lecithin, monoglycerides, and diglycerides are natural-derived compounds that are added to pet foods to act as emulsifying agents. In this capacity, they function to prevent separation of fat from other components of the diet, allowing greater contact between antioxidants and the lipid components in the food.

The natural-derived antioxidant formulations that are available for use in pet foods have improved greatly in recent years. However, they still have limited value when used as the only type of antioxidant in a commercially produced pet food because the concentration that must be included to provide an adequate level of protection is very high. Commercial pet foods undergo rigorous processing procedures that can include exposure to high heat, steam, and pressure. In addition, they must be protected from damaging oxidative reactions during varying lengths of storage. An effective antioxidant system must have high stability and retain its antioxidant functions after being subjected to the high heat, pressure, and moisture of food processing (i.e., have good "carry-through"). Most natural-derived antioxidants have poor carry-through, so an excess amount of the additive must be included in the food to compensate for high losses during processing. These additions are inefficient and add to the cost of the food.

When natural-derived antioxidants are used in pet foods, the products of choice are the mixed tocopherols, usually in combination with ascorbic acid and rosemary extract.[29,34] However, in most cases, these ingredients are used primarily to supplement the action of the synthetic antioxidants that are also included in the food. Because these natural-derived compounds tend to be significantly more expensive than synthetic antioxidants, it is difficult to attain the necessary level of natural-derived antioxidants without it becoming cost prohibitive.

Effective synthetic antioxidants for pet foods include butylated hydroxyanisole (BHA), butylated hydroxytoluene (BHT), tertiary butylhydroquinine (TBHQ), and ethoxyquin. BHA and BHT are approved for use in both human foods and animal feeds and have a synergistic antioxidant effect when used together. BHA and BHT have good carry-through and a high efficacy in the protection of animal fats, but they are slightly less effective when used with vegetable oils.[29] TBHQ is an effective antioxidant for most fats and is approved for use in human and animal foods in the United States. However, this compound has not been approved in Canada or Japan, or by the European Economic Community, so it is not usually used in pet foods that have an international market.[29] Ethoxyquin has been approved for use in animal feeds for more than 30 years and is also approved for use in human foods. It has been used by pet food manufacturers for more than 15 years. Like BHT and BHA, ethoxyquin has good carry-through, and it has an especially high efficacy in the protection of fats. Ethoxyquin is more efficient as an antioxidant than BHA or BHT, which allows lower levels of the compound to be included in the feed. It is especially effective in the protection of oils that contain high levels of PUFAs.[31]

In recent years there has been some concern about the safety of synthetic antioxidants, specifically ethoxyquin, in pet foods. One of the arguments against the use of this additive is the fact that ethoxyquin is used as an antioxidant in the rubber industry. The biochemical mechanism through which ethoxyquin prevents oxidation of rubber is exactly the same mechanism through which it works to protect the fat in pet foods. Similarly, BHA and BHT were both originally used to protect petroleum products from the oxidative changes that led to "gumming."[31] But the fact that a compound acts as an antioxidant in other situations does not preclude it from being an effective antioxidant in foods. Like most compounds, ethoxyquin, BHA, and BHT have multiple uses. A second criticism of ethoxyquin originated from the observation that in outdated editions of the *Merck Chemical Index,* ethoxyquin was listed as an insecticide and herbicide. The manufacturer included possible functions of this compound in a broad screening process that attempted to identify all possible applications of new products. But ethoxyquin has never been promoted or sold as an insecticide or herbicide, and the company eliminated these as possible uses for the product in 1983.[36]

Ethoxyquin has been included in feeds for animals since 1959, and its safety in foods has been extensively studied in rabbits, rats, poultry, and dogs. The original studies on which the FDA based approval for the inclusion of ethoxyquin in animal feeds included a 1-year chronic toxicity study in dogs. Data from this and other studies were used to determine a "safe tolerance level" of 150 parts per million (ppm) (150 milligrams [mg]/kg) of food.[37] Subsequently, the manufacturer of ethoxyquin conducted a 5-year, multigenerational study in dogs. The data from this study failed to show any adverse side effects of ethoxyquin when it was fed at a level of 300 mg/kg of the diet.[38] Most recently, an independent research facility conducted a study for the manufacturer of ethoxyquin on the effects of ethoxyquin upon the long-term health of dogs.[39] Two generations of male and female dogs were fed diets containing either 0, 180, or 360 parts per million of ethoxyquin for a period of 42 months. During this time, the dogs mated and produced viable litters of puppies. There were no effects of the antioxidant upon the health or fertility of the adult dogs, or upon the health, growth, or mortality of their resultant puppies. There are no studies that support the contention that ethoxyquin is responsible for the variety of health problems reported by pet owners to the FDA. The maximum allowable concentration of ethoxyquin in all animal feeds is 150 mg/kg of the finished product. The FDA has requested that pet food companies voluntarily limit the level of ethoxyquin to 75 ppm. The pet food industry is honoring this request and is also conducting further studies of the effectiveness of ethoxyquin as an antioxidant in pet food at levels between 30 and 60 ppm. All pet foods that contain this additive must include it (as a preservative) in the list of ingredients.

It is important for pet owners to recognize that almost all products that humans and animals consume become toxic when consumed at high enough levels. The inclusion of synthetic antioxidants in commercial pet foods is necessary for the protection of dietary fat from detrimental oxidative changes. The proper use of these compounds prevents the occurrence of rancidity and the production of toxic compounds in pet foods. In most cases, synthetic antioxidants are the best compounds to use because of their efficacy, good carry-through, and cost. In contrast, poor carry-through, instability, and high levels needed for effective protection make natural-derived antioxidants difficult to use as the only type of antioxidant in a pet food (Table 16-3).

Pet foods also contain some additives that are included expressly to contribute to characteristics of color, texture, or palatability. For example, coloring agents are often added to enhance consumer appeal. Some examples include carotenoid pig-

TABLE **16-3**

Common Antioxidants Used in Pet Foods

	Cost	Availability	Carry-Through	Effectiveness
Natural-Derived				
Mixed tocopherols	High	Low	Poor	Low
Ascorbic acid	High	Low	Poor	Low
Ascorbyl palmitate	High	Low	Poor	Low
Synthetic				
BHA	Low	Moderate	Good	High
BHT	Low	Moderate	Good	High
TBHQ	Low	Poor	Good	High
Ethoxyquin	Low	Good	Excellent	High

ments, iron oxide, tartrazine, sunset yellow, and allura red. Other coloring agents, such as nitrites, bisulfites, and ascorbate, are included to prevent discoloration of the pet food. As with human foods, an artificial color can be used in a pet food only if it has been accepted as safe by the FDA. Flavor ingredients are included in some pet foods to support label claims regarding flavor. AAFCO regulations require that the designated flavor be detectable by a recognized testing method.[12] A related group of additives are those included to enhance palatability. These compounds are usually sprayed onto the outside of dry pet foods to make the food more appetizing to pets. The most commonly used palatability enhancer is digest. The term *digest* refers to solutions that are produced through the enzymatic degradation of various types of meat or meat byproducts. This process is conducted under controlled conditions and is stopped when the protein in the mixture is partially digested. The resulting slurry of liquid is highly palatable to dogs and cats and is usually sprayed onto dry foods as an outer coating. In some cases, the digest is dried and added to the food as a powder following the application of a layer of fat. Digest can also be used as a means of designating the food's flavor. Other examples of palatability enhancers in commercial pet foods include garlic, onion, and various spices.

Finally, emulsifiers and thickening agents are important additives for the effect they have upon the pet food's texture. In canned pet foods, gums, glycerides, and modified starches are included for the production of a thick sauce or gravy. Examples of these ingredients are carrageenan, guar gum, gum arabic, and carboxymethylcellulose. These agents can also be sprayed onto the outside of a dry food so that when water is added to the food before feeding, they create a gravy or thick sauce.

C H A P T E R

17

Types of Pet Foods

The majority of pet owners in the United States feed their companion animals commercially prepared pet foods instead of homemade diets. Commercial products are available in several forms that vary according to the processing methods used, the ingredients included, and the methods of preservation. Foods can also be categorized according to their nutrient content, the purpose for which they are formulated, and the quality of ingredients they contain. One of the broadest classifications of commercial pet foods divides products according to processing method, methods of preservation, and moisture content; these categories are the dry, canned, and semimoist foods. Commercial products can be further categorized according to their quality and the marketing methods used to sell them. This chapter examines the various types of commercial pet foods, the advantages and disadvantages of each, and the use of homemade diets.

DRY PET FOODS

Dry pet foods contain between 6% and 10% moisture and 90% or more dry matter (DM).[10] This category of pet foods includes kibbles, biscuits, meals, and expanded products. Ingredients commonly used in dry pet foods include cereal grains, meat, poultry or fish products, some milk products, and vitamin and mineral supplements. A certain level of starch must be included in expanded products to allow proper processing of the product.

Kibbles and biscuits are prepared in much the same manner, although the shape of the product differs. In each case, all of the ingredients are mixed into a homogeneous dough, which is then baked. When biscuits are made, the dough is formed or cut into the desired shapes and the individual biscuits are baked much like cookies or crackers. When kibble is produced, the dough is spread onto large sheets and baked. After cooling, the large sheets are broken into bite-size pieces and packaged. Many dog and cat treats are baked biscuits, and a few companies still produce complete and balanced kibbles. Dry meals, the major type of dry pet food sold before 1960, are prepared by mixing together a number of dried, flaked, or granular ingredients.

The development of the extrusion process resulted in the almost complete replacement of meals and kibbles with extruded pet foods. The extrusion process produces expanded pet foods. This procedure involves mixing all of the ingredients together to form a dough, which is then cooked under conditions of high pressure and temperature. The machine that is used to cook and shape expanded foods is called an *extruder*. The dough moves very quickly through the extruder and is further mixed as it proceeds. The high temperatures, movement of the mixture, and rising pressure allows cooking to occur very rapidly (within 20 to 60 seconds). When the cooked dough reaches the end of the extruder, it exits through a die (small opening). The die forces the slightly soft product into the desired shape and a rotating knife cuts the forms into the desired kibble size. Extrusion causes rapid cooking of the starches within the product, resulting in increased digestibility and palatability. After cooling, a coating of fat or digest is usually sprayed on the expanded pellets (a process called "enrobing"). Hot air drying reduces the total moisture content of the product to 10% or less. Expanded products represent the most common type of dry pet food currently produced and sold in the United States.

The cooking process of extruded and baked dry foods improves the digestibility of the complex carbohydrates in the product and enhances the food's palatability. Heat treatment and storage can result in minor losses of some vitamins, so compensatory amounts of these nutrients are included by most manufacturers when the diet is formulated. The heat used in the extrusion process also sterilizes the product, and the low amount of moisture that is present in dry foods aids in the prevention of growth of bacteria or fungus.

The caloric density of dry pet foods typically ranges between 3000 and 4500 kilocalories (kcal) of metabolizable energy (ME)/kilogram (kg), or between 1300 and 2000 kcal/pound (lb) on a dry-matter basis (DMB). Dry cat foods are often slightly higher in energy density than dog foods. The energy density of dry pet foods is somewhat limited by the processing and packaging methods used. However, the majority of dry pet foods can fully supply for the energy needs of the majority of companion animals. Products that are formulated for adult maintenance will only be bulk limited if fed to hard-working or stressed dogs or puppies that have very high energy requirements. In these cases, "high performance" pet foods have been developed to meet the energy requirements of working dogs and growing puppies. Depending on the purpose of the food, the DM content of dry dog foods is between 8% and 22% fat and 18% and 32% protein (Table 17-1). Cat foods of all types contain slightly higher levels of protein than dog foods.

Dry dog foods are the most common type of pet food bought by pet owners in the United States.[2] In general, these products are more economical to feed than semimoist or canned foods, and they store well because of their low moisture content. Large quantities of these products can be bought at one time, and dry products have a reasonably long shelf-life when stored under proper conditions. Many pet owners prefer feeding dry foods because they can leave a bowl of food available to their pet at all times without worrying about spoilage. In some cases, dogs

TABLE **17-1**

Nutrient Content of Dry, Semimoist, and Canned Dog Foods

	AF Basis	DM Basis
Dry		
Moisture (%)	6-10	0
Fat (%)	7-20	8-22
Protein (%)	16-30	18-32
Carbohydrate (%)	41-70	46-74
ME (kcal/kg)	2800-4050	3000-4500
Semimoist		
Moisture (%)	15-30	0
Fat (%)	7-10	8-14
Protein (%)	17-20	20-28
Carbohydrate (%)	40-60	58-72
ME (kcal/kg)	2550-2800	3000-4000
Canned		
Moisture (%)	75	0
Fat (%)	5-8	20-32
Protein (%)	7-13	28-50
Carbohydrate (%)	4-13	18-57
ME (kcal/kg)	875-1250	3500-5000

AF, As fed.

and cats can be fed free-choice with a dry food and not overconsume. However, the high fat content and palatability of some of the foods marketed today preclude free-choice feeding for many dogs and cats. Dry pet food may also offer some dental hygiene advantages. The chewing and grinding that accompanies eating dry biscuits or pet food may aid in the prevention of plaque and calculus accumulation on teeth.[40]

A potential disadvantage of dry pet foods, when compared with semimoist or canned foods, is that dry foods may be less palatable to some dogs and cats. This disadvantage is especially true of foods that are low in fat or that contain poorly digestible ingredients. However, in recent years, dry pet foods that contain high-quality ingredients and moderate to high levels of fat have been developed and marketed. These foods are nutrient dense and highly palatable to most companion animals. Because of their high caloric density and digestibility, lower amounts of these diets need to be fed, which results in lower stool volume. This factor, plus the enhanced palatability, have made these new, higher fat dry foods popular with many pet owners.

Because ingredients that are primarily low in moisture are used to formulate dry pet foods, harsh or improper drying of the ingredients can cause a reduction in nutrient availability and the loss of nutrients. As a result, poor-quality dry foods may have very low digestibilities and nutrient availabilities. Companies that manufacture high-quality, premium products only use properly treated ingredients to ensure that the digestibilities of their products remain high after processing.

CANNED PET FOODS

There are two primary types of canned pet foods—those that provide complete and balanced nutrition and those that provide a dietary supplement or treat in the form of a canned meat or meat byproduct. Complete and balanced canned foods may contain blends of ingredients such as muscle meats, poultry or fish byproducts, cereal grains, texturized vegetable protein (TVP), and vitamins and minerals. Some of these products contain only one or two types of muscle meat or animal byproducts, with enough supplemental vitamins and minerals to make the ration nutritionally complete. The second type of canned food, often referred to as "canned meat products," consists of the same types of meat listed earlier but without supplemental vitamins and minerals. These foods are not formulated to be nutritionally complete and are intended to be used only as a supplement (or treat) to an already complete and balanced diet. For example, some pet owners add a small amount of canned pet food to their pet's complete and balanced dry food every day. The high fat content of the canned supplement enhances the texture and palatability of the pet's diet. Although many complete and balanced dry foods are also highly palatable and provide a balanced diet, some pet owners believe that a dry diet alone becomes boring or bland to their pet. Adding a spoonful or two of a product that looks like meat or stew makes many owners believe they are making the meal more enjoyable for their pet.

Canned pet foods are prepared by first blending the meat and fat ingredients with measured amounts of water. Measured amounts of dry ingredients are then added and the entire mixture is heated. Canning occurs on a conveyor line. Most pet foods are sold in either 3-, 6-, or 14-ounce (oz) cans. After filling, the cans are then sealed with a double seam, washed, and labeled with a manufacturer code and date. Pressure sterilization of canned products is called *retorting*. Temperatures and times for retorting vary with the product and can size, but typically, cans are held at around 250° Celsius (C) for 60 minutes. After exiting the retort, the cans are cooled under controlled conditions to ensure the sterility of the product and the integrity of the sealed cans. To designate the product, paper labels are then applied during the final step of production.

From a processing standpoint, there are three types of canned foods—loaf, chunks or chunks in gravy, and a chunk-in-loaf combination. Depending on the ingredients used, these products can vary greatly in nutrient content, digestibility, and availability.[41] In general, canned foods are more palatable and digestible than many dry pet foods, and they contain a higher DM proportion of protein and fat (see Table 17-1). The high heat and pressure involved in processing canned foods kills harmful bacteria and causes some nutrient losses. Manufacturers of high-quality products conduct the research necessary to determine the extent of these losses and then adjust their formulations to compensate for them. However, some companies may not properly consider the nutrient losses that occur during the canning process. Manufacturers that use the calculation method to substantiate their label claims are not required to account for these losses because the calculation method is completed before processing.

When measured on a DMB, the caloric content of canned pet foods generally ranges between 3500 and 5000 kcal/kg or about 1600 and 2300 kcal/lb. The fat content of canned pet foods ranges between 20% and 32%, and protein levels are usually between 28% and 50%. Most canned products contain a relatively small proportion of digestible carbohydrate when compared with that in other types of pet foods (see Table 17-1). Often, canned foods are also more expensive than dry pet foods. Although expense is often not a concern for owners of cats or small dogs, it can become significant when feeding large dogs or multiple pets. Nutrient and price comparisons between canned and dry pet foods should always be made on either a DMB or a caloric-density basis because canned foods contain a very large proportion of water (see p. 155). In the United States the moisture content of pet foods can be as high as 78%, or equal to the natural moisture content of the ingredients used, whichever is greater.[12] On average, canned pet foods contain about 75% water; this amount can be compared with dry pet foods, which contain approximately 6% to 10% moisture.[10]

Some advantages of canned pet foods include their extremely long shelf-life and high acceptability. The sterilization and sealing of the cans allows these products to be kept for long periods before opening, without the need for special storage considerations. Because of their nutrient content and texture, canned foods tend to be highly palatable to dogs and cats. However, this can be a disadvantage for some companion animals. Dogs and cats that have moderate to low energy requirements may be predisposed to the development of obesity when fed exclusively canned pet foods. If fed free-choice, the high palatability of these products can override an animal's inherent tendency to eat to meet its caloric requirements, resulting in the overconsumption of energy.

In recent years, gourmet-type canned cat foods have become especially popular. These products may or may not be nutritionally complete, and they contain primarily animal tissues such as fish, shrimp, tuna, or liver. These foods are often sold in small, one-serving or two-serving cans and appeal to owners' desires to give their cat "something special." There may be an inherent danger in the exclusive feeding of these products to some cats. More so than dogs, cats are susceptible to the development of fixed food preferences if fed a diet that contains a single type of ingredient for a long period. Some cats eventually accept only this one food item and will refuse to eat any other type or flavor of food.[42,43] If the food is not complete and balanced, nutrient imbalances may occur. Therefore, if canned foods are used with cats, it is advisable to feed complete and balanced rations that contain more than one principal ingredient. The gourmet products can be used as supplemental feeding, but they should not make up the entire diet. The high fat content of canned foods also makes these products calorically dense. Dogs and cats with increased energy needs may benefit from the increased energy that can be obtained from a lower volume of food.

SEMIMOIST PET FOODS

Semimoist pet foods contain 15% to 30% water and include fresh or frozen animal tissues, cereal grains, fats, and simple sugars as their principal ingredients. These products are softer in texture than dry pet foods, which contributes to their acceptability and palatability. Several methods of preservation are used to prevent contamination and spoilage of semimoist foods and permit an extended shelf-life. The inclusion of humectants such as simple sugars, glycerol, or corn syrup binds water molecules in the food and make them unavailable for use by invading organisms. Until 1992, propylene glycol was also used as a humectant in semimoist pet foods. However, the Food and Drug Administration (FDA) determined that this compound was a potential health risk to cats and has prohibited its use in cat foods. Further protection is provided by preservatives such as potassium sorbate, which prevents the growth of yeasts and molds. Small amounts of organic acids may also be included to decrease the pH of products and inhibit bacterial growth.

The high simple sugar content of many semimoist pet foods contributes to the palatability and digestibility of these products. Although dogs have been shown to enjoy the taste of simple sugars, cats are less likely to select sweet foods.[44,45] Semimoist pet foods that contain a high proportion of simple carbohydrates have digestibility coefficients that are similar to those of canned foods. However, because of their lower fat content, the caloric density of semimoist foods is usually less. The ME content of semimoist foods typically ranges between 3000 and 4000 kcal/kg on a DMB, or about 1400 to 1800 kcal/lb. Semimoist foods contain between 20% and 28% protein and between 8% and 14% fat on a DMB. The proportion of carbohydrate in semimoist foods is similar to that of dry foods (see Table 17-1). However, the carbohydrate in semimoist pet foods is largely in the form of simple carbohydrates, with a relatively small proportion of starch.

Semimoist pet foods appeal to some pet owners because they generally have less odor than canned foods, and many come in convenient single-serving packages. These foods are also available in a large variety of shapes and textures that often resemble different types of meat products, such as ground beef, meat patties, or chunks of beef. Although these different forms do not reflect nutrient content or palatability for the pet, they do appeal to the tastes of many pet owners. Semimoist foods do not require refrigeration before opening and have a relatively long shelf-life. The cost of these foods when compared on a DMB is usually between the cost of dry and canned products. However, products sold as single-serving packages are often comparable in price to canned pet foods. Because they are lower in energy density than canned foods, semimoist diets can be fed free-choice to some pets. However, these products dry out and lose appeal when left in a pet's bowl for an extended period of time.

SNACKS AND TREATS

Snacks and treats have become increasingly popular with pet owners in recent years. A survey conducted in 1965 showed that Nabisco's Milk Bones dominated the treat market, and the choice of snacks at that time was extremely limited. However, in less than 20 years, almost every major pet food company began marketing some type of dog or cat snack.[46] This increase can be theorized to reflect some of the changing roles that dogs and cats have had in our society within the last few decades. Pet owners purchase treats not because of their nutritional value but as a way of showing love and affection for their pets. Feeding and caring for a pet is a nurturing process, and giving pets "special" snacks generates the positive feelings that accompany nurturing and the expression of affection. Pet owners also give their dogs treats and snacks as training aids to reinforce desired behaviors, at times of arrival or departure, as a means of providing a sense of variety in the pet's diet, and as an aid to proper dental health.[47]

However, most pet owners buy pet treats for emotional reasons. Therefore palatability to the pet is of chief importance. Owners are less concerned with the nutritional value of a snack than they are with its appearance and palatability. In the early years, all dog treats were in the form of baked biscuits. Over time, different shapes, sizes, and flavors of biscuits were developed and marketed. Because treats are usually impulse buys, owners are more likely to try a new flavor or type of treat than they are to completely switch dog or cat food. To capitalize on this, manufacturers have continued to develop new types of dog and cat snacks. Today, treats can be categorized into four basic types—semimoist, biscuits, jerky, and rawhide products. Cat treats are usually in the form of either semimoist or biscuit products, while rawhides and jerky products are highly palatable to many dogs. Many treats are made to resemble foods that humans normally eat, such as hamburgers, sausage, bacon, cheese, and even ice cream. Examples of several popular treat concepts include snacks that are made with all-natural ingredients, that promote dental health, or that are made from livestock body parts such as ears, hooves, or even noses.

Although treats and snacks do not have to be nutritionally complete, a significant proportion of these products are formulated to be complete and balanced, and some carry the same nutritional label claims as dog and cat foods. In general, treats and snacks are highly palatable and cost significantly more than other types of pet foods when compared on a weight basis. Part of this cost is a reflection of the larger amounts of marketing effort and money directed toward making the product attractive to pet owners.[48] Although some snacks and treats can provide complete nutrition, they are not required to be nutritionally complete and are not intended for this purpose.

BRANDS OF PET FOODS

Popular

Brands of commercial pet foods can be classified into three general categories—popular, premium, and generic. The popular brands include foods that are marketed nationally or regionally and sold in grocery store chains. The companies that produce these foods devote a substantial amount of energy and finances to advertising, which results in a high name recognition of their products. The principal marketing strategies used to sell these products relate to the diet's palatability and its appeal to the pet owner.

Most popular brands are produced using variable formulations. This means that the ingredients included in a particular brand may vary from batch to batch, depending on ingredient availability and the cost to the manufacturer. For example, poultry meal may be the primary protein source in Happy Pal dog food the first time a pet owner purchases a bag. However, because of changes in market prices, the second bag may include lower amounts of poultry meal and higher amounts of other protein sources such as poultry byproduct meal or a cereal grain. When variable formulation is used, the guaranteed analysis panel will not change, but the source and the quality of the ingredients may be altered without notice. This alteration can result in variable product quality and digestibility and may cause gastrointestinal upset in some pets when a new bag of food is fed.

Some of the nationally marketed popular brands carry label claims that are verified through the Association of American Feed Control Officials' (AAFCO's) feeding trials. However, smaller manufacturers that produce and sell foods regionally often use the calculation method to validate label claims (see pp. 166-167). In general, popular brands of pet food tend to have lower digestibilities than most premium brands of foods, but they typically contain higher quality ingredients and have higher digestibilities than do the generic or private-label pet foods. Ingredients, palatability, and digestibility may vary significantly among brands, as well as among different products produced by the same manufacturer.

Premium

The term *premium pet foods* refers to products developed to provide optimal nutrition for dogs and cats during different stages of life. These foods are targeted toward companion animal owners, hobbyists, and professionals who are very involved with their animal's health and nutrition. In general, quality ingredients that are highly digestible and have good to excellent nutrient availability are used in these products.[41] Manufacturers of most premium pet foods formulate and market products for different stages of life and lifestyles. For example, dog foods have been developed for hard-working dogs (performance diets), adult dogs during maintenance, growing dogs of different sizes, and bitches during lactation and gestation. The companies that produce these products provide educational materials about companion animal nutrition and feeding to pet owners and professionals, and their foods are usually only available through pet supply stores, feed stores, or veterinarians.

In contrast to popular brands, most premium brands of pet food are produced using fixed formulations. This means that the manufacturer will not change the ingredients that are used in response to ingredient availability or market price. In addition, most manufacturers of these foods validate their label claims through AAFCO feeding studies as opposed to the calculation method. This validation guarantees the pet owner that the food has been adequately tested through actual feeding studies with animals. Premium pet foods are usually more costly on a weight basis because of the high-quality ingredients that are used and the level of testing that is conducted on the products. However, because these products are usually very digestible and nutrient dense, smaller amounts need to be fed, and the cost per serving is often comparable to many popular brands of pet food.

Generic or Private-Label

Generic pet foods are products that do not carry a brand name. These products are usually produced and marketed locally or regionally. One important consideration of the manufacturers of generic foods is producing a low-cost product. For this reason, inexpensive, poor-quality ingredients may be used, and few, if any, feeding tests are conducted. These products almost exclusively use the calculation method rather than AAFCO feeding trials to validate label claims of nutritional adequacy. Some products have not been formulated to be nutritionally complete and will not even carry a label claim.[44] Feeding studies with dogs have shown that generic products have significantly lower digestibilities and nutrient availabilities than popular and premium brands of food.[44] Poor-quality ingredients and a low fat content result in low palatability. Generic products represent the least expensive and typically the poorest quality of pet foods commercially available to pet owners.

Private-label pet foods are products that carry the house name of the grocery store chain or other store in which they are sold. Like generic pet foods, these products are usually produced on a least-cost basis. The only difference is that private-label foods are produced (or simply packaged and labeled) under a contract with the grocery store whose name they carry. Most are produced by the same companies that make generic products and may be similar in quality to generic pet foods. Private-label foods often claim to be comparable to premium foods, although they sell for a much lower price. As in any industry, "clone" products are marketed that may imitate the name, packaging, bag colors, and/or ingredient lists of premium foods.

Although the low cost may be appealing to some pet owners, there are several problems that may occur with generic and private-label pet foods. Because these foods may be produced using inexpensive ingredients and because minimal testing may be conducted, low nutrient availability can result in a product that is not actually complete and balanced. A study with growing puppies compared the effects of feeding a nationally produced, popular brand of dog food to three price brand (generic and private-label) foods.[49] The puppies that were fed the price brands required between 19% and 40% more food for each lb of body weight gained than those that were fed the national brand. Moreover, at the end of the 10-week growth study, puppies that were fed one of the price brands developed graying of the hair coat and had significantly reduced growth rates when compared with those in the other groups. These puppies also had significantly lower hemoglobin, packed cell, and serum albumin levels than the dogs that were fed the national brand. The graying of the hair coat was presumed by the investigators to be indicative of a deficiency in one or more essential nutrients. Digestibilities of diet DM, crude protein, crude fat, and nitrogen-free extract (an estimate of carbohydrate content) were lower in two of the price brand products as compared to the national brand. Protein digestibility was especially low, indicating that poor-quality protein sources were used and possibly that excessive heat caused damage to dietary protein during processing. Other studies have reported the occurrence of zinc-responsive dermatosis in dogs that were fed generic pet foods.[50,51,52] It is believed that the high proportion of plant products and phytate in generic foods binds dietary zinc, making it unavailable for absorption by the body. The inclusion of poor-quality meat and bone meals containing high amounts of calcium may exacerbate this problem, because high levels of calcium inhibit zinc absorption.[51] Problems with ingredient quality and variability, nutrient balance and availability, and the uncertainty of adequate testing and quality control generally make generic and private-label foods a poor choice for pet owners when selecting a commercial pet food.

HOMEMADE DIETS

Although the majority of pet owners in the United States enjoy the convenience, economy, and reliability of commercially produced pet foods, some owners still prefer to prepare homemade diets for their pets. If a homemade diet is going to be fed, the recipe must be guaranteed to produce a ration that is complete and balanced. One of the problems with preparing homemade pet foods is that many of the recipes that are available have not been adequately tested for nutrient content and availability. Once an adequate recipe is found, the ingredients that are purchased should conform as closely as possible to the recipe and should be consistent between batches of food. Most recipes allow the owner to prepare a relatively large volume at one time and freeze small portions for extended use. Ingredients should never be substituted or eliminated from the recipe because of the danger of imbalancing the ration. Pet owners should also be aware of the dangers of feeding single food items in lieu of a prepared diet. Foods that owners enjoy are not necessarily the most nutritious foods to feed to their pets. Homemade diets can provide adequate nutrition to companion animals provided that a properly formulated recipe is used, the correct ingredients are included, and the recipe is strictly adhered to on a long-term basis.

VETERINARY DIETS

In the past 2 decades, a host of human health claims have become associated with the consumption of certain types of foods, ingredients, and nutrients. Examples include the relationship between fiber consumption and dietary fat intake and certain heart and gastrointestinal health claims. As a direct result of this trend in human foods, companion animal nutritionists and pet food manufacturers have begun to investigate the use of diet and dietary ingredients for the nutritional management of disease conditions in dogs and cats. This has resulted in a rapid increase in the number of therapeutic, or veterinary, diets that are available to veterinarians and pet owners. These foods can be distinguished from pet foods formulated for healthy animals by their mode of sale and the manner in which they are labeled. Specifically, veterinary diets are sold only through veterinary clinics and are labeled for use only under the direction of a veterinarian.[53,54]

Companion animal professionals should critically evaluate any therapeutic diets that they are considering, paying specific attention to the type and quantity of research that supports the clinical benefits. Well-controlled, randomized clinical studies in which the diet was fed to pets with naturally occurring diseases are the most desirable.[55] Results from clinical trials can also be supported by studies performed in a laboratory or kennel setting that uses an appropriate model for the disease in question. In all cases, the diet or dietary component should be demonstrated to provide a realistic level of benefit and an acceptable level of risk to justify its use. Examples of veterinary diets that are currently available to small animal veterinarians include diets for animals recovering from trauma or severe illness, weight-loss formulations, diets for the nutritional management of kidney or gastrointestinal disease, and products for the diagnosis and management of food-induced allergies. As more knowledge is gained concerning the benefits of diet and certain nutrients for companion animal health, additional veterinary diets are expected to become available.

CHAPTER

18

Evaluation of Commercial Pet Foods

The large variety of commercial pet foods produced and sold in the United States can make the selection of a proper diet a complex and confusing process. The information presented earlier in this section illustrates the need for pet owners to critically evaluate a product before feeding it to their pets. Because many pet foods are intended to provide the only source of nutrition for a pet throughout its life, it is extremely important that owners select a product capable of providing optimal nutrition and promoting long-term health. The following chapter provides tools that companion animal owners and professionals can use to evaluate commercial pet foods. These criteria aid in distinguishing between products that are inadequate, acceptable, or optimal in their ability to provide proper nutrition to a companion animal (Box 18-1).

BOX **18-1**

Factors to Consider in the Evaluation of Pet Foods

Complete and balanced nutrition
Palatability
Digestibility
Metabolizable energy (ME) content
Feeding cost
Reputation of manufacturer
Dental health contribution
Taurine content (cats only)
Urine-acidifying ability (cats only)

COMPLETE AND BALANCED

The phrase "complete and balanced" means that a food contains all of the essential nutrients at levels that meet a pet's requirements. Because animals eat or are fed to meet their energy requirements, nutrient levels in the diet must be balanced so that when an animal meets its caloric needs, its requirements for all other nutrients are fulfilled at the same time. The regulations of the Association of American Feed Control Officials (AAFCO) allow pet food manufacturers to include the complete and balanced claim on their label if they have substantiated it through one of two possible methods. Option one requires that the pet food be successfully evaluated through a series of AAFCO-sanctioned animal feeding trials. Option two requires only that the food is formulated to meet the minimum and maximum levels of nutrients established by the AAFCO's *Nutrient Profiles* for dog and cat foods (see pp. 157-158). It is a common misconception that every pet food that carries the complete and balanced label claim has been proven to provide optimum nutrition through rigorous animal testing.[56] A pet food that has only been formulated on paper to meet the AAFCO's standards (option two) may not actually be complete and balanced when fed. Animal testing of pet foods is currently the best way to assess nutrient availability. These tests are capable of detecting problems and inadequacies in products that could not be detected when only chemical analysis or calculations are used.[57]

The first criterion that a pet owner should use when evaluating a food is a check for the complete and balanced claim. The life stages of the claim should correspond to the owner's intended use for the food (i.e., for adult maintenance, for all life stages, for performance). Pet food manufacturers are currently required to include the method of substantiation that was used for the complete and balanced claim on the pet food label. If a statement that AAFCO feeding trials were conducted is included, this means that the food was adequately tested through feeding trials with dogs and cats. However, if the statement merely claims that the food meets the AAFCO's *Nutrient Profiles,* this signifies that AAFCO feeding tests were not conducted. In these cases, the owner has no way of knowing whether or not the pet food in question has been adequately tested through feeding trials before it was marketed. Pet owners can contact the manufacturer directly and request information regarding the type of testing that has been conducted on the product. If the manufacturer does not support the complete and balanced claim through feeding trials that measure the long-term effects of feeding the food, then a product may not be adequate for long-term feeding.

PALATABILITY

The palatability and acceptability of a pet food are important because a food must be acceptable to the pet in order for it to provide optimum nutrition. A pet's daily intake of essential nutrients is the product of the quantity of food eaten and the concentration of available nutrients in the food. Because of this relationship, the amount of food that is eaten is as important as the food's nutrient and energy content. An unpalatable food will be rejected by a dog or cat regardless of the level or balance of nutrients that it contains. Similarly, a diet can be palatable but still not contain adequate levels of some nutrients. Contrary to popular belief, dogs and cats are not capable of detecting nutrient deficiencies or imbalances in their diets. Companion animals will continue to consume an imbalanced diet until the physiological effects of nutrient deficiencies or excesses cause illness or a reduction in food intake.

Palatability is defined in the pet food industry by the manner in which it is tested. The measure that is used is food intake, which is based upon the assumption that a greater intake of one food over another is an indication of higher palatability.[58] A particular food will be ranked higher in palatability than a second food if a greater volume of the first food is eaten by test animals.[59] Therefore palatability should not be considered to be an intrinsic property of the food, but rather a property of an animal's perception of the food and the tendency to select one particular food over another. Several factors have been shown to be important in determining food selection in dogs and cats. The primary senses that are involved are olfaction, taste, and touch.

The odor of a food is used by animals for the selection of acceptable foods and the rejection of dangerous or toxic foods. In dogs and cats, odor is very important in food selection, and feeding behavior can be altered by a food's smell alone.[60] This is due to the highly developed olfactory acuity of dogs and cats.[61] Smell is probably intrinsically linked to taste, which is the second important sense for food selection. The most abundant taste units on the tongues of dogs and cats are those that are sensitive to amino acids. These units are sensitive to specific groups of amino acids, and interestingly, some amino acids that are inhibitory in the cat tend to be either neutral or stimulating in dogs.[62] This preponderance of amino acid taste "buds," or units, in the mouths of dogs and cats may be explained by their carnivorous nature, which allows them to distinguish between meats of varying sources and qualities. Other differences between dogs and cats are seen in their preference for sweet foods. While dogs are capable of detecting simple sugars and many show a distinct preference for sweet foods, cats do not respond to simple sugars.[63] It has been speculated that this may reflect the strictly carnivorous diet of the cat and their lack of selective pressure for a need to detect plant foods. Although smell and taste are the primary senses used in food selection, dogs and cats also react to a food's shape and texture.

Food preferences of individual dogs and cats probably develop from a combination of genetic predisposition and experience. In palatability testing, individual experiences become important because dogs and cats may be very accepting of flavors or textures that they have been previously exposed to and may reject foods that are novel or have been associated with a negative experience. These factors have a strong influence on the results of palatability tests and are complicated by the fact that there are conflicting data concerning the effect of early learning on food preferences in dogs and cats. Early studies reported that limiting flavor experiences at an early age in puppies and kittens led to fixed food habits in which all novel foods were rejected.[64] When puppies and kittens were provided with foods of varying flavors and textures early in life, they showed an enhanced acceptance of novel food items. These results are in conflict with more recent work that found when puppies were fed a single type of canned diet from 7 to 16 weeks of age, they preferred a novel food to their normal diet.[60,65] Another study concluded that the two most important factors in food selection in young puppies were palatability and novelty.[66] It appears that both a pet's age and the duration of exposure to a singular food item or a variety of foods is important in determining a pet's reaction to novel foods.[58]

Several pet food properties directly affect palatability and food choice in dogs and cats.[67] The quality of ingredients and the way that they are cooked, processed, and stored significantly affects palatability. For example, grains and the starches they contain provide a desirable texture to dry pet foods when properly extruded and stored. However, grains will be perceived as highly unacceptable if mold growth has occurred or if the product has not been properly extruded. Poorly extruded starches cause food particles to have high bulk densities, which negatively affect the texture and chewiness of the product. Poorly processed or poorly stored foods may also contain high levels of oxidized oils and fats. The aldehydes produced by fat oxidation are highly unpalatable. Overprocessing of protein or the inclusion of poor-quality protein sources in a pet food can lead to byproducts that are perceived as unpalatable. Finally, the form and size of the food particles are important, especially to cats.

Because of the marketing value of highly palatable foods, most of the products currently sold are highly acceptable to pets. However, low-quality products may have decreased palatability as a result of the inclusion of poor-quality ingredients or harsh processing methods. Although not the only factors involved, proper processing, handling, and storage of pet foods containing high-quality ingredients contribute to a food's acceptability and palatability. Once an acceptable degree of palatability has been met, however, the owner must evaluate other diet characteristics that are important for the delivery of optimal nutrition. Because most commercial pet foods available today are very palatable to dogs and cats, problems of overconsumption and weight gain are much more common than are problems of diet rejection. Although palatability is important, it should not be used as the sole criterion when evaluating a food and should not be considered an indication of the food's nutritional adequacy.

DIGESTIBILITY

The digestibility of a pet food is an important criterion because it directly measures the proportion of nutrients in the food that are available for absorption. True and apparent digestibility can only be measured through controlled feeding trials (see pp. 167-168). The results of these trials provide digestibility coefficients for the food's dry matter (DM), crude protein, crude fat, and nitrogen-free extract (NFE), which is a measure of the carbohydrate fraction in a food. Studies of popular brands of dog foods report that the average digestibility coefficients for crude protein, crude fat, and NFE are 81%, 85%, and 79%, respectively.[68] A similar study with cats reports that popular brands of commercial cat foods have average digestibility coefficients of 78%, 77%, and 69% for crude protein, crude fat, and NFE, respectively. Premium pet foods usually have slightly higher digestibility coefficients than these values, and generic products have substantially lower digestibilities.[41,49] Digestibilities as high as 89%, 95%, and 88% for crude protein, crude fat, and carbohydrate, respectively, can occur in dry-type premium pet foods. In general, the ingredients used in pet foods are lower in digestibility than those in most foods consumed by humans. As the quality of ingredients included in the food increases, so will the food's DM and nutrient digestibility.

A pet food that is low in digestibility contains a high proportion of ingredients that cannot be digested by the enzymes of the gastrointestinal tract. These components pass through to the large intestine, where they are partially or completely fermented by colonic bacteria. Rapid or excessive bacterial fermentation leads to the production of gas (flatulence), loose stools, and (occasionally) diarrhea. In addition to these side effects, a greater quantity of a poorly digested food must be fed to the animal because the pet is absorbing a smaller proportion of nutrients from the feed. As the quantity of food that is consumed increases, rate of passage through the gastrointestinal tract also increases. A more rapid passage of food through the intestines further contributes to poor digestibility, high stool volume, and gas production. A pet food's digestibility is decreased by the presence of high levels of dietary fiber, ash, phytate, and poor-quality protein. Improper processing or excessive heat treatment can also adversely affect digestibility. In contrast, pet food digestibility is increased by the inclusion of high-quality ingredients and increased levels of fat, as well as the use of proper processing techniques.

In general, dogs and cats digest foods of animal origin better than those of plant origin. This difference is primarily the result of the presence of lignin, cellulose, and other components of fiber in plant ingredients. However, it is important for owners and professionals to recognize that low-quality animal products containing high amounts of skin, hair, feathers, and connective tissue are also not well digested by dogs and cats. Although a pet food that contains high-quality animal products has a higher digestibility than a plant-based food, pet foods that contain poor-quality animal ingredients may have lower digestibilities than plant-based products with similar nutrient profiles.[21]

Several studies have shown that the apparent digestibilities of the major organic nutrients in commercial pet foods are significantly higher for dogs than for cats.[24,69] Both the dog and the cat belong to the order Carnivora and are classified as simple-stomached carnivores. The cat is a very strict carnivore, but the dog is more omnivorous in nature. This difference is reflected in the abilities of the two species to digest certain types of dietary components. A study comparing the digestive capabilities of dogs and cats found that when fed the same dog or cat food, dogs had higher apparent digestibility coefficients and obtained more digestible nutrients per unit of food eaten than cats for almost all nutrients and types of foods.[69] It was suggested that some of these differences could be explained by a greater ability of the dog to digest dietary fiber. Recent data from studies of the fermentative capacities of canine and feline colonic microflora indicate that while both dogs and cats are capable of fermenting certain types of fiber, the cat is less tolerant of wide ranges of fiber fermentability than the dog.[70,71,72,73]

Regardless of differences in the digestive capabilities of dogs and cats, it is important to be aware that commercial pet foods can differ significantly in digestibility and nutrient availability. The labels of two products may have the same ingredient lists and guaranteed analysis panels, but when the products are fed, they may have different digestibilities. This variability will directly affect the ability of each diet to provide adequate levels of nutrients to an animal. A greater quantity of a poorly digested diet must be fed to an animal in order to meet its nutrient requirements. This fact is illustrated by a study with growing dogs that compared two commercial dry dog foods (R1 and R2) using feeding trials that followed the AAFCO feeding test protocols.[74] Chemical analysis of the two diets showed that they contained identical levels of nutrients. However, when fed to a group of dogs, the effect of each diet on growth and development was significantly different. Dogs that were fed the R2 diet grew significantly less and ate less food than did the R1-fed dogs. The R2-fed dogs became anorexic, had significantly lower body weights and body lengths, and showed poor coat quality and graying of the hair coat. These dogs also had depressed hemoglobin and hematocrit values and lower serum cholesterol, alkaline phosphatase, calcium, and phosphorus levels. The authors of the study concluded that the R2 diet had a lower palatability and that its nutrients were less available than those in the R1 diet. Subsequent digestibility trials found that the R2 diet was 18% lower in apparent digestibility than diet R1. In another study, digestibility trials of four commercial dog foods with identical guaranteed analysis panels showed that the national brand of food had a significantly higher digestibility than did the three price brands that were examined.[49] It is important to note that in both of these studies the analytical values obtained through chemical analysis provided no information that would indicate differences in the digestibility of the foods.

Currently, AAFCO regulations do not allow pet food manufacturers to include quantitative or comparative digestibility claims on their labels.[12] This information can only be obtained by actually feeding the food. Some pet food companies include digestibility data with the literature that they provide about their foods. Many manufacturers of premium brands of foods include this information with the educational materials they give to the retailers, pet supply stores, and veterinarians who sell their foods. However, most popular brands of pet food that are sold through grocery store chains do not provide information regarding digestibility. If digestibility information is not readily available, this information may be obtained by writing or calling the company directly. Pet owners should choose foods that have a DM digestibility of 80% or greater and should reject any foods that have digestibilities lower than 75%.

Buying a package of pet food and actually feeding it to a pet can also provide valuable information about a food's digestibility. A product that is highly digestible will produce low stool volumes and well-formed, firm feces. In addition, the fecal matter will not contain mucus, blood, or any recognizable components of the pet

TABLE **18-1**

Determination of Cost Per Serving

	ME Requirement		Kcal/kg		Quantity/Day	Price/kg	Price/lb	Cost/Day
Diet A	4500	÷	4500	=	1 kg (2.2 lb)	28 ¢	12.7 ¢	28 ¢
Diet B	4500	÷	3600	=	1.25 kg (2.75 lb)	25 ¢	11.4 ¢	31 ¢

food. Defecation frequency should be relatively low, and bowel movements should be regular and consistent. Normal growth rates and body weight should be easily maintained by the food without the need to feed excessive quantities, and long-term feeding should result in healthy skin and hair coat. Although these observations do not provide quantitative information about digestibility, they are a reasonably accurate measure of a diet's ability to supply absorbable nutrients to a companion animal.

METABOLIZABLE ENERGY CONTENT

The ME of a pet food represents the amount of energy that is available for an animal for use (see pp. 169-170). The energy density of pet foods is typically expressed as kilocalories (kcal) of ME per unit weight (kilogram [kg] or pound [lb]). ME can be determined either through feeding trials or, less accurately, through calculation using standard energy values for protein, carbohydrate, and fat (see Section 1, pp. 4-8).

Energy density should be considered when evaluating a pet food because it will directly affect the quantity of food that must be fed to meet the pet's energy requirement. For example, two dry dog foods that are advertised as performance diets for working dogs have ME values of 4500 kcal/kg (diet A) and 3600 kcal/kg (diet B). If a sled dog that is training in mild weather conditions requires 4500 kcal/day, it will need to consume 1 kg of diet A or 1.25 kg of diet B (Table 18-1). The consumption of 25% more of diet B is necessary to meet this dog's daily caloric requirement. Hard-working dogs and lactating bitches and queens all have high energy requirements. These requirements are often best met by feeding a food that is relatively high in energy and nutrient density. On the other hand, a diet with a lower energy density facilitates weight maintenance in adult pets that lead sedentary lifestyles. However, if the ME content of a pet food is too low, the quantity of food that the pet needs to eat in order to meet its requirement may exceed the physical capacity of the gastrointestinal tract. The consumption of an excessive quantity of food leads to increased rate of passage through the gastrointestinal tract and decreased digestibility. In general, pet owners should select a pet food that contains between 3000 and 5000 kcal/kg on a dry-matter basis (DMB), depending on the needs of the animal.

Before 1994, AAFCO regulations prohibited the inclusion of statements of caloric density on pet food labels. But in 1994 the AAFCO passed a regulation allowing voluntary label claims of ME content. This new regulation requires companies that include ME claims to substantiate the ME content through either a calculation method using modified Atwater factors or through data collected from a series of digestibility trials with animals. As in the case of the complete and balanced claim, the method that the company uses to substantiate the ME claim must be stated (see pp. 156-158). In addition to knowing the caloric density of the pet food, it is also helpful for pet owners to know the relative energy contributions that are provided by the carbohydrate, protein, and fat in the diet. The dietary proportion of fat should be higher for hard-working animals and lower for sedentary adult or elderly animals. Similarly, the proportion of calories supplied by soluble carbohydrate should be increased in diets that are intended for adult maintenance or for elderly animals.

FEEDING COST

As the quality of the ingredients included in a pet food increases, so does the cost to the manufacturer. Therefore, as a product's quality increases, so does its price per unit weight. When making price comparisons between foods, it is important to consider the cost of actually feeding the food as opposed to the cost per unit weight. The cost per serving of a high-quality product is often equal to or lower than that of an inferior product because a smaller quantity of the high-quality pet food is fed. Using the previous example, the price of diet A is $25 for a 40-lb bag and the price of diet B is $22 for a 40-lb bag. Although a bag of diet A is actually more expensive than that of diet B, the cost of feeding diet B is higher because of its lower energy density (see Table 18-1). When evaluating a food for the first time, owners can record the purchase date and the price of the food. When the package is empty, dividing the cost of the product by the number of days that the bag lasted provides the cost per day to feed that particular food. A second product with the same net weight can then be compared in the same manner.

REPUTATION OF THE MANUFACTURER

The reputation of the pet food manufacturer should always be considered when selecting a pet food. Companies that have a national reputation for producing consistent, high-quality products and devoting resources to consumer education about proper nutrition for companion animals should be selected. The inclusion of a toll-free phone number on the product's package indicates a company that welcomes inquiries about their products. In addition, the manufacturer's response to all inquiries should be timely, thorough, and direct. A pet food manufacturer should be expected to readily supply information about the pet food's ingredients, level of testing, digestibility data, ME content, and nutrient content. Pet food manufacturers that produce quality products are concerned with their reputations and with serving the needs and concerns of the pet owners who buy their pet foods. This concern will be evidenced by the company's accessibility to consumers and their response to questions about their products.

OTHER FACTORS

Several other factors may be considered when evaluating commercial pet foods. A cat food's taurine content should be assessed. The availability of taurine in a diet is influenced by a number of factors, including other nutrients and the type of processing that is used. Therefore the adequacy of the taurine level of a diet can only be assessed through actual feeding trials. Pet food manufacturers should be able to show that their product will maintain normal blood taurine levels in cats when it is fed on a long-term basis. Whole blood taurine should be maintained in adult cats at a level of 250 nanomole per milliliter (ml) or greater.[57,75] Generally, extruded dry foods that contain greater than 1000 mg/kg and canned cat foods that contain greater than 2000 to 2500 mg/kg on a DMB are adequate.[57,76]

Cat foods also should be evaluated with regard to their ability to produce an acidified urine. A urinary pH of 7 or higher is currently believed to be an important risk factor for the development of struvite-induced feline urolithiasis.[77] Feeding a diet that maintains a urinary pH between 6 and 6.8 when fed ad libitum inhibits the development of the struvite crystals that may cause this disorder. However, a diet that produces an overly acidified urine (less than 6) can put the cat at risk of metabolic acidosis and skeletal decalcification. Pet owners should select a diet that has been shown (through feeding trials) to produce a urine pH of between 6 and 6.8. Although magnesium was once implicated as an important risk factor for struvite urolithiasis, it is now known that magnesium levels in the diet only become significant when urinary pH is maintained at too high a level.[75,77] However, it is still wise to avoid products that have magnesium contents greater than 0.1% of the diet's DM. Currently, pet food manufacturers in the United States are not allowed to include information about urinary pH on the cat food label. This information can be obtained through educational literature produced by the company or by contacting the manufacturer directly.

Another factor that may be assessed is a pet food's ability to contribute to dental health in dogs and cats. It has been speculated that dry pet foods and hard biscuits may contribute to dental health because the abrasion involved in chewing reduces plaque and calculus formation (see Section 6, pp. 481-482).[78] In addition, there are numerous oral chewing devices available that are designed to improve dogs' dental health or maintain healthy gingivae. Most research indicates that diet alone is unable to maintain clinically healthy gingivae or prevent periodontal disease in the absence of regular tooth-brushing and other types of oral cleansing.[79,80] Although dry pet foods and the feeding of hard biscuits as treats may contribute to dental health and reduce calculus formation, feeding dry pet food should not be considered an alternative to regular dental care and teeth cleaning.[78]

The overall best judge of a commercial pet food is the animal itself. Once a pet food has been evaluated and selected, pet owners should feed the product for a minimum of 2 months before evaluating its total effect on their pet's health. A diet that provides good nutrition and adequate energy supports normal weight gain or weight maintenance, healthy skin, a shiny and healthy coat, normal fecal volume and consistency, and overall vitality in the pet. Signs of a poor diet include weight loss or poor growth, poor coat quality, the development of skin problems, and a lack of vigor. Whenever any of these signs are observed, a thorough examination by a veterinarian should be conducted. Although changing the diet may be warranted, other medical causes of these problems should always be investigated.

SECTION 3

KEY POINTS

- The pet food industry has grown tremendously since commercial pet foods were introduced in the United States in the early 1900s. In 1996, pet food retail sales amounted to $11.5 billion, and today there are over 300 companies producing more than 3000 brands of pet food. It is easy to see how choosing a proper diet for a pet can be confusing!

- There are numerous agencies involved in the pet food industry. These agencies have various roles. Some have regulatory authority, and others have advisory responsibility (see Table 14-1).

- Statements and claims made on pet food labels, and even the name of the food itself, are regulated by the Association of American Feed Control Officials (AAFCO). For example, AAFCO requires that such claims as "complete and balanced nutrition for all stages of life" must be substantiated either through feeding trials or by formulating the food to meet the AAFCO's *Nutrient Profiles* for dog and cat foods. If a product uses a flavor in its name (e.g., "Beefy Stew"), that flavor must have been detected by a recognized testing method.

- When looking at the pet food label, most consumers first read the guaranteed analysis panel. Here manufacturers report the *minimum percentages* of crude protein and crude fat and the *maximum percentages* of moisture and crude fiber. Consumers should be aware that these percentages do not represent actual amounts of protein and fat and that using these percentages to compare different products or brands can be misleading.

- The ingredient list can tell consumers the principal components of the pet food and whether the components are from plant or animal sources. If an animal-source ingredient is listed first or second in a canned pet food or within the first three ingredients of a dry food, the food can usually be assumed to contain animal products as its principal protein source. However, the ingredient list does not provide information about the quality of the ingredients.

- **Tip:** If different forms of the same ingredient are listed separately (e.g., kibbled wheat, ground wheat, wheat flour, flaked wheat, wheat middlings, wheat bran), consumers should be aware that the collective "wheat" content may be very high and actually make up a large percentage of the food's content.

- **Caveat emptor:** Purchasing a low-cost pet food may seem economically practical, but low-cost pet foods usually contain low-quality, less-digestible ingredients. Therefore more food must be fed to an animal to provide adequate nutrition than if the animal was being fed a high-quality, highly digestible food with greater nutrient availability. Thus the per-meal cost of the inexpensive food may be higher. Also, companies producing low-cost pet foods generally do not test the foods using AAFCO feeding protocols. Remember, buyers usually "get what they pay for."

- **Tip:** Additional information about the nutrient content of high-quality pet foods can be found in pamphlets obtained from the pet supply store or veterinarian where the food was purchased, or it can be obtained directly from the manufacturer. Reputable manufacturers will readily supply information, and many have toll-free telephone numbers listed on the package.

- Dry dog foods are the most common type of pet food purchased by consumers in the United States. Dry foods are economical and easy to store and feed, and they may be beneficial to dental hygiene. High-quality dry foods have high nutrient densities and digestibilities, meaning that less food can be fed, more nutrients will be absorbed and used, and stool volume will decrease.

- **Tip:** There are two primary types of canned pet foods—those that provide complete and balanced nutrition and those that do not. Complete and balanced canned foods contain vitamins and minerals in addition to muscle meats, poultry or fish byproducts, cereal grains, and/or texturized vegetable protein (TVP). Foods that are not complete and balanced do not contain all the necessary vitamins and minerals and should be considered as a dietary supplement only. Consumers should make sure they read the labels to determine if a canned food is complete and balanced for a pet's life stage and lifestyle.

- **Caution:** Feeding cats one type of "gourmet" cat food exclusively may result in the cat's refusal to eat any other type or flavor of food. Because these "gourmet" foods may or may not be nutritionally complete, nutrient imbalances may occur. When feeding a cat canned food, complete and balanced rations that contain more than one principal ingredient should be fed.

- Although generic or private-label (store brand) foods may appeal to pet owners because of their low cost, owners are cautioned that the cost is a reflection of the inexpensive, low-quality ingredients used and the lack of feed-trial testing. For example, one study comparing the effects of feeding generic and private-label foods versus a nationally produced popular brand to puppies showed that the puppies fed the generic and private label foods had graying of the hair coat and significantly reduced growth rates, as well as significant abnormalities of some blood values.

- Digestibility represents the proportion of nutrients in a food that is available for absorption into an animal's body. Commercial pet foods can differ significantly in digestibility and nutrient availability, even if two products have the same ingredient lists and guaranteed analysis panels.

SECTION 3

REFERENCES

1. Enterline WR: The production of extruded pet foods, *Pet Food Ind*, 26-30, July/Aug 1986.
2. Harlow J: US pet food trends. In *Proceedings of the Petfood Forum*, Chicago, 1997, Watts Publishing.
3. Phillips T: Top ten retail US pet food sales, *Pet Food Ind*, 4-8, Jan/Feb 1990.
4. Lazar V: Dog food history, *Pet Food Ind*, 40-44, Sept/Oct 1990.
5. Deshmukh AR: Regulatory aspects of pet foods, *Vet Clin Nutr* 3:4-9, 1996.
6. Phillips T: NRC profile, *Pet Food Ind*, 10-18, Mar/Apr 1992.
7. AAFCO pet food regulatory update. In *Proceedings of the Petfood Forum*, Chicago, 1997, Watts Publishing.
8. Dzanis DA: Regulatory update. In *Proceedings of the Petfood Forum*, Chicago, 1996, Watts Publishing.
9. Van Soest PJ: The uniformity and nutritive availability of cellulose, *Fed Proc* 32:1804-1808, 1973.
10. Burger IH, Blaza SE: Digestion, absorption and dietary balance. In *Dog and cat nutrition*, ed 2, Oxford, England, 1988.
11. Zimmerman J: How to do your own label review. In *Proceedings of the Petfood Forum*, Chicago, 1995, Watts Publishing.
12. Association of American Feed Control Officials: Pet food regulations. In *AAFCO official publication*, Atlanta, 1998, The Association of Feed Control Officials.
13. Lewis LD, Morris ML, Hand MS: Pet foods. In *Small animal clinical nutrition*, ed 3, Topeka, Kan, 1987, Mark Morris Association.
14. Weigel J: Changing values: reference vs. actual. In *Proceedings of the Petfood Forum*, Chicago, 1996, Watts Publishing.
15. Whitlock L: Ingredient changes: understanding the impact on your products. In *Proceedings of the Petfood Forum*, Chicago, 1995, Watts Publishing.
16. Wiernusz CJ, Shields RG, Van Vlierbergen DJ, and others: Canine nutrient digestibility and stool quality evaluation of canned diets containing various soy protein supplements, *Vet Clin Nutr* 2:49-56, 1995.
17. Bisset SA, Guilford WG, Lawoko CR, and others: Effect of food particle size on carbohydrate assimilation assessed by breath hydrogen testing in dogs, *Vet Clin Nutr* 4:82-88, 1997.
18. Wang X: *Effect of processing methods and raw material sources on protein quality of animal protein meals* (PhD thesis), Urbana, Ill, 1996, University of Ilinois.
19. Shields RG, Kigin PD, Izquierdo JA, and others: Counting calories: caloric claims—measuring digestibility and metabolizable energy, *Pet Food Ind*, 4-10, Jan/Feb 1994.
20. Fahey G, Hussein SH: The nutritional value of alternative raw materials used in petfoods. In *Proceedings of the Petfood Forum*, Chicago, 1997, Watts Publishing.
21. Case L, Czarnecki GL: Protein requirements of growing pups fed practical dry-type diets containing mixed-protein sources, *Am J Vet Res* 51:808-812, 1990.
22. Hill R: Soy in petfoods: myth vs. fact. In *Proceedings of the Petfood Forum*, Chicago, 1995, Watts Publishing.
23. Kendall PT, Holme DW: Studies on the digestibility of soya bean products, cereal, cereal and plant by-products in diets of dogs, *J Sci Food Agric* 33:813-820, 1982.
24. Kendall PT: Comparable evaluation of apparent digestibility in dogs and cats, *Proc Nutr Soc* 40:45a, 1981.
25. Hickman MA, Bruss MA, Morris JG, and others: Dietary protein source (soybean vs. casein) and taurine status affects kinetics of the enterohepatic circulation of taurocholic acid in cats, *J Nutr* 122:1019-1026, 1992.

26. Zuo Y, Fahey GC Jr, Merchen NR, and others: Digestion response to low oligosaccharide soybean meal by ileal cannulated dogs, *J Anim Sci* 74:2441- 2449, 1996.

27. Kunkle GA: Zinc-responsive dermatoses in dogs. In Kirk RW, editor: *Current veterinary therapy VII*, Philadelphia, 1980, WB Saunders.

28. Adams CR: Stability of vitamins in processed dog food, *Pet Food Ind*, 20-21, Jan/Feb 1981.

29. Papas AM: Antioxidants: which ones are best for your pet food products?, *Pet Food Ind*, 8-16, May/June 1991.

30. Shermer WD: Effective use of antioxidants: optimizing ingredient quality. In *Proceedings of the Petfood Forum*, Chicago, 1995, Watts Publishing.

31. Hilton JW: Antioxidants: function, types and necessity of inclusion in pet foods, *Can Vet J* 30:682-684, 1989.

32. Dziezak D: Preservatives: antioxidants—the ultimate answer to oxidation, *Food Tech* 9:94-102, 1986.

33. Coelho M, Parr J: The benefits of antioxidants. In *Proceedings of the Petfood Forum*, Chicago, 1996, Watts Publishing.

34. Reynhout GS, Berdahl DR: Natural antioxidant systems—experiences in the human food industry. In *Proceedings of the Petfood Forum*, Chicago, 1997, Watts Publishing.

35. Packer JE, Slater TF, Willson RL: Direct observation of a free radical interaction between vitamin E and vitamin C, *Nature* 278:737-738, 1979.

36. Coelho M: Ethoxyquin: science vs marketing, *Petfood Ind*, Sept/Oct 1995.

37. Dzanis DA: Safety of ethoxyquin in dog foods, *J Nutr* 121:S163-164, 1991.

38. Monsanto Chemical Company: *A five-year chronic toxicity study in dogs with santoquin: report to FDA*, 1964.

39. Monsanto Chemical Company: *Ethoxyquin backgrounder*, Dec 1996.

40. Samuelson AC, Cutter GR: Dog biscuits: an aid in canine tartar control, *J Nutr* 121:S162, 1991.

41. Kallfelz FA: Evaluation and use of pet foods: general considerations in using pet foods for adult maintenance, *Vet Clin North Am Small Anim Pract* 19:387-403, 1989.

42. Munson TO, Holzworth J, Small E, and others: Steatitis ("yellow fat") in cats fed canned red tuna, *J Am Vet Med Assoc* 133:563-568, 1958.

43. Griffiths RC, Thornton GW, Willson JE: Pansteatitis (yellow fat) in cats, *J Am Vet Med Assoc* 137:126-128, 1960.

44. Bartoshuk LM, Harned MA, Parks LTD: Taste of water in the cat: effect of sucrose preference, *Science* 171:699-701, 1971.

45. Houpt KA, Smith SL: Taste preferences and their relation to obesity in dogs and cats, *Can Vet J* 22:77-81, 1981.

46. Willard TR: Treats and new products, *Pet Food Ind*, 18-24, Sept/Oct 1984.

47. Morgan T: Treat trends, *Pet Food Ind*, 32-37, Sept/Oct 1997.

48. Lazarus C: Resealable treats, *Pet Food Ind*, 8-12, Nov/Dec 1996.

49. Huber TL, Wilson RC, McGarity SA: Variations in digestibility of dry dog foods with identical label guaranteed analysis, *J Am Anim Hosp Assoc* 22:571-575, 1986.

50. Miller WH Jr: Nutritional considerations in small animal dermatology. *Vet Clin North Am Small Anim Pract* 19:497-511, 1989.

51. Wolf AM: Zinc-responsive dermatosis in a Rhodesian Ridgeback, *Vet Med* 82:908-912, 1987.

52. Sousa CA, Stannard AA, Ihrke PJ, and others: Dermatosis associated with feeding generic dog food: 13 cases (1981–1982). *J Am Vet Med Assoc* 192:676-680, 1988.

53. Dzanis DA: When pet foods are drugs, *FDA Vet* 8:4-5, 1993.

54. Kronfeld DS: Health claims for pet foods: particulars, *J Am Vet Med Assoc* 205:174-177, 1994.

55. Polzin DJ: Good science: how do you know if a dietary recommendation is sound?, *Pet Food Ind*, 11-14, Nov/Dec 1996.

56. Dzanis DA: Complete and balanced? Substantiating the nutritional adequacy of pet foods: past, present and future, *Petfood Ind*, 22-27, July/Aug 1997.

57. Morris JG, Rogers QR: Evaluation of commercial pet foods, *Tijdschr Diergeneesk* 1:67S-70S, 1991.

58. Thorne CJ: Behaviour and palatability testing. In *Proceedings of the Petfood Forum*, Chicago, 1997, Watts Publishing.

59. Morris JG: The effect of nutrient content on dietary choice. In *Proceedings of the Petfood Forum*, Chicago, 1997, Watts Publishing.

60. Mugford RA: External influences on the feeding of carnivores. In Kare MR, Maller O, editors: *The chemical senses and nutrition*, New York, 1977, Academic Press.

61. Dodd GH, Squirre DH: Structure and mechanism in the mammalian olfactory system, *Symp Zoo Soc London* 45:35-36, 1980.

62. Boudreau JC, Sivakuma L, Do LT, and others: Neurophysiology of geniculate ganglion (facial nerve) taste systems: species comparisons, *Chem Senses* 10:89-127, 1985.

63. Beauchamp GA, Maller O, Rogers JG: Flavor preferences in cats: effects on sucrose preference, *Science* 171:699-701, 1977.

64. Kuo ZY: *The dynamics of behaviour development: an epigenetic view*, New York, 1967, Random House.

65. Mugford RA: Comparative and developmental studies of feeding in dogs and cats, *Brit Vet J* 133:98, 1977.

66. Ferrel F: Effects of restricted dietary flavour experience before weaning on postweaning food preferences in puppies, *Neurosci Biobehav Rev* 8:191-198, 1984.

67. Kestrel-Rickert D: What constitutes palatability?. In *Proceedings of the Petfood Forum*, Chicago, 1995, Watts Publishing.

68. Kendall PT, Holme DW, Smith PM: Methods of prediction of the digestible energy content of dog foods from gross energy value, proximate analysis and digestible nutrient content, *J Sci Food Ag* 3:823-828, 1982.

69. Kendall PT, Holme DW, Smith PM: Comparative evaluation of net digestive and absorptive efficiency in dogs and cats fed a variety of contrasting diet types, *J Small Anim Pract* 23:577-587, 1982.

70. Sunvold GD, Fahey GC Jr, Merchen NR, and others: Dietary fiber for cats: in vitro fermentation of selected fiber sources by cat fecal inoculum and in vivo utilization of diets containing selected fiber sources and their blends, *J Anim Sci* 73:2329-2339, 1995.

71. Sunvold GD, Titgemeyer EC, Bourquin LD, and others: Fermentability of selected fibrous substrates by cat faecal microflora, *J Nutr* 2721S-2722S, 1994.

72. Sunvold GD, Fahey GC Jr, Merchen NR, and others: Dietary fiber for dogs. IV. In vitro fermentation of selected fiber sources by dog fecal inoculum and in vivo digestion and metabolism of fiber-supplemented diets, *J Anim Sci* 73:1099-1109, 1995.

73. Visek WJ, Robertson JB: Dried brewer's grains in dog diets, *Proc Cornell Nutr Conf*, 40-49, 1977.

74. Sheffy BE: The 1985 revision of the National Research Council nutrient requirements of dogs and its impact on the pet food industry. In Burger IH, Rivers IPW, editors: *Nutrition of the dog and cat*, New York, 1989, Cambridge University Press.

75. Pet Food Industry: DVM recommendations: does your cat food earn them?, *Pet Food Ind*, 4, July/Aug 1990.

76. Morris JG, Rogers QR: Why is the nutrition of cats different from that of dogs?, *Tijdschr Diergeneesk* 1:64S–67S, 1991.

77. Tarttelin MF: Feline struvite urolithiasis: factors affecting urine pH may be more important than magnesium levels in food, *Vet Rec* 121:227-230, 1987.

78. Jensen L, Logan E, Finney O, and others: Reduction in accumulation of plaque, stain, and calculus in dogs by dietary means, *J Vet Dent* 12:161-163, 1996.

79. Gorrel C, Rawlings JM: The role of tooth brushing and diet in the maintenance of periodontal health in dogs, *J Vet Dent* 13:139-143, 1996.

80. Rawlings JM, Gorrel C, Markwell PJ: Effect of two dietary regimens on gingivitis in the dog, *J Small Anim Pract* 38:147-151, 1997.

4

FEEDING MANAGEMENT THROUGHOUT THE LIFE CYCLE

The previous sections have examined basic nutritional principles, the nutrient requirements of dogs and cats, and the different types of diets that can be fed to companion animals. Although knowledge of nutrient requirements and pet foods is essential, an understanding of feeding methods, feeding behavior, and dietary management is also necessary for the provision of optimal nutrition and care. The following section provides practical guidelines for feeding healthy dogs and cats throughout all stages of life. Proper dietary management and care that begins at birth and continues throughout life supports optimal health and vitality in companion animals and ultimately contributes to a quality life and a rewarding human/companion animal relationship.

This section examines feeding management for each stage of life and for different levels of physical activity. Guidelines are provided that help pet owners to properly select the best food for their particular dog or cat during each stage of life.

These recommendations provide a starting point for feeding dogs and cats. However, it is important to remember that every dog and cat is an individual. For example, two adult animals of the same breed, age, and relative size in the same household may have significantly different energy and nutrient needs. Pet owners should use general guidelines coupled with regular assessments of their pet's weight, health status, and vigor to evaluate the best way to feed their particular dog or cat.

CHAPTER

19

Feeding Regimens for Dogs and Cats

NORMAL FEEDING BEHAVIOR

An examination of the way that the wild ancestors of the dog and cat hunted and consumed food provides insight into the normal eating behaviors exhibited by domesticated pets. An obvious difference between the domestic dog and cat and their progenitors is that wild canids and felids were required to expend considerable amounts of energy locating and capturing prey and did not have a reliable and consistent source of nutrition. In contrast, our domestic pets are usually provided with a consistent source of palatable and nutritious foods. Despite this difference, domestic dogs and cat have retained certain behavior patterns that are associated with obtaining food and feeding.[1] Both dogs and cats are classified in the order Carnivora, but only cats are true carnivores; dogs are more omnivorous in nature. This difference is manifested by unique anatomical and metabolic characteristics, as well as in the differing ways the two species obtain and ingest food.

Dogs

The wolf, the dog's wild relative, obtains much of its food supply by hunting in a pack. Cooperative hunting behaviors allow the wolf to prey on large game that would otherwise be unavailable to a wolf hunting alone. As a result, most wolf subspecies tend to be intermittent eaters, gorging themselves immediately after a kill and then not eating again for an extended period of time. Competition between members of the pack at the site of a kill leads to the rapid consumption of food and the social facilitation of eating behaviors. Wolves and other wild canids also exhibit food hoarding behaviors; small prey or the remainder of a large kill are buried when food is plentiful and later dug up and eaten when food is not readily available.

BOX 19·1

Practical Feeding Tips: Methods to Decrease the Rate of Eating

Feed a less palatable diet.
Feed a dry-type pet food.
Add water to the dry food just before serving.
Train adult animals to eat only from their own bowl.
Feed puppies from several pans.

Like their ancestors, domestic dogs tend to eat rapidly. This tendency can be a problem for some dogs because it may predispose them to choke or swallow large amounts of air. If social facilitation is the cause of rapid eating, feeding the dog separately from other animals, thus removing the competitive aspect of mealtime, often normalizes the rate of eating. In other cases, changing the diet to a food that is less palatable or to one that is difficult to consume rapidly solves the problem. For example, some dogs readily gorge themselves on canned or semimoist foods but return to eating at a normal rate when fed a dry diet. If a dog attempts to eat dry food too quickly, adding water to the diet immediately before feeding decreases the rate of eating and minimizes the chance of swallowing large amounts of air.

Social facilitation is observed in domestic dogs that are fed together as a group. The presence of another animal at mealtime can stimulate a poor eater to consume more food. For example, pet owners often comment that their dog was a poor eater until a second dog was introduced into the family. Studies have shown that puppies and dogs usually consume more food when fed as a group, as compared with when they are fed alone.[2] If food is available at all times, the effects of social facilitation eventually become minimal. On the other hand, if dogs are fed their meals as a group, dominance interactions may occur. As a result, dominant animals obtain most of the food, and the subordinate pets receive less than their required amount. Training adult dogs to eat only from their own bowls or feeding young puppies with several pans of food is a way to eliminate this problem (Box 19-1).

Vestiges of the wolf's food hoarding behaviors are often observed in domestic dogs. It is not uncommon for dogs to bury bones in yards or, much to the owner's chagrin, to hide coveted food items in furniture or under beds. However, unlike their wild ancestors, many domestic dogs forget about these hidden caches and rarely return to dig them up.

The dog's ancestry suggests that an intermittent feeding schedule consisting of large meals interrupted by periods of fasting is the most natural way to feed dogs. However, when dogs are given free access to food, they will consume many small meals frequently throughout the day. This pattern is similar to that seen in cats, with the exception that dogs tend to eat only during the daytime.[2] It appears that the domestic dog is capable of adapting to a number of different feeding regimens. These regimens include portion-controlled feeding, time-controlled feeding, or free-choice (ad libitum) feeding. These regimens, and the advantages and disadvantages of each, are discussed later in this chapter.

Cats

It is common to think of the domestic cat as a descendant of the wild felids that prey on large, grazing animals. However, the primary ancestor of the cat is actually the small, African wild cat, *Felis libyca*. This cat's primary prey are small rodents about the size of field mice.[2] Therefore the immediate ancestor of the cat is not an intermittent feeder like the larger wild cats; rather, it is an animal that feeds frequently throughout the day by catching and consuming a large number of small rodents. Like the majority of wild felids, the African wild cat is a solitary animal, living and hunting alone for much of its life and interacting with others of its species only during mating season. This solitary nature has resulted in an animal that eats slowly and is uninhibited by the presence of other animals.

Most domestic cats consume their food slowly and do not exhibit social facilitation. If fed free-choice, cats nibble at the food throughout the day, as opposed to consuming a large amount of food at one time. Several studies of eating behavior in domestic cats have shown that if food is available free-choice, cats eat frequently and randomly throughout a 24-hour period.[3,4] It is not unusual for a cat to eat between 9 and 16 meals per day, with each meal having a caloric content of only about 23 kilocalories (kcal).[3,4] Interestingly, the caloric value of a small field mouse is approximately 30 kcal. It has been suggested that the eating behaviors observed in domestic cats are similar to those of feral domestic cats eating rodents or other small animals.[4,5,6] Like the dog, the cat is capable of adapting to several types of feeding schedules. Meal feeding may even be preferred by many owners and cats because it represents a time of pleasurable interaction, characterized by daily and familiar feeding routines of communication, petting, and handling.[7]

WHAT TO FEED

Pet owners have a choice of feeding one of three types of commercially prepared foods or a homemade formula. Most pet owners prefer the convenience, cost-effectiveness, and reliability of feeding commercial products. The decision of whether to feed a canned, semimoist, or dry commercial pet food can be made with an understanding of the advantages and disadvantages of each type of food (see Section 3, pp. 187-192). If a homemade diet is fed, care must be taken to ensure that a complete and balanced ration is prepared, that all ingredients and the final diet are stored safely to avoid spoilage, and that there is consistency of ingredients and nutrient content between batches of food. Surveys have shown that more than 90% of pet owners in the United States feed commercially prepared pet foods as the primary component of their pet's diet.[8] Therefore most of the discussion in this section concerns feeding commercial diets to pets; reference is made to homemade diets in special situations.

BOX 19-2

Factors to Consider When Selecting a Pet Food

Nutrient content and bioavailability
Palatability and acceptance
Effect on gastrointestinal tract functioning
Caloric density
Diet digestibility
Long-term feeding effects

One of the most important considerations when choosing a dog or cat food is the pet's stage of life and lifestyle. Nutrient and energy needs differ according to an animal's age, activity level, reproductive status, and health. As knowledge about these needs has been acquired, specific diets have been developed by pet food companies to efficiently meet the needs of pets during different ages and physiological states.

Several important factors must be considered when selecting a food for dogs and cats in all physiological states. Nutrient content and bioavailability are of primary importance:

- The food should provide all of the essential nutrients in adequate amounts and in the proper balance to meet the needs of the pet's lifestyle and stage of life.
- The food must supply sufficient energy to maintain ideal body weight or support optimal tissue growth. Caloric needs must be met when the food is fed in an amount that is well within the limits set by the animal's appetite and by the storage and digestive capacity of its gastrointestinal tract.
- The food must be appetizing to the pet and should be acceptable when fed as the primary diet over an extended period of time. The form and texture of the food must be appealing and should be able to be easily chewed and ingested.
- Feeding the pet food for extended periods of time should support proper gastrointestinal tract functioning and consistently result in the production of regular, firm, and well-formed stools.
- The long-term effects of feeding the food must be assessed. The food should support those measurements of vitality and health that are somewhat subjective, such as good coat quality, healthy skin condition, proper body physique and muscle tone, and high energy level (Box 19-2).

WHEN AND HOW TO FEED: FEEDING REGIMENS

There are three types of feeding regimens that may be used when feeding dogs and cats. These regimens are called free-choice (also called ad libitum or self-feeding), time-controlled feeding, and portion-controlled feeding. One method of feeding may be preferred over another, depending on the owner's daily schedule, the number of animals being fed, and the acceptability of the method by the pet or pets.

Free-choice feeding involves having a surplus amount of food available at all times. The pet is able to consume as much food as is desired at any time of the day. This type of feeding relies on the animal's ability to self-regulate food intake so that energy and nutrient needs are met. Dry pet food is most suitable for this type of feeding because it will not spoil as quickly as canned food or dry out as easily as semimoist products. However, even if dry food is used, the food bowl or dispenser should be cleaned and refilled with fresh food daily.

Compared with other feeding methods, free-choice feeding requires the least amount of work and knowledge on the part of the owner. The food and water supply is replenished only one time daily, and it is not necessary to determine the pet's exact daily requirements. If dogs are fed free-choice in a kennel setting, the kennel noise that usually occurs in response to mealtime is decreased or eliminated; this fact is considered a distinct advantage by many kennel owners. In addition, the constant presence of food in the kennel can help to relieve boredom that may be associated with confinement and to minimize undesirable behaviors such as coprophagy (stool eating) and excessive barking. Using free-choice feeding with a group of dogs that are housed together and have access to several food dispensers ensures that even the most subordinate dogs are able to consume adequate food, because there is always surplus food available.

When dogs are fed free-choice they tend to consume frequent, small meals throughout the day. This pattern may have an energy balance advantage because a greater meal-induced energy loss occurs when many small meals are consumed, as compared with when one or two large meals are eaten per day.[9] However, this loss is usually more than compensated for by the tendency of some dogs that are fed free-choice to increase their total daily food intake. This effect of a free-choice regimen can be an advantage for dogs or cats that are "poor keepers" and do not eat enough to meet their energy needs when fed one or two meals per day. Animals with very high energy needs may also benefit from consuming frequent meals on a free-choice regimen. Feeding numerous small meals per day is often prescribed for pets with dysfunctions in the ability to digest, absorb, or utilize nutrients, and for dogs who have a history of gastric dilatation. However, because free-choice feeding allows the animal rather than the owner to decide when it is time to eat, animals that require frequent feeding as a treatment for medical conditions are better fed on a portion-controlled, rather than a free-choice, basis.

Although free-choice feeding is convenient for the owner, problems such as anorexia or overconsumption may go undetected with this method. If an animal is sick, or if dominance hierarchies result in a submissive dog not being allowed to eat, a change in feed intake may not be noticed until the dog has lost substantial weight. If the decreased intake is the result of a medical problem, valuable time may be lost before the problem is diagnosed. The opposite situation, overconsumption and the development of obesity, is fairly common in pets that are fed free-choice. Although almost all animals are capable of eating to meet their caloric needs, the regulatory mechanisms that control food intake can be overridden if an animal is leading a relatively sedentary lifestyle and is fed a highly palatable and energy-dense food. In this situation, a dog or cat often consumes more energy than is required to meet its daily needs. In growing animals this can result in an accelerated growth rate and increased deposition of body fat; in adult animals it leads to obesity.

Most dogs and cats overconsume when they are first introduced to a free-choice feeding regimen. However, over time many animals adjust their intake to meet caloric needs. It is advisable to begin free-choice feeding by setting out a dish of food immediately after the dog or cat has consumed a meal. This extra food helps to prevent engorgement by the pet the first time that a surplus amount of food is available. The ability to adapt to free-choice feeding depends on the physiological state, energy level, temperament, and lifestyle of a pet. Although some adult dogs and cats maintain optimal weight and condition on this type of regimen, others habitually overeat and should not be fed free-choice.

Meal feeding involves controlling either the portion size or the amount of time that the pet has access to food. Similar to a free-choice regimen, time-controlled feeding relies somewhat on the pet's ability to regulate its daily energy intake. At mealtime, a surplus of food is provided and the pet is allowed to eat for a predetermined period of time. Most adult dogs and cats that are not physiologically stressed are able to consume enough food to meet their daily needs within 15 to 20 minutes. Although one meal per day can be sufficient for feeding adult pets during maintenance, providing two meals per day is healthier and more satisfying. There is some evidence that feeding once daily can lead to gastric changes associated with gastric dilatation in large breeds of dogs.[10] Moreover, feeding two times per day reduces hunger between meals and minimizes food-associated behavior problems, such as begging and stealing food.

As in the case of free-choice feeding, there are some dogs and cats that do not adapt well to time-controlled feeding. Pets that are very fastidious may not consume enough food within the allotted period. In contrast, other pets use the opportunity to eat voraciously throughout the allotted period. A time-controlled feeding program may actually exacerbate gluttonous behavior because pets quickly learn that they have to "beat the clock" whenever a meal is offered.

Portion-controlled feeding is the feeding method of choice in most situations. This procedure allows the owner the greatest amount of control over the pet's diet. One or several meals are provided per day, and they are premeasured to meet the pet's daily caloric and nutrient needs. As in the case of time-controlled feeding, many adult pets can be maintained on one meal per day, but providing two or more daily meals is preferable. Portion-controlled feeding enables the owner to carefully monitor the pet's food consumption and immediately observe any changes in food intake or eating behavior. The pet's growth and weight can be strictly controlled with this method by adjusting either the amount of food or the type of food that is fed. As a result, conditions of underweight, overweight, or inappropriate growth rate can be corrected at an early stage.

A disadvantage to portion-controlled feeding is that it demands the greatest time commitment and knowledge on the part of the owner. Guidelines for feeding are provided on the bags or containers of most pet foods; these can be used as a starting point when determining the amount to feed. Additional advice can be obtained from veterinarians, breeders, and pet food companies. The time commitment of portion-controlled feeding is usually not an issue with most pet owners unless very large numbers of animals are involved. Most owners coordinate their pets' meals with their own and find that mealtime becomes an enjoyable routine for both their pets and themselves.

DETERMINING HOW MUCH TO FEED

In all animals, food intake is governed principally by energy requirement. When companion animals are fed free-choice, the underlying control over the amount of food consumed is primarily the pet's need for energy. Although highly palatable or energy-dense foods can override the natural tendency to eat to meet energy needs, energy is still the dietary component that most strongly governs the amount of food consumed. When companion animals are fed on a portion-controlled basis, owners select a quantity of food based primarily on the pet's weight, thereby feeding to meet energy needs. If the pet gains too much weight (energy surplus), the owner decreases the amount that is fed. Conversely, if weight is lost, an increased amount of food is provided.

Commercial pet foods are formulated to contain the proper amount of essential nutrients when a quantity is fed that meets the pet's energy requirement. Balancing energy density with nutrient content ensures that when an animal's caloric needs are met, its needs for all other essential nutrients are met by the same quantity of food. Therefore the best way to determine how much to feed a particular animal is to first estimate the animal's energy needs and then calculate the amount of a particular pet food that must be fed to meet that need.

A number of factors affect a pet's energy requirement. These factors include age, reproductive status, body condition, level of activity, breed, temperament, environmental conditions, and health. When determining a pet's energy requirement, these factors are accounted for by adding or subtracting calories from the quantity of food that is determined to support the maintenance energy requirement of the adult pet. The maintenance requirement refers to the amount of kcal of energy per day necessary to support a normally active adult animal that is not reproducing and is living in a temperate climate. For example, energy needs during the latter stage of gestation in dogs and cats increase from 1.25 to 1.5 times the female's maintenance requirement. If an active 15-kilogram (kg) (33-pound [lb]) bitch normally requires 810 calories per day for maintenance, she would require approximately 1012 to 1215 kcal/day at the end of gestation. If a food containing 4500 kcal/kg (3.5 ounces [oz] per cup) is fed, this would correspond to approximately 2¼ cups of food per day (Table 19-1). The information presented later in this section provides

TABLE **19-1**

Determination of Quantity to Feed During Maintenance and Gestation (15-kg Dog)

	Energy Requirement (kcal of Metabolizable Energy [ME])		Energy Density*	Quantity (kg)			Lbs	Oz		Cups per Day
Maintenance	810	÷	4500	= 0.198	× 2.2	= 0.44	= 7.0	÷ 3.5**	=	2.25
Gestation	1112	÷	4500	= 0.247	× 2.2	= 0.54	= 8.6	÷ 3.5	=	2.50

*Energy density (kcal/kg) can be obtained from product literature or by contacting the pet food manufacturer.
**An 8-oz measuring cup contains approximately 3.5 oz. of dry food.

estimates for accounting for these factors when estimating the energy requirements of a given animal.

Another way to determine the amount to feed a dog or cat is to use the guidelines included on the commercial pet food label. All pet foods that carry the "complete and balanced" claim are required to include feeding instructions on the product label.[11] These guidelines usually provide estimates of the quantity to feed for several different ranges in body size. Such instructions provide only a rough estimate that can be used as a starting point when first feeding a particular brand of food. Adjustments in these estimates should be made based on the owner's knowledge of the individual animal and on the animal's response to feeding.

C H A P T E R

20

Pregnancy and Lactation

Proper feeding and care of reproducing animals is necessary for the health and condition of the dam and sire and for the viability, health, and growth of their offspring. It has been observed that successful gestation and lactation in companion animals is the result of a combination of factors. These factors include selection of healthy breeding animals, application of correct breeding management techniques, maintenance of a healthy environment, and the consistent and long-term provision of a proper diet.[12,13] Ideally, the correct feeding and management of reproducing animals begins during growth and development of the dam and sire and continues throughout mating, gestation, and lactation (Boxes 20-1 and 20-2).

PREBREEDING FEEDING AND CARE

The selection of breeding animals should include screening for any faults or anomalies that are believed to be genetically transmissible.[14,15] All animals should also undergo a thorough assessment of temperament, structure, and health before being admitted into a breeding program. Conformation shows and various types of working trials can be used by breeders to evaluate their animals and compare them to established breed standards. Once an adult dog or cat has been selected for breeding, a complete physical examination should be given, including a fecal check for internal parasites, serological tests for brucellosis and herpesvirus in dogs, and the administration of any required vaccinations.

Before breeding, both the sire and the dam should be in excellent physical condition, well-exercised, and not overweight or underweight. It is especially important that the dam be at optimum weight and in prime condition. If the dam is underweight, she may be unable to consume enough food during gestation to provide for her own nutritional needs as well as the needs of her developing fetuses. Lack of proper nutrition in the dam can result in decreased birth weight and increased neonatal mortality. Conversely, an overweight condition in the dam can lead to the development of very large fetuses and dystocia.

BOX 20-1

Practical Feeding Tips: Gestation

Feed a diet that is highly digestible and energy- and nutrient-dense.
Do not increase feed intake until fifth or sixth week of gestation.
Provide several small meals per day during late gestation.
Increase feed intake to approximately 1.25 to 1.5 times maintenance by the end of gestation.
Dams should gain no more than 15% to 25% of body weight by the end of gestation.
Dams should weigh 5% to 10% above normal body weight after whelping.

BOX 20-2

Practical Feeding Tips: Lactation

Feed a diet that is highly digestible and energy- and nutrient-dense.
Provide adequate calories to prevent excess weight loss.
Feed two to three times maintenance during peak lactation.
Provide free-choice feeding or several small meals per day during peak lactation.
Slowly reduce dam's intake after fourth week of lactation.
Provide clean, fresh water on a free-choice basis.

The queen or bitch should be fed a high-quality, highly digestible food that is adequate for gestation and lactation. Pet foods specifically formulated for gestation and lactation, performance diets, and high-quality puppy or kitten foods are recommended. If a change in diet is required, the new food should be introduced as soon as signs of proestrus are observed. Pet foods that have increased nutrient density are appropriate because of the increased nutrient requirements of reproduction. These needs can then be met without excess food consumption, thus avoiding the likelihood of gastrointestinal upset or weight loss. Changing to this diet early in the dam's reproductive cycle allows her to be fully adjusted to the new food when breeding takes place and prevents the need to abruptly change diets during either gestation or lactation.

During estrus, many bitches exhibit a slight depression in appetite. A study of 129 bitches showed an average decrease in food intake of 17% during estrus, with the lowest level of intake occurring at or around ovulation.[16] This short-term loss of appetite is natural and does not appear to affect fertility or litter size in normal bitches. In most dogs, appetite usually returns to normal within several days.

FEEDING MANAGEMENT DURING GESTATION AND PARTURITION

Bitches

In pregnant bitches, less than 30% of fetal growth occurs during the first 5 to 6 weeks of pregnancy. Although the fetuses are developing rapidly, they are very small until the last third of the 9-week gestation. As a result, there is only a slight increase in the dam's weight and nutritional needs during the first 5 to 6 weeks of gestation (Figure 20-1).[12,17] After the fifth week, fetal weight and size increase greatly for the remaining 3 to 4 weeks of gestation. In the dog, more than 75% of weight and at least half of fetal length is attained between the fortieth and fifty-fifth day of gestation.[17] Therefore optimal nutrition is imperative during the last few weeks of gestation to ensure optimal fetal growth and development.

If a bitch is at ideal weight at the time of breeding, no increase in food intake is necessary until the fifth or sixth week of gestation. Contrary to popular belief, a bitch should not receive a greater amount of food immediately after she has been bred. An increase of food at this time is unnecessary and could lead to excessive weight gain during pregnancy. It is not unusual for bitches to undergo a transient

FIGURE **20-1**

Weight gain pattern in bitches during gestation and lactation.

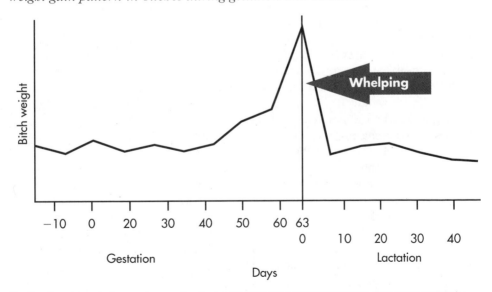

(From *Managing canine reproduction*, symposium proceedings, American College of Veterinary Internal Medicine, May 25, 1997. Used with permission.)

FIGURE **20-2**

Nutritional needs of the bitch during gestation and lactation.

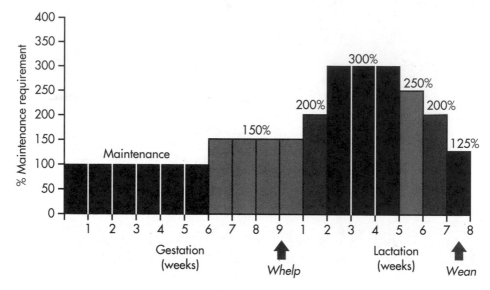

(From *Managing canine reproduction*, symposium proceedings, American College of Veterinary Internal Medicine, May 25, 1997. Used with permission.)

period of appetite loss at approximately 3 weeks of gestation. Like appetite depression that occurs during estrus, this change lasts for only a few days. After the fifth or sixth week of pregnancy, the bitch's food intake should be increased gradually so that at the time of whelping her daily intake is approximately 25% to 50% higher than her normal maintenance needs, depending on the size of the litter and the size of the bitch (Figure 20-2).[17] Her body weight should increase by approximately 15% to 25% by the time of whelping. Using the previous example, a bitch whose optimum weight is 15 kilograms (kg) (33 pounds [lbs]) should weigh between 17 and 19 kg (37 and 41 lbs) at the end of her pregnancy.

As the developing puppies increase in size, there is a reduction in the abdominal space available for expansion of the bitch's digestive tract after a meal. Therefore it is helpful to provide several small meals per day during the last few weeks of gestation so that abdominal space does not limit the bitch's ability to consume an adequate quantity of food. It is important to provide enough food during this period because dams that are underweight during middle and late gestation may have difficulty maintaining body condition and milk production after parturition. On the other hand, it is just as important not to overfeed pregnant bitches. Excessive intake and weight gain will be reflected in heavier fetuses and may result in complications at the time of whelping.

Mammary gland development and milk production occur 1 to 5 days before parturition, and many bitches refuse all food approximately 12 hours before whelp-

FIGURE 20-3

Weight gain pattern in queens during gestation and lactation.

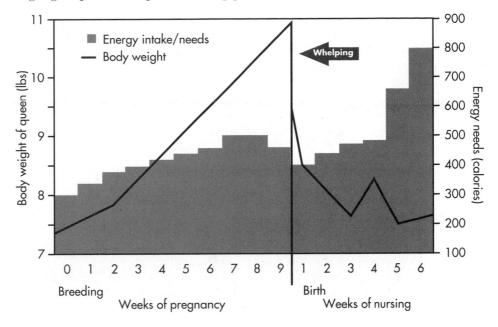

ing. A slight drop in body temperature, occurring 12 to 18 hours before the start of labor, is a fairly reliable indicator of impending parturition.

Once the bitch has whelped the litter and expelled all of the fetal placentas, and when her puppies are resting normally, she should be provided with fresh water and food. Most bitches will begin eating within 24 hours of whelping. If necessary, the dam's appetite can be stimulated by moistening her food with warm water. Adding water to the food also ensures that adequate fluid is consumed. If the bitch has been adequately prepared for lactation, she should have a postwhelping weight that is 5% to 10% above her prebreeding maintenance weight.

Queens

The weight gain pattern that occurs in pregnant queens is slightly different from that observed in bitches (Figure 20-3).[18] Although most of the bitch's weight increase occurs during the last third of gestation, pregnant queens exhibit a linear increase in weight beginning around the second week of gestation. A second difference between bitches and queens involves the type of weight that is gained during pregnancy. In dogs, almost all of the preparturition gain is lost at whelping.[19] In contrast, weight loss immediately following parturition in the cat accounts for only 40% of the weight that was gained during pregnancy. The remaining 60% of the queen's weight gain is body fat and is gradually lost during lactation. Thus it appears that the queen is able to prepare for the excessive demands of lactation by accumulating surplus body energy stores during gestation.

The queen should be fed a diet that is intended for reproduction throughout gestation and lactation. The amount of food she receives should be gradually increased, beginning during the second week of gestation and continuing until parturition (see Figure 20-3). At the end of gestation, the queen should be receiving approximately 25% to 50% more food than her normal maintenance needs. Because most cats adapt well to free-choice feeding, this is often the best way to provide the pregnant queen with adequate nutrition during pregnancy. The queen's weight gain should be monitored closely to prevent excessive weight gain during this time.

FEEDING MANAGEMENT DURING LACTATION

For both bitches and queens, the most important nutritional consideration during lactation is the provision of adequate calories. Ample energy intake allows for sufficient milk production and prevents drastic weight loss in the dam. Adequate water intake is also important for the production of a sufficient volume of milk. The stress that lactation imposes on the bitch or queen depends on the dam's nutritional status and weight at parturition, her litter size, and her stage of lactation. Dams with large litters and dams that have minimal body energy stores at parturition are at greatest risk for excessive weight loss and malnourishment during lactation.

Depending on the size of the litter, a bitch or queen will consume two to three times her maintenance energy requirement during lactation (see Figures 20-2 and 20-3). A general guideline is to feed 1.5 times maintenance during the first week of lactation, 2 times maintenance during the second week, and 2.5 to 3 times maintenance during the third to fourth week of lactation.[20] Another general rule of thumb for dogs suggests adding 100 kilocalories (kcal) of metabolizable energy (ME) per day to the bitch's normal maintenance diet for each lb of litter.[21] Peak lactation occurs at 3 to 4 weeks postpartum and is followed by the introduction of solid or semisolid food to the litter. After the fourth week, the amount of milk consumed by the puppies and kittens will decrease as their solid food intake gradually increases.

Lactation represents one of the greatest nutritional challenges to the animal. Many pet foods formulated for adult maintenance do not provide sufficient nutrient density for a bitch or queen during lactation. Research on lactating bitches found that when a diet containing approximately 4200 kcal/kg (1900 kcal/lb) was fed, little or no weight loss occurred during the entire period of lactation. However, bitches with four or more puppies fed a diet with a lower energy density (3100 kcal/kg) lost weight during lactation.[22] In addition to causing weight loss in the dam, energy deficiency during lactation may also affect the quantity of milk produced. If milk quantity is affected, compromised puppy and kitten growth and an increased risk of neonatal morbidity can result.

A highly digestible, nutrient-dense diet should be fed to all lactating queens and bitches, regardless of litter size. Premium pet foods that are formulated for performance or high activity are recommended because these foods are formulated to provide optimal levels of energy and nutrients to pets that are experiencing conditions of physiological stress. Even when a premium-quality food is fed, the quantity of food that the dam requires during peak lactation may exceed the capacity of her gastrointestinal tract. Therefore the daily ration should be divided into several meals or should be fed free-choice. After 3 weeks, it is advisable to feed the bitch and queen separately from the litter to prevent the puppies and kittens from consuming the dam's food.

Water is also of utmost importance during lactation. Inadequate fluid intake leads to a significant decrease in the quantity of milk produced. Fresh, cool water should always be readily accessible to the lactating queen and bitch.

By 3 to 4 weeks of age, puppies and kittens begin to be interested in solid food. At the same time, the dam's interest in nursing starts to decline. As this occurs, the dam's daily food intake should be slowly reduced. By the time that the puppies and kittens are of weaning age (7 to 8 weeks), the dam's food consumption should be less than 50% above her normal maintenance needs.

FEEDING THE DAM DURING WEANING

Bitches and queens begin to wean their puppies and kittens at approximately 6 to 10 weeks of age. Most breeders impose complete weaning by 7 to 8 weeks of age so that the puppies and kittens can be transferred to their new homes. Puppies and kittens that begin eating solid food at 3 to 4 weeks of age are usually consuming the major portion of their diet in the form of solid food by the time they are 7 to 8 weeks old.

If the dam continues to produce milk immediately before weaning, several days of limited feeding aid in decreasing milk production. If milk production is allowed to continue at a high level during weaning, there is an increased chance for the dam to develop mastitis. All food should be withheld from the dam on the day of weaning, provided she is in good physical condition. The dam's daily ration should then be gradually reintroduced at 25%, 50%, 75% and, finally, 100% of her maintenance level on successive postweaning days.

In general, bitches and queens lose some weight during lactation, but the amount should not exceed 10% of their normal body weight.[17] Proper feeding and management during gestation and lactation ensure that weight loss is minimized, even when large litters are raised. The condition of the bitch or queen at the time of breeding influences her ability to withstand the stresses of gestation and lactation and significantly affects her body condition at the end of the reproductive cycle. An animal who is in poor condition when bred loses greater amounts of weight than is desirable and will require an extended period of repletion after weaning. The repletion period allows the dam's body to regain stores of nutrients lost during gestation and lactation. In these cases, an energy- and nutrient-dense, highly digestible food should be fed until the queen or bitch has returned to optimal body condition.

SUPPLEMENTATION DURING GESTATION AND LACTATION

Some breeders regularly supplement their bitch's or queen's diet with calcium or calcium-containing foods, such as cottage cheese or other dairy products, during gestation and lactation. The added mineral is believed to ensure healthy fetal development during pregnancy and aid in milk production during lactation. It is also thought that calcium may prevent the onset of eclampsia after parturition.

But supplementation with calcium or any other mineral during pregnancy is not necessary for healthy fetal development as long as the dam is consuming a well-balanced, high-quality, commercial ration. In fact, some claim that excessive supplementation with calcium or vitamin D during pregnancy may cause soft-tissue calcification and physical deformities in developing fetuses.[23] Although calcium needs are high during both gestation and lactation, the bitch and queen normally obtain the additional nutrient requirements through consumption of higher amounts of the normal diet (see Section 5, pp. 342-343).

21

Nutritional Care of Neonatal Puppies and Kittens

 The young of dogs and cats are altricial, which means that puppies and kittens are born in a relatively immature state and are completely dependent upon the mother's care. The neonatal period is considered to be the first 2 weeks after birth, and it is a period of rapid development and growth. Preweaning mortality estimates for puppies and kittens are estimated to be as high as 40%, with the vast majority of deaths occurring during the neonatal period.[24] As more information has become available about the needs of newborns, it is apparent that proper nutritional support during this time is critical for maintaining health and preventing neonatal illness and mortality.

The first 36 hours of a puppy's or kitten's life are a critical time because the process of birth and the sudden environmental changes that newborns experience are very stressful. Therefore every effort should be made during this time to minimize stress and variations in the environment. A quiet, warm whelping/queening area should be provided, and human visitors outside of the immediate family should be prevented from disturbing the litter during the first few days.

COMPOSITION OF NATURAL MILK

Immediately after parturition, the dam produces a special type of milk called *colostrum*. Colostrum is vitally important for the provision of passive immunity to newborn puppies and kittens. Passive immunity is provided in the form of immunoglobulins and other immune factors that are absorbed across the intestinal mucosa of the newborns. Most of these factors are large, intact proteins. Once absorbed into the body, these factors offer protection from a number of infectious diseases.

In some species, such as humans, rats, rabbits, and guinea pigs, a significant proportion of passive immunity is acquired in utero. In contrast, puppies and kittens, like pigs, horses, and ruminant species, obtain the greatest proportion of maternally derived antibodies through the colostrum. These differences are due to the types of placentas found in different species, and they reflect the number of placental layers the antibodies must transverse to reach developing fetuses. The dog and cat have an endotheliochorial placenta consisting of four layers, which allows only about 10% to 20% of passive immunity to be transferred in utero. Therefore, for puppies and kittens, the major proportion of passive immunity is acquired after birth via the colostrum.

In older neonates and adult animals, normal digestive processes would result in the complete digestion of the immunological compounds found in colostrum, making them unavailable to the body as immune mediators. However, the intestinal mucosa of newborn dogs and cats is capable of absorbing intact immunoglobulins provided by colostrum. The time during which the newborn's gastrointestinal tract is permeable to the intact immunoglobulins in colostrum is very short. The term *closure* refers to the change in the gastrointestinal tract's absorptive capacity that precludes further absorption of large, intact proteins. The mechanisms behind closure are not fully understood, but they appear to be related to the increasing levels of circulating insulin that appear after the initiation of suckling.[25] This limits the ability of the neonatal intestine to absorb intact proteins to about the first 48 hours of life.[26] Therefore it is vitally important that newborn puppies and kittens receive adequate colostrum as soon as possible within the first 1 to 2 days after birth.

In addition to the immunological and nutritional benefits of colostrum, the volume of fluid ingested immediately after birth contributes significantly to postnatal circulating volume.[26] It is believed that a lack of adequate fluid intake shortly after birth may contribute to circulatory failure in newborns. Water turnover is also very high in newborn puppies and kittens, necessitating a consistent fluid intake to maintain normal blood volume throughout the neonatal period.[27] For this reason, the volume of milk produced by a bitch or queen is as important as its nutrient content.

Like the milk of many mammalian species, the milk of dogs and cats changes during lactation to effectively meet the needs of the developing young. Several forms of colostrum are produced during the first 24 to 72 hours after birth, after which the composition slowly transforms to mature milk. A recent study with cats found that the protein content of colostrum produced on the first day of lactation was very high (greater than 8%); however, protein rapidly declined to about half this value by the third day of lactation.[30] Protein concentration then slowly increased throughout lactation to reach a concentration of about 8%. Lipid concentration in cat milk followed a similar pattern. On the first day of lactation, the total lipid concentration was high—9.3%—but it rapidly decreased to 5.3% by the third day. Values then gradually increased until the forty-second day of lactation, after which they declined slightly.[29,30] In contrast, milk lactose concentrations in cat milk stay relatively constant throughout lactation. Also significant is the type of protein to be found in the milk. In cats, colostrum protein has a casein-to-whey ration of about 40:60.[30] This ratio shifts to a predominance of casein as colostrum changes to mature milk, with a final ratio of about 60:40. This change has been observed in the milk of other species and is significant because the amount of casein may affect protein digestion, mineral utilization, and the amino acid composition of the milk. Al-

TABLE **21-1**

Average Nutrient Composition of Mature Dog and Cat Milk

	Dog Milk	Cat Milk
Protein (%)	4-6	6.3-8.6
Lactose (%)	4-5	4
Fat (%)	4.5-5.2	5-9
Calcium (mg/L)	1600-1900	1500-2000
Magnesium (mg/L)	60	70-80
Iron (mg/L)	6-13	3-6
Zinc (mg/L)	7-10	5-7
Copper (mg/L)	1.7	1.3
Energy (kcal/L)	800	850-1600

Adapted from Lonnerdal B, Keen CL, Hurley LS, and others: Developmental changes in the composition of Beagle dog milk, *Am J Vet Res* 42:662-666, 1981; Adkins Y, Zicker SC, Lepine A, and others: Changes in nutrient and protein composition of cat milk during lactation, *Am J Vet Res* 58:370–375, 1997; and Keen CL, Lonnerdal B, Clegg MS, and others: Developmental changes in composition of cats' milk: trace elements, minerals, protein, carbohydrate and fat, *J Nutr* 112:1173-1769, 1982.

though the nutrient composition of colostrum produced between the first and third days of lactation has not been studied in the dog, it is possible that this species shows a similar pattern. Like cat milk, the fat and protein content of dog milk gradually increase throughout lactation[28,31] (Table 21-1).

Calcium concentrations in dog and cat milk are similar, increasing in both species over the course of lactation. The concentrations of protein and calcium in milk are highly correlated during lactation because casein has a high calcium-binding capacity.[28,29] The milk of both dogs and cats also has a relatively high iron concentration. These two species are similar to the rat and several marsupial species in their ability to concentrate iron in their milk at a level that is substantially higher than the concentration found circulating in plasma.[29,30,31] The high iron content in milk may reflect a high requirement for this mineral during the first few weeks of life. The concentration of iron is strongly influenced by the stage of lactation, with values increasing slightly during the first 2 days of lactation and then gradually declining. The magnesium content of cat milk is slightly higher than the magnesium content of dog milk (see Table 21-1).[30,31,32]

NORMAL DEVELOPMENT OF PUPPIES AND KITTENS

During the first few weeks of life, puppies and kittens should nurse at least four to six times per day. Infrequent or weak nursing often signifies chilling, illness, or congenital problems and should be attended to immediately by a knowledgeable breeder or veterinarian. The two primary activities of all newborns are eating and sleeping. The eyes of puppies and kittens open between 10 and 16 days after birth and their ears begin to function between 15 and 17 days after birth. Normal body temperature for puppies is 94° Farenheit (F) to 97° F for the first 2 weeks of life. Normal kitten temperature during this time is about 95° F. By 4 to 5 weeks of age, body temperatures have reached the normal adult temperature in both species (approximately 101.5° F).

Because puppies and kittens have no shivering reflex for the first 6 days of life, an external heat source is necessary. The dam is the best source of this warmth. After 6 days the puppies and kittens are able to shiver, but they are still very susceptible to chilling. Keeping the environment warm and free from drafts is of utmost importance during the first few weeks of life to prevent hypothermia. It is recommended that the environmental temperature be kept at 70° F during this period, assuming the dam is providing an adequate amount of warmth and protection to the newborns.[26] Newborns should be weighed daily during the first 2 weeks and then every 3 to 4 days until weaning. A helpful guideline is for puppies to gain between 1 and 2 grams (g) per day for every pound of anticipated adult weight for the first 3 to 4 weeks of life. For example, if the anticipated adult weight of a dog is 25 pounds (lb), the puppy should be gaining between 25 and 50 g/day (0.9 to 1.8 ounces [oz]). Kittens usually weigh between 90 and 110 g at birth and should gain between 50 and 100 g (1.8 to 3.5 oz) per week until they are 5 to 6 months of age.

Although there is limited information available concerning milk intake in nursing puppies and kittens, one study reported that Beagle puppies consume between 160 and 175 g of milk per day.[33] Naturally, puppies of larger breeds are expected to consume a greater volume of milk, with smaller breeds and kittens consuming less volume. Similarly, the volume of milk that a bitch produces varies with her size. German Shepherds produce about 900 g of milk per day in early lactation, with increases to a level of up to 1700 g/day during peak lactation.[34] In contrast, a much smaller breed, the Dachshund, produces between 100 and 180 g/day in early lactation. Other influences upon the volume of milk produced are litter size, age at which supplemental food is introduced, and age of weaning. In healthy puppies and kittens, the dam's milk supports normal growth until puppies and kittens are approximately 4 weeks old.[33] Supplemental feeding with commercial milk replacer should only be necessary with unusually large litters. After 4 weeks, milk alone no longer provides adequate calories or nutrients for continued normal development. At approximately the same time, puppies and kittens become increasingly interested in their environment and begin to spend more time awake and playing with each other. The time at which the dam's milk is no longer solely able to meet the nutrient needs of the offspring corresponds to the time at which the young are becoming interested in trying new foods.

INTRODUCTION OF SOLID FOOD

Supplemental food should be introduced at 3 to 4 weeks of age. A commercial food made specifically for weaning puppies or kittens can be used, or a thick gruel can be made by mixing a small amount of warm water with the mother's food. Cow's

BOX 21-1

Practical Feeding Tips: Introducing Solid Food to Puppies and Kittens

Begin introducing semisolid food at 3 to 4 weeks of age.
Feed a gruel of growth dry diet mixed with water.
Feed the gruel in a small, shallow dish.
Feed puppies and kittens several times per day; remove the bowl after 30 minutes.
Begin feeding dry food at 6 weeks of age.

milk should not be used to make the gruel because it has a higher lactose content than bitch's and queen's milk and may cause diarrhea. Puppies and kittens should not be fed a homemade "weaning formula." Although the foods that are used to make these formulas are of high nutrient value, homemade formulas are usually not nutritionally balanced or complete. The use of this type of formula should be avoided unless its exact nutrient composition is known.

The semisolid food should be provided in a shallow dish, and puppies and kittens should be allowed access to fresh food several times per day. The food should be removed after 20 to 30 minutes. At first, little food will be consumed, and the litter's major food source will continue to be the dam's milk. However, by 5 weeks of age, the young should be readily consuming semisolid food. The deciduous teeth erupt between 21 and 35 days after birth. By 5 to 6 weeks of age, puppies and kittens are able to chew and consume dry food. Nutritional weaning is usually complete by 6 weeks of age, although some bitches and queens continue to allow their young to nurse until 7 to 8 weeks of age or longer (Box 21-1). Recent studies of weaning in dogs indicate that puppies will continue to suckle at 7 weeks of age even when offered free access to solid food.[35] It is believed that the psychological and emotional benefits of suckling may be as important as the nutritional benefits in puppies that are older than 5 weeks of age. For this reason, complete weaning (behavioral weaning) should not be instituted until puppies and kittens are at least 7 to 8 weeks of age.

NUTRITIONAL CARE OF ORPHANS

The bitch and queen normally supply warmth, stimulus for elimination and circulatory functions, passive immunity, nutrition, maternal attention, and security to their puppies and kittens. Technically, an orphan is any young animal that does not have access to the milk or care of its mother. Circumstances that may render young puppies and kittens orphans include the death of the dam, the production of an inadequate quantity or quality of milk, or rejection of the young by the dam. Whatever the underlying cause, once puppies or kittens are orphaned they depend on humans for the provision of maternal care, proper nutrition, and a suitable

TABLE **21-2**

Proper Room Temperature for Orphan Puppies and Kittens

Age (weeks)	Temperature (F)
0-1	85°-90°
2-4	80°-85°
5-6	70°-75°
More than 6	70°

environment. Although it is difficult, if not impossible, to fully compensate for the absence of the dam, the use of proper diet, management techniques, and feeding techniques can result in the development of normal, healthy puppies and kittens.

Maintaining the Proper Environment

Orphaned animals must be kept in a warm, draft-free, and clean environment. Maintaining the appropriate temperature is of the utmost importance because chilling can decrease the survivability of newborns. When a bitch or queen is present, her body heat provides an excellent heat source and protection against drafts. In her absence, the ambient temperature must be increased. For the first week of life, the ambient temperature should be kept between 85° F and 90° F. This temperature can be decreased slightly to between 80° F and 85° F during the second to fourth weeks and to between 70° F and 75° F during the fifth week. After the litter reaches 5 to 6 weeks of age, a room temperature of approximately 70° F can be maintained (Table 21-2). Generally, newborn kittens and small puppies require slightly higher ambient temperatures than do large puppies. A heating pad or heat lamp may be used to provide heat, although a pad is often preferred because it allows for the maintenance of a normal day/night light cycle. Regardless of the type of heater used, the heat source should provide a temperature gradient within the whelping box so that the puppies and kittens can move to warmer or cooler areas as needed. Humidity must also be considered. If the environment is too dry, neonates are subject to dehydration. If dry heat is used to keep the whelping box warm, pans of water should be placed near the heaters to maintain room humidity. A relative humidity of approximately 50% is effective in preventing dehydration and maintaining moist nasal and respiratory passages in newborn puppies and kittens.[36] Drafts in the room can be controlled by providing a whelping box or incubator with high sides.

What to Feed

One of the greatest challenges involved in raising orphaned puppies and kittens is providing them with adequate nutrition. Because the best possible nutrition for young animals comes from their dam, foster mothering is the best solution for orphaned newborns. Unfortunately, a foster mother of the same species is usually not

TABLE **21-3**

Nutrient Composition of Milk from Various Species (%)

Species	Fat	Protein	Lactose	DM
Dog	5.0	5.0	4.5	22.8
Cat	7.0	7.5	4.0	18.5
Cow	3.8	4.7	4.7	12.4
Goat	4.5	4.6	4.6	13.0

Adapted from Baines FM, *J Small Anim Pract* 22:555-578, 1981. Adkins Y, Zicker SC, Lepine A, and others: Changes in nutrient and protein composition of cat milk during lactation, *Am J Vet Res* 58:370-375, 1997; and Keen CL, Lonnerdal B, Clegg MS, and others: Developmental changes in composition of cats' milk: trace elements, minerals, protein, carbohydrate and fat, *J Nutr* 112:1763-1769, 1982.

available. The alternative is to provide nutrition through a well-formulated milk replacer. A milk replacer will nourish the puppies and kittens for the first few weeks of life until their digestive and metabolic functions develop to the point at which solid food can be introduced. It is important that the chosen formula closely approximates the composition of the natural milk of the bitch or queen. Feeding a formula that is not similar in composition to the species' natural milk can result in diarrhea and digestive upsets and has the potential to compromise growth and development.

Several commercially produced canine and feline milk replacers are available. Most of these products are composed of cow's milk that has been modified to simulate the composition of bitch's and queen's milk (based on crude protein and crude fat levels). A comparison of the compositions of the milk of different species shows that bitch's and queen's milk have larger proportions of their calories from fat and protein and lower proportions from lactose than the milk of ruminant species such as the cow and goat. Although the percentages (by weight) of these nutrients only differ slightly, the more dilute composition of ruminant milk exacerbates the relative differences between these values. This is reflected by the lower dry matter (DM) content of goat's and cow's milk as compared to the milk of dogs and cats (Table 21-3).[37] When converted to a caloric basis, the lactose content of cow's milk is nearly three times that found in bitch's milk.[38] For this reason, puppies that are fed straight cow's milk will develop severe diarrhea.[26] Evaporated cow's milk is occasionally recommended for raising orphans because it has levels of protein, fat, calcium, and phosphorus that are similar to bitch's milk. However, the lactose content of evaporated milk is still much too high for young puppies.[38] In addition, recent evidence shows that the casein-to-whey protein ratio in cow's milk is not ideal for puppies, and cow's milk contains an excessive proportion of casein for neonatal kittens.[39]

There are numerous recipes available for the formulation of homemade milk replacers. Most of these use a combination of cow's or goat's milk and eggs. Eggs are added to increase the protein content and dilute the lactose concentration of the ruminant milk. Regardless of the popularity of a homemade formula, pet owners should be advised that most of these recipes were originally developed through trial-and-error techniques, and their actual nutrient compositions are not known. A published analysis of several commonly used homemade formulas found that these recipes contain a wide range of nutrient compositions.[38] Although some formulas seem to be adequate for feeding puppies and kittens, many contain a nutrient composition that is drastically different from that of natural bitch's and queen's milk. A homemade formula should only be used if its nutrient composition is known and if the formula has been proven to be safe and effective for raising orphaned puppies or kittens. If a well-researched product that is formulated for puppies and kittens is available, this is preferable to a homemade formula.

Commercial milk replacers are the preferred source of nutrition for orphans. A product that has been tested for the specific purpose of raising neonatal puppies and kittens should be selected. In addition, unlike homemade formulas, the nutrient content and the biological integrity of commercial preparations is guaranteed. However, some commercial formulas can vary in their ability to provide orphans with adequate nutrition and calories. For example, a study that compared feeding queen's milk, a commercial milk replacer for cats, and an experimental milk replacer to kittens ranging from 2 to 6 weeks of age found that the commercial product caused chronic diarrhea and the development of lens opacities and cataracts.[40] Suboptimal levels of the essential amino acid arginine in the commercial formula appeared to be the cause of the cataracts, and an unusually high crude fiber content may have been the cause of the diarrhea. When the kittens were switched to a growth diet at 6 weeks of age, the lens opacities resolved almost completely, and diarrhea subsided during the sixth week of feeding. More recently, research on the nutrient composition of dog and cat milk has led to the development of replacers that nearly match the nutrient profiles of natural milk and that promote growth rates that closely match those of nursing neonates.[41,42]

Because the Association of American Feed Control Officials (AAFCO) does not currently provide detailed guidelines for testing milk replacers, it is important for pet owners to obtain information from manufacturers about a replacer's nutrient composition, nutritional integrity, and feeding efficacy. Also, it is important to note that even a well-formulated commercial milk replacer cannot provide newborns with the antibodies that are normally found in colostrum. Therefore, if newborns are orphaned before they have received colostrum, extra care must be taken to maintain a clean environment and prevent the transmission of disease.

How Much to Feed

Calorie and fluid intake must be adjusted so that the puppies and kittens are able to consume enough formula to meet their nutrient needs for growth and, at the same time, not underconsume or overconsume fluid volume. During the first few weeks, the food intake of the neonate is largely limited by stomach volume. Most newborn puppies can handle only 10 to 20 milliliters (ml) of milk per feeding. Kittens are able to handle approximately $\frac{1}{3}$ to $\frac{1}{2}$ of this amount.[38] Therefore the concentration of the formula is extremely important. The milk replacer for puppies should have a caloric value of between 800 and 1000 kilocalories (kcal) of metabolizable energy (ME) per

TABLE **21-4**

Volume of Milk Replacer to Feed Orphan Puppies (General Guidelines)

Body Weight (oz)	Body Weight (g)	Volume/Day (oz)	Volume/Day (tbsp or cup)	Volume/Day (
5	140	1.5	3 tbsp	45
10	285	2.5	⅜ cup	75
20	570	5.0	⅝ cup	150
30	850	8.0	1 cup	235
50	1420	12.0	1½ cup	355
70	1990	17.0	2⅛ cup	505
100	2840	25.0	3⅛ cup	740

Data provided by Iams Technical Center, Lewisburg, Ohio, 1999, The Iams Company.

TABLE **21-5**

Volume of Milk Replacer to Feed Orphan Kittens (General Guidelines)

Body Weight (oz)	Body Weight (g)	Volume/Day (oz)	Volume/Day (tbsp or cup)	Volume/Day (g)
4	115	1.00	2.0	30
6	170	1.50	3.0	45
8	225	1.75	3.5	50
10	285	2.25	4.5	65
12	340	3.00	6.0	90
14	440	3.75	7.5	110

Data provided by Iams Technical Center, Lewisburg, Ohio, 1999, The Iams Company.

liter (L), a concentration that is similar to that of bitch's milk.[33] Queen's milk has a caloric density of approximately 850 to 1600 kcal ME/L.[30,38] If the energy concentration is lower than this, more feedings per day will be necessary to meet the neonate's needs. In this case, the intake of excess fluid would adversely affect water balance and may stress the immature kidneys. Conversely, if the energy density of the formula is too high, digestive upsets and diarrhea may occur.

There are various estimates of the caloric needs of newborn puppies. A generally accepted guideline suggests that during the first 3 weeks of life, orphaned puppies need to receive between 130 and 150 kcal of ME per kilogram (kg) of body weight per day. After 4 weeks of age, caloric needs increase to 200 to 220 kcal/kg of body weight.[33,38] Less is known about the optimal energy intake of newborn kittens, but one guideline suggests feeding 20, 25, 30, and 35 ml/100 g of body weight during the third, fourth, fifth and sixth week of life, respectively.[39] In all cases, these figures should be used only as guidelines because the individual requirements of puppies and kittens can vary greatly. Orphans should be weighed daily to ensure that they are receiving enough nourishment to support normal weight increases. General guidelines for determining the volume to feed are provided in Tables 21-4 and 21-5.

Once determined, the total volume of formula should be divided equally among the daily feedings. If the concentration of the formula is correct, neonates that are bottle-fed should be able to self-regulate their formula intake. Feeding orphans four to five times per day is usually practical, with the feedings spaced at even time intervals. This schedule is often reasonable for human caretakers, and it also allows the neonates to obtain their needed hours of uninterrupted sleep.

Methods of Feeding

Two possible methods may be used to feed orphaned puppies: bottle-feeding with a small animal nursing bottle or delivering the formula directly into the stomach using a stomach tube. If puppies and kittens are bottle-fed, they should be held in a natural nursing position with the head tilted slightly upward. The bottle should be held in a manner that minimizes air intake by the puppy or kitten. When bottle-fed, orphans usually reject the bottle when their stomachs are full. However, the correct volume of formula should still be estimated and measured for each feeding. This step aids in record keeping and minimizes the risk of overfeeding.

Many breeders prefer to use a feeding tube with orphans. This method of feeding is faster and, if conducted properly, reduces the risk of formula aspiration. The necessary equipment is an infant feeding tube attached to a syringe. For puppies and kittens that weigh less than 300 g (10 oz), a number 5 or 8 French-sized tube can be used. For larger puppies, a number 10 French tube is appropriate. The depth of insertion can be estimated by measuring the distance from the puppy or kitten's nose to the last rib. This length is marked on the tube and should be readjusted every 2 to 3 days to account for growth. The syringe is filled with a measured volume of warm formula, and extra air in the syringe and tube is expelled. To insert the tube, the puppy or kitten is held upright, the mouth is opened slightly and the tube is gently inserted over the tongue to the back of the throat. This contact will induce a swallow reflex, and the tube should pass easily down into the stomach. If any resistance is felt, this indicates that the tube may be in the trachea, and should be removed and reinserted. When the tube is inserted properly into the stomach, the puppy or kitten will be breathing normally and not crying or showing distress. Formula should be administered slowly over a 2- to 3-minute period. Because the neonate cannot self-regulate intake when tube-fed, formula volume must always be carefully measured to avoid overfeeding or underfeeding.

Fresh formula should be made up daily and warmed to approximately 100° F before feeding. A slightly restricted quantity of formula should be fed for the first two to three feedings; this allows gradual adjustment to the milk replacer. If puppies and kittens are overfed during the first few days, diarrhea may result, leading to dehydration and increased susceptibility to infection. After each feeding and several times daily, the anal/genital area of the newborns should be massaged gently with a damp cloth. This action simulates the dam's licking and stimulates urination and defecation. Grooming, cleaning, and feeding of the orphans should be conducted on a regular basis, and the box should be cleaned several times per day.

BOX 21-2

Practical Feeding Tips: Orphan Puppies and Kittens

Provide a warm, draft-free, clean environment.

Feed a milk replacer that closely approximates the nutrient composition of bitch's or queen's milk.

Estimate the correct amount of formula based on an animal's age and weight.

Divide the formula into four to five equal feedings per day.

Bottle-feed or use a feeding tube.

Weigh orphans regularly: one time per day for the first week and one to two times per week thereafter.

Introduce semisolid food at 3 to 4 weeks.

Wean to dry pet food by 6 to 10 weeks.

Orphans should be weighed regularly. There may be a small decrease in body weight during the first 2 to 3 days because of the restricted feeding of the new formula. After this, if a well-formulated milk replacer is used, growth will closely approximate that of dam-raised puppies and kittens.[41,42]

Orphans show an increased demand and tolerance for food once their eyes open and they are on their feet. At this time, a small shallow bowl of formula should be provided before each bottle-feeding. The puppies and kittens should be encouraged to lap formula from the bowl. The bowl of formula should not be left out for more than 20 or 30 minutes at a time. Once the litter readily initiates lapping at each meal, they can begin to take entire feedings from the bowl. In general, puppies adjust to lapping at an earlier age and more rapidly than kittens.

When the orphans are 3 to 4 weeks old, a gruel can be made using milk replacer and dry dog or cat food or a puppy or kitten weaning formula. Once semisolid food is introduced, fresh water should be available at all times. The thickness of the gruel can be gradually increased with time. This gradual change allows the puppies and kittens to become accustomed to chewing and swallowing solid food and enables their gastrointestinal tracts to adapt to the new food. By 6 to 8 weeks of age, puppies and kittens should be consuming normal dry food (Box 21-2).

22

Growth

 Most puppies and kittens are fully weaned from their dam and ready to be placed in their new homes by 7 to 9 weeks of age. For puppies, this represents an ideal time to enter a new home because the primary socialization period occurs between 5 and 12 weeks of age. At 7 weeks of age the puppies have spent sufficient time with their litter to allow proper canine socialization. The remainder of this important developmental period can then be spent bonding to their new owners. It is believed that cats also undergo a primary socialization period at approximately the same age. Although this period is not as well defined in kittens as it is in puppies, 7 to 9 weeks appears to be the best age for kittens to begin positive relationships with their new human companions.

DIETARY REQUIREMENTS OF GROWING DOGS AND CATS

The most rapid period of growth in dogs and cats occurs during the first 6 months of life. Medium breeds of dogs attain their mature size by approximately 12 to 18 months of age; smaller breeds and cats reach adult size by 8 to 12 months.[43,44] Large and giant breeds of dogs, such as German Shepherds, Rottweilers, Great Danes, and Newfoundlands, do not usually reach mature size and weight until they are 18 to 24 months of age. When they reach maturity, most dogs and cats have increased their birth weight by 40- to 50-fold. Thus an enormous amount of growth and development takes place in a relatively short period of time. Supplying a balanced diet during growth is crucial for an animal's adequate development and the attainment of normal adult size (Figures 22-1 and 22-2).

Puppies and kittens should be fed a diet that has been formulated for growth. The pet food should be guaranteed to be nutritionally adequate for growth or for all stages of life, as proven by the use of the Association of American Feed Control Officials' (AAFCO's) feeding trials (see Section 3, p. 200). Growth represents a period of rapid tissue accretion and development, which is reflected primarily by

FIGURE **22-1**

*A, Golden retriever at 6 months of age. **B, C,** and **D**, Same dog at 33, 54, and 88 months of age.*

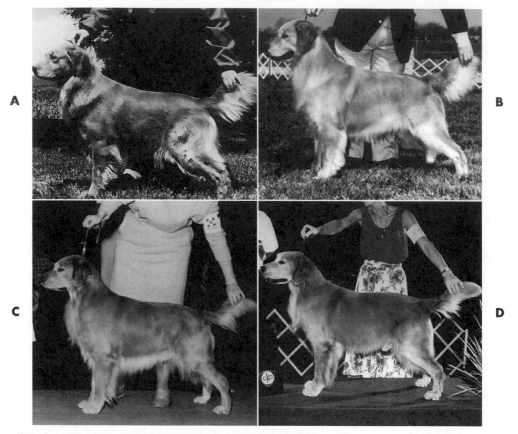

(CH Sun Dances Fibber MacGee, bred and owned by Sun Dance Kennels, Lisa and Jerry Halcomb.)

increased needs for energy and essential nutrients. Although their nutrient requirements reflect additional needs for growth, there is no current evidence that growing dogs and cats have requirements for nutrients that are not needed by adults.

Breed-Specific Nutrition?

While individual breeds of dogs and cats do not appear to have different nutrient requirements during growth, enormous variation does exist in the mature size and body weight of different breeds and types of dogs. For example, a 5 pound (lb) Chihuahua and a 150 lb Newfoundland both achieve complete development and

FIGURE **22-2**

Rate of weight gain in several dog breeds from 0 to 28 months.

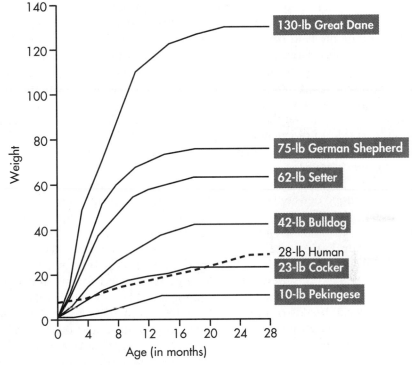

(Adapted from *Current veterinary therapy V*, Philadelphia, 1974, WB Saunders.)

growth within relatively similar periods of time. The 30-fold difference in mature size between these two dogs means that the Newfoundland's rate of growth and amount of tissue accretion far exceeds that of the Chihuahua. These enormous differences are not observed in cats, which vary relatively little in mature size. Because different breeds of dogs have different rates of growth and mature weights, the food that is fed during growth should reflect these differences. In recent years, pet food companies have recognized these differences and have developed dog foods that provide optimal nutrition for growing dogs of different mature sizes and weights. The two groups of dogs of greatest interest are the large and giant breeds and the small and toy breeds.

The genetic selection for breeds of dogs that have a large mature size concurrently selects for the potential to grow very rapidly.[45] Feeding these dogs diets that are very energy- and nutrient-dense or overfeeding during periods of rapid growth leads to maximal growth rates. However, numerous studies have demonstrated that a rapid growth rate is not compatible with optimal skeletal development and maturation.[46,47,48] Feeding dogs to achieve maximal rates of growth has been shown to contribute to the development of skeletal diseases such as osteochondrosis, hypertrophic osteodystrophy, and canine hip dysplasia. Besides energy, another nutrient that is important is calcium. Excessively high amounts of calcium in the diet or supplementation with this mineral negatively affects skeletal development in large breeds of dog (see Section 5, pp. 337-339).[48,49,50] These findings are in direct contrast to the commonly held belief that growing dogs benefit from supplementation with calcium. Because large and giant breeds of dogs may be genetically predisposed to developmental skeletal disorders and because they have the capacity for a rapid growth rate, a pet food designed to control the rate of growth and promote normal skeletal maturation is warranted. An appropriate diet contains a slightly lower energy density and fat than most puppy foods, a balanced level of high-quality protein, and a level of calcium and phosphorus that is approximately 30% less than puppy foods intended for small breeds of puppies. A recommended nutrient profile for a diet formulated for growth in large and giant breeds is one that contains 26% to 28% protein, 14% to 16% fat, 0.8% to 0.9% calcium, 0.6% to 0.8% phosphorus, and a caloric density between 350 and 365 kilocalories (kcal) per cup (see Section 5, pp. 335-337).[50,51,52]

Dogs of the small and toy breeds have higher energy requirements per unit of body weight than do the large and giant breeds. This occurs because basal metabolic rate is related to total body surface area. Small and toy breeds have higher ratios of surface area to body weight than do large breeds and so have higher energy needs per unit of weight (lb or kilogram [kg]). In addition to their relatively high energy needs, small breeds of puppies also have small stomachs that hold limited amounts of food. A dog food formulated for growing small and toy breeds should be higher in energy and nutrient density than a food formulated for large dogs, and it should contain ingredients that are highly digestible and available. The size and shape of the kibble pieces should be designed for small mouths to facilitate easy chewing and consumption.

Energy

Nutrient and energy needs during growth exceed those of any other stage of life except lactation. The energy needs of growing puppies, regardless of breed, are approximately twice those of adult dogs of the same size. After 6 months of age, these needs begin to decline as the animal's growth rate decreases. General guidelines for determining energy needs for growing dogs are provided in Table 22-1. Similarly, growing cats have energy needs that are significantly higher than are the maintenance needs of adult cats. Although moderately active adult cats require 50 to 60 kcal of metabolizable energy (ME) per kg of body weight, growing kittens need substantially more than this amount of energy during peak growth (Table 22-2).[53,54]

Protein

The protein requirement of growing puppies and kittens is higher than the protein requirement of adult animals. In addition to normal maintenance needs, young an-

TABLE 22-1

Calculation of Energy Requirements for Growing Dogs

Age	K Value	Example
Small and Medium Breeds		
6 to 11 weeks	375	7-lb puppy: $375 \times 3^{0.67} = 404$ kcal/day
3 to 4 months	350	14-lb puppy: $350 \times 6.4^{0.67} = 1214$
5 to 7 months	225	18-lb puppy: $225 \times 8.2^{0.67} = 921$
8 to 12 months	160	20-lb dog: $160 \times 9.1^{0.67} = 702$
Large and Giant Breeds		
6 to 11 weeks	340	16-lb puppy: $340 \times 7.3^{0.67} = 1288$
3 to 4 months	300	34-lb puppy: $300 \times 15.4^{0.67} = 1874$
5 to 7 months	200	50-lb puppy: $200 \times 22.7^{0.67} = 1620$
8 to 12 months	160	58-lb dog: $160 \times 26.4^{0.67} = 1434$
12 to 24 months	132	64-lb dog: $132 \times 29^{0.67} = 1260$

TABLE 22-2

Calculation of Energy Requirements for Growing Cats

Age	K Value	Example
6 to 19 weeks	250	3-lb kitten: $250 \times 1.4 = 350$ kcal/day
5 to 6½ months	130	5-lb kitten: $130 \times 2.3 = 299$
7 to 8½ months	100	6-lb kitten: $100 \times 2.7 = 270$
9 to 11 months	80	7-lb kitten: $80 \times 3.2 = 256$
12 months	60	8-lb cat: $60 \times 4.5 = 270$

imals also need more protein to build the new tissue that is associated with growth. Because young animals consume higher amounts of energy and thus higher quantities of food than adult animals, the total amount of protein that they consume is naturally higher. Pet foods fed to growing puppies and kittens should contain slightly higher protein levels than foods developed for maintenance only. More importantly, the protein included in the diet should be of high quality and highly digestible. This type of protein ensures that sufficient levels of all of the essential amino acids are being delivered to the body for use in growth and development. The actual percentage of protein in the diet is not as important as is the balance between protein and energy. The minimum proportion of energy that should be supplied by protein in the diet for growing dogs is 22% of the ME kcal, and the minimum for growing cats is 26%.[11] Optimal levels are between 25% and 29% of ME kcal for puppies and 30% and 36% for kittens.

Calcium and Phosphorus

Diets for growing dogs and cats should contain optimal, but not excessive, amounts of calcium and phosphorus. The AAFCO's *Nutrient Profiles* recommend that dog and cat foods formulated for growth contain a minimum of 1% calcium and 0.8% phosphorus on a dry-matter basis (DMB).[11] These recommendations are based upon diets containing 3500 and 4000 kcal/kg. Research studies have shown that the dog's requirements for calcium and phosphorus are actually less than these amounts.[50,51,55,56] However, the AAFCO's *Nutrient Profiles* include safety factors that account for differences in the availability of nutrients in pet foods and for individual differences between animals. Therefore this level ensures that all growing dogs and cats receive adequate levels of these essential nutrients.

Many commercially available pet foods contain slightly more than the recommended levels of calcium and phosphorus, so they will supply more than adequate amounts of calcium and phosphorus to growing pets.[57] In contrast, foods formulated for large breeds of growing dogs should contain lower percentages of calcium and phosphorus because of the lower energy densities of these diets and the need to carefully control calcium intake during growth. In addition, it is now known that small excesses of dietary calcium increase the likelihood of developmental bone diseases such as osteochondrosis and hypertrophic osteodystrophy (see Section 5, pp. 339-342). Dietary calcium and phosphorus supplements should never be added to a balanced, complete pet food that has been formulated for growing dogs or cats (see Section 5, pp. 337-343).

PET FOOD DIGESTIBILITY AND ENERGY DENSITY

Diet digestibility and energy density are important considerations when feeding growing pets because of the quantity of food necessary to meet the requirements for growth and development. Growing dogs and cats have higher requirements for energy and essential nutrients than adults, but they also have less digestive capacity, smaller mouths, and smaller and fewer teeth.[58] This is especially true for small and toy breeds of dogs. These differences limit the amount of food that a young animal can consume and digest within a meal or a given amount of time. If a diet is low in digestibility or energy density, a larger quantity must be consumed. The effects of low digestibility are exacerbated by the fact that as increasing amounts of a food must be fed, diet digestibility decreases further. When a poor-quality food with a low energy density is fed to growing puppies and kittens, the limits of the pet's stomach may be reached before adequate nutrients have been consumed. The result is compromised growth and impaired muscle and skeletal development. Young animals benefit from eating a food that is energy- and nutrient-dense because the volume of food intake need not be excessive and intake will not be limited by the size of the animal's stomach.

It is equally important that growing dogs and cats not be overfed. Overfeeding during growth leads to an accelerated growth rate and can predispose the animal to obesity later in life. In large breeds of dogs, an accelerated growth rate can contribute to the development of certain skeletal disorders (see Section 5, pp. 331-333). One of the most common causes of overnutrition in growing puppies and kittens is the addition of supplemental foods to a balanced diet that has been formulated for growth. Supplementation is unnecessary and may be detrimental; therefore it is not recommended (see Section 5, pp. 352-357).

FEEDING PROCEDURES DURING GROWTH

Once a puppy or kitten has been placed in a new home, the owner may wish to feed a pet food that is different from the food that was fed to the litter. If the pet's diet is going to be changed, the new food should be introduced very gradually. No dietary change should be made at all within the first few days that the puppy or kitten is in the new home. Moving to a new home and leaving the dam and litter mates is very stressful, and providing a brand new diet at the same time can exacerbate this stress. Most breeders send a small package of food along with the puppy or kitten. This food should be fed for the first few days that the animal is in the new home. After 2 or 3 days, the new food can be introduced by mixing it in quarter increments with the original diet. The proportion of the new food should be increased for 4 successive days until the puppy or kitten is consuming only the new diet.

Dogs

Proper feeding of young dogs supports normal muscle and skeletal development and a rate of growth that is typical for the dog's particular breed. All dogs grow and develop rapidly during the first year of life, but small and toy breeds reach maturity earlier than large breeds (see Figure 22-2). Overfeeding for maximal growth rate and early maturity should be avoided. Studies with rats have shown that overnutrition early in life results in an increased number of fat cells and higher total body fat during adulthood.[59,60] In contrast, other studies have shown that mild restriction of calories during growth results in significantly increased longevity.[61] Rapid growth rates are also related to developmental bone diseases in dogs. These effects have also been observed in other species such as humans, horses, poultry, and swine.[44,45,62,63,64,65,66]

When obesity occurs in a young animal there is often an increase in both the size and number of fat cells in the body. This condition, called *hyperplastic obesity,* is believed to be more resistant to treatment than is *hypertrophic obesity,* which involves only an increase in fat cell size.[67,68] The presence of additional numbers of fat cells results in a higher percentage of body fat, even if the animal is not yet overweight. Thus an animal with fat cell hyperplasia has a higher percentage of total body fat than an animal that weighs the same amount but has a normal number of fat cells.[59,69] Normal adipocyte hyperplasia occurs during specific critical periods of development in growing animals.[70,71] The exact age that these periods occur in dogs and cats is not known. However, data in other species indicate that adipose tissue growth normally occurs during either infancy or adolescence.[59,72,73] If these data are true for the dog and cat, it is probable that the level of nutrition provided to growing pets is of importance in determining the number of fat cells that the animal has at maturity.

It has been postulated that superfluous fat cell hyperplasia during the critical periods of adipose tissue growth may produce a long-term stimulus to gain excess weight in the form of excess adipocytes that require lipid filling.[74] The existence of excess numbers of adipocytes results in both an increased predisposition toward obesity in adulthood and an increased difficulty in maintaining weight loss when it occurs. This theory has been supported by several studies on laboratory animals showing that early overnutrition results in increased numbers of fat cells and increased total body fat throughout adult life.[59,60] The use of proper feeding techniques that allow judicious control of a growing dog's weight are therefore important for long-term weight control.

A second reason that overfeeding for maximal growth rate and development is not desirable relates to its potential to affect skeletal development. A concern for skeletal development is important when feeding large and giant breeds of dogs, which generally exhibit a higher incidence of developmental bone disorders. Some commonly diagnosed skeletal diseases in young dogs include hypertrophic osteodystrophy (metaphyseal osteopathy), osteochondrosis, panosteitis, and hip dysplasia.[75,76,77,78,79] Genetics plays a role in each of these disorders, but heredity is not completely responsible for their existence. For example, hip dysplasia has been estimated to have a hereditary component of approximately 40%, with environmental factors playing an important role in the expression of the disease.[80] Several studies support the theory that nutrition is one of the environmental factors that influences the development of these diseases. The two most important nutritional factors to be identified are supplementation with calcium and feeding an energy- and nutrient-dense diet at a level that supports a maximal growth rate (see Section 5, pp. 333-343).[43,77,78]

In contrast, feeding growing dogs moderately restricted levels of a well-balanced diet does not affect final body size or development.[44,45,49,51,78] Dogs that are fed restricted levels of food that support a slower growth rate still attain normal adult size, but they do so at a later age. It is advisable to feed growing dogs enough to attain an average, rather than a maximal, growth rate for the dog's particular breed. This goal can best be achieved through strict portion-controlled feeding, reduced dietary energy density, and the frequent assessment of growth rate, weight gain, and body condition.

Growing dogs have a very steep growth curve, and their total daily energy needs do increase as they grow. The amount of food that is fed should be adjusted in response to a weekly or biweekly assessment of the dog's body condition and weight.[78,81] A dog that is too thin has easily palpable ribs with little or no overlying fat layer. The tail base may be prominent, and the overhead profile will be an exaggerated hourglass. A dog that is overweight has a moderate to heavy layer of fat overlying the ribs. In very overweight puppies, the ribs may be difficult to even feel. There may be a thickening around the base of the dog's tail due to fat stored in that area. The dog's profile will show only a slight hourglass shape, and in very overweight dogs, there is no waist at all. Overweight dogs who are older than 6 months lose their abdominal tuck and may show abdominal distention. Growing dogs who are at their ideal weight have ribs that are easily palpable with just a thin layer of overlying fat. The bony prominences of the hips are easily felt but not prominent. The dog's profile from above has an hourglass shape with a well-defined waist. Owners should assess body condition regularly and adjust the amount of food that is fed to maintain the dog's ideal body condition throughout the growth period.

Portion-controlled feeding is the recommended feeding regimen for growing dogs. A high-quality, highly digestible food formulated for growth should be fed. The dog's daily portion of food should be divided into two to three meals per day until the dog is 4 to 6 months of age. After 6 months, two meals per day can be fed. Some large and giant breeds of dogs may benefit from three or more feedings per day as a precaution again the development of gastric dilatation volvulus (see Section 5, pp. 361-365). Free-choice feeding is not recommended for growing dogs because this type of feeding regimen makes it difficult to monitor and control weight gain and growth rate and has been associated with a greater incidence of developmental bone disease. Dogs should be fed on a portion-controlled basis until they have reached at least 80% to 90% of their adult weight.[35] If a pet owner eventually wishes to switch a dog to a free-choice regimen, this should be done only after the dog has achieved mature size.

Some breeders suggest feeding an adult maintenance food rather than a growth diet to large- and giant-breed puppies. It is thought that owners can more easily maintain a lower rate of growth for their dog by feeding an adult food because maintenance diets typically have lower energy densities than growth diets. However, adult maintenance foods are not formulated for growth, and their nutrients are not balanced with the energy of the diet for the needs of growing dogs. Because a growing puppy requires up to twice the amount of energy per day as an adult of the same weight, the puppy may need to consume a larger volume of an adult food to meet its energy needs. This may result in the inadvertent consumption of excess amounts of other nutrients (such as calcium). If very large volumes of food are fed to meet the puppy's energy needs, this can also lead to digestive upsets, gastric discomfort, or diarrhea. It is therefore best to choose a highly digestible growth diet in which the nutrient content has been thoroughly evaluated and that has an energy and nutrient density designed for a growing dog.

In addition to controlling food intake, owners should also provide regular periods of exercise for their growing dog. Exercise aids in the achievement of proper energy balance and supports normal muscle development. Young dogs should be exercised at a level that maintains a lean, well-muscled body condition throughout their growing period. Daily running, swimming, or retrieving for 20 to 40 minutes is adequate for most dogs. High-impact activities such as playing with other dogs, wrestling with owners, or prolonged periods of running should be strictly supervised and provided only in moderation. There is evidence that exercise that is overly vigorous or intense may predispose young dogs to skeletal abnormalities such as osteochondritis dissecans.[82] Care should always be taken to avoid excessive periods of exercise involving prolonged concussion to developing joints in growing dogs, especially dogs of the large or giant breeds.

Cats

Like dogs, growing cats should be fed to achieve normal growth and development. A high-quality, commercial cat food that has been proven to be adequate for growth through AAFCO feeding trials is recommended. Supplementation of this diet is not necessary and can be detrimental. Normal feline feeding behavior results in the frequent consumption of many small meals throughout the day.[2,3,4,6] If adequate exercise is provided, most growing cats can self-regulate their energy intake when fed free-choice and will not overeat. In general, excessive caloric intake and accelerated growth rate are not common problems in growing cats. However, if inadequate exercise is provided or a highly palatable diet is fed, excessive weight gain can result. In these situations, portion-controlled feeding should be used (Box 22-1).

BOX 22-1

Practical Feeding Tips: Growing Dogs and Cats

Feed a highly digestible, nutrient-dense food formulated for growth.

Meal-feed using a portion-controlled regimen.

Feed three to four meals per day until 4 to 6 months of age; feed two or more meals per day after 6 months.

Feed to achieve an average rate of growth for a pet's breed **and** to support a lean body condition.

Avoid overfeeding or underfeeding to promote maximal growth rate.

Feed a reduced-calcium diet to large- and giant-breed puppies.

Provide regular daily exercise.

Do not add nutrient supplements to a pet's balanced diet.

CHAPTER

23

Adult Maintenance

A dog or cat that has reached mature adult size and is not pregnant, lactating, or working strenuously is defined as being in a *maintenance state*. This category includes most of the dogs and cats kept as house pets. The major nutritional concerns during this period of life are the provision of a nutritionally complete and balanced diet that supplies the pet's daily nutrient needs. Feeding proper amounts of a high-quality, well-formulated diet throughout a pet's adult life contributes to optimal health and the maintenance of ideal body weight and condition.

Adult dogs should be fed a high-quality food formulated for adults and proven to be adequate for maintenance through long-term feeding trials. Although canned, semimoist, or dry food can be fed, dry foods are often preferred for this stage of life. In general, canned and semimoist foods have higher caloric densities on a dry-matter basis (DMB) than dry foods. When canned or semimoist foods are fed to adult dogs, they may contribute to the development of obesity if intake is not closely monitored. Dry dog foods are less calorically dense, and they can also help to maintain proper tooth and gum hygiene (see Section 6, pp. 481-482). Dry foods are also easier and more economical to feed to large groups of dogs than are other types of foods.

The availability of highly palatable pet foods coupled with the sedentary lives of many dogs has resulted in a high incidence of obesity in the adult dog population. It is estimated that 25% to 30% of American dogs and cats are either overweight or obese.[83,84,85] In contrast, one survey estimated that only about 2% of dogs are thin or moderately underweight.[83] The two most effective ways to prevent obesity in adult dogs are to provide daily exercise and to closely regulate food intake. Exercise can be in the form of daily walks or runs or several sessions of vigorous games such as fetch or hide and seek. Swimming is also an excellent form of exercise. Most dogs enjoy swimming if introduced to water at an early age and in a gradual manner. Monitoring an adult dog's daily food intake is best accomplished through portion-controlled feeding. Some dogs are able to self-regulate their food intake when fed free-choice. However, many dogs tend to overconsume and gain weight. Providing two or more premeasured meals at regular times each day is a simple way to carefully regulate a dog's food intake.

The guidelines printed on pet food labels provide an estimate of the amount needed to feed an average adult dog that is living indoors and provided with a moderate amount of exercise. Alternatively, an estimate of the amount to feed can be calculated using the pet's ideal body weight (see Section 2, pp. 83-88, and Table 9-2, p. 85). Although each of these approximations can be used as a starting point, every dog should be fed as an individual. Adjustments can be made depending on the pet's activity level, temperament, body condition, and weight status.[86] The recent development of body condition scoring systems for dogs and cats provides a reliable method for owners and veterinarians to use when assessing body condition in pets.[85,87,88] Because body weight alone is not necessarily a reliable indicator of a dog's body condition, these visual tools have been developed as aids for determining optimal body condition and for the diagnosis of obesity in companion animals. Examples of body scoring systems for dogs and cats are provided in Figures 23-1 and 23-2. The use of body scoring is discussed in detail in Section 5, pp. 313-317.

It is not necessary to feed a wide variety of foods to adult dogs. Most dogs are best maintained on a constant diet of a balanced pet food and a constant supply of fresh water. Changing the diet frequently can result in gastrointestinal tract upset with resulting diarrhea and/or vomiting. If a pet's diet is to be changed, the new food should be introduced slowly by mixing it in increasing amounts with the dog's original food over a period of 4 days.

Like dogs, adult cats should be fed a food proven to be adequate for maintenance. Cats are nonvoracious feeders and prefer to eat many small meals frequently throughout the day.[4,6] Many cats will adapt to free-choice feeding and can maintain their normal body weight on this type of regimen. Although any type of food can be fed to adult cats, dry cat foods are best suited for free-choice feeding because they keep fresh longer than other foods. In addition, cats are less likely to overconsume dry foods when fed free-choice. In general, cats that live entirely indoors have less opportunity or inclination to exercise than do cats who have access to the outdoors. As a result, indoor cats are more prone to obesity; therefore regular exercise should be encouraged. A visual body score chart can be used to evaluate an adult cat's body condition (see Figure 23-2). If an adult cat cannot maintain normal body condition on a free-choice regimen, portion-controlled feeding should be instituted.

FIGURE **23-1**

Assessment of body condition in the dog.

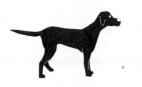 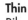

Thin
Ribs, lumbar vertebrae, and pelvic bones easily visible. No palpable fat. Obvious waist and abdominal tuck.

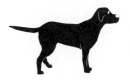

Underweight
Ribs easily palpable. Minimal fat covering. Waist is easily noted when viewed from above. Abdominal tuck evident.

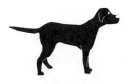

Ideal
Ribs palpable without excess fat covering. Waist observed behind ribs when viewed from above. Abdomen tucked up when viewed from the side.

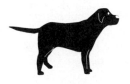

Overweight
Ribs palpable with a slight excess of fat covering. Waist is discernible when viewed from above but is not prominent. Abdominal tuck is apparent.

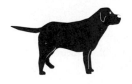

Obese
Ribs not easily palpable under a heavy fat covering. Fat deposits noticeable over lumbar area and at base of tail. Waist barely visible to absent. No abdominal tuck; may exhibit obvious abdominal distention.

FIGURE **23-2**

Assessment of body condition in the cat.

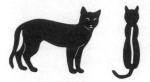

Thin
Ribs, lumbar vertebrae, and pelvic bones easily visible. Thin neck and narrow waist. Obvious abdominal tuck. No fat in flank folds; folds often absent.

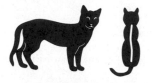

Underweight
Backbone and ribs easily palpable. Minimal fat covering. Minimal waist when viewed from above. Slightly tucked abdomen.

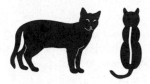

Ideal
Ribs palpable but not visible. Slight waist observed behind ribs when viewed from above. Abdomen tucked up; flank folds present.

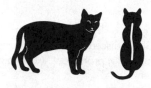

Overweight
Slight increase in fat over ribs but ribs still easily palpable. Abdomen slightly rounded; flanks concave. Flank folds hang down with moderate amount of fat; jiggle noted when walking.

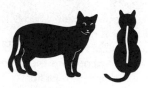

Obese
Ribs and backbone not easily palpable under a heavy fat covering. Abdomen rounded; waist barely visible to absent. Prominent flank folds that sway from side to side when walking.

24

Performance and Stress

 Dogs work with people in a variety of capacities, including acting as aids for the blind and the physically disabled, pulling sleds on arctic expeditions and races, herding and guarding sheep, hunting, and performing protection and drug detection tasks for the police and military. The type of training, level of exercise, and daily routine that a dog experiences vary with the type of work. In general, all working dogs have higher energy requirements than adult dogs during periods of normal maintenance. Depending on the type and intensity of work, modifications in the nutrient composition of the diet and changes in the daily feeding regimen of a working dog may be necessary.

ENDURANCE PERFORMANCE

Endurance performance in dogs, as in humans, involves prolonged periods of exercise at submaximal levels of exertion. Sled dogs working in cold environments represent the ultimate canine endurance athletes. These dogs have been used as the accepted mode of transportation in Alaska and surrounding territories for many years. During the Gold Rush of the late 1800s, prospectors traveled to the Yukon territory and used dogs to cross the northern tundra in search of gold. As mining camps and towns developed, sled dog trails were forged to connect coastal towns to interior camps. These trails provided the major transport routes for the provision of food and supplies to the camps. Although most of the mining camps are now mere ghost towns, dogs and dog sledding remain an integral part of the area's economy and culture. In addition to their importance in Alaska, sled dog teams have been used by explorers of the north and south poles. Robert Perry reached the North Pole via dog sled in 1909, and Roald Amundsen reached the south pole with his team of dogs in 1911. Throughout this century, sled dog teams have continued to provide transportation in certain areas of the world. In addition, mushing and sled dog racing have become popular outdoor sports for many dog enthusiasts. Today, sled dog races are held in many parts of the world, including Europe, Alaska, and several of the lower 48 states.

The Iditarod is one of the most well known and publicized long-distance sled dog races. Informally called the "the last great race on earth," the Iditarod is run every March, beginning in Anchorage and ending in Nome. The trail that is followed is symbolically designated to be 1049 miles long (1000 miles because it is at least that long, and 49 miles because Alaska was the forty-ninth state to be admitted to the union). Officially, the race distance is 1158 miles by the northern route or 1163 miles by the southern route. Because of its great length and the difficult terrain, the Iditarod represents the ultimate endurance test for the canine athlete. Dog teams average up to 100 miles per day in subzero temperatures and over difficult snow-covered terrain. Nutritionists and exercise physiologists interested in the care and nutrition of these dogs have used this race and similar long-distance sled dog races to collect valuable information about the energy, nutrient, water, and electrolyte needs of working dogs. This research has provided information for the development of diets that provide optimal nutrition for working dogs; it has also contributed to improved information about the proper care and husbandry of endurance-trained dogs.

Physiology

The type of work that occurs during endurance competitions differs from that performed during short races or sprinting events, such as greyhound racing or lure coursing. Greyhounds engage in brief, intense bouts of high-speed running, while sled dogs pull for several hours at a time at slower speeds. Metabolically, the energy necessary for short sprints is obtained primarily through anaerobic pathways and secondarily through aerobic metabolism. Energy for long endurance events is predominantly derived from aerobic metabolism. Fat and carbohydrate are the two principal fuels that supply energy to working muscle. During low-intensity (aerobic) exercise, fat is the most important fuel used. This is supplied by free fatty acids (FFAs) derived from muscle and other tissues. As the intensity of the exercise increases, a shift toward more anaerobic metabolism occurs, and carbohydrate becomes increasingly important as a source of energy. This carbohydrate is supplied by muscle glycogen and, as muscle glycogen becomes depleted, is supplemented by the production of glucose by the liver (gluconeogenesis). This metabolic response to different intensities of exercise and training has been observed in rats, humans, and dogs.[89,90,91,92,93] For example, a recent study showed that the rate of muscle glycogen utilization in a group of trained dogs completing an anaerobic test was almost 20-fold greater than rates observed in dogs during aerobic exercise.[94]

An examination of the types of muscles that are involved in endurance exercise provides information about the types of energy sources needed. The skeletal muscles of dogs contain three main types of muscle fibers: type I (slow twitch) and types IIa and IIb (fast twitch). Slow-twitch fibers have a high capacity for aerobic metabolism, and fast-twitch fibers can use both oxidative (aerobic) and anaerobic pathways.[95] The slow-twitch fibers use fatty acids and glucose for fuel and are believed to be important for endurance events. Although these fibers are found in all skeletal muscles, their numbers predominate in antigravity muscles such as the dog's anconeus and the quadratus muscles.[95,96] In general, endurance athletes have higher numbers of well-developed, slow-twitch fibers, and athletes involved in high-speed sprinting events have a higher proportion of fast-twitch fibers. Athletic conditioning is important for conditioning muscles and building muscle mass. In addition, athletic conditioning for endurance events increases the body's reliance upon fatty acid oxidation during submaximal bouts of exercise. This adaptation has been demonstrated in rats, humans, and dogs.[89,90] Recent evidence shows that the type of diet fed to dogs may also affect the use of fatty acids by working muscles, independent of the effects of training.[94,97]

Glycogen Loading

Although it is generally accepted that energy is the nutrient of most concern for working dogs, there has been much debate about the best way to supply energy in the diet. Increasing stamina and strength are goals for the nutritional programs of many human athletes. As a result, a great deal of research has been conducted concerning ways to supply fuel to long-distance runners and bikers.[89,98] Studies with humans have shown that an important limiting factor in prolonged exercise is the amount of glycogen present in the working muscles, and that the onset of fatigue is highly correlated with muscle glycogen depletion.[99,100] In addition, endurance for submaximal exercise can be increased by raising muscle glycogen stores and decreased by lowering muscle glycogen.[100,101] Therefore a major goal when feeding human endurance athletes is to either increase muscle glycogen stores or delay muscle glycogen depletion during periods of exercise.

The procedure of *glycogen loading* (also called *carbohydrate loading*) was developed for human athletes with the intent of increasing muscle glycogen stores before periods of prolonged exercise. Glycogen loading is accomplished by first depleting muscle glycogen through exhaustive exercise and/or consumption of a low-carbohydrate diet, followed by the consumption of a high-carbohydrate diet for 4 to 7 days.[100,102,103] The preliminary glycogen depletion phase results in *glycogen supercompensation* when the subject consumes a diet that is high in starch for several subsequent days. Glycogen stores in working muscles are significantly increased above normal levels when this regimen is followed by human athletes. The beneficial effects that higher initial glycogen stores have on endurance are believed to be the result of the availability of larger amounts of glycogen for anaerobic energy metabolism in the working muscles. In recent years, the first stage, glycogen depletion, has been shown to be unnecessary.[104,105] Today, many endurance athletes regularly consume a high-carbohydrate diet and concentrate on carbohydrate loading for the last few days prior to an endurance event.

Providing Energy for Working Dogs: Fat or Carbohydrate?

The two primary fuels for working muscle are muscle glycogen and FFAs. In the moderately active dog, approximately 70% to 90% of the energy for sustained work is derived from fat metabolism; only a small amount of energy is derived from carbohydrate metabolism.[106,107] However, until recently, little was known about fat and glycogen use in hard-working endurance dogs. Early field studies on sled dogs and laboratory studies on Beagles indicated that the ability to use fatty acids through aerobic pathways was more important than the use of muscle glycogen through anaerobic pathways.[89,108,109] In one study, a dog team that was fed a high-carbohydrate diet performed poorly and developed a stiff gait while racing. When the dogs were changed to a diet containing increased levels of fat and protein, performance improved and the observed lameness resolved.[110] The researchers suggested that feeding a high-carbohydrate diet to sled dogs may be responsible for the occurrence of a form of exertional rhabdomyolysis.[109,110] *Exertional rhabdomyolysis* is a disorder caused by rapid anaerobic metabolism of muscle glycogen, resulting in an accumulation of lactic acid. Lactic acid accumulation can have several adverse side effects, including damage to muscle-tissue membranes, edema, and inhibition of lipolysis and glycolysis.[111] These studies led to the theory that dietary fat is a preferred fuel for endurance in racing sled dogs.

Controlled studies in recent years have supported this hypothesis and have also provided important information regarding feeding management and training for racing sled dogs. Both the level of conditioning and the type of diet fed significantly affect energy use in working dogs. In a series of studies with 16 Alaskan Huskies, one group of dogs was fed a high-fat diet containing 60% of calories as fat, while the second group was fed a high-carbohydrate diet, containing 60% of calories as carbohydrate.[94,112,113] Standard aerobic and anaerobic tests on a treadmill were performed by the dogs prior to conditioning, after a 4-week aerobic training period, and again after a 4-week anaerobic training period. Results of the aerobic tests showed that both groups of dogs relied primarily upon FFAs and used little glycogen to complete the tests (Figures 24-1 and 24-2). Dogs that were fed a high-fat diet had significantly greater pre-exercise and post-exercise FFA concentrations when compared with dogs fed the high-carbohydrate diet, even before they were conditioned through training. The concentration of FFAs in the blood is a major determinant of fatty acid utilization by muscle, and it is an accepted indicator of fatty acid metabolism. These results indicate that feeding a high-fat diet to sled dogs before and during athletic training results in an enhanced ability to mobilize and use fat as a fuel.

A second controlled study examined the effect of diet on oxygen consumption (VO_2) max, mitochondrial volume, and maximal rates of fat oxidation in a group of endurance-trained Labrador Retrievers.[114] When dietary fat was increased from 15% to 60% of calories, dogs showed a 50% increase in VO_2 max and a 45% increase in maximal fat oxidation during aerobic exercise tests. These values indicate enhanced efficiency of fat utilization and capacity for aerobic work. Mitochondrial volume in muscles increased 50% in response to increasing fat in the diet. The authors suggest that stimulation of mitochondrial growth may be one mechanism through which feeding a high-fat diet improves aerobic work capacity and efficiency in endurance-trained dogs.

Although fat is the primary metabolic fuel for endurance dogs, and high-fat diets best supply this fuel, adequate muscle glycogen stores are still vitally important during exercise. As in other species, muscle glycogen depletion during prolonged

FIGURE 24-1

Muscle glycogen concentrations in trained and untrained dogs (aerobic tests). **A**, *Untrained, and* **B**, *aerobically trained.* HCD, *High-carbohydrate diet;* HFD, *high-fat diet;* mmole, *millimole.*

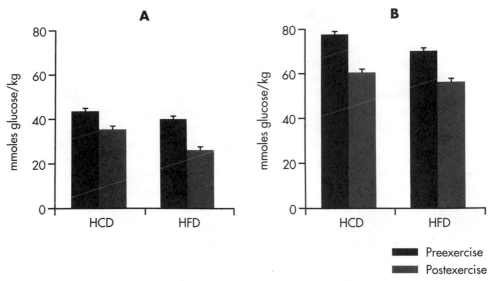

(From Reynolds AJ, Taylor CR, Hoeppler H, and others: The effect of diet on sled dog performance, oxidative capacity, skeletal muscle microstructure, and muscle glycogen metabolism. In Carey DP, Norton SA, Bolser SM, editors: *Recent advances in canine and feline nutritional research*, Iams International Nutritional Symposium, Wilmington, Ohio, 1996, Orange Frazer Press.)

FIGURE 24-2

Serum FFA concentrations in trained and untrained dogs (aerobic tests). **A**, *Untrained, and* **B**, *aerobically trained.* HCD, *High-carbohydrate diet;* HFD, *high-fat diet;* mmole, *millimole.*

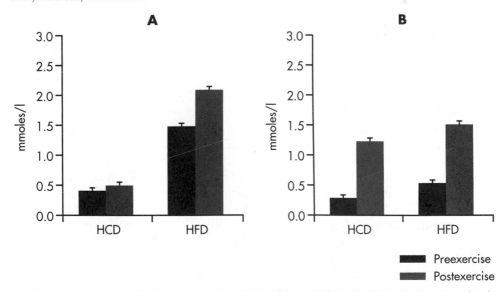

(From Reynolds AJ, Taylor CR, Hoeppler H, and others: The effect of diet on sled dog performance, oxidative capacity, skeletal muscle microstructure, and muscle glycogen metabolism. In Carey DP, Norton SA, Bolser SM, editors: *Recent advances in canine and feline nutritional research*, Iams International Nutritional Symposium, Wilmington, Ohio, 1996, Orange Frazer Press.)

exercise is associated with a decline in performance and fatigue in working dogs. The two factors that appear to have the greatest influence on muscle glycogen stores are athletic conditioning and diet (see Figure 24-1). In the study described previously, only small amounts of glycogen were used by dogs during the aerobic tests. However, some glycogen metabolism is always necessary to permit the continuation of FFA metabolism during aerobic work. In addition to this need, racing sled dogs experience periods of intense running near the end of races or when covering difficult terrain. To learn more about the needs of dogs during these periods, researchers also examined energy metabolism in sled dogs during bouts of intense anaerobic activity.[94] As in other species, dogs performing anaerobic tests rely heavily upon muscle glycogen as an energy source. In addition, completing a 4-week training period significantly increased the muscle glycogen levels in all dogs, regardless of the type of diet that was fed. While dogs that were fed a high-carbohydrate diet stored more muscle glycogen than those fed a high-fat diet, the carbohydrate-fed dogs also metabolized more glycogen to complete the anaerobic test. As a result, muscle glycogen levels at the completion of the standard anaerobic test were similar for all the dogs fed the two different diets. The researchers concluded that feeding high-fat diets to endurance-trained dogs not only prepares muscles to efficiently mobilize and use FFAs as an energy source, it also has a glycogen-sparing effect that can help to prolong glycogen use during distance racing.

Protein for Endurance Dogs

Current evidence indicates that endurance training and racing result in increased protein needs for dogs.[115] This increase is the result of both increased protein synthesis (anabolism) and a relatively small but significant increase in protein degradation (catabolism). Athletic conditioning results in adaptive physiological changes that facilitate efficient delivery of oxygen and nutrients to working muscles. These changes include increases in blood volume, red blood cell mass, capillary density, mitochondrial volume, and the activity and total mass of metabolic enzymes.[116,117] The increased tissue mass associated with athletic training must be supplied by additional protein in the diet. In addition, there is a slight but significant increase in protein catabolism during endurance exercise. This occurs because up to 10% of energy in exercising dogs can be derived from the metabolism of gluconeogenic amino acids.[118,119]

A recent study was conducted to determine optimal levels of dietary protein for sled dogs in training.[97] Diets supplying either 16%, 24%, 32%, or 40% of calories from protein were fed to sled dogs throughout a 12-week training period. Dogs that were fed 40% protein maintained a larger plasma volume and red blood cell mass during training than dogs fed diets containing less than 40% protein. The amount of protein in the diet also appeared to influence susceptibility to injury. While there were no injuries in any of the dogs that consumed the 32% or 40% protein diets, all of the dogs fed the 16% diet were injured at some point during the 12-week period, which kept them out of training for 2 or more days. It appears that the proportion of energy that is supplied by protein should be increased in the diets of endurance

BOX 24-1

Practical Feeding Tips: Endurance Performance

Feed a highly digestible, energy- and nutrient-dense diet (4500 kcal of ME/kg or greater).
Diet should contain:
   Calories from protein: 30% to 35%
   Calories from fat: 50% to 65%
   Calories from carbohydrate: 10% to 15%
   Omega-6:omega-3 fatty acid ratio between 5:1 and 10:1
   Moderately fermentable fiber: 3% to 7%
Provide continual access to clean, fresh water.
Feed two or more meals per day on a portion-controlled basis.
Feed the largest meal of the day after the day's training is complete.
Provide a meal 1.5 to 2 hours before training or an endurance event.
Feed a carbohydrate-containing supplement immediately after endurance exercise to promote glucose repletion.

Adapted from *Proceedings of the Performance Dog Nutrition Symposium,* Fort Collins, Colo, 1995, Colorado State University.

dogs in training to ensure adequate tissue accretion, prevent tissue loss, and possibly aid in the prevention of injury. Optimal protein concentrations of between 30% and 40% of calories are recommended in diets for endurance dogs (Box 24-1).

While providing enough protein in the diet is important, feeding a diet that contains more protein than the dog needs is neither necessary nor beneficial. Protein consumed in excess of the needs of tissue replacement and growth will be used as an energy source. Protein is one of the least desirable muscle energy fuels because it is inefficiently metabolized and cannot be stored in the body like fat or glycogen. Moreover, if muscle protein is used as an energy source, the dog's ability to support and maintain long bouts of muscular work may be impaired. The diet should supply adequate calories as fat and carbohydrate so that the protein that is fed can be used primarily for tissue protein synthesis and not for energy. For the canine athlete, the most efficiently used fuel appears to be fat, with carbohydrate supplying a smaller proportion of the calories in the diet.

Energy Needs of Sled Dogs

The total energy requirement of a endurance dog depends on the intensity and duration of the exercise and the environmental conditions in which the animal is working. Early research suggested that energy needs increase to between 1.5 and 2.5 times the normal maintenance requirements in dogs working in ambient temperatures.[120,121,122] Working in cold weather may further increase requirements by about 50%. Data for these estimates were collected from draft dogs that were covering relatively short distances and traveling at slower speeds than racing sled dogs.

FIGURE 24-3

Energy expenditure of sled dogs competing in a medium distance race (kcal/day).

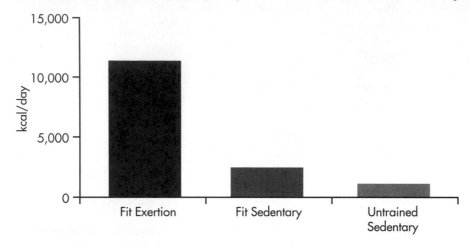

(From Hinchcliff KW, Reinhart GA, Burr JR, and others: Energy metabolism and water turnover in Alaskan sled dogs during running. In Carey DP, Norton SA, Bolser SM, editors: *Recent advances in canine and feline nutritional research,* Iams International Nutritional Symposium, Wilmington, Ohio, 1996, Orange Frazer Press.)

Typical dog teams used for hauling freight travel less than 20 miles per day at speeds of about 5 miles per hour. Energy needs for these dogs are estimated to be between 4000 and 8000 kilocalories (kcal)/day.[120,123]

In contrast, dogs trained for racing in long-distance sled races typically run 70 miles or more per day and travel at speeds of up to 9 miles per hour. A recent study found that racing sled dogs competing in a medium distance race (300 miles) expended an average of 11,200 kcal per day and consumed an average of 10,600 kcal/day (Figure 24-3).[124] These values are equivalent to burning 460 kcal/kilogram (kg) of body weight per day and consuming 440 kcal/kg of body weight per day. The researchers observed that the calculated values for sustained metabolic rate for these dogs appears to exceed previously predicted maximal values for mammals of their size. These extraordinarily high energy requirements and expenditures predicate the need to provide a diet that is energy-dense and highly digestive to allow the ingestion of needed calories in a volume of food that the dog's stomach and gastrointestinal system are capable of handling.

Water and Electrolyte Requirements

The same researchers who measured caloric intake and expenditure in racing sled dogs also examined water intake, water turnover, and electrolyte balance during medium- and long-distance races.[125,126,127,128] Dogs competing in a 300-mile race had a measured water turnover rate of approximately 250 milliliters (ml)/kg of body weight per day.[127] This is equal to about 5 liters (L) per day for an average-size sled dog. By comparison, sled dogs who were not racing had water turnovers of only

0.9 L per day. Dogs lose water primarily through respiration, urine, feces, and, to a very small degree, perspiration. The extremely high water loss in working sled dogs is primarily a result of increased urinary water loss. In all animals, urinary water loss is related to the obligatory urinary solute load, which in turn is affected by the quantity of food consumed and the composition of the diet.[129] Diets with a high protein concentration and/or large caloric intake result in higher obligatory solute loads. Because sled dogs consume up to 12,000 kcal/day when they are racing, they have extremely high solute loads and, as a result, very high obligatory urinary water losses. Dogs must be provided with fresh water frequently during racing to offset these losses and prevent dehydration.

Electrolyte balance is also an important consideration in exercising animals. Exercise-induced hyponatremia occurs in horses and humans and may be associated with clinical signs.[130,131] Decreases in serum sodium and potassium levels have also been observed in sled dogs during long-distance races.[128,129,132] While concentrations of these electrolytes usually remained within normal ranges and no clinical signs were reported, exercise-associated hyponatremia and total cation depletion have been observed in some dogs.[126,127] These changes appear to be attributable to the solute diuresis and urine sodium losses mandated by the large energy intake (and resultant solute loads) of racing dogs.[125,128] Urine osmolality did not change in response to exercise in the dogs studied. However, there was a shift in the type of solutes present in the urine. Urinary sodium, potassium, and chloride concentrations decreased, while urine urea concentration increased. Increased urinary urea is a direct result of the higher energy and protein intake of racing dogs. This change imposes significant increases in obligatory urinary water and sodium loss even in the face of renal cation conservation. Although decreases in serum cation concentration have not been associated with clinical signs in any of the dogs studied, these data indicate the importance of providing a diet that has an adequate level of sodium to racing sled dogs.

Glycogen Repletion after Exhaustive Exercise

Glycogen depletion is associated with fatigue and impaired performance in all species that have been studied.[109, 110, 133,134,135,136] As shown previously, feeding a diet that is formulated to spare glycogen is more successful than feeding a diet designed to increase muscle glycogen stores (i.e., glycogen loading) for endurance-trained dogs. However, glycogen depletion is still associated with fatigue and impaired performance in racing sled dogs.[137] In a typical medium- or long-distance race, sled dogs run for 4 to 6 hours at time, followed by a 2- to 4-hour rest period. During rest periods the dogs are usually provided with a high-fat, high-protein snack and are fed their full meal once they have finished running for the day. Because the diets of sled dogs are typically low in carbohydrates, glycogen depletion can occur when this feeding regimen is used, especially during events that involve successive days of racing or periods of intense running.

Studies conducted with human athletes show that the rate of muscle glycogen repletion after exhaustive exercise is substantially affected by the timing of carbohydrate ingestion.[138,139] If a carbohydrate supplement is ingested immediately after exercise, the rate of glycogen repletion for the first 2 hours is up to three-fold greater than if carbohydrate was not ingested. If ingestion of carbohydrate is delayed for 2 hours after exercise, the rate of glycogen repletion to working muscles is only half the rate observed when carbohydrate is consumed immediately after exercise. The mechanism believed to be responsible for this effect involves enhanced blood flow to muscles immediately following exercise. Exercise-induced blood flow to muscle results in increased glucose transport and, subsequently, enhanced glucose uptake and glycogen synthesis by the muscles. If carbohydrate intake is delayed, blood glucose level still increases, but the rate of muscle glycogen repletion is slowed.

A recent study was conducted on endurance-trained sled dogs to determine if carbohydrate feeding immediately after exercise was an effective means of muscle glycogen repletion between bouts of exercise.[137] Sled dogs were fed either a water and glucose polymer solution or water alone immediately after an exhaustive training run. Dogs that consumed the glucose polymer (1.5 grams [g]/kg of body weight) had significantly increased rates of muscle glycogen repletion when compared with dogs who were not supplemented (Figure 24-4). Plasma glucose levels increased significantly within 100 minutes of supplementation and were presumably responsible for enhanced delivery of glucose to muscles (Figure 24-5). Since many sled

FIGURE **24-4**

Muscle glycogen concentration in sled dogs before and after a 30 kilometer run.
Treatment A* = Water only following exercise; treatment B** = Water plus 1.5 g/kg
glucose polymer after exercise; treatment C** = Water only following exercise.
*Biopsied 1 hour before and immediately after exercise.
**Biopsied 1 hour before and 4 hours after exercise.

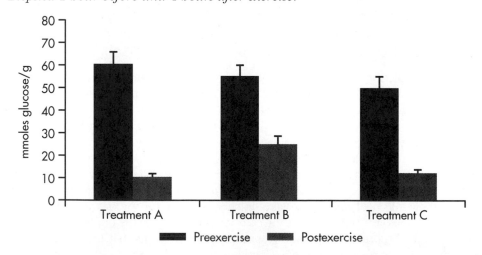

(From Reynolds AJ, Taylor CR, Hoeppler H, and others: The effect of diet on sled dog performance, oxidative capacity, skeletal muscle microstructure, and muscle glycogen metabolism. In Carey DP, Norton SA, Bolser SM, editors: *Recent advances in canine and feline nutritional research*, Iams International Nutritional Symposium, Wilmington, Ohio, 1996, Orange Frazer Press.)

dog races are multiple-day events, feeding dogs to support rapid repletion of muscle glycogen is expected to enhance performance. The practice of providing a glucose polymer as a carbohydrate supplement immediately after exhaustive exercise may be especially helpful when sled dogs are fed diets that supply most of their calories as fat and when bouts of exercise are separated by only a few hours.

Practical Feeding and Diets for Endurance Dogs

It is now evident that dietary fat is an important component in the diet of working dogs because of its ability to supply energy to working muscles. In addition to its beneficial effects upon aerobic metabolism, fat also has a significant influence upon a diet's energy density and digestibility. The most efficacious way to increase both energy density and diet digestibility is to supply energy in the form of high-quality fat. A study with Beagles demonstrated the importance of diet digestibility and fat content.[109] A group of dogs were fed either a commercial, dry diet formulated for maintenance or one of three highly digestible, high-fat diets. After a period of dietary adaptation, endurance was measured using a standard treadmill test. The dogs

FIGURE **24-5**

Blood glucose concentrations after exercise in sled dogs fed water or 1.5 g/kg glucose polymer.

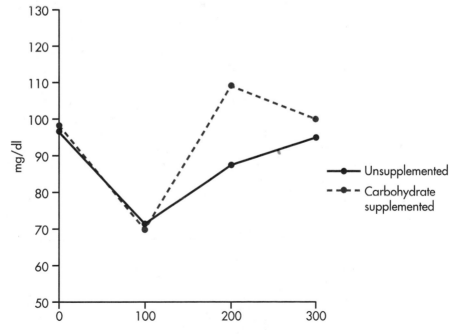

(From *Performance Dog Nutrition Symposium*, Dayton, Ohio, 1995, The Iams Company. Used with permission.)

fed the maintenance diet experienced exhaustion after 103 minutes, but the dogs fed the more energy-dense, highly digestible diets did not experience exhaustion until they had run for a significantly longer period (137 minutes). Analysis of these data showed that performance level in the Beagles was positively correlated with diet digestibility and the intake of digestible fat.

An animal with increased energy needs must consume a great deal of food to meet those needs. During long-distance racing, dogs' extremely high energy needs require the intake of a large volume of food. If the diet is low in digestibility, a large amount of dry matter (DM) must be ingested, and intake may be limited by the dog's gastric capacity and its ability to digest and assimilate large boluses of food. Therefore, in addition to the need for a high fat content as an energy source, high digestibility is necessary to limit the total volume of food that the dog must consume at each meal. Although some maintenance diets can supply enough energy if consumed in large enough quantities by working dogs, they may become bulk-limiting and thus limit performance in hard-working dogs. Diets formulated for working dogs should contain high quality sources of protein, fat, and carbohydrate to ensure high digestibility and availability of nutrients and minimize the volume of food that must be fed to meet a dog's needs.

Feeding practices that are best suited for hard-working dogs are designed to minimize gastrointestinal expansion during bouts of work and maintain a high work capacity throughout the session of exercise. Dogs should be fed on a portion-controlled basis so that the trainer can strictly regulate the timing and the size of meals. The main meal of the day should be fed after the day's session of training to allow adequate digestion of food. If possible, at least two meals should be provided per day, and a small meal can be provided 1.5 to 2 hours before endurance activity. High-fat/high-protein snacks can be fed during rest periods between bouts of running during distance races, while a carbohydrate-containing drink or food can be fed immediately after exhaustive periods of work.

Depending upon the type of work and the environmental conditions, water losses can increase by ten- to twenty-fold during exercise.[128,129] Therefore it is important that dogs are provided with water at frequent intervals throughout a session of work. Even mild dehydration can lead to reduced work capacity, decreased strength, and hyperthermia.[140] Working dogs should be given frequent opportunities to drink small amounts of fresh water during periods of extended work. In addition, water can be added to meals as a method of increasing water intake during periods of heavy training or racing. This practice prevents the development of even mild dehydration. Cool water is preferable because it is more palatable to most dogs and is more effective in helping to cool the body.[141]

SPRINT RACING PERFORMANCE

The exercise that sprint-racing dogs engage in is substantially different from that required of endurance sled dogs. Greyhound races are extremely short, sprinting events. In the United States, racing takes place on an oval tract and involves distances between $\frac{5}{16}$ and $\frac{3}{8}$ of a mile. During a race, dogs reach speeds of 36 to 38 miles per hour, but they maintain this speed for only 30 to 40 seconds. It is known that brief, intense periods of exercise preclude the mobilization and delivery of fatty acids and the adequate oxygenation of tissue necessary for aerobic metabolism.[142] As a result, the primary source of energy for this type of exercise is the anaerobic metabolism of carbohydrate. Both muscle glycogen and circulating blood glucose supply energy to muscles during brief bouts of intense work.[143] This process differs from endurance exercise, in which FFAs and a small amount of glycogen supply energy to the working muscles. Postrace biochemical data collected from racing Greyhounds indicate that the greyhound relies primarily on anaerobic metabolism for energy.[144,145,146] Blood lactate levels increase dramatically from prerace values of 8 milligrams (mg)/deciliter (dl) to postrace values of 220 mg/dl, which reflects the significant contribution of anaerobic metabolism of carbohydrate to the energy demands of the race.[144] It appears that the Greyhound is well adapted to this type of work because both lactate levels and blood pH return to normal values within 1 hour of the race.[145] Training also increases the body's ability to metabolize accumulated lactic acid following an intense bout of exercise.[147]

Studies with human athletes indicate that dietary modification is more effective in influencing endurance athletes than sprinters. This may be a result of the fact that two factors that influence endurance during prolonged periods of exercise are the body's ability to use fat for energy and the quantity of glycogen stored in the working muscles. As discussed previously, both of these factors can be influenced by diet. Sprinters, on the other hand, rapidly use muscle glycogen and circulating glucose through anaerobic metabolism. A study with human runners showed that although the practice of glycogen loading increased the amount of exercise time until exhaustion, it did not appear to influence running speed at the beginning of the race.[98]

Although short-term, anaerobic energy metabolism may not be readily influenced by diet, it is still important that racing dogs receive diets that are energy dense and highly digestible. Feeding a diet that has been formulated for performance ensures that DM intake during racing or training is not excessive. The diet fed to racing Greyhounds should also contain moderate to high levels of digestible fat and protein and a moderate amount of highly digestible carbohydrate. Carbohydrate supplementation after intense bouts of exercise may also be helpful in enhancing the repletion of muscle glycogen stores.[137]

WEATHER EXTREMES

Adverse weather conditions in the form of extreme cold or heat result in increased energy needs in dogs and cats. This increase can be quite substantial depending on the severity of the weather. A study of dogs living in an arctic environment showed that an increase in energy intake of 70% to 80% was necessary for the dogs to maintain normal body temperatures without experiencing weight loss.[148] Dogs are capable of a significant level of cold-induced thermogenesis, a mechanism involving an increase in metabolic rate during exposure to a cold environment. The increased metabolic rate produces additional body heat that is used to maintain body temperature.

Although the increased energy needs of dogs in arctic environments are very great and result in large increases in daily energy intake, dogs housed outside during moderately cold weather also experience a degree of cold-induced thermogenesis. A study on Labrador Retrievers and Beagles showed that as environmental temperatures decreased from 59° Farenheit (F) (thermal neutral zone) to 47° F, the dogs' metabolizable energy (ME) intake increased and remained high until the ambient temperature was increased.[149] During the cold period, there was a slight decrease in mean body weight despite increased energy intake. Results from this study indicate that an average increase in ME intake of 25% is necessary to maintain body weight in dogs housed in cool conditions. This figure can be used as a general guide for increasing the ME intake of dogs that are housed outdoors during the winter months. However, factors such as the dog's size, its coat type and length, the type of shelter that is provided, and weather conditions such as wind and drifting snow significantly influence the amount of food needed by dogs housed in cold environments.[150] For example, a study on Beagles, Labrador Retrievers, and Siberian Huskies found that the ME requirements of Siberian Huskies are less affected by fluctuations in environmental temperature than are the ME intakes of Beagles and Labrador Retrievers.[151] It appears that the double coats of Huskies act as a protective barrier to insulate them against large fluctuations in environmental temperature.

The energy needs of dogs and cats also increase with high environmental temperatures and humidities. The exposure to high ambient temperature causes an increase in the amount of energy that must be used to cool the body. Working dogs in humid environments experience slight increases in energy needs; at the same time they often exhibit a reduction in appetite.[152] Therefore it is important to provide dogs working in hot environments with a diet that is high in caloric and nutrient density so that nutritional needs may be met without the consumption of large quantities of food. It is also especially important that cool water be provided continuously in warm or humid environments.

STRESS

Working animals are exposed to a variety of stresses, such as intense physical exertion, weather extremes, and psychological strain. Although repeated, low levels of tolerable stresses are believed to be a necessary component of training and improved performance, severe stress can result in a breakdown in performance.[108] Signs of severe stress in dogs include apathy, depression, anorexia, and a reluctance to work. It has been suggested that some of the side effects of severe stress in working dogs include diarrhea and dehydration, exertional rhabdomyolysis, lower bowel bleeding, anemia, and metatarsal fractures.[86] However, no controlled research studies have been conducted on working dogs to substantiate these claims.

External influences such as training regimen, housing conditions, environmental temperature and humidity, and the type of training methods that are used greatly influence the degree of stress that an individual animal experiences. Internal influences on stress include an animal's temperament, age, physical capabilities, and nutritional status. The provision of a well-balanced, high-quality diet formulated for working dogs helps to prevent the onset of severe stress, but it cannot compensate for other adverse conditions in a dog's life. In other words, a sound nutritional program is extremely important for hard-working animals, but it will never counteract the detrimental effects of the stress produced by poor training or care.

The major nutritional considerations for working dogs experiencing stress are energy density and diet digestibility. In addition to these dietary modifications, many breeders, exhibitors, and trainers believe that stressed dogs must also receive supplements of certain vitamins and minerals. However, there is no evidence to suggest that working dogs require higher amounts of these nutrients. Supplemental vitamin C was first advocated as an aid in the relief of various stress conditions in human athletes because plasma ascorbate levels were found to decline during stress.[108] This practice was then extended to working animals. However, several controlled studies on human athletes have demonstrated that vitamin C supplementation has no beneficial effect on either anaerobic or aerobic work capacity.[153] Studies examining the effects of supplementation with other vitamins have shown a similar lack of results. Research investigating the specific effects of supplemental vitamins and minerals on performance in working and stressed dogs must be conducted before any valid recommendations can be made. If a diet is nutritionally balanced and a dog is consuming enough to meet its energy needs during work, supplemental vitamins and minerals should not be necessary.

CHAPTER

25

Geriatrics

Improvements in the control of infectious diseases and in the nutrition of dogs and cats in recent years has resulted in a gradual increase in the average lifespan of companion animals. While the maximum lifespan of a given species remains relatively fixed, the average lifespan within a population can be significantly affected by genetics, health care, and nutrition. Currently, it is estimated that more than 40% of dogs and 30% of cats in the United States are at least 6 years of age, and approximately 30% of these pets are 11 years or older.[154,155] The increased number of geriatric pets and the understanding that most of these dogs and cats have been cherished family members for many years necessitates increased attention to the care and proper nutrition of this portion of the companion animal population. Nutritional goals for aging pets are to slow or prevent the progression of metabolic changes associated with aging, minimize clinical signs of aging, and enhance the pet's quality of life and, if possible, life expectancy.

NORMAL PHYSIOLOGICAL CHANGES THAT OCCUR WITH AGING

In general, dogs of different mature body size and conformation age at different rates.[156] The maximum lifespan of the dog is estimated to be about 27 years, and the average lifespan is approximately 13 years.[157,158] Small breeds of dogs live significantly longer than large and giant breeds.[159] Therefore, breed and adult size must be considered when determining whether or not a dog is geriatric. General guidelines divide dogs into four categories based upon adult size, with smaller dogs considered elderly at a later age than larger dogs (Table 25-1). Cats appear to age more slowly than most dogs and do not show breed differences in aging or longevity.[160] The average lifespan of the domestic cat is approximately 14 years, and its maximum lifespan may be as high as 25 to 35 years.[157] Healthy cats are considered to be geriatric when they are approximately 10 to 12 years old.

TABLE **25-1**

Suggested Ages for Geriatric Dogs and Cats

Species/Size	Age Considered Geriatric
Dogs	
5 to 20 lbs	11.5 years
21 to 50 lbs	11.0 years
51 to 90 lbs	9.0 years
Greater than 90 lbs	7.5 years
Cats	12.0 years

TABLE **25-2**

Age-Related Changes in Laboratory Values for Dogs*

Unchanged	Decreased	Increased
Alanine aminotransferase	Albumin	Globulin
Blood urea nitrogen	Albumin:globulin ratio	Platelets
BUN:creatinine ratio	Creatinine	Neutrophils
Cholesterol	Hematocrit	Serum potassium
Creatine kinase	Hemoglobin	Serum sodium
Eosinophils	Lymphocytes	Serum triglycerides
Gamma-glutamyl-transferase	Red blood cells	
Lactate dehydrogenase	Serum calcium	
Magnesium		
Serum chloride		
Total bilirubin		

*Data collected from 36 young and old Fox Terriers (1.8 vs. 11.5 years) and Labrador Retrievers (1.5 vs. 9.6 years) (From Hayek MG: Age-related changes in physiological function in the dog and cat: nutritional implications. In Reinhart GA, Carey DP, editors: *Recent advances in canine and feline nutrition,* vol 2, Iams Nutrition Symposium Proceedings, Wilmington, Ohio, 1998, Orange Frazer Press).

Biological effects of aging on the body include a gradual decline in the functional capacity of organs, beginning shortly after the animal has reached maturity. Recent preliminary studies have shown age-related changes in laboratory values for the dog and cat (Tables 25-2 and 25-3).[161,162] The clinical significance of these changes is not known and may not be relevant in many cases. Moreover, the limited number of animals that were examined preclude using these data to make generalized conclusions about age-related changes to blood chemistry and cell data. However, these data do indicate that multiple physiological systems are affected by the normal aging process and that aging in healthy animals is accompanied by changes in laboratory values.

Different systems of the body age at different rates, and the degree of compromised function that must occur before clinical signs are seen depends on many factors in a pet's life. Although one pet may exhibit severe pathological effects of ag-

TABLE **25-3**

Age-Related Changes in Laboratory Values for Cats*

Unchanged	Decreased	Increased
Eosinophils	Alanine aminotransferase	Cholesterol
Hematocrit	Alkaline phosphatase	Globulin
Lymphocytes	Aspartate aminotransferase	Monocytes
Neutrophils	Albumin	
Serum potassium	Albumin: globulin ratio	
	Creatinine kinase	
	Hemoglobin	
	Serum calcium	
	Serum phosphorus	
	White blood cells	

*Data collected from 40 young and old cats (0.9 vs. 8.9 years) (From Hayek MG: Age-related changes in physiological function in the dog and cat: nutritional implications. In Reinhart GA, Carey DP, editors: *Recent advances in canine and feline nutrition,* vol 2, Iams Nutrition Symposium Proceedings, Wilmington, Ohio, 1998, Orange Frazer Press).

ing by 7 years, another may exhibit no clinical signs even at 12 years. It is also not unusual for more than one chronic disease to be present in a single geriatric pet. This variability necessitates that older animals be assessed as individuals, using functional changes in body systems rather than chronological age to categorize them with the elderly population.

Metabolic Effects

An animal's resting metabolic rate (RMR) naturally slows with aging. This decline is caused primarily by changes in the pet's body composition, specifically a loss of lean body tissue. Normal aging in all animals is associated with decreases in lean body tissue (muscle) and total body water and an increase in the proportion of body fat. A decline in body water accompanies the loss of lean body tissue because lean tissue contains 73% water, while adipose tissue contains only 15%. Age-related changes in body composition may differ for dogs and cats. A study comparing young and old dogs reported that the body fat content of young dogs was between 15% and 20%, while that of older dogs was between 25% and 30%.[163] In contrast, the body fat content of adult, normal weight cats has been reported to be between 8% and 13%, but it was not shown to change significantly between the ages of 1 and 9 years.[164] However, recent data collected from a colony of young and old cats and dogs found that the body mass of young cats averaged 30% and increased to 35% in cats that were older than 7 years (Table 25-4).[165] The higher body fat in the recent study may reflect the increased incidence of obesity among cats today or a difference in feeding regimen and body weight in the different groups of cats studied. In dogs, fat body mass index increased from a mean of 18% in dogs less than 1.5 years to 27% in dogs older than 7 years of age. In both dogs and cats, the percentage of lean body mass declined with age.

TABLE 25-4

Body Composition in Young and Old Cats and Dogs*

	Lean Body Mass (%)	Fat Body Mass (%)	Bone Body Mass(%)
Young Cats	69	30	1
Old Cats	64	35	1
Young Dogs	79	18	3
Old Dogs	70	27	3

*Data collected from 40 young (less than 1.5 years) and old (greater than 7 years) cats and 36 young (less than 1.5 years) and old (greater than 7 years) Fox Terriers and Labrador Retrievers (The Iams Technical Center, Lewisburg, Ohio, 1998).

Lifestyle factors must be considered when assessing the metabolic rate and energy needs of older pets. While some pets voluntarily reduce their physical activity as they become older, others remain active and athletic well into their later years. It is estimated that total daily energy requirements may decrease by as much as 30% to 40% during the last third of a pet's lifespan as a result of both reduced activity and decreased metabolic rate.[166] However, because physical activity helps to offset age-associated losses of lean body tissue, the RMR in older pets who are very active may not decrease significantly. Therefore, while RMR and energy needs generally decrease with aging, pets must be assessed individually to determine whether or not a decrease in energy intake is warranted.

Changes in the Integument

The skin loses elasticity and becomes less pliable with age as a result of increased calcium content and pseudoelastin in the elastic fibers. This loss of elasticity is often accompanied by hyperkeratosis of both the skin and the follicles. Follicles may atrophy, resulting in areas of hair loss. The loss of pigment cells in the hair follicles and reduced activity of the enzyme tyrosinase results in the production of white hairs, often observed around the muzzle and face of older dogs and cats. The incidence of skin neoplasia also increases with age. The median age for the development of skin tumors is about 10.5 years in dogs and 12 years in cats.[167]

Changes in the Gastrointestinal System

It has been suggested that a number of changes take place in the gastrointestinal tract as animals age. These include reduced salivary and gastric acid secretions and decreased villus size, cellular turnover rate, and colonic motility.[155] Although it has been theorized that the aging of the gastrointestinal tract leads to a decreased ability to digest and absorb nutrients, studies on healthy older dogs and cats show conflicting results. A study comparing the digestive efficiency of 1-year-old Beagles to elderly Beagles (10 to 12 years old) found no difference in the older dogs' ability to digest and absorb nutrients.[168] Similarly, a later study reported no significant difference in digestibility coefficients measured in young adult Beagles and very old Beagles (16 or 17 years old).[169] In contrast, a recent study found no significant differences in protein, fat, or energy digestibility between young (less than 6 years old) and old (greater than 8 years old) dogs, but there was a trend toward reduced digestibility coefficients in the older group of dogs.[170]

Fewer studies have been conducted with geriatric cats. However, data that are available indicate that aging changes in the digestive capabilities of cats may be more significant than those observed in dogs. Although one study reported no significant differences in digestive efficiency between young adult cats and cats that were older than 10 years of age, the older group of cats had a lower mean fat digestibility coefficient (0.80) than the young group (0.88).[171] This trend has been supported by subsequent studies.[170,172] When six different age groups of cats were studied, protein digestibility decreased slightly and fat digestibility decreased significantly with increasing age.[170] Together these two trends led to a highly significant linear relationship between age and a decline in dietary energy digestibility. The oldest group of cats (12 to 14 years) had significantly lower digestibility coefficients for energy than all of the younger age categories. Interestingly, these older cats (12 to 14 years) were able to maintain normal weight by consuming more food than the younger cats. These results suggest that cats are capable of self-regulating their intake very precisely, even in the face of reduced digestive capacities. Although not determined in this study, possible underlying causes for age-related decreases in digestive capability include reductions in pancreatic enzyme secretion or bile acid secretion in elderly cats. These data indicate that a slight to moderate reduction in gastrointestinal functioning may occur in some healthy older pets. While these changes may not severely affect health, they should be considered when formulating or selecting diets for geriatric dogs and cats.

Changes in the Urinary System

A decline in renal function is observed in humans after the fourth decade of life.[173] Changes include reduced renal plasma flow, reduced glomerular filtration rate, and decreased ability to concentrate urine and acidify urine. Similarly, certain strains of laboratory rats show age-related deterioration of kidney morphology and function.[174] Because chronic renal failure is a major cause of illness and mortality in geriatric cats and is one of the four leading causes of death in old dogs, the effects of normal aging on the canine and feline kidney have been studied.[175,176,177] One of the first studies evaluated clinical changes in renal function in a colony of Beagles over a period of 13 years.[178] Results showed that nephrosclerosis was the most frequently diagnosed kidney lesion in older dogs. The data from this study also indicated that normal kidney aging may lead to nephron loss of up to 75% before clinical or biochemical signs occur in older dogs. Pets with less than 75% loss are usually clinically normal but may be more susceptible to renal insult than younger animals still possessing renal reserve capacity.[179]

In contrast, another study that compared nutrient utilization and metabolism in young and old Beagles reported no loss of renal functioning associated with aging.[168]

These results were supported by a recent study that examined the effects of aging and dietary protein intake on renal function and morphology in aging dogs.[180] All of the dogs were between 7 and 8 years old at the start of the study and were uninephrectomized to reduce renal mass by 50%. This procedure was included in the study design because a reduction of renal mass makes residual renal tissue more vulnerable to insult and would be expected to exacerbate any effects of aging or diet. Over a 4-year period, none of the dogs showed a decline in renal functioning. Age-related changes to the kidneys included the development of moderate renal lesions, but these were not affected by diet and did not significantly affect renal functioning. When the dogs in this study were compared with young dogs that had been uninephrectomized, the older dogs had compensatory responses to uninephrectomy that were indistinguishable from those of the young dogs. However, the older dogs did show a blunted renal response to a protein meal when compared with younger dogs. Results of these studies illustrate the importance of evaluating geriatric patients as individuals when assessing renal function. Aging alone is not associated with decline in renal functioning or chronic renal disease.

When renal disease does occur in older pets, it directly affects nutrition and dietary management because clinical kidney insufficiency is associated with weight loss, muscle wasting, altered plasma protein profiles, decreased caloric and nutrient intake, intestinal malabsorption, and reduced assimilation and use of nutrients. The accumulation of the metabolic products of protein, of which urea is the most abundant, is believed to further contribute to the development of the clinical and physiological abnormalities of renal failure. Dietary modification attempts to minimize the accumulation of these end products in the bloodstream while still supplying adequate energy and protein to maintain weight and minimize the muscle wasting associated with old age and compromised renal function (see Section 6, pp. 462-471).

Changes in the Musculoskeletal System

Old age is accompanied by a decline in the percentage of lean body mass and bone mass. Both the number and size of muscle cells decrease with age, and the cortices of the long bones become thinner, dense, and brittle. This may be due in part to inadequate absorption of calcium in the intestine of some older pets. Arthritis commonly occurs in older pets and obesity can compound the effects of arthritis. The presence of joint pain may also affect the pet's desire and ability to eat. Decreased appetite, leading to weight loss, is occasionally observed in severely arthritic pets. Along with medical therapy, there are several new neutraceuticals available that may be of aid in the management of arthritis in older pets.

Changes in the Cardiovascular System

Heart-related disease is a fairly common cause of morbidity in older pets and is estimated to occur in up to 30% of aged dogs.[181] The incidence in cats is not known, but it is thought to occur less frequently.[182] Cardiac output decreases by as much as

30% between midlife and old age.[166] Maximal heart rate and oxygen consumption during exercise also decrease significantly. Recent studies comparing young and old dogs' cardiovascular responses to exercise found that aging of the cardiovascular system results in a loss of organ reserve and adaptability, which is presumed to lead to cardiovascular disease in some older dogs.[183] In animals with adult onset heart disease, fibrosis and myocardial necrosis eventually interfere with normal conduction pathways and result in arrhythmias. Normal vascular changes of aging include hyaline thickening of the media of the blood vessels and increased deposition of calcium in the intima of the aorta and the media of the peripheral arteries.[183,184] All of these changes contribute to a progressive increase in the workload of the heart, which can eventually lead to the development of congestive heart disease or heart failure.

Changes in the Special Senses

Old age may result in a general reduced reaction to stimuli and partial loss of the sensations of vision, hearing, and taste. Nuclear sclerosis or cataracts of the lens are frequently seen in older dogs and cats. A decrease in taste acuity may lead to decreased interest in food, reduced intake, and weight loss in some older pets.

Changes in Behavior

The most common behavioral problems that occur in old dogs and cats are related to or secondary to degenerative disease and other geriatric changes.[185,186,187] Several of these behavioral changes may affect a pet's ability or desire to obtain adequate nutrition. For example, pets suffering from the chronic pain of arthritis may become increasingly irritable and reluctant to engage in any type of activity, including eating. On the other hand, the development of diabetes mellitus in dogs is often accompanied by a ravenous appetite. Because diabetic pets are usually overweight to begin with, the desire to consume large amounts of food further exacerbates this condition.

Depression or pathological mourning as a result of the loss of a beloved housemate or owner can result in severe anorexia in older pets. If prolonged, this anorexia can lead to weight loss and increased susceptibility to illness. Changes in the social structure of the family, usually because of the introduction of another pet, may also cause elderly dogs or cats to change their eating patterns. In some instances, social facilitation may cause an abrupt increase in intake, predisposing the pet to obesity. In other cases, intimidation by the new pet may cause the older animal to suddenly decrease food intake.

One of the most noticeable changes in the behavior of geriatric pets is their resistance to a change in daily routine. A move to a new residence, the introduction of a new pet, or a change in the owner's work schedule may be met with depression, alterations in elimination patterns, and/or changes in eating habits. It is important to be aware that geriatric cats are particularly predisposed to behavior problems when their environment is altered.[186] Introducing changes gradually and allowing the elderly pet sufficient time to adapt is often effective in minimizing stress and preventing the occurrence of behavioral problems.

NUTRIENT CONSIDERATIONS FOR OLDER PETS

Aging pets have a need for the same nutrients that were required during earlier physiological states. However, the quantities of nutrients required per unit of body weight may change, and the way in which nutrients are provided to the pet may require modification. Such changes usually depend on changes in energy require ments and the presence or degree of degenerative disease. Nutrients that may be of specific concern in aging dogs and cats are discussed in the following sections.

Energy

The reduction in the metabolic rate and physical activity of geriatric pets results in a decreased total daily energy requirement. It has been estimated that inactivity alone may cause a decrease of up to 20% of the pet's total daily energy requirement.[182] This decrease, coupled with the natural slowing of basal metabolic rate, can result in a total reduction in energy needs of up to 30% to 40%.[166] A recent controlled study of energy needs in older dogs and cats found that as cats and dogs age, their requirement for energy significantly declines.[170] Dogs that were older than 8 years consumed approximately 18% fewer calories than breed-matched dogs less than 6 years of age. While the effect in cats was less pronounced, a decline in energy requirements with age was also seen. However, it is important to note that the oldest group of cats (12 to 14 years) actually consumed a greater quantity of food to compensate for their reduced capacity to digest fat and protein in the diet.

Elderly pets vary greatly in their energy needs, depending on individual temperament, presence of degenerative disease, ability to digest and assimilate nutrients, and amount of daily exercise. Caloric intake should be carefully monitored in older pets to ensure adequate intake of calories and nutrients while at the same time preventing the development of obesity. Dogs and cats that are between 7 and 9 years of age are beginning to age and are at the highest risk for obesity. Therefore pet owners and veterinarians should carefully monitor the dietary intake and weight status of these pets to ensure that their intake matches their energy needs as they begin to decline. This is most easily accomplished by selecting a diet that is formulated to be less energy-dense, while still providing optimal levels of essential nutrients.

Protein and Amino Acids

The decrease in lean body mass that occurs with aging results in a loss of the protein reserves that can normally be used by the body during reactions to stress and illness. Stress triggers nervous, metabolic, and hormonal adaptations that allow the body to adapt to adverse stimuli. The mobilization of body protein is a characteristic physiological response to stress. Older animals are subject to a high incidence of disease and stress and are therefore especially vulnerable if their ability to react is compromised. It is important that geriatric pets be provided with high-quality protein at a level that is sufficient to supply the essential amino acids needed for body maintenance needs and to minimize losses of lean body tissue.

Studies conducted with human subjects have shown that the efficiency of protein use is slightly lower in the elderly than in young adults. The amount of available energy in the form of egg protein required for nitrogen balance was reported to be 4% in young men, but it increased to 6% in elderly men.[188] Similar results have been reported in dogs. An early study compared the protein requirements in young and old animals.[189] The ratio of liver and muscle protein to deoxyribonucleic acid (DNA) was measured and used as an estimate of body protein reserves. Results showed that protein/DNA ratios were maximized when young adult dogs were fed a semipurified diet containing 12.4% protein. Old dogs, on the other hand, required 18.8% protein to maximize body protein reserves. However, this increased need does not appear to be caused by reduced digestive capacity. A study that compared the digestive capabilities of 12-year-old dogs to 1-year-old dogs found no difference in the ability of old dogs to digest protein and other nutrients from four different diets when compared with young adult dogs.[168,190]

A recent study examined the effects of feeding graded levels of dietary protein to groups of young and geriatric dogs.[191] The dogs were fed isocaloric diets containing either 16%, 24%, or 32% crude protein for a period of 8 weeks. At the end of the feeding period, whole body protein turnover and rates of protein synthesis and degradation were measured using administration of the tracer amino acid ^{15}N-glycine.[192] When all data were considered, the authors estimated that the minimum dietary protein requirement of the geriatric dog is between 16% and 24% when supplied as a high-quality chicken byproduct meal. However, the data also indicated that additional benefits may be provided to geriatric dogs if they are fed a diet containing more than 24% protein. This was evidenced by the minimization of incremental differences between protein synthesis and degradation when the dogs were fed diets containing increased protein. This change may allow for an effective increase or maintenance of muscle mass in geriatric individuals by supplying a continual source of essential amino acids needed for tissue repair and immunocompetence.

Aging pets should be fed diets with a percentage of calories from protein that is slightly higher than the minimum necessary for adult maintenance. In addition to having diminished protein reserves, the decreased total energy needs of the older pet may result in the need to slightly increase the proportion of protein calories in the diet. Premium pet foods formulated for adult maintenance or for geriatric pets contain high-quality protein sources and therefore can provide an adequate level and quality of protein to older pets (see Section 3, pp. 194-195). However, pet food brands that contain minimal amounts of protein from poor-quality sources may not be capable of providing adequate protein nutrition. Similarly, energy-dense foods with reduced levels of protein that are formulated for dogs and cats with existing kidney failure do not supply appropriate levels of protein for healthy elderly pets.

Much controversy still exists concerning dietary protein and renal function in older animals. As discussed previously, decreased renal functioning is a normal occurrence with aging in humans, rats, and to some degree, dogs and cats. As a direct result of this knowledge, and because of a series of studies conducted on rats, some investigators once recommended that all elderly pets receive moderately reduced protein diets in an attempt to prevent or minimize the progression of kidney dysfunction.[193] However, it is also important that healthy, geriatric dogs and cats receive adequate amounts of high-quality protein to minimize losses of body protein reserves and satisfy maintenance protein needs. Although a reduction in protein intake affects the expression of clinical signs of chronic renal failure once a certain level of dysfunction has occurred, there is no evidence to support a systematically reduced protein level in the diets of healthy older pets. It is recommended that the protein in the diet of geriatric dogs should not be restricted simply because of old age. Rather, elderly pets should receive diets containing optimal levels of high-quality protein. If chronic renal disease is diagnosed, moderate protein restriction and other dietary modifications are implemented as needed (see Section 6, pp. 462-471).

Fat

It has been theorized that the increase in the percentage of body fat that occurs with aging is partially a result of an increasing inability of the body to metabolize lipids.[190] Slightly decreasing the amount of fat in the diet may benefit geriatric dogs and cats, provided that the fat that remains in the diet is both highly digestible and rich in essential fatty acids (EFAs). A decrease in the proportion of calories contributed by fat also decreases the diet's energy density. This is an advantage for older pets with reduced energy needs.

There is also recent evidence that aging is associated with a gradual decline in the ability to desaturate EFAs.[194,195,196] This change appears to be due to decreased activity of desaturase enzymes, most specifically delta-6-desaturase.[197] Recent evidence from old and young Beagles and Labrador Retrievers found significant age-related differences in serum levels of arachidonic and eicosapentaenoic acid.[198] The data from this preliminary study indicated that there also may be breed-specific, age-related differences in the ability to elongate omega-3 and omega-6 fatty acids. An important unsaturated fatty acid that is affected by alterations in delta-6-desaturase activity is gamma-linolenic acid. Gamma-linolenic acid is an omega-6 fatty acid that has important roles in the maintenance of healthy skins and coats. Because older pets may have a diminished ability to produce gamma-linolenic acid from dietary linoleic acid, a pet food supplemented with this fatty acid may be beneficial.

Vitamins and Minerals

No controlled research has been conducted that examines the vitamin requirements of geriatric dogs and cats. However, it has been suggested that moderate increases in requirements for potassium, the B vitamins, and fat-soluble vitamins A and E may occur if polyuria or subclinical decreases in absorption occur.[193,199] There are currently no data available that support this theory. The development of decreased glucose tolerance with age may cause a slight increase in the requirement for the B vitamins necessary for carbohydrate use. However, a deficiency of these vitamins has never been demonstrated in older pets.

Recent evidence shows that, similar to other species, the immune system of the dog declines with age.[161,200,201] Studies have demonstrated age-related declines in mitogen stimulation, chemotaxis, and phagocytosis in dogs.[201] Similar to changes in fatty acid metabolism, the rate of age-related decline may be different for different breeds of dogs.[202] These data demonstrate an age-related decline in immunity that may increase the susceptibility of geriatric animals to infectious diseases. The potential exists to influence this rate of decline with nutrients that enhance the canine immune response, specifically antioxidants such as vitamin E, beta carotene, or lutein. Although further research is needed, preliminary studies show that these nutrients have beneficial effects on the canine and feline immune systems.[203,204,205] Geriatric diets that incorporate increased levels of vitamin E, as well as the carotenoid compounds beta carotene and lutein, may be helpful in enhancing the immune systems of geriatric pets.

Supplemental dietary phosphorus should not be fed to older pets. Diets high in this mineral have been shown to contribute to kidney damage in human subjects by increasing blood flow and filtration through the glomerulus and promoting calcium and phosphorus deposition in the kidneys.[206,207] There is also evidence in dogs and cats that excess phosphorus in the diet may contribute to the progression of kidney disease and may indirectly contribute to an increase in parathyroid hormone levels by causing a reduction in serum calcitriol levels.[182,208,209,210] Although the effects of high-phosphorus diets on kidney function in healthy geriatric dogs and cats are not known, it is prudent to avoid an excess of this mineral in the diet (see Section 6, p. 458).

Sodium in dog and cat foods has received attention because of the concern about this nutrient in human diets. Some commercial pet foods contain as high as 2% sodium, even though the actual sodium requirement of dogs and cats is much lower than this. However, at levels of 2% or greater, intake of the diet is self-limiting. Pets will not consume diets that contain excessively high amounts of sodium.[11] At levels below 2%, sodium has not been shown to cause disease in healthy dogs. Therefore the sodium content in the diet of healthy elderly pets should not be of concern, provided the level is within the recommended range of 1% or less on a dry-matter basis (DMB).

FEEDING MANAGEMENT AND CARE OF OLDER PETS

Major objectives of the feeding and care of geriatric dogs and cats should be to maintain health and optimal body weight, slow or prevent the development of chronic disease, and minimize or improve clinical signs of diseases that may already be present. Routine care for geriatric pets should involve adherence to a consistent daily routine, regular attention to normal health care procedures, and periodic veterinary examinations for assessment of the presence or progression of chronic disease. Stressful situations and abrupt changes in daily routines should be avoided. If a drastic change must be made in an older pet's routine, attempts should be made to minimize stress and accomplish the change in a gradual manner.

Optimal body weight can be maintained and obesity prevented through the judicious control of caloric intake and adherence to a regular exercise schedule. Although many adult dogs and cats are able to maintain normal body weights when fed free-choice, this may no longer be possible as the pet ages. Decreasing energy needs may lead to obesity in some older pets if a free-choice regimen is continued. It is recommended that geriatric dogs and cats be fed at least two to three small meals per day, rather than one large meal. Feeding several small meals per day promotes improved nutrient use and may decrease feelings of hunger between meals.[211] The timing and size of meals should also be strictly regulated. A regular schedule minimizes alimentary stress and supports normal nutrient digestion and use. Fresh water should be available at all times to older dogs and cats.

Geriatric cats and some older dogs may become very particular about their eating habits. The pet's willingness to eat new foods may decrease. It may be necessary for owners to provide an especially strong-smelling or highly palatable food to their older cat.[211] Other dogs and cats may accept only one particular brand or flavor of food. If possible, pet owners should accommodate these needs, provided that the preferred food can provide adequate nutrition to the pet.

If a chronic disease state that requires specific nutrient alterations is present (e.g., diabetes, renal disease, congestive heart failure), the pet should be fed a diet that is appropriate for the management of the disorder. Healthy older pets can be fed a diet that contains high-quality ingredients, moderate to high levels of high-quality protein, and moderately reduced amounts of fat. Many commercially available premium pet foods formulated for adult maintenance or for geriatric pets are suitable. Lower quality pet foods are not generally recommended for elderly pets because some of these products provide poorly available nutrients.

Proper care of the teeth and gums is important for geriatric pets. If an owner is unable or unwilling to regularly examine and brush a pet's teeth, yearly descaling by a veterinarian is necessary to prevent buildup of dental calculus and the development of periodontal disease. Dental problems can lead to decreased food intake, anorexia, and systemic disease if not treated promptly in older animals.

Regular and sustained periods of physical activity help to maintain muscle tone, enhance circulation, improve alimentation, and prevent excess weight gain. The level and intensity of exercise should be adjusted to an individual pet's physical and medical condition. Many dogs, if healthy and maintained in good condition, can enjoy running and playing active games with their owners well into old age. Almost all older dogs benefit from and enjoy two 15- to 30-minute walks per day. Although most cats do not readily accept walking on a lead, playing games with older cats can be an acceptable form of exercise (Box 25-1).

BOX 25-1

Practical Feeding Tips: Elderly Companion Animals

Provide regular health checkups at least two times per year.

Avoid sudden changes in daily routine or diet.

Feed a diet that contains high-quality protein and is specifically formulated for geriatric pets.

Use portion-controlled feeding to prevent obesity; feed to maintain ideal body weight.

Provide a moderate level of regular exercise.

Maintain proper care of teeth and gums.

When necessary, provide a therapeutic diet to manage or treat disease.

SECTION 4

KEY POINTS

- Competitive (rapid) eating, a characteristic of the dog's ancestor, the wolf, can cause choking or excessive food intake in domestic dogs. Feeding dogs alone or changing the diet can help.

- In contrast to dogs, most cats eat slowly. If fed free-choice, cats will eat small meals frequently and randomly throughout a 24-hour period.

- The type of feeding regimen used depends on several factors: the owner's schedule, the number of animals being fed, and the pet's acceptance of the feeding method. For dogs, portion-controlled feeding is the method of choice in most situations.

- Although free-choice feeding has some advantages, owners should evaluate pets fed through this method for the development of problems such as anorexia, overconsumption, or difficulties due to social hierarchies within groups of dogs.

- Commercial pet foods balance nutrient content and energy density, thus ensuring that when an animal's caloric needs are met, its needs for all other essential nutrients are also met.

- Determining how much to feed a dog or cat is based on age, reproductive status, body condition, level of activity, breed, temperament, and environmental conditions. Commercial pet food labels provide general guidelines, but every pet must be evaluated and fed as an individual.

- During pregnancy, supplementation with calcium or any other mineral is not necessary or recommended if a well-balanced, commercial ration is fed.

- Within the first 24 hours after birth, colostrum provides intact immunoglobulins, thereby protecting puppies and kittens from a number of infectious diseases. The nutrient content of colostrum differs significantly from mature milk, and its intact immunoglobulins provide passive immunity to the neonates.

- Orphaned puppies and kittens represent a challenge to an owner. Once orphaned, they must depend on humans for maternal care, proper nutrition, and a suitable environment. Maintaining proper warmth, normally provided by body heat from the bitch or queen, is critical to ensure survival of the newborn puppies and kittens. Close attention should be paid to temperature guidelines and methods of providing a warm environment.

- There are a number of commercial milk replacers available. One that matches a dam's milk in composition and performance should be chosen. However, none can provide the immune protection of colostrum. Thus, if the animals are orphaned before they received colostrum (within the first 24 hours after birth), they will be more susceptible to infectious disease.

- To support the growth of new tissues, pet foods for growing puppies and kittens should have a slightly higher protein content than foods fed for adult maintenance.

- Contrary to popular belief, calcium and phosphorous supplements are not necessary for growing pets and can be harmful in large and giant breeds of dogs, contributing to the development of certain developmental skeletal disorders.

- Hyperplastic obesity is an increase in both the size and number of fat cells. Hypertrophic obesity is an increase in fat-cell size. As has been found in other species, it is possible that if young, growing animals are overnourished, they may be predisposed to obesity at maturity.

- Although heredity certainly plays a role in the development of certain skeletal disorders, studies have identified diet supplementation with certain nutrients and/or feeding an energy- and nutrient-dense diet at a level that supports maximal growth rate as other contributing factors.

- An endurance study showed that a highly digestible, high-fat diet can provide the extra energy needed by working dogs and contribute positively to endurance performance.

- It is well known that carbohydrate intake, or loading, in humans provides the necessary energy for performing athletes. However, a similar effect has not been observed in working dogs.

- Working dogs should be fed using the portion-controlled method, with the main meal of the day provided after the period of exercise. In general, hardworking dogs should be fed two to three meals per day, with a small meal fed 1.5 to 2 hours before the exercise.

- In contrast to working dogs, racing Greyhounds draw energy from the anaerobic metabolism of carbohydrates; muscle glycogen and circulating blood glucose fuel muscles during their brief periods of intense work. Although such short-term energy metabolism may not be strongly influenced by diet, racing dogs should be fed energy-dense, highly digestible diets that have been formulated for performance.

- As a general guideline, an average increase of 25% of a dog's metabolizable energy (ME) intake is necessary to maintain body weight in dogs housed in cool conditions (less than 59° Farenheit [F]).

- Advances in health care and nutrition are leading to increased longevity for companion animals. Paralleling the events of aging in humans, geriatric cats and dogs experience many of the same changes. The functioning efficiency of body systems and organs declines, the resting metabolic rate (RMR) decreases, and pets reduce their physical activity. As a result, energy requirements may decrease significantly.

- **The Protein Controversy**: Contrary to popular belief, protein in the diets of geriatric dogs should not be restricted simply because the dog is old. Attempts to prevent or minimize the natural decline in kidney function associated with aging by reducing protein consumption may lead to a negative nitrogen balance and losses of body protein reserves. Although protein reduction does have a significant positive effect on clinical signs of chronic renal failure once a certain level of dysfunction has occurred, protein should not be arbitrarily restricted in a generally healthy older pet.

- **Tip**: Exercise and nutrition can be adapted to fit a geriatric pet's needs. More frequent feedings (two or more times a day) aid digestion and help the pet avoid feelings of hunger. Fast games of fetch can be replaced by one or two 15- to 30-minute walks each day.

SECTION 4

REFERENCES

1. Thorne CJ: Understanding pet response: behavioural aspects of palatability. In *Proceedings of the Petfood Forum*, Chicago, 1997, Watts Publishing.
2. Houpt KA: Ingestive behavior: the control of feeding in cats and dogs. In Voith VL, Borchelt PL, editors: *Readings in companion animal behavior*, Trenton, New Jersey, 1996, Veterinary Learning Systems.
3. Mugford RA: External influences on the feeding of carnivores. In Kare MR, Maller O, editors: *The chemical senses and nutrition*, New York, 1977, Academic Press.
4. Kanarek RB: Availability and caloric density of diet as determinants of meal patterns in cats, *Physio Behav* 15:611-618, 1975.
5. Hart BL, Hart LA: *Canine and feline behavioral therapy*, Philadelphia, 1985, Lea and Febiger.
6. Kane E, Morris JG, Rogers QR: Acceptability and digestibility by adult cats of diets made with various sources and levels of fat, *J Anim Sci* 53:1516-1523, 1981.
7. Bradshaw JW, Cook SE: Patterns of pet cat behaviour at feeding occasions, *Appl Anim Behav Sci* 47:61-74, 1996.
8. Doyle Dane Bernback International: DDB study documents belief in animal rights, *Pet Food Ind*, 20-22, Mar/Apr 1984.
9. Leblanc J, Diamond P: The effect of meal frequency on postprandial thermogenesis in the dog (abstract), *Fed Proc* 44:1678, 1985.
10. Wingfield WE: *Proceedings of the Colorado State University Annual Conference for Veterinarians*, 1978, Colorado State University.
11. Association of American Feed Control Officials: *Official publication*, Atlanta, 2000, The Association of American Feed Control Officials.
12. Lepine A: Feeding management of the reproductive cycle, *Proc North Amer Vet Conf*, 27-29, 1997.
13. Lawler DF, Bebiak DM: Nutrition and management of reproduction in the cat, *Vet Clin North Am Small Anim Pract* 16:495-519, 1986.
14. Smith CA: New hope for overcoming canine inherited disease, *J Am Vet Med Assoc* 204:41-46, 1994.
15. Giger U: Diagnosis and management of hereditary disease in the dog, *Proc Soc Theriogen*, 152-154, 1996.
16. Bebiak DM, Lawler DF, Reutzel LF: Nutrition and management of the dog, *Vet Clin North Am Small Anim Pract* 17:505-533, 1987.
17. Moser D: Feeding to optimize canine reproductive efficiency, *Probl Vet Med* 4:545-550, 1992.
18. Loveridge GG: Bodyweight changes and energy intake of cats during gestation and lactation, *Anim Tech* 37:7-15, 1986.
19. Holme DW: Practical use of prepared foods for dogs and cats. In *Dog and cat nutrition*, New York, 1982, Pergamon Press.
20. Kronfeld DS: Nature and use of commercial dog foods, *J Am Vet Med Assoc* 166:487-493, 1975.
21. Mosier JE: Nutritional recommendations for gestation and lactation in the dog, *Vet Clin North Am Small Anim Pract* 7:683-692, 1977.
22. Ontko JA, Phillips PH: Reproduction and lactation studies with bitches fed semi-purified diets, *J Nutr* 65:211-218, 1958.
23. Lewis LD, Morris ML, Hand MS: Dogs: feeding and care. In *Small animal clinical nutrition*, Topeka, Kan, 1987, Mark Morris Associates.
24. Hoskins JD: Puppy and kitten losses. In *Veterinary pediatrics: dogs and cats from birth to six months*. Philadelphia, 1995, WB Saunders.
25. Donovan SM, Odle J: Growth factors in milk as mediators of infant development, *Annu Rev Nutr* 14:147-167, 1994.

26. Fisher EW: Neonatal diseases of dogs and cats, *Br Vet J* 138:277-284, 1982.

27. Lepine A: Nutrition of the neonatal puppy, *Proc North Am Vet Conf*, 27-29, 1997.

28. Lonnerdal B, Keen CL, Hurley LS, and others: Developmental changes in the composition of Beagle dog milk, *Am J Vet Res* 42:662-666, 1981.

29. Keen CL, Lonnerdal B, Clegg MS, and others: Developmental changes in composition of cats' milk: trace elements, minerals, protein, carbohydrate and fat, *J Nutr* 112:1763-1769, 1982.

30. Adkins Y, Zicker SC, Lepine A, and others: Changes in nutrient and protein composition of cat milk during lactation, *Am J Vet Res* 58:370-375, 1997.

31. Lonnerdal B, Keen CL, Hurley LS: Iron, copper, zinc and manganese in milk, *Ann Rev Nutr* 1:149-174, 1981.

32. Lonnerdal B: Lactation and neonatal nutrition in the dog and cat, *Proc North Am Vet Conf*, 13-16, 1997.

33. Oftedal OT: Lactation in the dog: milk composition and intake by puppies, *J Nutr* 114:803-812, 1984.

34. Russe I: Laktation der Hundin, *Zentralbl Veterinarmed* 8:252-282, 1961.

35. Malm K, Jensen P: Weaning in dogs: within—and between—litter variation in milk and solid food intake, *Appl Anim Behav Sci* 49:223-235, 1996.

36. Monson WJ: The care and management of orphaned puppies and kittens, *Vet Tech* 8:430-434, 1987.

37. Monson WJ: Orphan rearing of puppies and kittens, *Vet Clin North Am Small Anim Pract* 17:567-576, 1987.

38. Baines FB: Milk substitutes and the hand rearing of orphan puppies and kittens, *J Small Anim Pract* 22:555-578, 1981.

39. Lepine AJ: Nutrition of the neonatal canine and feline, In Reinhart GA, Carey DP, editors: *Recent advances in canine and feline nutrition,* vol 2, Iams Nutrition Symposium Proceedings, Wilmington, Ohio, 1998, Orange Frazer Press.

40. Remillard RL, Pickett JP, Thatcher CD, and others: Comparison of kittens fed queen's milk with those fed milk replacers, *Am J Vet Res* 54:901-907, 1993.

41. Lepine AJ, Kelley RL, Bouchard G: Effect of feline milk replacers on growth and body composition of nursing kittens (abstract), *Proc Am Coll Vet Intern Med Forum*, 737, 1998.

42. Kelley RL, Lepine AJ, Bouchard G: Effect of milk composition on growth and body composition of puppies (abstract), *FASEB Proc* 12:A837, 1998.

43. Douglass GM, Kane E, Holmes EJ: A profile of male and female cat growth, *Comp Anim Pract* 2:9-12, 1988.

44. Allard RL, Douglass GM, Kerr WW: The effects of breed and sex on dog growth, *Comp Anim Pract* 2:15-19, 1988.

45. Lepine AJ: Nutritional influences on skeletal growth of the large-breed puppy, *Proc North Amer Vet Conf*, 15-18, 1998.

46. Hedhammer A, Wu F, Krook L, and others: Overnutrition and skeletal disease: an experimental study in growing Great Dane dogs, *Cornell Vet* 64(suppl 5):1-159, 1974.

47. Kealy RD, Olsson SE, Monti KL, and others: Effects of limited food consumption on the incidence of hip dysplasia in growing dogs, *J Am Vet Med Assoc* 201:857-863, 1992.

48. Dammrich K: Relationship between nutrition and bone growth in large and giant dogs, *J Nutr* 121:S114-S121, 1991.

49. Hazewinkel HAW, Goedegebuure SA, Poulos PW, and others: Influences of chronic calcium excess on the skeletal development of growing Great Danes, *J Am Anim Hosp Assoc* 21:377-391, 1985.

50. Goodman SA, Montgomery RD, Fitch RB, and others: Serial orthopedic examinations of growing Great Dane puppies fed three diets varying in calcium and phosphorus. In Reinhart GA, Carey DP, editors: *Recent advances in canine and feline nutrition,* vol 2, Iams Nutrition Symposium Proceedings, Wilmington, Ohio, 1998, Orange Frazer Press.

51. Lepine AJ: Nutritional management of the large breed puppy. In Reinhart GA, Carey DP, editors: *Recent advances in canine and feline nutrition,* vol 2, Iams Nutrition Symposium Proceedings, Wilmington, Ohio, 1998, Orange Frazer Press.

52. Nap RC, Hazewinkel HAW, Vorrhout G, and others: The influence of the dietary protein content on growth in giant breed dogs, *J Vet Comp Orthop Trauma* 6:1-8, 1993.

53. Kendall PT, Blaza SE, Smith PM: Comparative digestible energy requirements of adult Beagles and domestic cats for body weight maintenance, *J Nutr* 113:1946-1955, 1983.

54. Loveridge GG: Factors affecting growth performance in male and female kittens, *Anim Tech* 38:9-18, 1987.

55. Jenkins KJ, Phillips PH: The mineral requirements of the dog. II. The relation of calcium, phosphorus and fat levels to minimal calcium and phosphorus requirements, *J Nutr* 70:241-250, 1960.

56. Gershoff SN, Legg MA, Hegsted DM: Adaptation to different calcium intakes in dogs, *J Nutr* 64:303-311, 1958.

57. Kallfelz FA, Dzanis DA: Overnutrition: an epidemic problem in pet practice?, *Vet Clin North Am Small Anim Pract* 19:433-466, 1989.

58. Earle KE: Calculations of energy requirements of dogs, cats and small psittacine birds, *J Small Anim Pract* 34:163-183, 1993.

59. Faust IM, Johnson PR, Hirsch J: Long-term effects of early nutritional experience on the development of obesity in the rat, *J Nutr* 110:2027-2034, 1980.

60. Johnson PR, Stern JS, Greenwood MRC, and others: Effect of early nutrition on adipose cellularity and pancreatic insulin release in the Zucker rat, *J Nutr* 103:738-743, 1973.

61. Ross MH: Length of life and caloric intake, *Am J Clin Nutr* 25:834-838, 1972.

62. Saville PD, Lieber CS: Increases in skeletal calcium and femur thickness produced by under nutrition, *J Nutr* 99:141-144, 1969.

63. Dluzniewska KA, Obtulowicz A, Koltek K: On the relationship between diet, rate of growth and skeletal deformities in school children, *Folia Med Cracov* 7:115-126, 1965.

64. Wise DR, Jennings AR: Dyschondroplasia in domestic poultry, *Vet Rec* 91:285-286, 1972.

65. Reiland S: The effect of decreased growth rate on frequency and severity of osteochondrosis in pigs: an experimental investigation, *Acta Radiol* 358:179-196, 1978.

66. Wyburn RS: A degenerative joint disease in the horse, *N Zealand Vet J* 25:321-322, 335, 1977.

67. Hirsch J, Knittle JL, Salans LB: Cell lipid content and cell number in obese and non-obese human adipose tissue, *J Clin Invest* 52:929-934, 1966.

68. Bjorntorp P, Sjostrom L: Number and size of fat cells in relation to metabolism in human obesity, *Metabolism* 20:703-706, 1971.

69. Faust IM, Johnson PR, Stern JS, and others: Diet-induced adipocyte number increase in adult rats: a new model of obesity, *Am J Physiol* 235:E279-E286, 1978.

70. Bertrand HA, Lynd FT, Masoro EJ, and others: Changes in adipose mass and cellularity through the adult life of rats fed ad libitum or a life-prolonging restricted diet, *J Gerontol* 35:827-835, 1980.

71. Hirsch J, Knittle JL: Cellularity of obese and non-obese adipose tissue, *Fed Proc* 29:1516-1521, 1970.

72. Etherton TD, Wangsness PJ, Hammers VM, and others: Effect of dietary restriction on carcass composition and adipocyte cellularity of swine with different propensities for obesity, *J Nutr* 112:2314-2323, 1982.

73. Lewis DS, Bertrand HA, Masoro EJ: Pre-weaning nutrition on fat development in baboons, *J Nutr* 113:2253-2259, 1983.

74. Vasselli JR, Cleary MP, van Itallie TB: Modern concepts of obesity, *Nutr Rev* 41:361-373, 1983.

75. Grondalen J: Arthrosis in the elbow joint of young rapidly growing dogs. VI. Interrelation between clinical, radiographical and pathoanatomical findings, *Nord Vet Med* 34:65-75, 1982.

76. Kuhlman G, Biourge V: Nutrition of the large and giant breed dog with emphasis on skeletal development, *Vet Clin Nutr* 4:89-95, 1997.

77. Grondalen J: Metaphyseal osteopathy (hypertrophic osteodystrophy) in growing dogs: a clinical study, *J Small Anim Pract* 17:721-735, 1976.

78. Richardson DC, Toll PW: Relationship of nutrition to developmental skeletal disease in young dogs, *Vet Clin Nutr* 4:6-13, 1997.

79. Richardson DC: The role of nutrition in canine hip dysplasia, *Vet Clin North Am Small Anim Pract* 22:529-541, 1992.

80. Willis MB: Hip scoring: a review of 1985-1986, *Vet Rec* 118:461-462, 1986.

81. Armstrong PH, Lund EM: Changes in body composition and energy balance with aging, *Proc Sym Health Nutr Geriatr Dogs,* 11-15, 1996.

82. Slater MR, Scarlett JM, Donoghue S, and others: Diet and exercise as potential risk factors for osteochondritis dissecans in dogs, *Am J Vet Res* 53:2119-2124, 1992.

83. Edney ATB, Smith AM: Study of obesity in dogs visiting veterinary practices in the United Kingdom, *Vet Rec* 118:391-396, 1986.

84. Scarlett JM, Donoghue S, Saidla J, and others: Overweight cats: prevalence and risk factors, *Int J Obesity* 18:S22-S28, 1994.

85. Laflamme D: Development and validation of a body condition score system for dogs, *Canine Pract* 22:10-15, 1997.

86. Rainbird AL: Feeding throughout life. In Edney ATB, editor: *Dog and cat nutrition*, Oxford, England, 1988, Pergamon Press.

87. Laflamme DP, Kealy, RD, Schmidt DA: Estimation of body fat by body condition score, *J Vet Int Med* 8:154A, 1994.

88. Laflamme DP, Schmidt DA, Deshmukh A: Correlation of body fat in cats using body condition score or DEXA, *J Vet Int Med* 8:214, 1994.

89. Bergstrom J, Hermansen L, Hultman E, and others: Diet, muscle glycogen and physical performance, *Acta Physiol Scand* 71:140-150, 1967.

90. Issekutz B JR, Miller HI, Paul P: Aerobic work capacity and plasma FFA turnover, *J Appl Physiol* 20:293-296, 1965.

91. Miller H, Issekutz B, Rodahl K: Effect of exercise on the metabolism of fatty acids in the dog, *Am J Physiol* 205:167-172, 1963.

92. Paul P, Issekutz B, Miller HI: Interrelationship of free fatty acids and glucose metabolism in the dog, *Am J Physiol* 211:1313-1320, 1966.

93. Conlee RK, Hammer RL, Winder WW, and others: Glycogen repletion and exercise endurance in rats adapter to a high fat diet, *Metabolism* 39:289-294, 1990.

94. Reynolds AJ, Fuhrer L, Dunlap HL, and others: Effect of diet and training on muscle glycogen storage and utilization in sled dogs, *J Appl Physiol* 79:1601-1607, 1997.

95. Armstrong RB: Distribution of fiber types in locomotory muscles of dogs, *Am J Anat* 163:87-98, 1982.

96. Guy PS, Snow DH: Skeletal muscle fibre composition in the dog and its relationship to athletic ability, *Res Vet Sci* 31:244-248, 1981.

97. Reynolds AJ: Effect of diet on performance, *Proc Perform Dog Nutrit Symp*, Fort Collins, Col, 1995, Colorado State University.

98. Karlsson J, Saltin B: Diet, muscle glycogen and endurance performance, *J Appl Physiol* 31:203-206, 1971.

99. Hermansen L, Hultman E, Saltin B: Muscle glycogen during prolonged, severe exercise, *Acta Physiol Scand* 71:129-139, 1967.

100. Sherman WM, Costill DL, Fink WJ, and others: Effect of exercise-diet manipulation on muscle glycogen and its subsequent utilization during performance, *Int J Sports Med* 2:114-118, 1981.

101. Fielding RA, Costill DL, Fink WJ, and others: Effects of pre-exercise carbohydrate feedings on muscle glycogen use during exercise in well-trained runners, *Eur J Appl Physiol* 56:225-229, 1987.

102. Ahlborg BJ, Bergstrom J, Brohult J: Human muscle glycogen content and capacity for prolonged exercise after different diets, *Forvarsmedicin* 3:85-89, 1967.

103. Bergstrom J, Hultman E: A study of glycogen metabolism during exercise in man, *Scan J Clin Lab Invest* 19:218-228, 1967.

104. Blom PCS, Costill NK, Vollestad NK: Exhaustive running: inappropriate as a stimulus of muscle glycogen supercompensation, *Med Sci Sports Exercise* 19:398-403, 1987.

105. Sherman WM, Costill DL, Fink WJ, and others: Effect of exercise-diet manipulation on muscle glycogen and its subsequent utilization during performance, *In J Sports Med* 2:114-118, 1981.

106. Therriault DG, Beller GA, Smoake JA, and others: Intramuscular energy sources in dogs during physical work, *J Lipid Res* 14:54-61, 1973.

107. Paul P, Issekutz B: Role of extramuscular energy sources in the metabolism of the exercising dog, *Am J Physiol* 22:615-622, 1976.

108. Downey RL, Kronfeld DS, Banta CA: Diet of Beagles affects stamina, *J Am Anim Hosp Assoc* 16:273-277, 1980.

109. Hammel EP, Kronfeld DS, Ganjam VK, and others: Metabolic responses to exhaustive exercise in racing sledge dogs fed diets containing medium, low and zero carbohydrate, *Am J Clin Nutr* 30:409-418, 1976.

110. Kronfeld DS: Diet and the performance of racing sledge dogs, *J Am Vet Med Assoc* 162:470-473, 1973.

111. Sahlin K: Effect of acidosis on energy metabolism and force generation in skeletal muscle. In Knuttgen HG, Vogel JA, Poortmans J, editors: *Biochemistry of exercise*, Champaign, Ill, 1983, Human Kinetics Publishers.

112. Reynolds AJ: The effect of diet and training on energy substrate storage and utilization in trained and untrained sled dogs, In *Nutrition and physiology of Alaskan sled dogs*, abstracts of a symposium at the College of Veterinary Medicine, 1992, Ohio State University.

113. Reynolds, AJ, Fuhrer L, Dunlap HL, and other: Lipid metabolite responses to diet and training in sled dogs, *J Nutr* 124:2754S-2759S, 1994.

114. Reynolds AJ, Hoppler H, Reinhart GA, and others: Sled dog endurance: a result of high fat diet or selective breeding? *FASEB J*, 1995.

115. Adkins TO, Kronfeld DS: Diet of racing sled dogs affects erythrocyte depression by stress, *Can Vet J* 23:260-263, 1982.

116. Kronfeld DS, Hammel EP, Ramberg CF Jr, and others: Hematological and metabolic responses to training in racing sled dogs fed diets containing medium, low, or zero carbohydrate, *Am J Clin Nutr* 30:419-430, 1977.

117. Querengaesser A, Iben C, Leibetseder J: Blood changes during training and racing in sled dogs, *J Nutr* 2760S-2764S, 1994.

118. Hinchcliff KW, Olson J, Crusberg C, and others: Serum biochemical changes in dogs competing in a long distance sled race, *J Am Vet Med Assoc* 202:401-405, 1993.

119. Gollnick PD: Energy metabolism and prolonged exercise. In Lamb DR, Murray R, eds: *Perspectives in exercise science and sports medicine*, vol 1, Carmel, Ind, 1988, Benchmark Press.

120. Orr NWM: The feeding of sledge dogs on Antarctic expeditions, *Br J Nutr* 20:1-11, 1966.

121. Gannon JR: Nutritional requirements of the working dog, *Vet Ann* 21:161-166, 1981.

122. Orr NWM: The food requirements of Antarctic sledge dogs. In Graham-Jones O, editor: *Canine and feline nutritional requirements*, Oxford, England, 1965, Pergamon Press.

123. Wyatt HT: Further experiments on the nutrition of sledge dogs, *Brit J Nutr* 17:273-279, 1963.

124. Hinchcliff KW, Swenson RA, Schreier CJ, and others: Metabolizable energy intake and sustained energy expenditure of Alaskan sled dogs during heavy exertion in the cold, *Am J Vet Res* 58:1457-1462, 1997.

125. Hinchcliff KW, Swenson RA, Burr JR, and others: Exercise-associated hyponatremia in Alaskan sled dog: urinary and hormonal responses, *J Appl Physiol* 83:824-829, 1997.

126. Hinchcliff KW, Swenson RA, Schreier CJ, and others: Effect of racing on serum sodium and potassium concentrations and acid-base status of Alaskan sled dogs, *J Am Vet Med Assoc* 210:1615-1618, 1997.

127. Hinchcliff KW: Energy and water expenditure. In *Proc Perform Dog Nutrit Symp*, Fort Collins, Col, 1995, Colorado State University.

128. Hinchcliff KW, Reinhart GA, Burr JR, and others: Effect of racing on water metabolism, serum sodium and potassium concentrations, renal hormones, and urine composition of Alaskan sled dogs. In Reinhart GA, Carey DP, editors: *Recent advances in canine and feline nutrition,* vol 2, Iams Nutrition Symposium Proceedings, Wilmington, Ohio, 1998, Orange Frazer Press.

129. Kohn CW: Composition and distribution of body fluids in dogs and cats. In Dibartola S, editor: *Fluid therapy in small animal practice*, Philadelphia, Penn, 1992, WB Saunders.

130. Surgenor S, Uphold RE: Acute hyponatremia in ultra-endurance athletes, *Am J Emerg Med* 12:441-444, 1994.

131. Schott HC, MeGlade KS, Molander HA, and others: Body weight, fluid, electrolyte, and hormonal changes in horses competing in 50- and 100-mile endurance rides, *Am J Vet Res* 58:303-309, 1997.

132. Burr JR, Bradley DM, Vaughn DM, and others: Serum biochemical values in dogs before and after competing in long-distance races, *J Am Vet Med Assoc* 211:175-179, 1997.

133. Bergstrom J, Hultman E, Roch-Norlund AE: Muscle glycogen synthetase in normal subjects: basal values, effect of glycogen depletion by exercise and of a carbohydrate rich diet following exercise, *Scand J Clin Lab Invest* 29:231-236, 1972.

134. Bergstrom J, Hultman E: Muscle glycogen synthesis after exercise: an enhancing factor localized to the muscle cells in man, *Nature* 210:309-310, 1966.

135. Armstrong R, Saubert C, Sembrowich W: Glycogen depletion in rat skeletal muscle fibers at different intensities and duration of exercise, *Pflugers Arch* 352:243-256, 1974.

136. Hodgson DR, Rose RJ, Allent JR, and others: Glycogen depletion patterns in horses competing in day two of a three day event, *Cornell Vet* 75:366-374, 1985.

137. Reynolds AJ, Carey DP, Reinhart GA, and others: The effect of post exercise carbohydrate supplementation on muscle glycogen synthesis in trained sled dogs, *Am J Vet Res* (submitted and accepted), 1998.

138. Ivy JL, Miller W, Power V: Endurance improved by ingestion of a glucose polymer supplement, *Med Sci Sports Exerc* 15:466-471, 1983.

139. Ivy JL, Katz AL, Cutler CL, and others: Muscle glycogen synthesis after exercise: effect of time of carbohydrate ingestion, *J Appl Physiol* 64:1480-1485, 1988.

140. Gisolfi CV: Water and electrolyte metabolism in exercise. In Fox EL, editor: *Nutrient utilization during exercise,* Columbus, Ohio, 1983, Ross Laboratories.

141. Fink WJ, Greenleaf JE: Fluid intake and athletic performance. In Haskell W, Scala J, Whittam J, editors: *Nutrition and athletic performance: proceedings of a conference on nutritional determinants of athletic performance,* 1981.

142. Askew EW: Fat metabolism in exercise. In Fox EL, editor: *Nutrient utilization during exercise,* Columbus, Ohio, 1983, Ross Laboratories.

143. Saltin B, Karlsson J: Muscle glycogen utilization during work of different intensities. In *Muscle metabolism during exercise,* vol 2, New York, 1971, Plenum Press.

144. Bjotvedt G, Weems CW, Foley K: Strenuous exercise may cause health hazards for racing Greyhounds, *Vet Med* 79:1481-1487, 1984.

145. Rose RJ, Bloomberg MS: *Responses to sprint exercise in the Greyhound: effects on hematology, plasma biochemistry and muscle metabolism,* International Greyhound Symposium, Orlando, Fla, 1983.

146. Dobson GB, Parkhouse WS, Weber SW, and others: Metabolic changes in skeletal muscle and blood of Greyhounds during 800-m track sprint, *Am J Physiol* R513-R519, 1988.

147. Donovan DM, Brooks GA: Endurance training affects lactate clearance not lactate production, *Am J Physiol* 244:E83-E92, 1983.

148. Durrer JL, Hannon JP: Seasonal variations of intake of dogs living in an arctic environment, *Am J Physiol* 202:375-378, 1962.

149. Blaza SE: Energy requirements of dogs in cool conditions, *Can Pract* 9:10-15, 1982.

150. Campbell IT, Donaldson J: Energy requirements of Antarctic sledge dogs, *Br J Nutr* 45:95-98, 1981.

151. Finke MD: Evaluation of the energy requirements of adult kennel dogs, *J Nutr* 121:S22-S28, 1991.

152. McNamara JH: Nutrition for military working dogs under stress, *Vet Med Small Anim Clin* 67:615-623, 1972.

153. Williams MH: Vitamin supplementation and physical performance. In Fox EL, editor: *Nutrient utilization during exercise*, Columbus, Ohio, 1983, Ross Laboratories.

154. Goldston RT, Notesworthy GD, Willard MD, and others: *Establishing a geriatrics management program*, St Louis, 1996, Ralston Purina.

155. Venn A: Diets for geriatric patients, *Vet Times,* May 1992.

156. Goldston RT: Introduction and overview of geriatrics. In Goldston RT, editor: *Geriatrics and gerontology of the dog and cat*, Philadelphia, 1995, WB Saunders.

157. Brace JJ: Theories of aging, *Vet Clin North Am Small Anim Pract* 11:811-814, 1981.

158. Macdougall DF, Barker J: An approach to canine geriatrics, *Brit Vet J* 140:115-123, 1984.

159. Deeb BJ, Wolf NS: Studying longevity and morbidity in giant and small breeds of dogs, *Vet Med* (suppl 7):702-709, 1994.

160. Griffith BCR: The geriatric cat, *J Small Anim Pract* 9:343-355, 1968.

161. Strasser A, Niedmuller H, Hofecker G, and others: The effect of aging on laboratory values in the dog, *J Vet Med* 40:720-730, 1993.

162. Hayek MG: Age-related changes in physiological function in the dog and cat: nutritional implications. In Reinhart GA, Carey DP, editors: *Recent advances in canine and feline nutrition,* vol 2, Iams Nutrition Symposium Proceedings, Wilmington, Ohio, 1998, Orange Frazer Press.

163. Meyer H, Stadfeld G: Investigation on the body and organ structures of dogs. In *Nutrition of the dog and cat,* Oxford, England, 1980, Pergamon Press.

164. Munday HS, Earle KE, Anderson P: Changes in body composition of the domestic shorthaired cat during growth and development, *J Nutr* 124:2622S, 1994.

165. Hayek MG, Davenport GM: Nutrition and aging in companion animals, *J Anti Aging Med* 1:117-123, 1998.

166. Mosier JE: Effect of aging on body systems of the dog, *Vet Clin North Am Small Anim Pract* 19:1-13, 1989.

167. MacDonald J: Neoplastic diseases of the integument. In *Proc Am Anim Hosp Assoc*, 17-20, 1987.

168. Sheffy BE, Williams AJ, Zimmer JF, and others: Nutrition and metabolism of the geriatric dog, *Cornell Vet* 75:324-347, 1985.

169. Buffington CA, Branham JE, Dunn GC: Lack of effect of age on digestibility of protein, fat and dry matter in Beagle dogs. In Burger IH, Rivers JPW: *Nutrition of the dog and cat*, Waltham Symposium #7, Cambridge, Mass, 1989, Cambridge University Press

170. Taylor EJ, Adams C, Neville R: Some nutritional aspects of ageing in dogs and cats, *Proc Nutr Soc* 54:645-656, 1995.

171. Anantharaman-Barr HG, Gicquello P, Rabot R: The effect of age on the digestibility of macronutrients and energy in cats. In *Proc Brit Small Anim Vet Assoc Cong*, Birmingham, England, 164, 1991.

172. Taylor EJ, Adams C, Coe S, and others: The effects of aging on the digestion of the cat. In *Proc of the First Cong Europ CNVSPA-FECAVA*, 309-310, 1995.

173. Brown WW, Davis BB, Spry LA: Aging and the kidney, *Arch Int Med* 146:1790-1796, 1986.

174. Bertaini T, Zoja C, Abbate M, and others: Age-related nephropathy and proteinuria in rats with intact kidneys exposed to diets with different protein content, *Lab Invest* 60:196-204, 1989.

175. Debartola SP, Rutgers HC, Zack PM: Clinicopathologic findings associated with chronic renal disease in cats: 4 cases (1973-1984), *J Am Vet Med Assoc* 190:1196-1202, 1987.

176. Polzin DJ: Topics in general medicine: general nutrition; the problems associated with renal failure, *Vet Med* 82:1027-1035, 1987.

177. Bronson RT: Variation in age at death of dogs of different sexes and breeds, *Am J Vet Res* 43:2057-2059, 1982.

178. Cowgill LD, Spangler WL: Renal insufficiency in geriatric dogs, *Vet Clin North Am Small Anim Pract* 11:727-749, 1981.

179. Kaufman GM: Renal function in the geriatric dog, *Comp Cont Ed Pract Vet* 6:108-109, 1984.

180. Finco DR, Brown S, Crowell W, and others: Effects of aging and dietary protein intake on uninephrectomized geriatric dogs, *Am J Vet Res* 55:1282-1290, 1994.

181. Hamlin RL: Managing cardiologic disorders in geriatric dogs. In *Proc Geriatr Med Symp*, 14-18, 1987.

182. Markham RW, Hodgkins EM: Geriatric nutrition, *Vet Clin North Am Small Anim Pract* 19:165-185, 1989.

183. Strasser A, Simunek M, Seiser M, and others: Age-dependent changes in cardiovascular and metabolic responses to exercise in Beagle dogs, *Zentralbl Veterinarmed A* 44:449-460, 1997.

184. Bright JM, Mears E: Chronic heart disease and its management, *Vet Clin North Am Small Anim Pract* 27:1305-1329, 1997.

185. Horwitz DA: Diagnosing and treating behavior problems in senior dogs. In *Senior Care/Vet Econ* (suppl), 54-63, Nov 1998, The Iams Company.

186. Houpt KA, Beaver B: Behavioral problems of geriatric dogs and cats, *Vet Clin North Am Small Anim Pract* 11:643-652, 1981.

187. Landsberg G, Ruehl W: Geriatric behavioural problems, *Vet Clin North Am Small Anim Pract* 27:1537-1559, 1997.

188. Zanni E, Calloway DH, Zezulka AY: Protein requirements of elderly men, *J Nutr* 109:513-524, 1979.

189. Wannemacher RW, McCoy JR: Determination of optimal dietary protein requirements of young and old dogs, *J Nutr* 88:66-74, 1966.

190. Sheffy BE, William AJ: Nutrition and the aging animal, *Vet Clin North Am Small Anim Pract* 11:669-675, 1981.

191. Davenport GM, Williams CC, Cummins KA, and others: Protein metabolism and aging. In Reinhart GA, Carey DP, editors: *Recent advances in canine and feline nutrition,* vol 2, Iams Nutrition Symposium Proceedings, Wilmington, Ohio, 1998, Orange Frazer Press.

192. Assimon S, Stein T: ^{15}N-glycine as a tracer to study protein metabolism in vivo. In Nissen S, editor: *Modern methods in protein nutrition and metabolism*, San Diego, 1992, Academic Press.

193. Branam JE: Dietary management of geriatric dogs and cats, *Vet Tech* 8:501-503, 1987.

194. Bolton-Smith C, Tavendale R, Woodward M: Evidence for age-related differences in the fatty acid composition of human adipose tissue, independent of diet, *Eur J Clin Nutr* 51:619-624, 1997.

195. Lorenzini A, Hrelia S, Biagi PL, and others: Age-related changes in essential fatty acid metabolism in cultured rat heart myocytes, *Prostaglandins Leukotrienes Essen Fatty Acids* 57:143-147, 1997.

196. Dinh L, Durand G, Dumont O, and others: Comparison of recovery of previously depressed hepatic delta-6-desaturase activity in adult and old rats, *Ann Nutr Metab* 39:117-123, 1995.

197. Biagi PL, Bordoni A, Hrelia S, and others: Gamma-linolenic acid dietary supplementation can reverse the aging influence on rat liver microsome delta-6-desaturase activity, *Biochem Biophys Acta* 1083:187, 1991.

198. Reinhart GA, Vaughn DM, Hayek MG and others: Effect of age on canine hepatic delta-6 and delta-5 desaturase activity (abstract), *J Anim Sci* 75 (suppl):227, 1997.

199. Laflamme D: Nutritional management, *Vet Clin North Am Small Anim Pract* 27:1561-1577, 1997.

200. Meydani SM, Hayek MG: Vitamin E and aging immune response, *Clin Geriatr Med* 11:567-576, 1995.

201. Greeley EH, Kealy RD, Ballman JM, and others: The influence of age on the canine immune system, *Vet Immunol Immunopath* 55:1-10, 1996.

202. Hayek MG, Kearns RJ, Turek JT, and others: Effect of age and dietary omega-5:omega-3 fatty acid ratio on the immune response of Fox Terriers and Labrador Retrievers.

203. Meydani SN, Hayek MG, Wu D, and others: Vitamin E and immune response in aged dogs. In Reinhart GA, Carey DP, editors: *Recent advances in canine and feline nutrition,* vol 2, Iams Nutrition Symposium Proceedings, Wilmington, Ohio, 1998, Orange Frazer Press.

204. Chew BP, Park JS, Wong DS, and others: Importance of beta-carotene nutrition in the dog and cat: uptake and immunity. In Reinhart GA, Carey DP, editors: *Recent advances in canine and feline nutrition,* vol 2, Iams Nutrition Symposium Proceedings, Wilmington, Ohio, 1998, Orange Frazer Press.

205. Chew PB, Wong TS, Park TS and others: Role of dietary lutein in the dog and cat. In Reinhart GA, Carey DP, editors: *Recent advances in canine and feline nutrition,* vol 2, Iams Nutrition Symposium Proceedings, Wilmington, Ohio, 1998, Orange Frazer Press.

206. Hostetter TH, Rennke HG, Brenner BM: Compensatory renal hemodynamic injury: a final common pathway of residual nephron destruction, *Am J Kidney Dis* 1:310-314, 1982.

207. Walser M: Does dietary therapy have a role in the predialysis patient?, *Am J Clin Nutr* 33:1629-1637, 1980.

208. Finco DR, Brown SA, Crowell WA, and others: Effect of phosphorus/calcium-restricted and phosphorus/calcium-replete 32% diets in dogs with chronic renal failure, *Am J Vet Res* 53:157-163, 1992.

209. Brown SA, Crowell WA, Barsanti JA: Beneficial effects of dietary mineral restriction in dogs with marked reduction of functional renal mass, *J Am Soc Nephrol* 1:1169-1179, 1991.

210. Ross LA, Finco DR, Crowell WA: Effects of dietary phosphorus restriction on the kidneys of cats with reduced renal mass, *Am J Vet Res* 43:1023-1026, 1982.

211. Care of old cats, *Feline Pract* 13:3-40, 1983.

SECTION

5

FEEDING PRACTICES: PROBLEMS, FADS, AND FALLACIES

Previous sections have examined nutrient requirements of dogs and cats, types of pet foods that can be fed, and proper feeding management practices throughout the lifetime of the healthy pet. Several decades ago, before much was known about the nutritional needs of dogs and cats and before nutritionally balanced pet foods were produced, nutrient deficiencies were a common occurrence in companion animals. Today, pet foods that provide complete nutrition and have the potential to promote optimal health are readily available to pet owners and professionals. As a direct result of advances in scientific knowledge and in the formulation of commercial pet foods, the occurrence of serious nutrient deficiencies in companion animals has become extremely rare. Feeding management problems are now more likely to result in problems of overnutrition rather than undernutrition. The provision of surplus calories, supplementation with excess amounts of certain vitamins and minerals, and feeding young dogs to promote a

301

rapid rate of growth are all practices that can result in developmental disease and chronic health problems. Less commonly, deficiencies or toxicities of certain vitamins can occur because of the presence of inhibitory substances in the food or improper feeding practices. This section focuses on problems and fallacies of feeding management that can cause nutrient imbalances and impair the health of growing and mature companion animals. These problems include obesity, feeding for a high rate of growth, supplementation with certain nutrients, deficiencies and excesses of certain vitamins, feeding inappropriate food items to pets, and common nutrition myths.

26

Obesity

 Obesity is currently the most common nutritional disorder that occurs in companion animals in the United States. Surveys have reported incidence rates of between 24% and 34% in adult dogs.[1,2,3,4,5] One of the most recent studies collected information on almost 130,000 dogs and cats from 55 private veterinary practices in 33 states.[2] Results showed that 27% of dogs were judged to be overweight or obese. The proportion of overweight/obese pets peaked during middle age (greater than 45%), while geriatric pets and young adults were much less likely to be obese. In addition, dogs that are overweight when they are adolescents are more likely to be overweight or obese as adults.[5] It can be theorized that the incidence of obesity in dogs has increased because a sedentary lifestyle has become the norm rather than the exception for many dogs. In addition, the provision of highly palatable and energy-dense foods may further contribute to the energy imbalance that leads to obesity.

Until recently, it was generally believed that obesity in cats was less prevalent. One of the first surveys conducted reported an incidence rate of only 9% in pet cats.[2] However, the incidence of obesity in cats appears to have increased dramatically within the past 10 years. Recent studies of house cats reported that between 25% and 40% of the cats seen by veterinarians were considered to be either overweight or obese.[2,6,7] Increased popularity of the cat as a house pet, decreased daily activity of cats that are confined indoors, and increased availability of highly palatable cat foods are all factors that may be responsible for the dramatic increase in the incidence of obesity in cats in the United States.

EFFECTS

Obesity is defined as the excessive accumulation of fat in the adipose storage areas of the body.[8] A body weight that is more than 15% to 20% above normal is generally considered to be indicative of obesity. Health problems in human subjects begin to increase when weight reaches 15% or greater above ideal body weight.[1,9,10] Dogs and cats that are overweight also have an increased risk of chronic health problems. These include hyperinsulinemia, glucose intolerance, and diabetes.[11] Obese dogs and cats may exhibit glucose intolerance and abnormal basal insulin and insulin response curves. When body weight is reduced, glucose intolerance often improves to near-normal values.[12] It has been postulated that obesity in dogs, as in humans, modulates glucose and insulin homeostasis, resulting in hyperinsulinemia and various degrees of glucose intolerance. It is very likely that persistent hyperinsulinemia caused by obesity is an important factor in the eventual development of diabetes mellitus in overweight pets.

Obesity may contribute to the development of pulmonary and cardiovascular disease. Excess weight puts a strain on the circulatory system because increased cardiac workload is required to perfuse the increased tissue mass. This increased workload may cause additional strain on a heart that is already weakened by fatty infiltration. The physical effects of carrying excess weight also contribute to exercise and heat intolerance, joint and locomotor problems, and the development of arthritis.[13] A recent 5-year study of the effects of food intake and body weight on the occurrence and severity of osteoarthritis in the hip joints of Labrador Retrievers found that ad libitum feeding and increased body weight were significantly correlated with an increased incidence and severity of osteoarthritis.[14] Another study reported that female dogs who were obese prior to a diagnosis of breast cancer had a significantly increased risk of death from this disease when compared with the risk in dogs who were underweight at the time of diagnosis.[15] The health risks of obesity in cats have also been studied recently.[16] Overweight cats are significantly more likely to develop diabetes mellitus, locomotor problems, and nonallergic skin problems when compared with cats of normal weight. Other potential risks included hepatic lipidosis, compromised cardiac and immune function, and increased risk of premature death. Finally, obese dogs and cats also have an increased surgical and anesthetic risk, and they experience an increased incidence of morbidity and mortality following surgical procedures.

TYPES

The basic problem of obesity involves an increased mass of body fat produced either by an enlargement of fat cell size alone (hypertrophic obesity) or by an increase in both fat cell size and fat cell number (hyperplastic obesity). Pets that develop hyperplastic obesity are generally believed to be difficult to treat and have a poor long-term prognosis. Normal adipocyte hyperplasia occurs during specific critical periods of development. In most species, these periods occur during early growth and occasionally during puberty.[17] Once adulthood is reached, the number of fat cells does not normally increase further. Overfeeding during adulthood results in an increase in fat cell size, but no change in fat cell number. Although conditions of extreme and prolonged overfeeding can result in fat cell hyperplasia in some animals, the majority of cases of adult onset obesity are a result of fat cell hypertrophy alone.[18,19]

The body has the capacity to add new adipocytes, but it is not able to reduce its existing adipocyte number. This phenomenon, called the "ratchet effect," indicates that body fat can always increase, but it cannot decrease below a minimum level that is set by the total number of adipocytes and their need to remain lipid-filled. This fact is of importance when considering growth rate and weight gain in young, developing dogs and cats. Data from several studies with laboratory animals show that overnutrition during growth results in increased numbers of fat cells and total body fatness during adulthood.[20,21] Superfluous fat cell hyperplasia during the critical periods of adipose tissue growth may produce a long-term stimulus to gain excess weight in the form of excess adipocytes.[9] The greater number of fat cells results in both an increased predisposition toward obesity in adulthood and an increased difficulty in maintaining weight loss when it occurs. Therefore the reason that hyperplastic obesity is difficult to treat is that the excess fat cells maintain a stimulus for lipid deposition and are resistant to reductions in fat content below a certain level. Persistent overnutrition during development in growing dogs and cats may result in both hypertrophy and hyperplasia of adipocytes, leading to the development of obesity. The potential for an animal to produce excess numbers of fat cells during specific critical periods illustrates the importance of proper weight control throughout growth.

CAUSES

The fundamental underlying cause in all cases of obesity is an imbalance between energy intake and energy expenditure that results in a persistent energy surplus. Excess energy is stored primarily as fat, resulting in weight gain and a change in body composition. Although the problem of obesity appears very simple in terms of energy balance, a multitude of underlying causes exist, not all of which are completely understood. Moreover, the development of obesity in an individual dog or cat can be the result of several separate influencing factors occurring simultaneously (Box 26-1).

Factors that may contribute to the development of obesity can be classified as having either an endogenous or an exogenous origin. Endogenous factors include

BOX 26-1

Factors Contributing to Obesity in Companion Animals	
Endogenous Factors	**Exogenous Factors**
Age, sex, and reproductive status	Voluntary activity level
Presence of hormonal abnormalities or hypothalamic lesions	External influences on food intake
	Diet composition and palatability
Genetic predisposition	Living environment and type of lifestyle

the animal's age, sex and reproductive status, hormonal abnormalities, hypothalamic lesions, and genetic predisposition. Exogenous factors include voluntary activity level, external influences on food intake, diet composition, food palatability, and type of lifestyle. Most cases of companion animal obesity are a result of overfeeding, underexercising, or a combination of the two.[22,23] It is important to recognize that each of these situations may be a result of either external or internal aberrations. For example, a dog may consume excess food because the diet that is being fed is highly palatable and of high caloric density (exogenous stimuli). On the other hand, the cause would be of endogenous origin if the overeating was in response to lesions involving the satiety center located in the ventral medial hypothalamus.[24,25] The various causative factors that may be involved in the development of obesity are discussed in the following section.

Decreased Energy Expenditure

An animal's energy expenditure can be divided into three major components: resting metabolic rate (RMR), voluntary muscular activity, and meal-induced thermogenesis (see Section 2, pp. 75-77). Although the importance in companion animals is not known, a fourth component, adaptive thermogenesis, may also contribute to energy expenditure. An abnormally low RMR, meal-induced thermogenesis, and adaptive thermogenesis have all been studied as possible causes of weight gain in animals and humans. Studies measuring RMR have not supported the claim that obese individuals gain weight because they possess abnormally low RMR values.[26,27,28] In fact, the RMR of most obese subjects is actually higher than that in subjects of normal weight. Although the state of obesity is characterized primarily by excessive amounts of body fat, overweight animals also have increased amounts of lean body tissue. The elevated RMR accompanying obesity is accounted for by this increased, respiring tissue mass.[29] When the RMR is expressed in relationship to the total amount of lean body mass in obese animals, it is within a normal range.[26,27]

Subnormal meal-induced thermogenesis in an animal would result in lower energy expenditure than would normally be expected after the ingestion of a meal.[30] The long-term result of such a deficit would be a slightly positive energy balance, leading to an increased propensity toward weight gain. Although such a defect in a pre-obese animal would account for only a small number of calories per day, it may affect long-term energy balance and contribute to the development of obesity. However, studies with human subjects have shown that a defect in meal-induced thermogenesis could not singularly account for the large increases in weight that are seen in obese subjects.[31]

The existence of adaptive thermogenesis in several species of small mammals is widely accepted. However, the inference that other species can adapt to periods of overconsumption by increasing energy expenditure through changes in adaptive thermogenesis is still very controversial. If adaptive thermogenesis is present in species other than small rodents, it is possible that a defect in the response to overfeeding may be of importance in the development of obesity in some individuals. However, the paucity of well-controlled studies, coupled with the publication of

conflicting results, leads to the conclusion that adaptive thermogenesis in response to overeating is probably not a major contributing factor to the development of obesity in companion animals.

Reduced voluntary activity is the most important contributor to decreased energy expenditure in overweight companion animals. In today's society, most dogs are kept as companions and house pets rather than as active, working partners to their human owners. Cats are also experiencing decreased activity levels. Many cats lead sedentary, indoor lives rather than having the run of farms and neighborhoods as in the past. Additional factors that influence the voluntary activity level of dogs and cats are breed, temperament, age, type of lifestyle, reproductive status, and the presence of certain chronic illnesses or developmental disorders. In normal animals experiencing moderate levels of exercise, physical activity contributes approximately 30% of the body's total energy expenditure.[32] Decreased voluntary activity results in a direct reduction of this energy expenditure and can also affect a pet's daily food intake. Research studies have shown that completely sedentary animals actually consume more food and gain more weight than do animals that experience moderate activity levels.[33] It appears that inactivity below a certain level cannot be entirely compensated for by an adequate decrease in food intake. As a result, animals that are maintained at or below this minimum activity level will consume more than their energy needs and inevitably gain weight.

Endocrine Disorders

Two endocrine disorders that may influence body weight in companion animals are hypothyroidism and hyperadrenocorticism. Hypothyroidism results in a decreased RMR, which may in turn cause a predisposition for obesity. This disorder is diagnosed when clinical signs are observed and plasma levels of one or both of the thyroid hormone variants thyroxine (T_4) and triiodothyronine (T_3) are found to be below normal. Idiopathic atrophy of the thyroid gland is the most common cause of hypothyroidism in dogs.[34] This disorder occurs most frequently in middle-aged and older dogs, and certain breeds show a higher incidence than the general population. These breeds include Golden Retrievers, Doberman Pinschers, Irish Setters, Boxers, Old English Sheepdogs, Miniature Schnauzers, Airedale Terriers, and some Spaniel breeds.[34,35] Spayed females are also more likely to develop the disorder than other dogs.[36] Hypothyroidism can occur in cats, but it is much less common and has not been well documented.[37]

Clinical signs of hypothyroidism include lethargy, a dulled mental attitude, and easy fatigability.[38,39] Common skin changes include alopecia; the development of a dry, coarse coat; and skin hyperpigmentation. Cold sensitivity, exercise intolerance, and weight gain are clinical signs that result directly from the decreased RMR associated with hypothyroidism. However, only a small percentage of dogs exhibit all of these signs, and when obesity is seen, it is usually moderate.[39,40] Assessment of thyroid hormone levels should always be included in the differential diagnosis of obesity in companion animals. However, hypothyroidism is probably responsible for only a small percentage of cases of overt obesity in pets.

Hyperadrenocorticism (Cushing's syndrome) can also result in increased body size. This disorder is caused by the production of excess corticosteroids by the adrenal cortex. It is most common in middle-aged and older dogs, and breed predilections have been observed in Poodles, Dachshunds, Boxers, Brussels Griffons, and Boston Terriers.[34] Cushing's syndrome can occur in cats, but it is quite rare.[35] The primary clinical signs of this disorder include polyuria, polydipsia, lethargy, hair loss, and the development of a pendulous abdomen.[35,41] True obesity occurs in approximately 50% of the cases, although the presence of an enlarged abdomen may be perceived to be obesity by some pet owners. Diagnosis is based on adrenal function tests, which will differentiate between Cushing's-induced obesity and obesity as a result of other causes.

Effects of Neutering

Early survey studies reported that neutered male and female pets were more likely to be overweight than were intact animals.[4,42] Recent studies have supported these observations, showing that intact adult pets generally weigh less than neutered animals of the same breed and size.[43,44,45,46,47] The underlying cause of this difference is probably a combination of physiological and environmental factors. Veterinarians usually encourage clients to castrate or spay their pets before they become sexually mature. As a result, many dogs and cats are neutered between 6 months and 1 year of age. This period corresponds to a natural decrease in the pet's growth rate and energy needs. If owners are not aware of this change and continue to feed their pet the same amount of food, excess weight gain will result. Because spaying and neutering often occur just before maturity, the change in sexual status may be erroneously blamed for a weight gain that was actually the result of diminished energy needs and excess food intake.

Increasing age and a change in sexual status are also associated with a decrease in voluntary physical activity. In general, puppies and kittens are more active than adult animals. If an individual dog or cat naturally decreases its activity level as it reaches maturity, the consumption of the same quantity of food will result in weight gain. In addition, intact animals display sexually motivated behaviors that increase the amount of energy expended as physical activity. Male dogs and cats have an inclination to roam and fight with other males, and intact females increase their physical activity and roaming behavior during estrus.

Reproductive status can also affect voluntary food intake and RMR. Many female dogs and cats spontaneously decrease their food intake during estrus, and the cause of this change has been attributed to estrogen. A study with dogs examined the influence of estrus on voluntary food intake in 12 Beagle bitches.[43] Results showed that there was a tendency for females to decrease food consumption during the week that they were in estrus. The study's authors also examined food intake patterns in ovariohysterectomized and sham-operated bitches. Over a period of 90 days, the ovariohysterectomized bitches gained significantly more weight and consumed greater amounts of food than did the sham-operated controls. The authors attributed the difference in weight gain to an increase in food intake and a decrease in voluntary activity. Similar results have been reported in cats. Two recent studies found that male and female cats increased voluntary food intake after neutering and consumed more food than their intact counterparts.[46,47] However, another study compared intact male cats with neutered male cats and found that neutered males ate less but gained more weight than did intact males. This difference was theorized to be the result of decreased physical activity and increased efficiency of energy use that occurred with the loss of testosterone in the neutered animals.[45] A pet's RMR also seems to be affected by neutering. When RMR was measured using respiratory indirect calorimetry in neutered and intact cats, heat coefficients were greater in intact male and female cats than in neutered animals.[44] Intact males had heat coefficients that were 28% higher than those of neutered males, and intact females had heat coefficients that were 33% higher than those of neutered females. These results can be interpreted to mean that neutered male cats may require 28% fewer calories, and females 33% fewer calories, than their intact counterparts.

In recent years, early-age neutering (at 8 to 16 weeks of age) has become more common because of the benefits to pet population control and possibly to pet health. Recognition of the safety of these procedures for puppies and kittens led the American Veterinary Medical Association to approve a 1993 resolution supporting the concept of early-age neutering. However, one concern has been the potential of early-age neutering to influence a pet's tendency to become obese. A recent study compared metabolic rates and the development of obesity in cats that were surgically neutered at 7 weeks of age, surgically neutered at 7 months of age, or left intact.[44] All of the cats in the study were fed ad libitum until they were 2 years of age and were assessed regularly for body condition, metabolic rate, and glucose tolerance. Because body weight alone is not an accurate predictor of obesity, body condition scores were assigned and body mass index was calculated. The body condition scores and body mass indices of the neutered males and females were significantly higher than those in the intact animals, indicating that neutered animals were more obese than intact animals. However, no differences were observed between animals neutered at 7 weeks of age and those neutered at 7 months of age. These results, along with those reported in dogs, indicate that early-age neutering presents the same level of risk of weight gain as does neutering at the traditional age of 6 to 9 months.[44]

Old Age

As an adult animal ages, lean body mass declines, resulting in decreased RMR and total daily energy needs. The loss of lean body mass is exacerbated if aging is accompanied by a decrease in voluntary activity. The total daily energy needs of an average-sized, 7-year-old dog may decrease by as much as 20% when compared with its needs as a young adult. If food intake does not decrease proportionately with decreasing energy needs as an animal ages, weight gain results.

Genetic Predisposition

Several types of genetic obesity have been shown to exist in laboratory animals.[48,49,50] Studies have also indicated that there is a genetic component to obesity in some human subjects.[51,52,53] The fact that certain breeds of dogs have a dispro-portionately high incidence of obesity indicates that genetics may be a contributing factor in this species as well. Early studies identified Cocker Spaniels, Labrador Retrievers, Shetland Sheepdogs, and the small Terrier breeds as having a high incidence of obesity, while Boxers, German Shepherd Dogs, Fox Terriers, and the sight Hound breeds had a relatively low incidence.[4,54] A more recent survey study reported that Labrador Retrievers and Shetland Sheepdogs, as well as Golden Retrievers, Cocker Spaniels, Dachshunds, Miniature Schnauzers, Springer Spaniels, Chihuahuas, Basset Hounds, and Pugs were most likely to be overweight or obese.[2] It is theorized that the genetic tendency toward obesity originally had survival value for the dog in its wild state because those animals who efficiently stored excess energy as fat were better able to tolerate long periods of food deprivation.[54] No data have been reported concerning breed predilections to obesity in pet cats, but as purebred cats become increasingly popular, such predilections may also be identified in this species.

Alterations in Food Intake

Food intake is regulated in all animals by a complex system involving both internal physiological controls and external cues. Internal signals that affect appetite, hunger, and satiety include mechanical stimulation from the gastrointestinal tract; physiological responses to the sight, sound, and smell of food; and changes in plasma concentrations of specific nutrients, hormones, and peptides. External stimuli include factors such as food availability, the presence of other animals, the timing and size of meals, a food's composition and texture, and diet palatability. The external cues that affect food intake are probably most important in the regulation of food intake and the development of obesity in companion animals.

The most important external factor is feeding pets highly palatable diets that may induce some animals to overconsume. Studies with laboratory animals have shown that when rats are offered a highly palatable diet, they overeat and become obese.[55] This effect has been observed with high-fat diets, calorically dense diets, and "cafeteria" diets, which provide a large variety of highly palatable food items.[56] Long-term exposure to highly palatable foods in human subjects also leads to permanent increases in body weight, fat cell size, and fat cell number.[9] Although an endogenous predisposition to obesity and increased efficiency of weight gain may occur in some animals, the largest portion of weight gain observed when animals are fed highly palatable diets is a direct result of overconsumption.[56] Studies with human subjects have demonstrated that the quantity of food consumed varies directly with its palatability, and palatability does not appear to interact with levels of food deprivation. In other words, if food is perceived to be very appealing, an individual tends to eat more of it, regardless of the initial level of hunger.[57]

Palatability is an important diet characteristic that is heavily promoted in the marketing of commercial pet foods. Many pet owners select a product based on their own perceptions of the food's appeal and their pet's acceptance of the diet, rather than on indicators of nutritional adequacy. Semimoist foods and treats contain variable amounts of simple sugars and other humectants that contribute to palatability. Canned pet foods and some premium dry foods are high in fat content. Fat contributes to both the palatability and caloric density of the food. Feeding pets highly palatable foods on an ad libitum basis may contribute to both the development and the maintenance of obesity because many pets readily overconsume these foods. Similarly, the common practice of feeding a variety of table scraps and other appealing treats to dogs and cats can induce many pets to overeat and gain excessive amounts of weight.

A retrospective study of dietary patterns in adult female dogs found that up to 50% of calories were supplied to some dogs as table scraps, particularly those dogs of the toy breeds.[6] In addition, a recent study found that dogs that were reported to be overweight or obese were more frequently fed canned grocery store pet food or a homemade diet when compared with dogs that were judged to be at their ideal body weight.[2] Table scraps and some homemade diets that are fed to pets can also contain a high proportion of their calories from fat and thus can contribute to a caloric imbalance.

The social setting of meals also influences eating behavior. Most pets increase food intake when consuming food in the presence of other animals.[25,58] This process is called *social facilitation* and is usually more pronounced in dogs than in cats. In most pets, social facilitation causes a moderate increase in food intake and an increased rate of eating. In some, the increase in food intake in response to another animal's presence can be extreme enough to singularly cause weight gain.[25]

Similarly, meal frequency affects both food intake and metabolic efficiency. An increase in the number of meals per day results in increased energy loss to meal-induced thermogenesis (see Section 2, p. 76). There is also evidence in humans indicating that a decrease in lipogenesis (fat tissue synthesis) occurs when multiple meals are fed, as compared with consuming the same number of calories in only one or two meals.[59] However, if several meals are provided per day, portions must be strictly controlled. Increased feeding frequency often causes increased voluntary intake, thereby offsetting any metabolic benefits of multiple meals.

A final external factor that may be a contributing cause of obesity in companion animals is the nutrient composition of the diet. Nutrient composition affects both the efficiency of nutrient metabolism and the amount of food that is voluntarily consumed. When fed ad libitum, high-fat diets promote weight gain and obesity.[60] Although most animals decrease the volume of intake of a high-fat diet in an attempt to balance energy needs, the greater caloric density of the diet and its increased palatability usually cause a total increase in energy intake. Additionally, the metabolic efficiency of converting dietary fat to body fat for storage is higher than is the efficiency of converting dietary carbohydrate or protein to body fat. Therefore, if an animal is consuming more than its caloric requirement of a particular diet and if the excess calories are provided by fat, more weight will be gained than if the excess calories are coming from either carbohydrate or protein.

The caloric distribution of fat, carbohydrate, and protein is very important in determining a diet's potential contribution to weight imbalance in dogs and cats. As

FIGURE **26-1**

Recommended caloric distribution of dog foods (expressed as a percentage of ME calories).

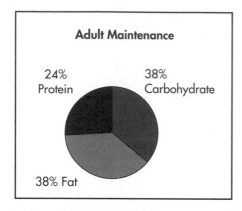

Adult Maintenance

24%
Protein

38%
Carbohydrate

38% Fat

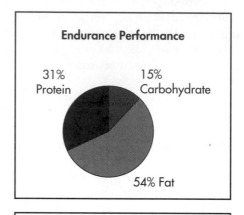

Endurance Performance

31%
Protein

15%
Carbohydrate

54% Fat

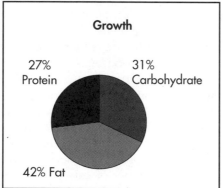

Growth

27%
Protein

31%
Carbohydrate

42% Fat

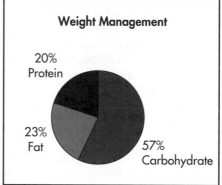

Weight Management

20%
Protein

23%
Fat

57%
Carbohydrate

the percentage of metabolizable energy (ME) calories from fat increases in a pet food, the ability of the diet to meet the high energy demands of a hard-working dog also increases. However, if this diet is fed to a dog that does not need it, weight gain may occur if intake is not strictly monitored. A diet that contains a low percentage of ME from fat will aid in weight loss or in the maintenance of normal body weight in a sedentary adult animal. The selection of a pet food should therefore match the proportion of ME contributed by fat to the animal's lifestyle and activity level (Figure 26-1).

DEVELOPMENT

Two stages occur during the development of obesity: the dynamic phase and the static phase. During the initial dynamic phase, an animal consumes more energy than it expends, and the surplus energy is deposited as both body fat and lean body tissue. As the dog or cat gains weight, its RMR increases proportionately to the increase in lean body mass. Eventually the increased RMR, coupled with the increased energy expenditure that is needed to move a larger body size, offsets the caloric surplus. At this point, zero energy balance is achieved, and the animal stops gaining weight. The static phase of obesity occurs when the animal is no longer gaining weight but achieves energy balance and maintains its overweight condition for a prolonged period of time.

If the initial dynamic phase occurs at a young age or if the energy surplus is extreme, fat cell hyperplasia occurs along with fat cell hypertrophy. Research in other species has shown that hyperplastic obesity is more resistant to treatment than is simple hypertrophic obesity.[20,21] The presence of additional numbers of fat cells results in a higher percentage of body fat. Therefore an animal with fat cell hyperplasia has a higher proportion of body fat than does an animal that weighs the same amount but has a normal number of fat cells. This difference affects energy expenditure and the ability to lose weight and maintain the loss when it occurs.

DIAGNOSIS

The diagnosis of obesity in companion animals should always include a veterinary examination for the presence of edema, ascites, hypothyroidism, hyperadrenocorticism, and diabetes mellitus.[61] After these diseases have been ruled out, a comparison of the pet's current weight with previous weight measurements or with its weight shortly after reaching adulthood may be indicative of abnormal weight gain. In some cases involving purebred dogs and cats, a comparison of the pet's body weight with the weights suggested by the breed's standard may also be a useful guideline for determining ideal body weight (Table 26-1; also see Appendix 2, pp. 553-556).

Estimating *percent body fat* is the most accurate method of diagnosing obesity. Ultrasound provides a noninvasive, rapid method for estimating subcutaneous fat, but it is not yet practical in most clinical settings.[62] Likewise, measurements of total body density are very accurate but usually not feasible.[42] In recent years, dual energy x-ray absorptiometry (DEXA) has been shown to provide a very accurate measurement of total body fat and lean body mass.[63] This procedure has been used extensively in research settings to determine the body composition of many species, including dogs and cats.[64,65,66] However, DEXA is neither practical nor economical for use by practicing veterinarians. The most practical method for assessing excess body fat and obesity in dogs and cats is palpating the thickness of tissue overlying the rib cage, lumbar area, and tail base, and the thickness along the ventral abdomen.[22,67] If a dog or cat is too thin, the ribs will be easily seen. An animal of normal weight will have barely visible ribs that can be easily felt when palpated. An overweight animal's ribs will not be visible and an overlying layer of fat can be felt. The pet is diagnosed as grossly obese if the ribs cannot be felt at all.

For practicing veterinarians and pet owners, visual assessment of the pet using a subjective body condition scoring system is an accurate and easily administered method. Several systems are available to practitioners and pet owners, all of which

TABLE 26-1

Standard Weights of Popular Breeds of Dogs

Breed	Male (lbs)	Female (lbs)
Basset Hound	65-75	50-65
Beagle (13")	13-18	13-16
Beagle (15")	17-22	15-20
Boxer	55-70	50-60
Chihuahua	2-6	2-6
Chow Chow	45-50	40-50
Cocker Spaniel	25-30	20-25
Collie	65-75	50-65
Dachshund, Miniature	8-10	8-10
Dachshund, Standard	16-22	16-22
Dalmation	50-65	45-55
Doberman Pinscher	65-80	55-70
English Springer Spaniel	49-55	40-45
German Shepherd	75-90	65-80
Golden Retriever	65-75	55-65
Labrador Retriever	65-80	55-70
Maltese	4-6	4-6
Miniature Schnauzer	16-18	12-16
Pekingese	10-14	10-14
Pomeranian	4-7	3-5
Poodle, Standard	50-60	45-55
Poodle, Miniature	17-20	15-20
Poodle, Toy	7-10	7-10
Rottweiler	80-95	70-85
Shetland Sheepdog	16-22	14-18
Shih Tzu	12-17	10-15
Siberian Husky	45-60	35-50
Yorkshire Terrier	4-7	3-6

involve subjective ranking of body composition based upon visual assessment and palpation (Figures 26-2 and 26-3).[68,69,70] Recent studies have shown that body scoring systems provide a highly reliable method for the diagnosis of obesity and are predictive of a pet's percent body fat.[69,70] Comparisons of body composition data collected using DEXA with assessments of body condition using a nine-point system revealed significant and positive correlations between body condition scores and percent body fat in both dogs and cats.[69,70] Interestingly, although the predictive value of the scoring system was the same for both male and female pets, females of both species had a higher percentage of body fat than males who were assigned the same body condition score.

FIGURE **26-2**

Assessment of body condition in the dog.

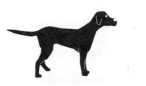 **Thin**
Ribs, lumbar vertebrae, and pelvic bones easily visible. No palpable fat. Obvious waist and abdominal tuck.

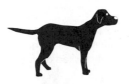 **Underweight**
Ribs easily palpable. Minimal fat covering. Waist is easily noted when viewed from above. Abdominal tuck evident.

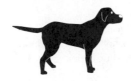 **Ideal**
Ribs palpable without excess fat covering. Waist observed behind ribs when viewed from above. Abdomen tucked up when viewed from the side.

 Overweight
Ribs palpable with a slight excess of fat covering. Waist is discernible when viewed from above but is not prominent. Abdominal tuck is apparent.

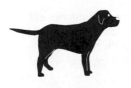 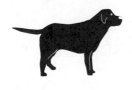 **Obese**
Ribs not easily palpable under a heavy fat covering. Fat deposits noticeable over lumbar area and at base of tail. Waist barely visible to absent. No abdominal tuck; may exhibit obvious abdominal distention.

Body condition scoring involves the assessment of several different areas of the body. Dogs and cats who are at their ideal body weight should have an hourglass shape when viewed from above, showing an observable waist behind the ribs (see Figures 26-2 and 26-3).[47] In heavily coated animals, the waist should be easily palpated beneath the pet's hair coat. The loss of a waist as a result of excess fat between the muscles of the abdominal wall and the presence of a pendulous abdomen as a result of fat accumulation in intraabdominal sites are both indicative of

FIGURE 26-3

Assessment of body condition in the cat.

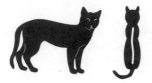

Thin
Ribs, lumbar vertebrae, and pelvic bones easily visible. Thin neck and narrow waist. Obvious abdominal tuck. No fat in flank folds; folds often absent.

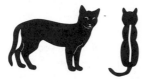

Underweight
Backbone and ribs easily palpable. Minimal fat covering. Minimal waist when viewed from above. Slightly tucked abdomen.

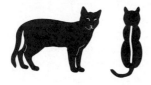

Ideal
Ribs palpable but not visible. Slight waist observed behind ribs when viewed from above. Abdomen tucked up; flank folds present.

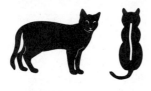

Overweight
Slight increase in fat over ribs but ribs still easily palpable. Abdomen slightly rounded; flanks concave. Flank folds hang down with moderate amount of fat; jiggle noted when walking.

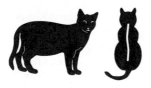

Obese
Ribs and backbone not easily palpable under a heavy fat covering. Abdomen rounded; waist barely visible to absent. Prominent flank folds that sway from side to side when walking.

excess body fat. Dogs have a tendency to develop fat deposits over the thorax and spine and around the base of the tail, while cats often accumulate fat just anterior to the inguinal region. In addition, overweight cats develop folds of skin and underlying fat in the flank area. Subjective evaluation of the animal's gait, exercise tolerance, and overall appearance can also be used to support a diagnosis of obesity.

The development of visual body condition assessment tools is also of benefit to pet owners. Veterinary practitioners can use illustrative charts to teach clients to monitor their pets' weights and body conditions. Standardized visual aids are important because an owner's perception of his pet's weight is often inaccurate. A survey of dog owners found that when clients were asked to identify whether their dog was overweight, underweight, or at an appropriate body weight, approximately 30% to 40% of owners of overweight dogs felt their dog was at an appropriate body weight.[69,70] However, when cat owners and veterinarians were asked to select overweight cats from a series of illustrations of cats' silhouettes, owners and veterinarians were in close agreement as to which animals were overweight. Because some owners may be unable or reluctant to recognize weight gain or obesity in their own pet, the use of body condition charts may be helpful to veterinarians as a tool to teach about ideal body weight and to convince some owners of their pet's need to lose weight.

MANAGEMENT

The short-term goal of the treatment of obesity is to reduce body fat stores. This goal relies on the induction of a negative energy balance. Negative energy balance can be accomplished by restricting dietary intake, stimulating total energy expenditure, or a combination of the two.[71] The long-term goal of treatment is for the pet to attain its ideal body weight and maintain this weight for the remainder of its life.

Dogs and cats that are 15% or more above their ideal body weight should be placed on a strict weight loss program. When initiating such a program, the determined rate of weight loss should be high enough to ensure a noticeable change within several weeks, yet low enough to minimize excessive hunger and the loss of lean body tissue. Because of the large variation in size and degree of obesity in individual animals, a recommended percentage of body weight loss per week should be used rather than a set quantity of weight loss. Studies with humans have shown that weekly rates of loss that are greater than 2% to 3% of body weight are unhealthy because lean body tissue losses are too great.[72] Conversely, if the rate of loss is too low (0.5% or less), pet owners may lose interest and motivation because results will not be observed for several weeks. Therefore a goal of 1% to 2% per week is recommended for most pets. In most cases, this translates to a program that will span about 8 to 12 months. For example, an adult dog with an ideal body weight of 25 kilograms (kg) (55 pounds [lbs]) that actually weighs 30 kg (66 lbs) should lose between 0.3 and 0.6 kg (0.7 to 1.3 lbs) per week. A starting point of about 1 lb of weight loss per week can be used as a target loss when calculating this dog's energy needs for the weight loss program; this can be adjusted as needed based upon the dog's current intake or its response to the caloric restriction (Table 26-2 and Box 26-2).

Three important components should be included in all weight reduction programs: behavior modification, exercise, and dietary modification. Dietary modification and exercise create an energy deficit that will result in weight loss. Behavior

TABLE 26-2

Energy Requirements for Weight Loss in Dogs and Cats

Dogs				
Current Weight (lbs)	Current Weight (kg)	ME* (kcal/day)	60% of ME (kcal/day)	Amount** (cups/day)
5	2.3	231	138	0.40
10	4.5	362	217	0.62
15	6.8	477	286	0.82
20	9.1	580	348	0.99
25	11.4	674	404	1.16
30	13.6	759	455	1.30
35	15.9	842	505	1.44
40	18.2	922	553	1.58
45	20.5	999	599	1.71
50	22.7	1069	642	1.83
55	25.0	1141	684	1.96
60	27.3	1210	726	2.07
65	29.5	1275	765	2.18
70	31.8	1340	804	2.30
75	34.1	1404	843	2.41
80	36.4	1467	880	2.52
85	38.6	1526	916	2.62
90	40.9	1586	952	2.72
95	43.2	1646	987	2.82
100	45.5	1704	1022	2.92
105	47.7	1759	1055	3.01
110	50.0	1815	1089	3.11
115	52.3	1871	1122	3.21
120	54.5	1923	1154	3.30

*Dogs: ME = 132 × (weight$_{kg}$)$^{0.67}$ Cats: ME = 60 × (weight$_{kg}$)

**Calculated for a pet food with a caloric density of 3500 kcal/kg and weight density of 3.5 oz/cup. Adjustments must be made for foods with higher or lower densities.

modification can be helpful in changing the owner's and the pet's behavior, which will aid in weight loss and the prevention of weight regain.

Behavior Modification

Behavior modification techniques are designed to change habits of the owner that may have contributed to the pet's initial weight gain. Such habits include providing the pet with high-calorie table scraps, providing a highly palatable and

TABLE 26-2, cont'd

Energy Requirements for Weight Loss in Dogs and Cats

Cats				
Current Weight (lbs)	Current Weight (kg)	ME* (kcal/day)	60% of ME (kcal/day)	Amount** (cups/day)
4	1.8	108	75.6	0.22
5	2.3	138	96.6	0.28
6	2.7	162	113.4	0.32
7	3.2	192	134.4	0.38
8	3.6	216	151.2	0.43
9	4.1	246	172.2	0.49
10	4.5	270	189.0	0.54
11	5.0	300	210.0	0.60
12	5.4	324	226.8	0.65
13	5.9	354	247.8	0.71
14	6.4	384	268.8	0.77
15	6.8	408	285.6	0.82
16	7.3	438	306.6	0.88
17	7.7	462	323.4	0.92
18	8.2	492	344.4	0.98
19	8.6	516	361.2	1.03
20	9.1	546	382.2	1.09

BOX 26-2

Calculation of Energy Needs for a Weight Loss Program

Target Weight Loss per Week

Ideal body weight = 25 kg (55 lbs)
Actual body weight = 30 kg (66 lbs)
Target weight loss per week = 30 kg × 2% = 0.6 kg/week (1.3 lbs)
This dog should lose approximately 1.3 lbs per week when placed on a weight loss program.

Caloric Requirement for Weight Loss

ME requirement (moderately active adult) = $132 \times W_{kg}^{0.67}$
$(30 \text{ kg})^{0.67} \times 132 = 1288.9$ (approximately 1289 kcal/day)
Caloric restriction for weight loss = 1289 × 0.60 = 773.4 kcal/day
Volume of food to feed
    Diet A (400 kcal/cup) = 773/400 = 1.9 cups per day
    Diet B (300 kcal/cup) = 773/300 = 2.57 cups per day

energy-dense food free-choice, encouraging or allowing begging, and frequently feeding dog biscuits and treats.[23] Some changes that can be instituted include keeping the pet out of the kitchen while meals are being prepared, decreasing the number of treats given per day or feeding treats formulated for weight control, breaking treats into small pieces and giving only a small piece at a time to the pet, providing attention and petting instead of food treats, keeping the pet out of the dining room during mealtimes, eliminating all "people foods" from the diet, and maintaining the pet on a portion-controlled feeding regimen. Establishing a strictly regulated schedule so that all meals are provided at the same time each day can also help to eliminate begging.[23]

Exercise

The inclusion of moderate, regular exercise in the treatment of obese pets affects body weight in several ways. Increased activity has the direct benefit of raising daily energy expenditure and thus contributing to the energy deficit that is necessary for weight loss. An increase in exercise also aids in the regulation of food intake. Studies with animals and humans have shown that caloric intake varies proportionally with energy expenditure during moderate to high levels of exercise. However, reduction of activity to a completely sedentary level results in increased food intake and eventual weight gain.[73,74] It appears that the normal physiological regulators of caloric intake do not function properly below a certain minimum level of physical activity, and an uncoupling of the relationship between energy expenditure and energy intake occurs. Even a small change in an overweight pet's activity level may be beneficial because of the possibility that normal physiological controls of food intake may be restored when activity increases.

Exercise also causes desired changes in body composition. Regular and continued exercise results in a higher proportion of lean tissue to fat tissue. Because an animal's RMR is directly related to the amount of lean body tissue that it has, increasing lean tissue contributes to the maintenance of a normal RMR during weight loss. Even during moderate weight loss programs, between 10% and 25% of weight loss comes from lean tissue.[75,76] As a result, a decline in RMR naturally occurs in response to caloric restriction, resulting in a decreased rate of weight loss over time. The inclusion of regular exercise along with caloric restriction minimizes or completely eliminates this decline in the RMR, allowing continued weight loss throughout the program and aiding in the prevention of weight regain.[77,78]

Physical activity should always be initiated at a low level with animals that are accustomed to a completely sedentary lifestyle. Twenty minutes of legitimate exercise three to five times per week is a good start. Daily exercise is ideal. Both the duration and the intensity of the exercise can be increased as the animal begins to lose weight and increases its exercise tolerance. Daily walking, running, or playing of fetch and other games are recommended forms of exercise for dogs. Although it is difficult to induce an increase in physical activity in some cats, many will enjoy walking outside on a harness or chasing and playing with toys. Whatever the cho-

important that the exercise program is regular an̲
span of the pet.

sen activity, it is important that the exercise program is regular and continues throughout the lifespan of the pet.

Diet

The third and most important component of a weight loss program for dogs and cats is caloric restriction. The first step to be taken when planning a diet is to weigh the pet and set a goal for weight reduction (see Table 26-2 and Box 26-2). An estimate of the pet's caloric requirement for maintenance of body weight should then be calculated. Feeding a diet that provides 60% to 70% of the calories necessary to maintain current body weight usually results in adequate weight loss.[79,80] Once a daily caloric intake for weight loss is calculated, the number should be compared to the number of calories that the pet is currently consuming. Caloric intake information can be obtained by requiring the owner to record all of the pet's food intake for several days. If the number of calories that has been estimated for weight reduction is not sufficiently lower than the number of calories that the pet is currently consuming each day, further adjustments will be necessary to ensure that the caloric deficit results in a desired rate of weight loss.

Although dogs can lose weight and maintain health on energy deficits as low as 40% of maintenance requirements, recent studies show that RMR and associated indicators of metabolic rate such as serum T_3 levels decrease significantly with increased caloric restriction.[79,81] In one study, RMR decreased up to 25% in dogs fed calorie-restricted diets.[81] It appears that dogs whose caloric intake is restricted to less than 60% of calories may be predisposed to weight rebound because of the effects of severe caloric restriction upon metabolic rate.

It is even more important to conservatively restrict calories in overweight cats. Cats should not be fed less than 60% of their maintenance energy requirement (MER) at the start of the weight loss program. Severe caloric restriction in this species results in increased losses of lean body tissue and lower losses of body fat, and it may also predispose cats to the development of hepatic lipidosis (see Section 6, pp 473-474).[82,83,84] Excess losses of lean body tissue may be related to the cat's inability to conserve nitrogen when fed limiting amounts of protein (see Section 2, pp. 105-111). Because of the cat's higher protein requirement and its inability to adapt to restricted protein, providing sufficient dietary protein is especially important.[85] Because some obese cats do not lose weight when fed a moderately restricted diet, a useful approach is to begin the weight loss program by feeding 75% of MER and evaluate weight and body condition for 2 weeks. If the loss is not adequate, restriction can be reduced to 50% of MER, again monitoring for a 2-week period. If the cat still does not lose weight, restriction can be further reduced to 25% MER. Because of the cat's tendency to develop hepatic lipidosis, veterinary monitoring should be an essential part of the weight loss program.

At a level of 60% to 70% of ME, most pets will lose between 1% and 2% of their total body weight per week. For example, the estimated daily caloric requirement of a 66-lb dog is 1289 kilocalories (kcal). Caloric restriction to 60% of this requirement equals 773 kcal/day. If a food that contains 400 kcal per 8-ounce (oz) cup is fed, this dog should receive about 2 cups of food per day. A caloric deficit of 3500 kcal is necessary to lose 1 lb of body fat. Therefore this amount of food should result in a loss of approximately 1 lb per week. If exercise is included in the program, the additional energy deficit will be accounted for by increased energy expenditure, and a slightly greater weight loss will be seen (see Table 26-2 and Box 26-2).

During the weight loss program, the pet should be weighed once each week, and a record or graph of weight loss should be kept. Caloric intake can be adjusted as the pet loses weight (see Table 26-2). If possible, follow-up veterinarian visits should be made every 2 to 3 weeks to record progress. Portion-controlled feeding should be used, even if a commercially prepared, reducing diet is fed. Portion-controlled feeding allows strict monitoring of a pet's total food intake and removes the opportunity for the pet to spontaneously increase its intake of a reduced-energy food. It may also be helpful to feed several small meals per day rather than one or two large meals. This practice may decrease signs of hunger and increase the energy losses of meal-induced thermogenesis.[86] Once the target weight has been reached, the daily volume of food can be slowly increased until an amount that maintains ideal body weight is provided.

Types of Diets for Weight Loss   Some pet owners include a great number of treats and table scraps in their pet's daily ration. When this is the case, simply eliminating all of the extra tidbits and restricting the pet's intake to 70% to 80% of its body weight requirement may lead to adequate weight loss. This is the preferred method to use with pets who are only slightly overweight, are exercised regularly, and have well-motivated owners.

When this type of caloric restriction is instituted, pets will naturally be hungrier than usual, and begging behaviors may increase proportionately. In addition, weight loss may be relatively slow due to the smaller caloric deficit. This may lead to poor compliance as owners will fail to see an appreciative weight change within several weeks. The lower limit of this type of dietary regimen, in terms of the caloric deficit, is set by the nutrient requirements of the dog or cat. Because a normal maintenance diet is being fed, it is imperative that the quantity provided is sufficient to meet the pet's total nutrient requirements. Commercial pet foods that are formulated for adult maintenance contain adequate amounts of protein, fat, vitamins, and minerals to meet the needs of an animal at normal weight who is consuming adequate calories. If the volume of a maintenance diet is reduced too drastically in an effort to limit calories, nutrient deficiencies may develop. Commercially prepared foods with reduced energy densities are formulated to contain adequate levels of nutrients while supplying less calories. Therefore, in cases of moderate to severe obesity or when owners are not strongly motivated to change their habits, a change of diet to a commercially prepared diet with a reduced energy density is recommended for weight reduction.

Several commercial pet foods that meet total nutrient requirements have been formulated to provide fewer calories than most adult maintenance foods. These reduced-calorie diets are divided into two distinct types: those that are low in fat and high in digestible, complex carbohydrate, and those that are high in indigestible fiber. Some high-fiber reducing diets also have a reduced level of fat, while others contain amounts of fat that are similar to or greater than those found in maintenance diets (Tables 26-3 and 26-4).

The reduction of dietary fat in diets for weight loss is effective for several reasons. Fat increases both the caloric density and the palatability of pet foods, and it promotes increased metabolic efficiency of body fat deposition.[32,87] On a weight basis, fat provides more than twice the calories of carbohydrate or protein. Therefore, decreasing the fat content of a pet food decreases caloric density and may slightly decrease palatability. In addition, carbohydrate and protein are potent stimulants for the secretion of insulin, while dietary fat is much less important as an insulin secretagogue. Because increased circulating insulin enhances the utilization of energy and metabolic rate, a diet that is high in carbohydrate and low in fat promotes energy utilization and metabolic rate.[88]

Commercial, low-fat diets contain between 8% and 11% fat on a dry-matter basis (DMB). This percentage is equivalent to 18% to 26% of the calories in a diet with

TABLE **26-3**

Low-Fat/High-Fiber vs. Low-Fat/High-Carbohydrate Reducing Diets

	Fat (%)	Crude Fiber (%)	Energy Density (kcal/cup)	ME Energy (% of Gross Energy)	Fecal Score (1-5)*	Fecal Volume (g/day)
Diet A	7.0	14.2	250	67.3	3.9	162.4
Diet B	9.7	3.0	270	87.8	4.5	46.5

*Fecal Score: 1 = Watery, diarrhea; 5 = Firm, compact.

Data provided by Iams Technical Center, Lewisburg, Ohio, 1993.

TABLE **26-4**

Nutrient Compositions of Several Reduced-Calorie Dog Foods

Food	Carbohydrate*	Fat*	Protein*	Fiber†	ME (kcal/kg)	Comments
A	57	21	22	14.0	2800	↑↑Fiber, ↓Fat
B	70	14	16	10.0	3000	↑Fiber, ↓↓Fat, ↓Protein
C	66	13	21	4.0	3300	↓↓Fat
D	62	21	17	10.0	3300	↑↑Fiber, ↓Fat, ↓Protein
E	36	37	27	4.0	3400	↔Fat, ↓CHO
F	66	20	14	5.5	3500	↑Fiber, ↓Fat, ↓Protein
G	48	30	22	3.5	3500	↓Fat
H	57	23	20	2.0	3800	↓Fat, ↓Fiber

*Percentage of ME kcal.

†Percentage by weight.

an energy density of 3500 kcal/kg. The decreased proportion of fat is low enough to reduce the caloric density of the food but high enough to still provide adequate palatability and the required amounts of essential fatty acids. Most pet foods that are marketed for weight reduction or for sedentary pets have decreased levels of fat. However, significant differences occur in the amounts of indigestible fiber, digestible carbohydrate, and protein that these foods provide (see Table 26-4).

Adult maintenance diets for pets with normal activity levels contain between 30% and 50% of their calories from digestible carbohydrate. Diets that are formulated for the weight maintenance of inactive dogs or for weight reduction for overweight dogs contain levels that are greater than 50%. High-quality, digestible carbohydrate provides an excellent source of energy in low-fat pet foods and has less than half of the caloric density of fat. Increasing the proportion of carbohydrate in the diet has the added advantage of inducing a higher dietary thermogenic response.[88,89,90] In other words, a high proportion of dietary carbohydrate contributes to higher energy expenditure by increasing the amount of heat loss as a result of meal ingestion. Pet foods that replace fat with complex carbohydrate without adding additional fiber retain the level of digestibility of the higher-fat products, but they contain less total calories (see Table 26-3 and Figure 26-1). Corn and rice are both excellent sources of digestible carbohydrate for pet foods. An added advantage to a low-fat diet that is high in complex carbohydrates is that, unlike reducing diets that are high in dietary fiber, it does not result in increased fecal volume or defecation frequency (see Table 26-3, diet B).

Recent studies have evaluated the efficacy of feeding low-fat, low-fiber diets to overweight and obese cats for the purpose of weight reduction.[91,92] When pet cats who were up to 40% overweight were fed a low-fiber, moderate-fat, reducing diet to provide 60% of their calculated MER, all the cats lost significant amounts of weight, and more than half reached 90% of ideal body weight within 18 weeks.[91] Cats that were greater than 30% above their ideal body weight at the start of the study took longer than 4 months to achieve targets weights, but they still lost weight consistently throughout the study. In a subsequent study, a group of obese cats were fed a low-fat, low-fiber diet restricted to intakes that were calculated to achieve 1.5% body weight loss for a 16-week period.[92] The diet contained 9.2% fat, 1.9% fiber and 33.5% high-quality protein. Fat contributed 23% of the ME calories in the diet. Cats lost an average of 21% of their body weight and 49% of their body fat. DEXA body composition analysis showed that lean body mass decreased only slightly, leading to a mean final body condition that was lower in fat and higher in lean tissue. Ultrasound-guided liver biopsies were obtained at the start and periodically throughout the study to monitor the effect of caloric restriction upon the development of hepatic lipidosis. Liver histology showed no lipid infiltration, indicating that the weight loss program did not present a risk for the development of hepatic lipidosis. Results of these studies indicate that a low-fiber, low-calorie diet for cats can effectively and safely result in weight losses in overweight pets.

An alternate way that the caloric density of a diet can be decreased is by diluting calories through the addition of indigestible fiber (see Table 26-3, diet A, and Table 26-4). Several commercial reducing diets are marketed that contain low levels of fat and unusually high amounts of dietary fiber. The rationale behind these products is that the increased bulk and decreased digestibility of the diet will contribute to satiety and cause a decrease in voluntary energy consumption and assimilation. The use of fiber has its origins in human weight reduction programs. However, there are conflicting data regarding the effects of fiber on food consumption in both human subjects and companion animals. Although certain types of dietary fiber may increase feelings of satiety in humans on a per-meal basis, most subjects (if allowed) will spontaneously overconsume high-fiber diets to meet their energy needs.[93,94,95] Moreover, long-term studies indicating the clinical benefits of dietary fiber in weight loss programs for human subjects are lacking.[96,97]

There are also variable and inconsistent results with companion animals. Studies with dogs and cats have examined the effects on short-term satiety of feeding high-fiber diets, measured through intake of a challenge meal.[97,98,99,100] This procedure involves providing test animals with a high-fiber diet that is periodically followed by the offer of an additional meal later in the day. The premise is that if satiety is induced by increased fiber, dogs will consume less of the challenge meal, compared with dogs who are fed a normal maintenance diet. Although variable results are reported, in most cases feeding pets a high-fiber diet did not significantly affect the volume of food that was ingested from a challenge meal offered later in the day. Interpretation of the results are often confounded by factors such as the amount of food fed prior to the challenge meal, the time that the animals are allowed access to food, and the interval after the last feeding. In a recent study, dogs fed a diet containing 10% crude fiber, 2.7% soluble fiber, and reduced fat consumed fewer total calories per day.[99] However, this difference was due to a dilution effect of the daily diet that was fed on a portion-controlled basis, not to reduced consumption of the challenge meal. When offered the challenge meal, dogs fed the high-fiber diet consumed the same volume of food as control dogs who were not fed the high-fiber, low-fat diet. As a result, when total calories consumed were calculated, the dogs fed the high-fiber, low-fat diet consumed fewer calories, principally because the energy density of the diet that was fed was significantly lower. The differences were due to portion-controlled feeding of a diluted diet, and it is questionable whether any significant effect upon satiety was induced. Other researchers have investigated whether the type of fiber that is fed is important.[97,98] When diets containing either soluble or insoluble fiber were fed to dogs, neither type of fiber significantly affected satiety in energy-restricted dogs. Although satiety remains a difficult phenomenon to measure and assess in companion animals, it appears that preoccupation with high-fiber diets for the treatment of obesity is not warranted or supported by current scientific evidence.

Optimal levels of dietary fiber are necessary in the diets of all pets, regardless of weight. Fiber is needed for proper functioning of the gastrointestinal tract and as a source of short-chain fatty acids (SCFAs) for intestinal cells. However, the weight-reducing effect of high levels of indigestible fiber in the diet is highly questionable, and excessive fiber intake can produce a number of adverse side effects. High intakes of dietary fiber cause decreases in nutrient digestion and availability through interference with absorption of lipids, calcium, zinc, and iron, and increased losses of fecal energy and nitrogen.[101,102,103,104,105] If a diet is simultaneously high in indigestible fiber and low in fat or other nutrients, it is possible that long-term feeding may result in nutrient deficiencies. Feeding restricted amounts for the purpose of weight loss increases this risk.

Increasing nonfermentable (insoluble) fiber also affects fecal production and defecation frequency. Results of studies with dogs have shown that providing more than 10% of dietary dry matter (DM) as fiber causes increased fecal production.[106] Fecal quality is also affected by the type of fiber that is used.[107,108] When high amounts of nonfermentable fiber are included in the diet, feces are dry and hard, which may lead to constipation. In contrast, if too much fermentable fiber is fed, this can lead to loose, watery stools and even diarrhea. Excess fiber consumption also causes increased gas production and defecation frequency. Although not usually a health risk, these latter side effects are certainly disagreeable to most pet owners (see Table 26-3).[109] In addition, some high-fiber diets appear to have reduced palatability, especially for cats.[110] This may induce further reductions in intake, leading to nutrient deficiencies or weight loss that is too rapid.

Like any reduced-calorie diet, high-fiber pet foods may be effective for weight control if portions are strictly controlled. However, the undesirable side effects of high-fiber, low-fat diets and their potential to decrease the availability of essential nutrients make them a poor choice for long-term caloric restriction. On the other hand, a weight loss diet that contains a reduced level of fat and a high proportion of digestible carbohydrate achieves the desired reduction in caloric density without sacrificing diet digestibility or nutrient availability (see Table 26-3, diet B).

Protein Content of Weight Loss Diets The significantly reduced protein content of some low-calorie, high-fiber pet foods may be of concern (see Table 26-4, foods B, D, and F). Research in humans has shown that fecal nitrogen increases with increasing levels of dietary fiber.[102,104] Fractionization studies indicate that the increased nitrogen is largely associated with bacterial mass, either as bacterial products, mucosal cell debris, or unabsorbed intestinal secretions. Another source of the increased fecal nitrogen may be unavailable protein complexes present within the fiber itself. The cooking and processing of high-fiber foods can result in the formation of Maillard products, polymerization products of certain carbohydrates and amino acids that become unavailable for absorption.

Research conducted with dogs and cats has shown that some types of fiber also significantly decrease apparent nitrogen digestibility in these species.[103,109] In one study, as levels of the soluble fiber carrageenan were increased in the diet from 0% to 20%, apparent crude protein digestibility decreased from 89.3% to 77.3% in dogs and from 85.6% to 77.2% in cats.[103] On the other hand, increasing the level of dietary cellulose did not affect protein digestibility in either group of animals. Additional data have shown that purified cellulose has a slightly negative effect on protein digestibility in adult dogs. When increasing levels of cellulose were added to a complete and balanced diet, no significant differences in protein digestibility occurred between individual diets, but there was a significant linear relationship between increasing dietary cellulose and apparent nitrogen digestibility.[109] Because certain types of dietary fiber may interfere with protein metabolism in dogs and cats, diets that contain increased levels of indigestible fiber and reduced levels of protein are not recommended for weight loss.

As discussed previously, a major goal of a weight loss program for pets is to minimize the loss of lean body tissue while supporting the loss of body fat. In general, higher rates of weight loss result in greater losses of lean body tissue. Limiting dietary protein can further exacerbate losses of lean body tissue. Dietary protein during weight loss is an especially important consideration in cats because cats have higher activities of protein-catabolizing enzymes in the liver and are unable to reduce the activities of these enzymes in the face of a reduction in dietary protein intake.[111,112] Moreover, compromised protein intake during weight loss or periods of anorexia has been identified as a possible factor in the development of feline idiopathic hepatic lipidosis.[113,114] Recent studies have shown that when caloric intake is calculated to provide a weight loss of between 1.5% and 3% per week, a protein intake of between 3.0 and 4.5 g/kg body weight per day is sufficient to prevent the development of hepatic lipidosis and to maintain greater than 85% of lean body mass in cats.[83,92,115] For example, when a low-fiber, low-fat diet containing 33.5% high-quality protein was fed at 60% of maintenance, cats safely lost weight and maintained a normal proportion of lean body tissue.[92] Dog foods formulated for weight loss can contain slightly lower levels of protein. A protein content of between 20% and 26% is recommended, provided the protein source is of high quality and is highly digestible.

Feeding Regimen   When any type of reduced-calorie food is used for weight loss in dogs and cats, strict portion-controlled feeding should always be used. Most dogs and cats, given the opportunity, merely increase the volume of food that they eat in an effort to keep energy intake the same. The advantage of feeding a reducing diet is that fewer calories can be consumed in a larger volume of food and there is less risk of causing a nutrient imbalance during restricted feeding of the diet. For example, if a reducing pet food that contains 300 kcal/cup is fed, the dog used in the previous example would receive 2½ cups of food a day rather than 2 cups (see Box 26-2). This larger volume of food may result in a greater feeling of satiety and less tendency to beg or steal food. Moreover, these pet foods are specifically formulated by pet food manufacturers to provide balanced nutrition while lowering the amount of calories being consumed.

Total Fasting as a Treatment for Weight Loss

Total fasting or starvation is another type of caloric restriction that can be used for weight reduction in dogs. However, fasting can have both immediate and long-term negative consequences. These consequences include excessive losses of lean body tissue, decreased intestinal mass surface and activity, and the potential for an increased proportion of body fat if weight is regained in the long term.[13] Because owners and veterinarians are capable of exerting total control over a pet's daily caloric intake, there are very few situations in which fasting as a cure for obesity is warranted. In addition, it is important to recognize that unlike dogs, cats are incapable of tolerating starvation. Fasting obese cats results in excessive losses of lean body tissue and increased hepatic fat deposition, which may lead to hepatic lipidosis (see Section 6, pp. 473-474). Therefore this type of dietary restriction should never be used with obese cats and only in extreme cases with obese dogs.

Metabolic changes that occur during fasting are adaptive processes that shift the brain's substrate use from primarily glucose to ketones.[116] In humans these metabolic shifts are accompanied by the development of ketosis, metabolic acidosis, accelerated urinary excretion of ammonia, and hyperuricemia.[117,118] These changes are responsible for many of the adverse side effects and health complications that accompany total fasting in human subjects. However, dogs do not develop ketosis, increase urinary ammonia excretion, or show a change in uric acid metabolism during prolonged starvation.[119] A study with adult dogs reported that blood ketone concentrations in fasted animals were less than 0.5 millimole (mmol)/liter (L) following a total fast of 2 weeks. In contrast, blood ketone levels in fasted human subjects increase from 5 to 8 mmol/L within only 1 week.[120,121] Liver function tests also remained normal in dogs during prolonged fasting.[120] The ability of the dog to greatly increase gluconeogenesis from glycerol and consequently maintain normoglycemia may be responsible for the dog's ability to adapt very quickly and efficiently to starvation and to develop fewer adverse side effects.

Fasting as a treatment should only be considered when the degree of obesity poses a significant health risk to the dog and the owner is poorly motivated to institute any type of caloric restriction. Hospitalization is required and may continue for as long as 6 to 8 weeks, depending on the severity of the pet's condition. During the fast, daily vitamin and/or mineral supplements should be provided to prevent nutrient deficiencies, and water should always be available. When the desired body weight has been attained, refeeding to a maintenance level can be introduced slowly over a period of several days. Follow-up veterinary visits should be scheduled so that weight maintenance can be monitored and, if necessary, the pet's daily ration readjusted.

There are several disadvantages to the use of fasting as a weight loss method, and these should always be considered before its implementation. Many pet owners are opposed to the use of starvation because they feel that it is inhumane. Others may not want to incur the cost of hospitalization. The effect that starvation has on body composition is also an important consideration. Although dogs can metabolically tolerate fasting, they still lose a greater proportion of lean body tissue when starvation is used for weight reduction as compared with the use of moderate caloric restriction.[121,122] A study with obese human subjects found that protein loss was two-fold to five-fold greater in fasted subjects than in subjects who were fed a restricted calorie diet for weight loss.[123] This loss of lean body tissue is not selective. Unrestricted expenditure of lean tissue for energy can result in tissue damage, particularly to the heart muscle.[13,124] In addition to this health risk, the loss of excessive amounts of lean body tissue during starvation may also predispose the dog to later weight regain. Physiological pressure to regain lean body mass can stimulate increased hunger and food intake, leading to the repletion of fat stores along with lean tissue stores.[122] Because the owner is not directly involved in the weight loss process, obesity recurrence is more likely after a program of starvation than if a more conservative, in-home treatment was used. As stated previously, fasting as a treatment for obesity is not recommended in the majority of cases and should only be used as a "last resort" measure.

MAINTAINING A REDUCED STATE AFTER WEIGHT LOSS

The dietary and exercise habits established during the treatment of obesity must be maintained for dogs and cats even after caloric restriction for weight loss has ended. The pet should be fed a well-balanced, complete food designed for adult maintenance and should continue with the level of daily exercise that was included in the weight loss program. Pet owners should avoid reverting to old habits such as feeding table scraps, providing a large number of treats, or allowing begging behaviors. Some pets can be fed a normal adult maintenance pet food once they have reached ideal body weight. However, others easily gain weight when fed these foods. A low-fat diet that is high in complex carbohydrates containing less calories but adequate nutrients for adult maintenance is suggested for weight maintenance in these pets. In all cases, portion-controlled feeding twice daily is the feeding schedule that should be used.

PREVENTION

Although a variety of different factors may contribute to the development of obesity, the two most important causes are overfeeding and underexercising. Obesity in pets can be successfully treated. However, the ideal situation is to prevent its occurrence in the first place. Veterinarians, veterinary staff, and breeders can have a large influence on the prevention of obesity in dogs and cats. Opportunities to advise clients and pet buyers regarding appropriate feeding management for new puppies and kittens occur during routine visits and when owners are first deciding upon a particular pet.

In human subjects, hyperplastic obesity, signified by the presence of an abnormally high number of adipose cells, is difficult to treat and has a poor long-term prognosis. The development of hyperplastic obesity usually takes place during growth and often leads to obesity in adult life. Although hyperplastic obesity has not been extensively studied in dogs and cats, it is assumed that the prognosis is similar to that in other species. It is possible that overnutrition in a young dog or cat sets the stage for a lifelong battle with obesity. It is imperative that adequate nutrients and calories for optimal growth be provided to young dogs and cats. However, feeding excess amounts of a calorically dense food may stimulate adipocyte hyperplasia and lead to an abnormally high rate of growth and weight gain. Growing pets should be fed an amount of food that promotes a normal growth rate and a lean body condition. Some pets are able to self-feed and will not overeat. However, many young dogs and cats overeat as a result of boredom, competition with other animals, or the availability of a highly palatable food. In the majority of cases, portion-controlled feeding should be used, and the pet's weight and rate of gain should be strictly monitored. Daily exercise should be started when pets are young, and it should be continued throughout life.

During adulthood, portion-controlled feeding, regular exercise, and avoidance of the development of bad habits are the conditions necessary to prevent obesity. As pets age, their energy requirements naturally decrease. Exercise tolerance also decreases as pets get older, and these changes may predispose older pets to weight gain. Maintaining moderate levels of exercise and possibly changing the pet's diet to a ration that is low in energy density can help to prevent obesity in later years (Box 26-3).

BOX 26-3

Practical Feeding Tips: Management of Obesity in Dogs and Cats

Develop a program that will produce a target weight loss of 1% to 2% of total body weight per week.

Select an appropriate diet for weight loss.

Restrict caloric intake to 60% to 70% of ME for current body weight.

Eliminate all table scraps and treats. Change feeding habits that contribute to overeating and obesity.

Include a program of moderate, daily exercise.

After desired weight loss has been achieved, adjust intake to maintain ideal body weight.

Prevent weight regain by continuing regular exercise and strictly monitoring caloric intake.

C H A P T E R

27

Overnutrition and
Supplementation

EFFECTS OF OVERNUTRITION DURING GROWTH

Improper feeding practices during growth are associated with several developmental skeletal disorders in dogs. It has been reported that almost one fourth of dogs visiting veterinary practices are diagnosed with musculoskeletal disorders.[125] The incidence in dogs that are less than 1 year of age is about 22%, and more than 90% of these cases are thought to be influenced by nutritional factors.[126] Specifically, free-choice feeding of diets that are nutrient- and energy-dense or supplementation with certain nutrients during growth are important factors in the etiology of these disorders. Skeletal diseases are most prevalent in the large and giant breeds, and their onset is usually associated with periods of rapid growth (Figure 27-1). The most common of these disorders are canine hip dysplasia (CHD), osteochondrosis, and hypertrophic osteodystrophy (HOD) (also called metaphyseal osteopathy).

Developmental Skeletal Disorders

CHD is a biomechanical disease of the coxofemoral joint, characterized by incongruity between surfaces of the head of the femur and the acetabulum. The degree of subluxation and joint laxity determines the severity of the disease, and affected dogs range from being asymptomatic throughout life to being severely crippled at a young age. Over time, the subluxation causes remodeling of the joint, typified by shallowing of the acetabulum, flattening of the femoral head, and development of osteoarthritis.

CHD is the most frequently encountered orthopedic disease in veterinary medicine.[127] It is generally accepted that its etiology is multifactorial, involving a strong genetic component and a number of potential environmental factors.[128,129] Of these, diet and growth rate are believed to be important. Specifically, growth during the

FIGURE **27-1**

Representative growth curves of several dog breeds.

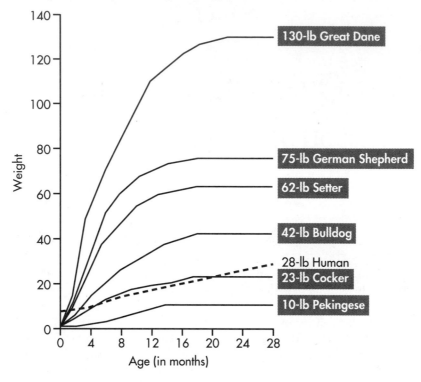

(Adapted from *Current Veterinary Therapy V*, Philadelphia, 1974, WB Saunders.)

period from 3 months to 8 months of age is critical in the development of CHD. Early studies have shown that dogs with excessive weight gain during this period have a higher frequency and more severe degenerative changes than dogs that grew at rates equal to or below the breed standard.[130]

Osteochondrosis is characterized by a focal disruption in endochondral ossification, which causes impaired maturation of cartilage. It can occur in both the physis and epiphysis of growth cartilage and at multiple points throughout the skeleton. In growing dogs, osteochondrosis of the articular epiphyseal cartilage most commonly occurs in the shoulder, stifle, hock, and elbow. Subsequent to the development of osteochondrosis, acute inflammatory joint disease or degenerative joint disease develops when the cartilage joint surface is disrupted. A common manifestation of osteochondrosis is osteochondritis dissecans (OCD). This occurs when a segment of articular (joint) cartilage is separated from the underlying bone and subchondral bone is exposed to synovial fluid. As with CHD, the etiology of osteochondrosis appears to be multifactorial. Identified risk factors include age, gender, breed, rapid growth rate and excessive weight gain, and nutrient excesses (particularly of calcium).[131,132] Breeds that demonstrate the highest incidence of this disorder include Great Danes, Labrador Retrievers, Newfoundlands, and Rottweilers.[131]

HOD occurs primarily in the large and giant breeds of dogs and is characterized by excessive bone deposition and retarded bone resorption. The distal ulna, radius, and tibia are most commonly affected. Radiographically, an irregular, translucent zone initially appears in the metaphysis and is separated from the growth plate by an excessively dense band of bone. As the disease progresses, additional bone is deposited outside of the periosteum, and soft-tissue swelling and subperiosteal hemorrhages develop around affected metaphyseal areas. The dog exhibits acute pain and swelling, lameness, intermittent pyrexia, and occasional anorexia. The observed swelling is due to both fibrous thickening of the periosteum and the deposition of new periosteal bone. HOD primarily affects dogs that are growing rapidly, and the initial signs are typically seen when dogs are between 3 months and 6 months of age.

Most forms of developmental skeletal disease are influenced by genetics, but heredity cannot fully explain their occurrence. For example, a heritability coefficient of 40% has been suggested for CHD.[133,134] This means that approximately 60% of the influencing factors are environmental in nature. Although it is difficult to identify all of the environmental components involved in these disorders, research studies have indicated that nutrition plays an important role. A number of nutrients have been examined, including energy, protein, vitamin C, fat, carbohydrate, and calcium. The data indicate that the two most important nutritional factors in the development of skeletal disease in dogs are excess caloric intake during growth and a high calcium intake.

ENERGY INTAKE AND GROWTH RATE

Excess energy intake during growth commonly occurs as a result of feeding a high-quality, growth diet to a young dog on a free-choice basis or feeding excess amounts of food on a portion-controlled basis. Some owners believe that puppies should be kept "plump" in appearance, and that a rotund puppy is a healthy puppy. However, when puppies are fed excessive amounts of a balanced diet, growth rate is maximized before excess weight in the form of fat is gained. As a result, a growing dog that appears to be slightly overweight is usually growing at a maximal rate. Studies with dogs, humans, and other species have shown that the consumption of excess calories resulting in a maximal or an above-average growth rate is not compatible with optimal skeletal development.[135,136,137,138]

An extensive study conducted with growing Great Danes found that generalized overnutrition contributed to the development of orthopedic problems in this breed.[137] Two groups of growing puppies were fed a highly palatable, energy-dense food throughout growth. The first group was fed free-choice, and the second group was fed amounts of food that were restricted to two thirds of the intake of the first group. The dogs that were fed free-choice grew significantly faster than did the dogs fed restricted amounts of food.

Moreover, bone tissue was significantly affected by the rapid growth rate. A variety of skeletal abnormalities were observed in the dogs that were fed free-choice, including enlargement of the costochondral junctions and the epiphyseal-metaphyseal regions of long bones, hyperextension of the carpus, and sinking of the metacarpophalangeal and metatarsophalangeal joints. The affected dogs exhibited varying degrees of lameness and pain when palpated. It was concluded that generalized overnutrition, in the form of excess energy, protein, calcium, and phosphorus, caused an increased growth rate in these dogs that contributed to abnormal skeletal development.

Additional work has been conducted with growing dogs of several other large breeds, including German Shepherds, Golden Retrievers, and Labrador Retrievers. In one study, a group of puppies that had high parental frequencies of hip dysplasia were examined. The incidence and severity of dysplasia was greater in puppies that had rapid growth rates as a result of increased caloric intake, as compared with those that were fed restricted amounts of food.[130] Similarly, when a group of puppies was hand-reared at a reduced rate of growth, they developed a very low incidence of hip dysplasia. In contrast, a control group that was fed to allow a much higher growth rate showed a very high incidence of hip dysplasia.[139,140]

A recent, well-controlled study with a group of 48 Labrador Retrievers reported that growing dogs that were fed 25% less food than dogs who were fed free-choice had significantly less hip joint laxity at 30 weeks of age and a lower incidence of hip dysplasia at 2 years of age.[141] The dogs in the study were fed a balanced diet that was formulated for growth, and radiographic criteria established by the Orthopedic Foundation of America (OFA) were used to evaluate the dogs' hips. Of the dogs in the free-choice group, 16 of 24 developed CHD, compared with 7 of the 24 dogs in the limited-feeding group.[138] The dogs were kept on their respective dietary regimens until they were 5 years of age and were regularly examined radiographically for the presence of osteoarthritis.[141] Osteoarthritis was observed in the hips of 7 of the 24 free-choice dogs by the time they were 1 year old, while none of the limited-feeding dogs showed osteoarthritis at 1 year. The effects of the feeding regimen remained statistically significant throughout the remainder of the 5-year study. When the dogs were 5 years old, 12 of the 23 remaining free-choice dogs (52%) and only 3 of the 23 limited-feeding dogs (13%) had radiographic signs of osteoarthritis. Moreover, the degree of osteoarthritis was more severe in free-choice dogs than in the restricted-feeding dogs. A significant and positive correlation was also found between body weight at 5 years of age and the presence of osteoarthritis in the hip joints.

The skeletal system of dogs is most susceptible to physical and metabolic stressors during the first 12 months of life. It is theorized that abnormal skeletal development during periods of rapid growth results from overloading the growing skeleton with prematurely increased muscle mass and body weight.[142] This theory is supported by the fact that rapidly growing male dogs of the large and giant breeds are more frequently affected than are smaller females. There also appears to be a correlation between increasing body size and the occurrence of the lesions associated with osteochondrosis.[141,142] A comparison between the bones of large and small breeds of dogs during periods of rapid growth shows that the bones of large breeds are relatively less dense than are the bones of small breeds at similar stages of development. Bones of large breeds have a thinner cortex, larger medullary cavity, and a less dense spongiosa.[143,144] It is thus possible that the bones of large dogs during growth are not as strong as those of smaller dogs during the same period. This may be the basis for the genetic predispositions toward skeletal abnormalities in the large and giant breeds. Recent evidence suggests that mechanical stress on the joints caused by excessive weight throughout growth and into maturity also contributes to the development of osteoarthritis.[142]

Overnutrition also has direct effects that negatively affect skeletal development. Studies with Great Danes have shown that overnutrition stimulates accelerated skeletal growth.[143] Great Dane puppies were fed a diet formulated for growth from weaning to 6 months of age. Puppies in one group were fed free-choice (ad libitum) and puppies in the second group were restricted to 70% to 80% of the amount consumed by the first group. As in previous studies, dogs fed ad libitum weighed significantly more than the restricted group at 6 months of age. Bone measurement data showed that accelerated skeletal growth, in the form of increased size and volume of bone, contributed significantly to the increased weight. The male dogs that experienced overnutrition also showed an increased rate of bone remodeling, resulting in enlarged bones with relatively low densities and low resistance to the greater weight they were required to bear. It appears that if a large dog is allowed to attain its maximal growth rate by consuming excess amounts of a balanced diet, the accelerated growth rate creates a rapidly growing skeleton that is less strong and less able to withstand the biomechanical stresses of the greater muscle mass and body weight that are put on it. Not only do these dogs weigh more, but their bones are less able to handle the added weight. The end result is the development of aberrations in ossification, damage to developing cartilage and growth plates, and premature closure of growth plates. Most often this manifests as osteochondrosis, but these changes may also be involved in the onset of several other developmental skeletal diseases.

Feeding for Optimal Growth Rate

The final skeletal height of a dog is strongly influenced by genetics. Providing adequate, but not excessive, amounts of a balanced diet enables an animal to achieve its potential size but at a slower rate than if excess food is provided.[145] Feeding an energy-dense, nutrient-balanced food at a level that promotes a high rate of growth decreases the time it takes the dog to attain adult size and can contribute to abnormal skeletal development. However, feeding restricted amounts of a balanced food to achieve a slower growth rate results in an animal of the same size, but at a later point in time. Allowing the skeleton to develop slowly eliminates the biomechanical stresses of excess weight and the changes in bone development associated with rapid growth.

The best way to attain a moderate growth rate is to strictly monitor body weight during growth and to feed to attain a lean body condition (see Figure 26-2, p. 315, and Box 27-1). The chief contributor to rapid growth and weight gain is dietary energy. Because fat is much more energy-dense than protein or carbohydrate, high-fat diets contribute significantly to excess energy intake. In recent years, several commercial foods have been specifically formulated for large-breed puppies. These foods are generally lower in energy density than many puppy foods, include highly available nutrients, and contain a moderate level of calcium (see pp. 339-343). A general recommendation is to select a food that has a moderately reduced energy content (between 3.8 and 4.2 kilocalories [kcal]/gram [g] of dry food) and between 14% and 17% fat (34% to 38% of calories as fat).[126,146] Calcium levels should be between 0.8% and 1.5%. Although dietary protein was once identified as a potential contributor to skeletal abnormalities, studies have shown that varying levels of dietary protein between 12% and 30% does not influence the occurrence or severity of osteochondrosis.[147] A dog food formulated for growing large-breed dogs should contain a minimum of 22% high-quality protein, with an optimum level of between 26% and 28% (23% to 26% of calories).[126,147,148]

Large- and giant-breed dogs should always be fed on a portion-controlled basis during growth. Free-choice feeding is not recommended because it increases the risk of spontaneous overconsumption and is not conducive to monitoring daily intake. In addition, ad libitum feeding appears to affect several hormonal regulatory systems of growth.[126,149] Circulating levels of insulin-like growth factor-1, thyroxine (T_4), and triiodothyronine (T_3) were found to be higher in growing dogs that were fed ad libitum when compared with levels in dogs that were fed on a portion-controlled basis. It is theorized that ad libitum feeding promotes enhanced metabolic processes that could positively influence growth rate. Portion-controlled feeding allows the owner to feed an amount of food that maintains optimum growth rate and body condition and adjust the dog's intake as energy needs change during growth.

The amount to feed can be estimated from guidelines provided on the food's package and then adjusted to attain ideal body condition (see Figure 26-2, p. 315). Because growing large- and giant-breed dogs have very steep growth curves, their

BOX **27-1**

Practical Feeding Tips: Feeding Growing Dogs to Decrease the Risk of Developmental Skeletal Disease

Select a complete and balanced dog food that has been formulated for growth in large and giant breeds.

Feed this food throughout the first 1 to 2 years of life.

Use a portion-controlled feeding regimen and carefully measure the amount of food that is fed each day.

Provide an amount of food that will support an average rate of growth for a dog's breed.

Provide an amount of food that will maintain a lean body condition throughout growth.

Strictly monitor weight gain and body condition until the dog reaches maturity.

Do not supplement the diet with minerals, vitamins, or additional foods.

intake requirements can change dramatically over short periods of time. Therefore, puppies should be weighed and evaluated at least once every 2 weeks. Young puppies should be fed three to four meals per day until they are 4 months old and two meals per day thereafter. A well-formulated growth diet should be fed throughout growth. For large and giant breeds, this corresponds to the first 16 to 24 months of life, depending upon the dog's breed and adult size.

CALCIUM SUPPLEMENTATION

Supplementing a pet's diet during growth and other periods of physiological stress is a common but risky practice. Calcium is a nutrient that is often added to the diets of dogs and, less commonly, to the diets of cats. The reason most often cited for calcium supplementation relates to its essential role in normal skeletal growth and development. Supplements such as dicalcium phosphate and bone meal are added to a growing dog's diet during growth spurts or when problems such as hyperextension of the carpus or sinking of the metacarpophalangeal joints occur. Professional breeders may encourage all of their puppy buyers to routinely supplement the pet's diet with calcium during the entire first year of life as a prophylactic measure. Some breeders believe that calcium supplementation is not only necessary for proper bone development but that it also prevents the development of certain skeletal disorders. In addition, dogs' diets are occasionally supplemented with minerals during gestation and lactation. Supplemental calcium and phosphorus are believed by some to ensure healthy fetal development during pregnancy, aid in milk production during lactation, and prevent the onset of eclampsia after parturition. Regardless of the good intentions, there are potential risks when excessively high levels of calcium are either included in the diet itself or added to an adequate and balanced diet. Excess dietary calcium can produce deficiencies in other nutrients and has the potential for causing several serious health disorders in dogs.

Supplementation during Growth

Research has shown that normal growth in puppies can be supported by a calcium intake of 0.37% available calcium or 0.6% total calcium.[148] The Association of American Feed Control Officials' (AAFCO's) *Nutrient Profiles* for dog foods sets minimum levels for calcium of 0.8% for growth and reproduction and 0.5% for adult maintenance. The profile also mandates a maximum level of 2.5% calcium in all dog foods. This maximum level was included because published data have indicated that excess calcium during growth may contribute to abnormal skeletal development.[150,151] Studies indicate that a high level of calcium in the diet is associated with the occurrence of osteochondrosis, enlarged joints, dropped hocks, splayed feet, angular limb deformities, Wobbler's syndrome, and stunted growth.[137,150,151]

In 1985 studies were undertaken with the purpose of determining the effect of varying levels of dietary calcium upon the occurrence of developmental skeletal disease in growing Great Danes.[150,152] An experimental diet was formulated that met the recommendations of the 1974 National Research Council's (NRC's) *Nutrient Requirements for Dogs*. Both the control group and the experimental group of dogs received this diet throughout growth. In addition, the experimental group received calcium carbonate supplementation to achieve a level of 3.3% in the diet, which is three times the amount recommended by the NRC.[153,154] Results showed that excessive calcium intake resulted in chronic hypercalcemia and hypophosphatemia. Skeletal differences between the control and experimental dogs included a higher percentage of total bone volume, retarded bone maturation, retarded bone remodeling, and a decreased number of osteoclasts (bone resorption cells) in the dogs receiving calcium supplementation. This group also showed a higher incidence and severity of the cartilage irregularities associated with osteochondrosis at the distal and proximal humeral cartilages. Clinically, calcium-supplemented dogs exhibited retained cartilage cones, severe lateral deviation of the feet, and the radius curvus syndrome previously described.[155]

The mechanism through which calcium exerts these effects relates to the homeostatic control of blood calcium and phosphorus levels. Excessive calcium intake in young dogs results in transient hypercalcemia and hypophosphatemia.[150] The hormone calcitonin is secreted in response to elevated serum calcium and lowers the plasma calcium to normal levels. Calcitonin produces its effects by decreasing bone resorption and retarding cartilage maturation in developing bone. The chronic suppression of bone resorption results in a gradual thickening and increased density of cortical bone. In growing dogs, this change interferes with normal bone remodeling. The deposition of excessive subperiosteal bone that results may cause the clinical signs of HOD and Wobbler's syndrome, and the chronic effects of calcitonin on cartilage maturation may result in the eventual detachment of the articular cartilage that is seen in OCD.[150] Because of their rapid periods of growth and their predisposition to skeletal disorders, large and giant breeds of dogs are especially susceptible to the pathological effects of excess calcium consumption. However, it is postulated that these changes also occur in smaller breeds at a subclinical level, resulting in an infrequent diagnosis of disease.[129]

The effect of excess dietary calcium and endogenous vitamin D formation on calcitonin-producing cells of the thyroid gland has also been examined.[156] Growing Beagles were given 2.3 g of supplemental calcium per day and exposed to daily sunlight. After 70 days, the thyroid glands of the supplemented dogs contained significantly increased proportions of calcitonin-producing C cells and decreased proportions of thyroid follicles, as compared with those of control dogs. The authors of the report concluded that high dietary calcium intake caused thyroid C-cell hyperplasia, which would suggest the occurrence of chronic hypercalcitoninism in these dogs. Additionally, electron microscopy of the thyroid C cells of dogs fed excess calories, protein, and calcium showed that these cells were releasing larger amounts of calcitonin than were the C cells of dogs fed restricted diets.

A complicating factor involved in calcium nutrition in dogs is that young dogs do not appear to have a mechanism that will protect them from absorbing large amounts of calcium when there are excessive concentrations in the diet. Dietary calcium is absorbed across the intestinal epithelium through either active transport or passive diffusion. The active transport mechanism is saturable, carrier-mediated, and depends on the animal's vitamin D status. The second mechanism is a nonsaturable, diffusional transfer that is directly dependent on the concentration of available calcium in the intestinal lumen. Studies of humans and laboratory animals have shown that nonsaturable passive diffusion is the predominant pathway for calcium absorption in neonates and young animals.[157] In adults, the percentage of calcium that is absorbed from the diet varies between 10% and 90%, depending on the composition of the food, the calcium content of the diet, and the physiological state of the animal.[158]

A study with growing dogs found that 45% of dietary calcium was absorbed when a normal level of calcium was fed (1.1% of the diet's dry matter [DM]).[159] The percentage of calcium absorption increased to 80% when the level of calcium was decreased to 0.55%. However, when the calcium level was increased to 3.3%, 45% of the calcium was still absorbed. As a result, calcium balance was significantly more positive in the dogs fed a high level of the mineral when compared with the balance in the dogs that were fed either normal or low concentrations. The mineral content of cortical and cancellous bone was greater in the high-calcium dogs, and there was decreased bone turnover and remodeling of the skeleton. As dogs age and reach maturity, they appear to be able to adapt to high calcium intakes by decreasing the proportion that is absorbed. Because young dogs lack this ability and also have rapidly developing and changing skeletons, they are especially susceptible to the adverse effects of high dietary calcium.

Diets containing excessively high amounts of calcium are also capable of causing a relative zinc deficiency in dogs.[160,161] High levels of calcium and other minerals, such as iron and copper, interfere with zinc absorption, possibly through competition for absorption sites or by acting as intestinal ligands.[162,163] Although adult animals can be affected, these effects have been most frequently observed in growing dogs. A controlled study found that puppies fed balanced diets containing excess supplemental calcium developed zinc deficiency within 2 to 3 months.[160] Clinical signs included impaired growth rate, anorexia, conjunctivitis, and the development of a dull, coarse hair coat. Desquamating skin lesions that are characteristic of zinc deficiency were also observed on the abdomen and extremities. Clinical cases of zinc deficiency have also been reported. Three separate litters of puppies developed zinc-responsive dermatosis when fed diets containing two to three times the NRC requirement for calcium. When supplemented with oral zinc, all puppies showed dramatic improvement within 7 to 10 days.[161]

Dietary Calcium Recommendations (Large and Giant Breeds)

Studies have shown that excess calcium consumption negatively influences skeletal development in large and giant breeds of dogs. Therefore, recommendations are needed for optimal dietary calcium concentrations for these breeds. A recent study of growing Great Danes examined the effects of three levels of dietary calcium: 0.48%, 0.8%, and 2.7%.[164] Each diet contained 26% protein and 14% fat, as well as sufficient phosphorus to provide a consistent calcium:phosphorus ratio of 1.2:1.0.

Puppies were assigned to the three diets at the age of weaning, and they were fed the experimental diets for 18 months. The experimental diets had a reduced caloric density and were formulated for large-breed puppies. After weaning and throughout the study, dogs were fed twice daily on a time-controlled regimen. Response criteria included growth rate and body conformation, bone mineral content, incidence of skeletal disease, and gait analysis.

During the first 5 months, the dogs consuming the moderate-calcium diet and the high-calcium diet grew faster than puppies consuming the low-calcium diet. After 5 months of age, the high-calcium group's growth rate declined. At the end of the study, these puppies were the leanest group with respect to body conformation. The low-calcium dogs grew more slowly, and by the end of the study they were slightly smaller in size than the dogs in the other groups.[146]

Results of dual energy x-ray absorptiometry (DEXA) measurements showed a significant positive effect of dietary calcium on bone mineral content (Table 27-1).[164] The effects of increased calcium on bone mineral content were evident in puppies as early as 2 months of age and continued to be significant until the puppies were 7 months old. After 7 months, bone mineral content gradually became similar among the three groups. By the time the pups were 12 months old, the differences were minimal, and at 14, 16 and 18 months no further effects of calcium intake upon bone mineral content were observed.

Body conformation and incidence of lameness followed a similar pattern.[165] Puppies fed the high-calcium diet had abnormal crouched posture by the time that they were 6 months old and accounted for 86% of the clinical lameness found in the study (Figure 27-2). Gait analysis studies showed that while none of the dogs fed either the low-calcium or the high-calcium diets had satisfactory gait symmetry on every examination, three of the four dogs examined in the moderate-calcium group were found to have satisfactory gait symmetry on every examination.[166]

The results of this ongoing study indicate that the mechanisms of calcium homeostasis that prevent puppies from absorbing excess amounts of calcium are not fully functional in Great Danes until they are about 7 months of age. Therefore the food that is fed to puppies from weaning and throughout growth should con-

TABLE **27-1**

Bone Mineral Content of Great Danes Fed Three Different Levels of Dietary Calcium

Age (months)	Low Calcium (g)	Moderate Calcium (g)	High Calcium (g)
2	77.55[b]	83.27[b]	110.38[a]
6	905.06[b]	1066.63[c]	1201.87[c]
12	1768.64[b]	1916.68[a,b]	2072.70[a]
14	2031.21	2069.72	2132.20

[a,b,c]Values within a row with different superscripts differ (P<0.5).

FIGURE **27-2**

*Lateral and rear view comparisons of normal and abnormal conformation in Great Danes fed moderate **(A)** and high **(B,C)** levels of calcium.*

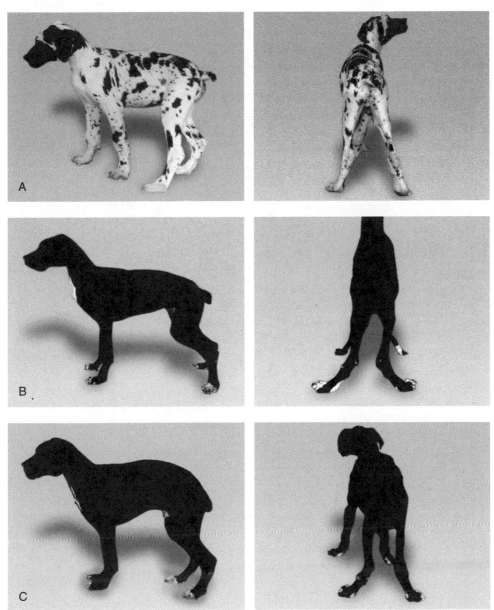

(From Goodman SA, Montgomery RD, Fitch RB, and others: Serial orthopedic examinations of growing Great Dane puppies fed three diets varying in calcium and phosphorus. In Reinhart GA, Carey DP, editors: *Recent advances in canine and feline nutrition*, vol 2, Iams Nutrition Symposium Proceedings, Wilmington, Ohio, 1998, Orange Frazer Press.)

tain adequate but not excessive calcium. A calcium level slightly lower than 1% appears to be beneficial for large-breed puppies. While 0.4% is too low, a level of 0.8% is optimal. Because changes in mineral composition in response to dietary calcium are present as early as 2 months of age and skeletal problems can be present by 5 to 6 months, the large-breed growth diet should be introduced at weaning.

Some breeders suggest feeding an adult maintenance rather than a commercial puppy food to large- and giant-breed puppies. However, because some maintenance diets are lower in energy density than growth diets, the dog must be fed a higher volume of the maintenance diet to meet its energy needs. If the calcium level in the adult diet is similar to that in the puppy food (e.g., 1.1%), then the total calcium the puppy consumes when fed the maintenance diet will actually be greater.[126,167] Likewise, if a growing dog is fed an appropriate amount of a high-quality pet food formulated for growth, supplementation with calcium is unnecessary and contraindicated. If a pet owner is feeding the pet a food that appears to contain inadequate or unavailable levels of calcium, switching the dog to a high-quality commercial diet is safer than attempting to correct the imbalance in the poor diet through supplementation.

Calcium Supplementation during Gestation and Lactation

Supplementation with calcium or any other mineral is not necessary for normal fetal development during pregnancy or for normal milk production during lactation. Although calcium needs do increase during these two physiological states, the dam's requirements are met by consuming increased amounts of a complete and balanced diet. In addition to being unnecessary for fetal bone development and milk production, supplemental calcium is also not effective in the prevention of puerperal tetany.

Puerperal tetany, or *eclampsia*, is a disease that most commonly occurs in small breeds of dogs at parturition or 2 to 3 weeks later. The disease is caused by a failure of the bitch's calcium-regulating mechanisms to maintain serum calcium levels when calcium is being lost via milk during lactation. Serum calcium decreases to less than 7 milligrams (mg)/deciliter (dl), and ataxia, muscular tetany, and convulsive seizures occur. Standard treatment is intravenous administration of calcium borogluconate.[168]

A similar hypocalcemic syndrome occurs after parturition in cows. It has been shown in this species that the consumption of a diet that is high in calcium during pregnancy actually increases the incidence of the disorder, but that a diet that is moderate to low in calcium decreases its incidence.[169,170] It is believed that a relative hypercalcemia resulting from high calcium intake during pregnancy exerts negative feedback on parathyroid hormone synthesis and secretion. This feedback decreases both the body's ability to mobilize calcium stores from bone and its ability to increase calcium absorption in the intestine. When calcium is suddenly needed for lactation, these regulatory mechanisms are unable to adapt quickly enough to the sudden calcium loss. The calcium that is available is diverted preferentially to milk production, and serum calcium decreases. Additional research concerning the effect of supplemental calcium during pregnancy on the incidence of this disorder needs to be conducted in dogs. However, it is currently recommended that if a bitch is being fed a high-quality, commercial food that has been designed for feeding through gestation and lactation, calcium supplementation is not necessary and is probably contraindicated.

ASCORBIC ACID (VITAMIN C) SUPPLEMENTATION

Companion animals do not have a requirement for dietary ascorbic acid. Like most species, dogs and cats produce endogenous ascorbic acid in the liver from either glucose or galactose. Therefore, unless there is a high metabolic need or inadequate amounts are being synthesized by the body, a dietary source of ascorbic acid is unnecessary in these species. The body requires ascorbic acid for the hydroxylation of the amino acids proline and lysine in the formation of the structural protein collagen. Collagen is the primary constituent of osteoid, dentine, and connective tissue fibers, and it is produced in quantity by osteoblasts during skeletal growth and development.

The practice of supplementing the diets of growing dogs with ascorbic acid can be traced back to a report that compared the development of HOD in young dogs with the bone abnormalities associated with scurvy (vitamin C deficiency) in humans.[171] It was theorized that an endogenous deficiency of ascorbic acid in dogs was responsible for the development of HOD. HOD occurs primarily in rapidly growing puppies of large-breed dogs. It is characterized by excessive bone deposition and retarded bone resorption and occurs most often in the distal ulna, radius, and tibia. The mandible may also be affected in some dogs.[172] Affected dogs exhibit acute pain and swelling in the metaphyseal regions of the long bones, intermittent pyrexia, and, occasionally, anorexia.[173]

Radiographic examinations of dogs with HOD and humans with scurvy both show radiotranslucent zones in affected metaphyses and eventual subperiosteal hemorrhages. Studies adding supportive evidence for a role of ascorbic acid in HOD reported decreased levels of ascorbic acid in the plasma and urine of dogs with HOD.[174,175,176] However, later evidence showed that a very crucial difference between HOD in dogs and scurvy in humans had been overlooked by the early investigations.[177] HOD is characterized by osteopetrosis, involving excess bone deposition in the metaphysis and periosteum and retarded bone resorption. Scurvy, on the other hand, is an osteoporotic condition, involving the demineralization of bone caused by impaired collagen formation by osteoblasts in the developing skeleton. This major difference provides strong evidence that the two conditions are not the same disorder.

More importantly, controlled studies of the efficacy of supplemental ascorbic acid as a therapeutic treatment for HOD have not supported the claim that low levels of dietary ascorbic acid are a causal agent for HOD in dogs.[175,178] A study with growing Labrador Retrievers found that supplementation with 500 mg of ascorbic acid/day from weaning to 4½ months of age had no effect on the development of skeletal disorders.[179] Both groups of dogs in the study were fed a highly palatable, energy-dense diet on a free-choice regimen. Dogs in both the supplemented and the nonsupplemented groups developed skeletal lesions indicative of HOD. In addition, supplemented dogs were found to have higher levels of circulating serum calcium. It was postulated that this "relative hypercalcemia" may have led to elevated calcitonin levels. As discussed previously, persistent hypercalcitoninism has the potential to contribute to the bone changes observed in many of the developmental skeletal disorders in young dogs. It was concluded that supplemental ascorbic acid has no preventive effect and may even exacerbate the development of certain skeletal lesions in growing dogs.

Like CHD and osteochondrosis, HOD is more likely to be caused by overnutrition leading to a high rate of growth than to an endogenous lack of ascorbic acid (see pp. 333-337). Alternatively, it has recently been theorized that HOD may be a vaccine-related illness or may be associated with immune compromise during certain periods of life.[178,180,181]

Although the original attention awarded to ascorbic acid status in dogs pertained specifically to HOD, this association was expanded, without scientific support, to include several other developmental bone disorders. These disorders included CHD and osteochondrosis. As a result, many breeders and professionals habitually began supplementing growing dogs' diets with ascorbic acid in the hope of preventing the onset of these diseases. However, there is no evidence to support the claim that supplemental ascorbic acid can prevent the development of either of these disorders in growing dogs.

In addition to being unwarranted, ascorbic acid supplementation in dogs and cats may be detrimental. Excess ascorbic acid is excreted in the urine as oxalate, and high concentrations of oxalate have the potential to contribute to the formation of calcium oxalate uroliths in the urinary tract. A more practical and scientifically supported route to preventing the development of skeletal diseases in dogs includes selective breeding practices, promotion of moderate growth rates in puppies, and feeding a high-quality, balanced, commercial ration that contains optimal amounts of protein, moderately reduced fat, and moderate amounts of calcium, without added supplements (see Box 27-1 and Box 27-2).

BOX **27-2**

Common Misconceptions about Feeding Large- and Giant-Breed Puppies

Vitamin and mineral supplements should be fed during growth.
Good foods to add to the puppies' food are eggs, milk, cheese, and yogurt.
Calcium carbonate is a recommended and safe calcium supplement for dogs.
Vitamin C tablets should be given daily.
Vitamin E supplementation ensures a healthy coat.
High dietary protein causes skeletal disease.
Large- and giant-breed puppies should be fed a low-protein diet (less than 15% protein)
Puppy foods should not be fed to large- and giant-breed puppies.
It is a good idea to add a tablespoon of corn oil or safflower oil to the puppies' food.
Feeding kelp granules or powder enriches a dog's natural coat color.
Adding cod liver oil to the diet is necessary during cold weather.
Daily fruits and vegetables should be provided in addition to the dog's normal diet.

C H A P T E R

28

Vitamin Deficiencies
and Excesses

 Although serious deficiencies of vitamins are highly unusual in pets today, select deficiencies and toxicities can occur as a result of improper feeding practices. Feeding excessive levels of foods that contain marginal levels of vitamin E and high amounts of polyunsaturated fatty acids (PUFAs) can lead to vitamin E deficiency in cats. Also, feeding cats foods that contain too much vitamin A can lead to toxicity. Thiamin deficiency can be induced by feeding raw fish, and biotin deficiency can be caused by feeding raw egg whites. Both raw fish and raw egg whites contain inhibitory substances. These problems are described in detail in this chapter.

VITAMIN E DEFICIENCY IN CATS: PANSTEATITIS

A condition called *pansteatitis* (yellow fat disease) occurs in cats that are fed diets containing marginal or low levels of alpha-tocopherol (vitamin E) and high amounts of unsaturated fatty acids. An animal's vitamin E requirement is directly affected by the level of unsaturated fatty acids present in the diet. As the level of PUFAs increases, the need for vitamin E also increases. For example, a diet that contains high levels of fish oil may cause a three-fold to four-fold increase in a cat's daily requirement for alpha-tocopherol.[182] If inadequate amounts of vitamin E are fed, dietary and body fat undergo oxidative degradation, leading to the formation of peroxides and hydroperoxides. The accumulation of reactive peroxides in the cat's adipose tissue results in pansteatitis, which is characterized by chronic inflammation and yellow-brown discoloration of body fat.

Clinical signs of pansteatitis in the cat include anorexia, depression, pyrexia, and hyperesthesia of the thorax and abdomen. The cat may demonstrate changes in behavior and agility and develop a poor or roughened hair coat.[183,184] Palpation of subcutaneous and intraabdominal fat deposits is painful to the cat and reveals

BOX 28-1

Signs of Pansteatitis in Cats

Depression and anorexia

Hyperesthesia (sensitivity to touch) of the chest and abdomen

Reluctance to move and decreased agility

Presence of abnormal fat deposits under the skin and in the abdomen

Dietary history that includes items that are high in unsaturated fats and low in vitamin E

the presence of granular or nodular fat deposits. Information concerning the animal's dietary history should be involved in the diagnosis, but confirmation of diagnosis is provided by histological examination of a fat biopsy sample. The fat of cats with pansteatitis is very firm and deep yellow to orange in color, with a diffuse inflammatory response.[183,185] The orange pigment (commonly referred to as *ceroid*) is believed to be an intermediate polymerization product of unsaturated fatty acids that have undergone peroxidation. The peroxidation occurs as a result of insufficient intracellular antioxidants, specifically vitamin E (Box 28-1).

Early cases of pansteatitis occurred almost exclusively in cats that were fed a canned, commercial, fish-based food made primarily of red tuna.[183,186] Later cases occurred in cats that were fed diets consisting wholly or largely of canned red tuna or fish scraps.[185,187] Red tuna packed in oil contains high levels of PUFAs and low levels of vitamin E. The addition of large amounts of fish products to a cat's diet appears to be the primary cause of pansteatitis in pet cats.

Treatment of pansteatitis involves the elimination of fish from the cat's diet and its replacement with a well-balanced, high-quality, commercial cat food. Dietary changes may be difficult in cats that have become accustomed to eating only a single food item. This problem has been most commonly reported in cats that received only red tuna as the principal component of their diet for an extended period of time.[185,186] Along with correction of the diet, vitamin E (alpha-tocopherol) should be administered orally at a dose of 10 to 25 international units (IU) twice daily for 5 to 7 days.[185,188] Corticosteroid therapy may also be used to decrease inflammation and reduce pain. Prognosis for recovery from pansteatitis is usually very good, but it may be slow in advanced cases.

VITAMIN A TOXICOSIS IN CATS: DEFORMING CERVICAL SPONDYLOSIS

Feeding excess amounts of the fat-soluble vitamins can be toxic to dogs and cats. This is not generally seen as a practical problem, except in the case of vitamin A. Vitamin A toxicosis has been reported most often in cats that are fed diets composed exclusively of liver or other organ meats. Although it is no longer a common practice because of the availability of commercial pet foods, some pet owners still feed their cats a diet consisting exclusively of liver, milk, and various table scraps. This practice is usually the result of well-meaning but poorly informed pet owners who believe that cats, being carnivores, will thrive on an all-meat or all-liver diet. Although many nutrients in these diets are imbalanced, one of the most serious problems that can occur is vitamin A toxicosis.

The pathological result of vitamin A excess in cats is the development of a syndrome called *deforming cervical spondylosis*. The effects of vitamin A on bone growth and remodeling result in the development of bony exostoses (outgrowths) along the muscular insertions of cervical vertebrae and the long bones of the forelimbs. Over time, these bony processes cause pain and difficult movement.[189] Vitamin A–induced skeletal disease is not a practical problem in dogs, but it has been produced experimentally. Studies have shown that extremely high intakes of vitamin A in growing dogs result in decreased length and thickness of long bones, premature closure of epiphyseal growth plates, and the development of osteophytes and periosteal reactions.[190] However, more recent studies with dogs have shown that feeding up to 400,000 IU/kilogram (kg) of dry matter (DM) to puppies, or as high as 787,000 IU/kg of DM to adult dogs, for periods of 6 months or 1 year caused no signs of toxicity and did not adversely affect bone density measurements.[191,192]

Initial clinical signs of deforming cervical spondylosis in cats include anorexia, weight loss, lethargy, and an increasing reluctance to move. Cats become unkempt in appearance and are less interested or able to groom themselves. As the disease progresses, a very characteristic postural change is observed; cats adopt a marsupial-like sitting position, holding the front legs elevated off the ground. They also often walk with their hind limbs flexed, and ventriflexion of the head is decreased or altogether absent. A fixed-stare expression is often observed, probably as a result of the cat's inability to turn its head to see. Lameness in one or both of the front limbs is seen in the later stages.[189,193] Development of exostoses occurs primarily in the first three joints of the cervical vertebrae and joints of the forelegs. It has been theorized that the normal movements involved in a cat's regular licking and grooming practices result in these predilection sites. Chronic intoxication with vitamin A appears to increase the sensitivity of the periosteum to the effects of low levels of trauma and repetitive movements that would normally be insufficient to cause an inflammatory response (Box 28-2).[193]

Experimental studies show that the level of vitamin A required to produce skeletal lesions within only a few months' time is between 17 and 35 micrograms (μg)/gram (g) of body weight.[193] A 1-kg (2.2 pound [lb]) kitten would have to consume a minimum of 17,000 μg (56,000 IU) of vitamin A per day to attain this level. According to the National Research Council's (NRC's) current *Nutrient Requirements for Cats*, a 1-kg kitten requires approximately 50 μg of vitamin A per day (1000 μg/kg of dry diet).[182] The toxic dose of vitamin A necessary to produce acute toxicity is therefore more than 300 times the kitten's daily requirement. An adult cat weighing 5 kg (11 lbs) would have to consume at least 85,000 μg of vitamin A daily to reach this toxic level. The daily vitamin A requirement for an active 5-kg adult

BOX 28-2

Signs of Deforming Cervical Spondylosis in Cats

Anorexia and weight loss
Increased lethargy and reluctance to move
Persistent lameness in one or both front legs
Decreased ability to self-groom
Decreased ventriflexion of the head
Posture changes by adopting a "marsupial-like" sitting position
Dietary history that includes items that contain a high concentration of vitamin A

cat is approximately 80 μg/day. Therefore an adult cat would have to consume 1000 times its daily requirement of vitamin A to achieve toxic levels. It is indisputable that a cat will never consume this level if it is receiving a nutritionally balanced, commercial pet food.

It would also be difficult for a cat to consume this high a level of vitamin A while being fed an all-liver diet. Beef liver contains approximately 160 μg (530 IU)/g.[194] An adult cat consuming 6 ounces (oz) of liver per day would be ingesting only 27,200 μg of vitamin A per day, quite a bit less than the levels described by researchers.[193] However, all of the case studies reported in the literature found that deforming cervical spondylosis developed in cats that were fed liver diets.

There are two possible explanations for this discrepancy. First, it is known that the livers of production animals vary greatly in vitamin A content.[194] The level of 160 μg of vitamin A/g in beef liver is an average, not an absolute, value. Second, and more importantly, all of the case studies that have been reported occurred in adult cats that had been fed liver diets for long durations.[195,196] The experimental work that has been conducted involved much higher levels of vitamin A and produced signs of toxicity in very short periods of time. At lower doses of vitamin A, cervical spondylosis appears to develop slowly over the lifetime of the cat, and clinical signs of the disease do not become evident until much later in adult life. This conclusion is supported by the fact that the average age for the diagnosis of cervical spondylosis in pet cats is 4.25 years.[189] Therefore the reported level of vitamin A required to produce toxicity in the cat (17 to 35 μg/g of body weight) may be realistic for the experimental production of acute toxicity, but the level that can produce deforming cervical spondylosis if excess vitamin A is consumed by pet cats for long durations of time is probably substantially lower.

Regular supplementation of a cat's diet with liver, even if it is added to a balanced diet, has the potential to cause skeletal problems if the practice is continued for several years. When liver is fed exclusively, vitamin A toxicosis may occur concurrently with nutritional secondary hyperparathyroidism because of the low-calcium, high-phosphorus content of organ meats.[196] Cod liver oil fed as a supplement also has the potential to induce vitamin A toxicity. Adding 1 tablespoon (tbsp) of cod liver oil to a cat's food twice daily will result in an intake of approximately 10,000 μg of additional vitamin A per day. Fish liver oils are also excessively high in vitamin D, and excessive supplementation may result in the combined effects of vitamin A and vitamin D toxicosis.

The treatment of vitamin A toxicosis in cats includes removing the source of excessive vitamin A from the diet, replacing the source with a complete and balanced pet food, and providing supportive therapy. The prognosis is guarded because resolution of skeletal lesions may never be complete. In addition, if the cat has been fed a liver diet for a long time, the change to a balanced pet food may be difficult, since many cats develop a fixed food preference and refuse to eat any other diet.

THIAMIN DEFICIENCY

Certain types of fish contain an enzyme called *thiaminase* that destroys thiamin (vitamin B_1). Consumption of these types of fish has been shown to cause thiamin deficiency in a variety of species. Experimental studies with cats have produced signs of thiamin deficiency within 23 to 40 days of consuming diets composed solely of raw carp or raw salt-water herring.[197] The subcutaneous administration of thiamin to affected cats resulted in recovery in all cases. Although both carp and herring can cause thiamin deficiency, perch, catfish, and butterfish do not show thiaminase activity. Other common types of fish that contain thiaminase include whitefish, pike, cod, goldfish, mullet, shark, and flounder. However, it is not known whether the thiaminase levels present in these fish are sufficient to produce deficiency in animals.[198]

Thiaminase is a heat-labile enzyme and is denatured by normal cooking temperatures. As a result, the potential for thiamin deficiency exists only when uncooked fish is fed.

Although thiamin deficiency is uncommon in dogs and cats, clinical cases have been reported. Cats appear to be more susceptible because of their high requirement for this vitamin in the diet and because of the tendency of pet owners to feed cats unconventional diets.[197,199] Most cases have been the result of feeding cats diets that contained a large proportion of raw fish.[197,200] Similarly, a group of sled dogs that was fed a diet consisting of frozen, uncooked carp developed clinical signs of thiamin deficiency after a 6-month period. The addition of oatmeal, a dry dog food, and 100 milligrams (mg) of thiamin per day to the diets of the affected dogs resulted in complete recovery within 2 months.[201]

Because thiamin is essential for normal carbohydrate metabolism, the central nervous system is severely affected by a deficiency of this vitamin. Initial clinical signs of deficiency include anorexia, weight loss, and depression. As the deficiency progresses, neurological signs of ataxia, paresis, and, eventually, convulsive seizures develop. The terminal stage is characterized by severe weakness and prostration and eventually leads to death.[201,202] A diagnosis of thiamin deficiency in dogs and cats is made based on clinical signs and the dietary history of the animal. Elevated plasma pyruvate and lactate concentrations are also useful in confirming a diagnosis.

Treatment includes elimination of raw fish from the diet; its replacement with a well-balanced, commercial pet food; and thiamin therapy. Thiamin should be administered intravenously or subcutaneously at a dose of 75 to 100 mg twice daily until neurological signs subside.[199] Oral thiamin supplementation should also be administered for several months following the initial clinical episode.[201] In most affected pets, these clinical signs will decrease within several days. However, if severe neurological damage has occurred, the pet may never make a full recovery. A permanent intolerance of physical exercise and some degree of persistent ataxia occasionally occurs in animals that have recovered from thiamin deficiency.

BIOTIN DEFICIENCY

Biotin is essential as a coenzyme for a number of carboxylation reactions involved in fatty acid, amino acid, and purine metabolism (see Section 1, p. 38). Dietary deficiencies of this vitamin are not generally a problem in dogs and cats because it is believed that these species are able to obtain most, if not all, of their requirement through synthesis by intestinal microbes.[154,182] However, deficiencies have been produced experimentally through prolonged antibiotic therapy or by feeding a diet containing raw egg white.[203,204,205] Egg white contains avidin, a secretory protein produced by the hen's oviduct during formation of the egg. When consumed, avidin combines with biotin in the intestine and prevents biotin absorption. The avidin in egg white is so effective in this capacity that feeding raw egg white has been used to experimentally induce biotin deficiency in laboratory animals.

Signs of biotin deficiency in dogs and cats include the development of scaly dermatitis, alopecia, and, eventually, diarrhea and anorexia.[204,206] Although egg white has the capacity to induce a biotin deficiency in companion animals, the danger of this occurring is slight. The fact that the yolk of the egg contains large quantities of biotin offsets the potential risk of causing a biotin deficiency when the entire egg is fed.

Furthermore, cooking denatures avidin and destroys its biotin-binding ability. Practically speaking, the only potential danger to companion animal nutrition would be regular supplementation of a pet's diet with only the white of the raw egg. Although egg is an excellent source of protein and provides a number of essential nutrients, it is wise to limit the amount fed to companion animals. In addition, feeding raw eggs is not recommended due to the risk of bacterial contamination.

29

Common Nutrition Myths

Like any science, nutrition has a number of "old wives' tales" and myths about the feeding of dogs and cats. Some of these myths and feeding fads have their origins in scientific fact, but the facts have been exaggerated, obscured, or misapplied. Other myths have arisen from nutritional misinformation perpetuated by a lack of scientific proof or disproof and by the pervasive desire to find easy solutions to medical or behavioral problems through diet. Although some nutritional myths cause no harm to pets, others have the potential to adversely affect health or contribute to a dietary imbalance. A number of commonly held myths are discussed in this chapter, as is scientific research that addresses these beliefs (Table 29-1).

TABLE **29-1**

Summary of Common Nutritional Myths

Myth	Supporting Research	Disputing Research	Conclusion (True/False)
Feeding brewer's yeast or thiamin repels fleas	Human studies that were poorly controlled	Two studies with dogs	False
Feeding garlic or onion repels fleas	None reported	None reported; reports of onion toxicity in dogs	False
Diet causes acute, moist dermatitis ("hot spots")	None reported; diet may play indirect role in some cases	Supportive evidence for other causes	False
Certain diets cause the coat to turn red in dogs	None reported	Supportive evidence for other causes	Probably false
Components in the diet cause GDV	None reported	Multiple studies	False
Ethoxyquin causes health problems	None reported	Several long-term studies with dogs and other species	False
High-fat pet foods cause hyperlipidemia	None reporting diet as a primary cause	Supportive evidence for other causes	False

FEEDING "PEOPLE FOODS" TO DOGS AND CATS

Some pet owners enjoy feeding their dogs and cats "people foods" for the same reasons that they like to give them treats and snacks. Providing a special treat is a way of showing affection and love, and adding table scraps and other choice food items to a pet's diet is believed to enhance the pet's enjoyment of the meal. Although some human foods are unsuitable for companion animals and should not be fed at all, others only become detrimental if they make up too high a proportion of the pet's diet. Some pet owners insist on feeding at least small amounts of "people foods" to their companion animals. If these foods are to be fed, proper guidelines should always be followed (Box 29-1).

Table Scraps

The amount of table scraps that are added to a pet's diet should be strictly limited. Although the owner may eat a very nutritious and well-balanced diet, the nutritional requirements of dogs and cats are not the same as for humans. In addition, most owners add only the choice scraps from their meals to their pet's dinner bowl, such as fat trimmings and leftover meat, and they leave the vegetables and grains behind. The table scraps that end up in the pet's bowl may be very tasty (and much appreciated), but they usually do not provide balanced nutrition. If table scraps are fed to pets, they should never make up more than 5% to 10% of the pet's total daily caloric intake.

BOX **29-1**

Practical Feeding Tips: Adding "People Foods" to a Pet's Diet

The addition of extra foods should be limited to no more than 5% to 10% of the pet's daily caloric requirement.

Any meat, fish, or poultry that is fed should be well cooked, and all bones should be removed.

The use of milk and cheese should be strictly monitored. Some adult dogs and cats are lactose intolerant and cannot efficiently digest dairy products.

The exclusive use of any single food item should be avoided, even when adding it to the pet's diet in very small amounts.

Correction of the nutrient imbalances of a poor diet by adding table scraps should not be attempted.

Vitamin and/or mineral supplements are unnecessary when a complete and balanced pet food is fed, and they can be detrimental to health.

Pet owners should be aware of the development of unwanted behavior problems, such as begging during mealtimes and stealing food.

The addition of all extra foods should be discontinued if weight gain, gastrointestinal tract upset, or signs of nutrient imbalance are seen.

Meat and Poultry

Some owners believe that because cats and dogs are carnivorous in nature, they should be able to survive on an all-meat diet. However, the muscle tissue of meat and poultry alone cannot supply complete nutrition to companion animals. Both of these high-protein foods are deficient in calcium, phosphorus, sodium, iron, copper, iodine, and several vitamins. It is true that, in the wild, the ancestors of dogs and cats survived on freshly killed meat. However, the fact that they consumed their *entire* prey, including bones, organs, and intestinal contents, is often overlooked. Like other supplemental foods, the addition of meat and poultry to the diet should be strictly limited because of their potential to imbalance the pet's diet (Table 29-2).

TABLE **29-2**

Nutrient Composition of a Performance Dry Dog Food with Added Proportions of Beef (Dry-Matter Basis)*

Nutrient	Dry Dog Food	75% Dog Food/25% Beef†	50% Dog Food/50% Beef	25% Dog Food/75% Beef
Protein	34%	39%	46%	55%
Fat	23%	24%	25%	26%
Carbohydrate	35%	30%	23%	14%
Crude fiber	1.9%	1.6%	1.3%	0.75%
Calcium	1.3%	1.1%	**0.87%**	**0.53%**
Phosphorus	1.0%	0.89%	**0.73%**	**0.53%**
Calcium:phosphorus ratio	1.3:1	1.2:1	1.2:1	1:1
Potassium	0.87%	0.89%	0.92%	**0.96%**
Sodium	0.60%	0.53%	0.44%	0.31%
Magnesium	0.11%	0.09%	0.08%	**0.06%**
Iron	215 mg/kg	183 mg/kg	142 mg/kg	**85 mg/kg**
Vitamin A	21,700 IU/kg	18,500 IU/kg	14,400 IU/kg	8600 IU/kg
Vitamin D	1950 IU/kg	1670 IU/kg	1290 IU/kg	**770 IU/kg**
Vitamin E	153 IU/kg	130 IU/kg	100 IU/kg	**60 IU/kg**
Thiamin	19.5 mg/kg	16.7 mg/kg	13 mg/kg	7.7 mg/kg
Riboflavin	25 mg/kg	21 mg/kg	16.5 mg/kg	10 mg/kg
Niacin	64 mg/kg	55 mg/kg	42 mg/kg	25 mg/kg
Metabolizable energy (ME)	4700 kcal/kg	4800 kcal/kg	5000 kcal/kg	5200 kcal/kg
Caloric Distribution				
Protein	27%	31%	35%	41%
Fat	45%	45%	47%	48%
Carbohydrate	28%	24%	18%	10%

*Imbalanced nutrients are expressed in bold print. Nutrient levels were compared to the Association of American Feed Control Officials' (AAFCO's) *Nutrient Profiles* and corrected for differences in energy density.

†Beef = fresh ground round.

Fish

Most cats and some dogs love the taste of fish. Advertising campaigns used by some pet food companies have convinced people that cats prefer the taste of fish over many other food items. In reality, cats enjoy fish to about the same degree that they enjoy several other high-protein foods. Although fish is a good source of protein for dogs and cats, it does not supply complete nutrition. In general, most types of deboned fish are deficient in calcium, sodium, iron, copper, and several vitamins. Some types of fish also contain small bones that are difficult to remove before cooking. These bones may easily lodge in a pet's throat or gastrointestinal tract and cause perforation or obstruction.

Tuna is a type of fish that is commonly fed to cats because it is readily available and inexpensive. Canned tuna packed in oil contains high levels of polyunsaturated fatty acids (PUFAs). The excessive intake of these oils can result in a vitamin E deficiency as a result of their high polyunsaturated fat and low vitamin E content. In the cat, this can eventually manifest as a condition called pansteatitis or "yellow fat disease." Signs of pansteatitis include decreased appetite, lethargy, elevated temperature, and tenderness and pain in the chest and abdomen.[185,186] Treatment includes eliminating fish from the cat's diet and replacing it with a well-balanced, high-quality commercial cat food (see pp. 345-346).

Raw fish should never be fed to pets. Certain types of fish, such as carp and herring, contain a compound that destroys thiamin, a B vitamin, and may cause a thiamin deficiency.[197,198] (see pp. 349-350). There is also the potential for parasite transmission when raw fish is fed. If any type of fish is added to a companion animal's diet, it should always be well cooked, and only very small amounts should be fed.

Liver

Liver is an excellent source of iron, protein, copper, vitamin D, and several B vitamins. However, like other single food items, it is not a nutritionally complete food. Liver is severely deficient in calcium and excessively high in vitamin A. Both of these nutritional imbalances can cause bone disorders. Vitamin A toxicity has been shown to develop slowly over a period of years in cats that were regularly fed fresh liver as their primary dietary protein source.[207,208,209] The bone deformities of vitamin A toxicity form gradually and may go undetected for several years. Severe and irreversible crippling eventually occurs, and diagnosis is often too late to be of any help (see pp. 346-349).[210,211] Although small amounts of liver added to a cat's diet are not harmful, liver as a primary component of the diet should be avoided.

Milk and Dairy Products

Almost all cats and dogs love the taste of milk. Although milk and dairy products are excellent sources of calcium, protein, phosphorus, and several vitamins, excessive intake may cause diarrhea in young and adult pets. Milk contains the simple sugar lactose. Lactose requires breakdown in the intestinal tract by the enzyme lactase. Some cats and dogs do not produce sufficient amounts of lactase to handle the large quantity of lactose present in milk. Lack of sufficient lactase results in an inability to completely digest milk and subsequently causes digestive upsets and diarrhea. Dairy products such as cheese, buttermilk, and yogurt contain slightly lower levels of lactose. Even though these products may be more easily tolerated, they still have the potential for causing diarrhea and dietary imbalances. Most pets can tolerate and enjoy an occasional bowl of milk, but like all supplementation, the practice of feeding milk should be strictly limited.

Dairy products should not be used as a supplemental source of calcium or protein. As discussed previously, excess dietary calcium can contribute to the development of skeletal disorders in growing dogs and is not helpful in preventing eclampsia in lactating dams (see pp. 337-343). Although dairy products do supply high-quality protein, they contain deficiencies and excesses of other nutrients and may contribute to a dietary imbalance if large amounts are added to an otherwise adequate diet.

Oils and Fats

Cod liver oil, vegetable oils, and animal fats are occasionally added to pets' diets to improve the taste of the diet or to supply additional vitamins. It is true that fish oils are excellent sources of vitamin A, vitamin D, and the omega-3 fatty acids. However, both of these vitamins are toxic when consumed in excess. Because vitamins A and D are stored in the liver, the effects of excess intake are cumulative and develop over long periods. The daily addition of 1 or 2 tablespoons (tbsp) of cod liver oil (or another vitamin A supplement) to a small pet's diet has the potential of eventually developing into a toxicity problem. In addition, oversupplementation with fat may result in either obesity or an eventual decrease in the quantity of food that is consumed. Food intake may decrease because energy needs will be met with a lower quantity of food. Deficiencies of other nutrients may then develop. Excessive intake of dietary fat may also cause digestive problems in some pets.

Some owners add fat to their pets' diets with the intention of improving coat quality. Dogs have a requirement for the essential fatty acid linoleic acid and possibly for alpha-linolenic acid, and cats require these fatty acids plus dietary arachidonic acid. Animals that are deficient in essential fatty acids will develop poor coat quality and skin problems. Pet food of inferior quality or foods that have been stored too long may contain inadequate levels of these fatty acids. However, if a high-quality pet food is being fed, adding fat or oil should not be necessary. In most cases, diet is not the principal cause of skin problems or poor coat quality in companion animals. More probable causes of skin disorders include internal and external parasitic infections, allergies, and various hormonal imbalances. If a coat or skin problem persists in a dog or cat, even when a high-quality food is fed, a veterinarian should be consulted.

Chocolate

Most dogs enjoy sweet flavors, including the taste of chocolate. Cats, on the other hand, are much less likely to find sweet foods palatable.[54] Chocolate contains a methylxanthine called theobromine, which is toxic to dogs when consumed in large quantities. Three methylxanthine compounds are commonly found in human foods; these are caffeine, theophylline, and theobromine. Caffeine is most abundant in coffee, tea, and cola beverages, and theophylline is found primarily in tea. Theobromine is the most abundant methylxanthine, found in cocoa and chocolate products. The main sites of action of xanthine compounds in the body are the central nervous system, cardiovascular system, kidneys, smooth muscle, and skeletal musculature. Theobromine in particular acts as a smooth muscle relaxant, coronary artery dilatator, diuretic, and cardiac stimulant.

Although it is not a common clinical problem, theobromine toxicity in dogs can be life-threatening when it occurs. Toxicity studies have shown that, when compared with several other species, the dog is unusually sensitive to the physiological effects of theobromine. This sensitivity appears to be the result of a lower rate of theobromine metabolism, resulting in a longer half-life in the bloodstream and tissues. After a single dose, the half-life of theobromine in the plasma of adult dogs is approximately 17.5 hours.[212] In comparison, theobromine's half-life in human subjects is 6 hours; in rats it is only 3 hours.[213,214] It has been theorized that the extended half-life in dogs may potentiate acute toxicity reactions to theobromine after the consumption of foods containing chocolate.[212]

Signs of theobromine toxicity in dogs include vomiting, diarrhea, panting, restlessness, increased urination or urinary incontinence, and muscle tremors. These signs usually occur about 4 to 5 hours after the dog has consumed the food containing chocolate. The onset of generalized motor seizures signifies a poor prognosis in most cases and often results in death.[215,216,217] Theobromine toxicity is treated by inducing vomiting as soon as possible. An activated charcoal "shake" given by gastric lavage may aid in decreasing the quantity of the drug that is absorbed into the bloodstream. Unfortunately, there is no specific systemic antidote for theobromine poisoning.

Although few controlled studies on the level of theobromine that constitutes a toxic dose have been conducted in dogs, data from long-term studies and case reports indicate that toxicity can occur when a dog consumes a dose of 90 to 100 milligrams (mg)/kilogram (kg) of body weight or more.[217] Factors such as individual sensitivity to theobromine, mode of theobromine administration, presence of other foods in the gastrointestinal tract at the time of ingestion, and variations in theobromine content between chocolate products cause wide variations in the susceptibility of individual dogs to chocolate poisoning. Chocolate products differ greatly in their theobromine content and, therefore, in their ability to produce theobromine poisoning.

Chocolate liquor, commonly called baking or cooking chocolate, is the base substance from which all other chocolate products are produced. The average level of theobromine in baking chocolate is about 1.22%.[218] A 1-ounce (oz) square contains approximately 346 mg of theobromine. Therefore, if a medium-sized dog weighing 25 pounds (lbs) (11 kg) consumed 3 oz of baking chocolate, a potentially fatal dose of 94 mg of theobromine/kg would be ingested. Commercial cocoa (unsweetened) has an average theobromine content of 1.89%, which is the highest theobromine content of all commonly consumed chocolate products. However, dogs are less likely to consume baking chocolate or cocoa powder than other sweeter chocolate products. The addition of sugar, cocoa butter, and milk solids to baking chocolate to produce sweet chocolates results in a significant dilution of theobromine content. For example, the level of theobromine in semisweet choco- late pieces is 0.463%. A 25-lb dog would have to consume approximately ½ lb of semisweet chocolate to reach a potentially toxic level of 95 mg/kg. Similarly, milk chocolate contains 0.153% theobromine. The ingestion of approximately 1½ lbs of milk chocolate would result in a potentially lethal dose for a 25-lb dog.

Dogs generally love the taste of chocolate, and owners occasionally give choco- late candy or foods containing chocolate to their dogs as a special treat. If a dog's intake of chocolate is strictly limited to occasional small treats, there is no danger of theobromine toxicity. All of the published case studies of theobromine toxicity in dogs have been the result of a pet accidentally ingesting a large amount of choco- late.[215,216,217] If given the opportunity, many pets will readily overconsume chocolate. Therefore all chocolate foods should be stored in areas inaccessible to pets.

MYTH: FEEDING BREWER'S YEAST
OR THIAMIN REPELS FLEAS

The use of either brewer's yeast or the B-vitamin thiamin (one of the yeast's com- ponents) as a repellent for external parasites has been advocated for many years. This practice can be traced back to several studies with human subjects that were conducted during the 1940s. In one study, when subjects were given oral doses of 100 to 200 mg of thiamin per day, it was reported that they experienced lower num- bers of mosquito bites and decreased severity of dermatological reactions.[219] An- other early study reported that benefits were observed when infants and children with severe flea infestations were treated with 10 mg of thiamin per day.[220] How- ever, neither of these studies were well controlled, and several subsequent studies with humans have failed to show any significant effect of thiamin supplementation on insect infestations.[221]

Companion animal owners and professionals, anxious to find safe and conve- nient means for controlling flea and mite infestations, quickly adapted this practice for use in dogs and cats. However, there is no evidence to indicate that feeding thi- amin or brewer's yeast has a repellent effect on fleas or mites in these species. Two controlled studies have reported that neither brewer's yeast nor thiamin repelled fleas or mosquitos in dogs. In the first study, dogs that were fed 14 grams (g) per day of active or inactive brewer's yeast had the same weekly flea counts as did a group of dogs that were not supplemented.[222] In the second study, neither flea counts nor the number of flea bites on dogs were affected by supplementation with 100 mg of thiamin per day.[221] Although supplementing pet's diets with brewer's yeast is probably not harmful, it is not effective in either repelling or controlling flea populations in homes or on the skin of companion animals.

MYTH: FEEDING GARLIC OR ONION REPELS FLEAS

Feeding either of these two food items will certainly make a pet's breath smell, but it will not have any effect on fleas. Moreover, feeding large amounts of onion to dogs or cats can be toxic. Excess consumption of onions results in the formation of Heinz bodies on circulating red blood cells, which ultimately results in the development of hemolytic anemia. In severe cases, this anemia can be fatal.[223,224,225] The toxic compound in onions that is responsible for this effect is n-propyl disulfide. Signs of hemolytic anemia produced by onion toxicity include diarrhea, vomiting, depression, fever, and dark-colored urine. Although vomiting and diarrhea may be immediate, the remaining signs usually appear 1 to 4 days following the ingestion of the onion. If onion toxicity is suspected, veterinary care should be sought immediately. Many dogs love the taste of onions and may overconsume if given the opportunity. Therefore onion-containing foods should be fed only in small amounts to dogs and cats, and they certainly should not be expected to have an effect on flea infestations.

MYTH: DIET CAUSES ACUTE MOIST DERMATITIS ("HOT SPOTS")

Acute moist dermatitis is a condition that is commonly referred to as "hot spots" because it frequently occurs during warm months of the year and because the lesions that develop are inflamed and feel hot to the touch. This disease is most commonly seen in breeds of dogs that have very dense, heavy coats, and it may be related to poor ventilation of the skin or improper grooming to remove matted hair and debris. Hot-spot lesions can develop within just a few hours. The lesions are usually first noticed as a patch of missing hair. A round, red, moist area that is extremely painful rapidly develops. The area often has a yellowish center surrounded by a reddened ring of inflammation. Self-trauma occurs in the form of biting and scratching at the affected area because the lesions are usually intensely pruritic. If not treated, the spots can spread to other areas of the body.

Any factor that causes irritation, pruritus, or self-trauma can lead to acute moist dermatitis. Allergic reactions, external parasites, skin infections, an unhealed injury, or improper grooming can all initiate self-trauma and the development of a hot spot. It is believed by some pet owners that a diet that is too "rich" or too high in protein is the cause of hot spots. However, there is no evidence that a relationship exists between acute moist dermatitis and protein levels in the diet.[226] Diet may play a role if it produces a severe fatty acid deficiency or if the pet has a food-induced allergy. Fatty acid deficiencies can occur when improperly formulated or improperly stored pet foods are fed and are characterized by a number of dermatological signs (see Section 2, pp. 96-97). Food-induced allergies may indirectly cause a hot spot to develop because allergies typically cause intense pruritus, which in turn may lead to self-trauma (see Section 6, p. 446). However, both of these conditions occur very infrequently. The most common underlying cause of acute moist dermatitis in dogs appears to be flea-bite hypersensitivity and other allergic skin diseases.[226]

MYTH: CERTAIN DIETS CAUSE COAT COLOR TO TURN RED IN DOGS

In recent years, dog show enthusiasts have become concerned with a problem that is commonly called "red coat". This term refers to a perceived change in coat color from almost any normal base color to a red or reddish brown. This change is of greatest concern to, and in fact has only been reported by, individuals who exhibit and/or breed dogs. It is the belief of some that a component or components in the diet is the cause of this malady. Several different brands of premium dog foods have been implicated. The specific brand that is targeted apparently depends on the part of the country where the owner lives and the breed of dog that is being discussed.

One of the difficulties in investigating this problem has been the inconsistency and infrequency of its occurrence. Interestingly, when pet food companies have attempted to investigate red coat, they have found that very few of the cases are first-person complaints. In most cases, the complainant did not actually own the dog or dogs that turned red but had heard of a case through friends or breeders. Secondly, there is still no precise definition of the red coat problem. The condition that one owner observes and calls red coat may not be the same that another interprets as the same problem. Although the perceived occurrence of red coat among dog show enthusiasts is quite high, the actual occurrence of the problem in dogs is extremely low. As a result, the number of actual dogs that have been available for investigators to study has been very small.

An understanding of normal coat color development is necessary to completely understand the potential causes of a change in coat color in a dog. An individual hair takes between 6 and 8 weeks to grow. Once mature, the hair enters a resting phase and remains dormant for weeks or months before being shed to make room for a new hair. The color of a dog's hair is determined by the type and amount of pigment that is deposited in the growing hair while it is in the hair follicle. Specialized pigment-producing cells within the follicle secrete either yellow-red pheomelanin or black-brown melanin that is then deposited within the actual hair. Other genetic factors affect the distribution of pigment within the hair shaft, the dilution or masking of color, and the distribution of color in different areas of the body. These factors result in the wide variety of coat colors that are seen in different breeds of dogs. In addition to genetics, other factors that may affect the color of the hair during either its growth or resting cycle include medications, topical substances, aging, environment, and diet.

A change in the color of a hair may be produced in one of two possible ways. A systemic factor may cause a change in the color of hairs while they are still in the hair follicle (e.g., a change in the pigment-producing cells). Within the hair, this type of change would be expected to extend from the skin surface outward toward the hair tip, and the portion of the hair that is affected would depend on the length of time that the influencing factor was in effect. For example, if the change was only in effect for 2 weeks, the color change would appear as a band of color on the length of the hair shaft. Because individual hairs within the entire coat are at different stages of development, the red color in the hair coat would be dispersed throughout the coat at different levels on each hair shaft. By definition, this type of change in coat color would take weeks to months to appear or disappear. Also, because hair growth occurs randomly throughout the coat, it would be expected that any change in color would not be uniform, but would occur in only the hairs that were growing at the time that the influencing factor was present. Resting hairs would not be affected by any factor that affected a change in coat color in the growing hairs.

The second way that a change in coat color can occur is through the deposition of a substance on the outside of the hair shaft. This change could involve substances that are either applied by the dog's owner, secreted by the dog's skin, or licked onto the hair by the dog. This type of change would involve the entire length of the hair shaft, and all of the hairs within a region would be affected. Therefore the appearance of this type of coat-color change would be significantly different from the appearance of the coat if a systemic factor was in effect.

There are several known factors that can affect hair coat color in dogs and could be responsible for imbuing a red hue to the coat. Aging of hair naturally causes a change in color. As a hair approaches the end of its resting period and is ready to be shed, black hairs turn reddish to reddish brown. This change occurs primarily near the tip of the hair, with the base of the hair remaining black. However, in some cases, especially when hairs are retained for a long period without shedding, the entire shaft may turn red. When the dog sheds its coat, these hairs are removed, and a return to normal color is seen. In addition to the age of the hair, exposure to sunlight can also cause black hairs to turn red. When this occurs, the change in color usually affects variable portions of the ends of the hairs. The color of the hair at the base (near the dog's skin) remains black.

Topically applied dips or shampoos that contain insecticides can also turn hair a red hue. This effect can be seen with any natural coat color, but it will be most noticeable in white or light-colored dogs. When an applied agent is the cause, the change in color will be uniform throughout the hair shaft. Similarly, frequent shampooing, using certain types of rinses, and blow drying can all alter hair coat color.

Finally, a commonly observed cause of coat-color change in dogs is porphyrin staining. Porphyrin is a substance found in the tears and saliva of dogs that turns red when exposed to sunlight. It is a normal end product of hemoglobin metabolism and is the substance responsible for the reddish staining that is seen around the eyes of some breeds of dogs. Dogs that lick excessively will also deposit porphyrins on their coat, causing these areas to stain red. Licking associated with allergic reactions or other dermatological problems may cause reddening of the coat.

In these cases, the entire length of the hair in certain regions of the body will be affected.

Although a number of different factors are known to cause coat-color changes in dogs, a connection between diet and red coat has never been demonstrated. Copper deficiency can cause hypopigmentation of the coat that may manifest as a reddening or graying of the hairs. However, other clinical signs accompany this deficiency, including anemia, skin lesions, and the development of a rough, dull hair coat.[227] The anemia of copper deficiency eventually causes clinical illness in affected dogs. It is highly unlikely that a dietary imbalance of any nutrient is the cause of the red coat problem in dogs. When a nutrient is deficient or in excess, multiple systems of the body are usually involved, and clinical signs other than just a change in coat color will develop.

The few cases of red coat that have been examined have been found to have an identifiable underlying cause. These causes have included exposure to sunlight, staining with porphyrin, the presence of old hairs that have not been shed, and a coexisting dermatological disease.[228] Although more research involving coat-color changes in dogs and cats needs to be conducted, it appears that nutrition is not the cause of the red coat problem in dogs that have been studied.

MYTH: TYPE OF DIET OR COMPONENTS IN THE DIET CAUSE GASTRIC DILATATION–VOLVULUS

Gastric dilatation–volvulus (GDV), commonly referred to as *bloat,* is a life-threatening disorder characterized by rapid and abnormal distention of the stomach (dilatation). This disorder is often, but not always, accompanied by rotation of the stomach along its long axis (volvulus). Dilatation occurs when gas and secretions accumulate within the stomach and are not expelled because of the occlusion of both the cardiac and pyloric sphincters. The condition rapidly worsens as the distended and rotated stomach places pressure on the major abdominal blood vessels, the portal vein, and caudal vena cava. This pressure causes a loss of blood flow to the stomach and other vital organs, decreased cardiac output, and the development of shock. At this point the dog's condition rapidly deteriorates, and if the GDV is not corrected quickly, shock and tissue damage become severe and death ensues. In addition, cardiac arrhythmias are observed in up to 40% of dogs with GDV and can cause death within weeks or months following apparent recovery from GDV.[229] Diagnosis is usually based on clinical signs, with radiographs used to distinguish between GDV and gastric dilatation without gastric torsion. Although the course of GDV can be quite variable among dogs, this disorder should always be treated as a medical emergency.

Bloat most often affects large, deep-chested dogs. The breeds that have been identified as being most susceptible include the Great Dane, Saint Bernard, Weimaraner, Irish Setter, Gordon Setter, Standard Poodle, and Basset Hound.[230]

Although rare, the disorder can also occur in small breeds of dogs and cats.[231,232] A dog that is developing GDV will exhibit acute abdominal pain and distention, and it will often whine, pace, salivate, and appear anxious. The dog may attempt to vomit but will be unable to regurgitate any stomach contents. As the problem progresses, hypovolemic shock occurs, characterized by pale mucous membranes, a rapid and weak pulse, increased heart rate, and weakness. In all cases, veterinary care must be provided immediately.

Initial treatment of GDV involves decompression of the stomach and treatment for shock. Surgical intervention is usually also necessary and involves derotation and repositioning of the stomach, followed by prophylactic measures that help to prevent recurrence. Surgery also allows assessment of the damage to the stomach and other organs. Even with treatment, prognosis is often guarded. In a retrospective study of almost 2000 cases, the case fatality rate was 33.6% in dogs treated for GDV at veterinary teaching hospitals.[230] The strongest prognostic indicator appears to be the extent of gastric necrosis that has occurred. Death occurs either during surgery because of irreversible shock or within several days of surgery as a result of cardiac complications or gastric necrosis.[233,234] While nonsurgical treatment is associated with a high rate of recurrence, the use of gastroplexy to surgically stabilize the stomach has been shown to significantly reduce recurrence and postoperative mortality.[233,235,236]

GDV is considered to have a multifactorial etiology. Potential influencing factors that have been studied include genetic predisposition, dietary management practices, diet type and composition, and intrinsic abnormalities such as elevated serum gastrin or altered gastric motility. Studies have examined most of these theories, and a growing body of evidence is available concerning the underlying causes of this disorder. Because a pet's diet is a factor that owners have some measure of control over, the theories that identify diet as an underlying cause have received an inordinate amount of publicity and attention. In addition, the results of studies that have examined the role of diet in GDV have often been misinterpreted or misrepresented. The end result is much confusion for pet owners, breeders, and some professionals about the actual role of various factors in the onset of GDV.

Genetics plays an important role in GDV to the degree that body type and structure are inherited characteristics. A recent study reported that the two most important risk factors affecting a breed's predisposition for development of GDV are a relatively high chest depth-to-width ratio and a large adult size.[237] Together, chest conformation and body size account for 76% of the variability in breed risk for GDV. Subsequent studies with Irish Setters have shown that there is a positive and significant correlation between increasing chest depth-to-width ratio and an individual dog's risk for developing GDV.[238] Moreover, chest depth-to-width ratios were found to be significantly influenced by genetics, suggesting that it may be possible to reduce the incidence of GDV through selective breeding.[239] Studies of the genetics involved in GDV are complicated by the fact that it is often difficult or impossible to separate these effects from environmental influences such as husbandry practices, medical care, and feeding management. However, dogs that inherit a large, deep-chested body type have an increased susceptibility to this disease, and this confor-mation appears to have a high heritability in some breeds of dogs.

Recent studies identified several additional risk factors for GDV.[240,241] While some of these, such as breed and conformation, are characteristics that are inher-ent to a particular dog, others are environmental factors over which owners have at least some measure of control. In one study, a group of 101 dogs that had acute episodes of GDV were individually matched with dogs of the same age, breed, and size. Comparisons of the two groups showed that physical characteristics that sig-nificantly increased an individual dog's risk of GDV included gender, body weight, and temperament. Specifically, male dogs who were underweight and were deter-mined to have a nervous or fearful temperament were at higher risk for eventually developing GDV. In contrast, a study of 74 Irish Setters with GDV and a group of matched controls found that the risk of GDV was not associated with gender or tem-perament in that breed.[241] The differences between these two studies may reflect differences between the general population of dogs and the subpopulation of a specific breed (Irish Setters). In both studies, however, the most significant precip-itating factor identified was an episode of environmental change or a stress-inducing event within several hours preceding the onset of clinical signs. In the Irish Setters that were studied, two precipitating risks that were identified were recent kenneling and a recent car journey.

Several nutritional factors have been found to influence a dog's risk for GDV.[240,242] These include consuming only one meal per day, having a fast rate of eating, and experiencing aerophagia while eating. On the other hand, feeding table foods, having snacks available between meals, and adding canned food to a dog's diet all decreased the risk of GDV. This second group of practices all contribute to a more frequent meal schedule and are assumed to result in a decreased volume of food being fed during a single meal. These findings are in agreement with earlier reports that the majority of cases of GDV occur when the dog has recently con-sumed a large meal or quantity of water.[242]

The mechanism through which meal frequency affects gastric health may have to do with the volume of food that is fed. A study with Irish Setters reported that dogs fed one large meal per day throughout growth developed larger, heavier stom-achs than did dogs fed three meals per day during the same period.[242] Dogs that were fed once daily also had greater gastric distention than did dogs fed multiple meals, but no differences in gastric motility were seen between the two groups. The investigators concluded that feeding one time per day, rather than feeding multiple small meals per day, may contribute to changes associated with GDV in suscepti-ble dogs. It has also been postulated that strenuous exercise, stress, or excitement may also be contributing factors, especially before or after a meal or a large volume of water is consumed.

Composition of the diet or type of diet that is fed has received much attention as a possible cause of GDV, but there are little actual data to support this theory. Dry dog foods have been implicated because of the belief that they absorb water and expand while in the stomach, causing an abnormal amount of gastric disten-tion. Another theory proposes that cereal-based, dry diets delay gastric emptying when consumed and contribute to the accumulation of gas in the stomach. The presence of soybean products in pet foods has also been proposed as a causative factor. It has been theorized that soy provides a fermentative substrate for *Clostridium* bacteria within the stomach, which produces the gas responsible for GDV. A study with large breeds of dogs compared the effects of feeding a dry cereal-based; canned meat; or canned, cereal-based diet on gastric motility and the rate of gastric emptying. Results showed no significant effect of diet on gastric function in any of the dogs that were studied.[243]

Another study reported that intragastric moistening of ingested dry dog food also failed to produce the stomach distention characteristic of GDV.[244] A clinical study involving 240 dogs that had been treated for GDV did not find any correlation between the type of food that was fed and the occurrence of GDV.[245] Lastly, although there is some disagreement, the fermentation theory has been largely refuted by the observation that the gas found in the stomachs of dogs with GDV is made up primarily of atmospheric gas, indicating that swallowed air is usually the source of the gas, not fermented stomach contents.[246,247] Production of fermentative gas in the stomach of dogs with GDV can occur after death and may lead to the erroneous conclusion that this gas was the initial cause of the disorder. Studies of postmortem tissue decomposition have been unable to demonstrate that the presence of *Clostridium* bacteria in the stomach is primary to the disease, rather than secondary. Currently, the studies that are available support the conclusion that GDV is not a dietary disorder per se, and that its development is not related to any component in pet foods nor to the type of food that is fed.

The final group of theories involves intrinsic factors that affect gastric motility and gastric emptying. Emptying of the stomach is delayed in dogs that have had GDV.[248] One theory proposed that chronically elevated levels of the hormone gastrin could contribute to these changes in gastric function. Delayed gastric emptying is a direct effect of gastrin. However, studies with dogs that had been treated for GDV reported no differences in serum gastrin levels between these dogs and healthy control dogs.[249] Other studies have shown that the stomachs of dogs that have recovered from GDV have electrical (neural) activity that results in abnormal muscular contractions. These abnormal contractions lead to premature closure of the pylorus, gastric retention of solids, and delayed gastric emptying.[249] It is currently proposed that GDV may be the result of a functional defect that prevents normal gastric motility and emptying. This inherent defect may predispose the dog to an atonic stomach and, possibly, to the stretching of the gastrohepatic ligament that is necessary for the development of GDV. Other contributing factors include hereditary predisposition, body size, temperament, feeding one meal per day, swallowing air while eating (aerophagia), and overeating.

Although the type of diet and components within the diet are not causal factors in GDV, several feeding management practices can be used to help prevent GDV in dogs that are susceptible or have a history of GDV. In other words, although what the dog eats does not appear to affect the occurrence of GDV, how the dog is fed and the feeding environment can be managed to minimize the chances of GDV. Portion-controlled meal feeding should be used. Several small

BOX 29-2

Practical Tips: Prevention of GDV in Susceptible Dogs

Use portion-controlled meal feeding as the feeding regimen.

Feed several small meals per day to prevent overfilling of the stomach.

Do not allow the consumption of a large volume of water immediately before or after eating or exercise.

Feed susceptible dogs separately from other animals. If possible, supervise mealtimes.

Do not provide exercise for 1 hour before and 3 hours after meals.

Minimize stress and environmental changes.

If signs of GDV are observed, seek veterinary assistance immediately.

meals should be fed per day, as opposed to one large meal, to prevent overfilling of the stomach. Similarly, although fresh water should be available at all times, dogs should not be allowed to drink a large volume of water before or after eating or after exercise. Because dogs often increase their rate of eating or the amount that they eat when in the presence of other dogs, all susceptible dogs should be fed separately, and any stress that may be associated with the feeding environment should be minimized. If possible, feeding times should be scheduled so that the dog is supervised and can be observed for 1 to 2 hours after meals. Lastly, although exercise as a predisposing factor has not been confirmed, it is prudent to withhold exercise for 1 hour before and at least 3 hours after feeding. All dogs that have a susceptible body type or a history of GDV should be carefully monitored for signs of GDV. If signs are seen, veterinary care should be sought immediately (Box 29-2).

MYTH: ETHOXYQUIN CAUSES REPRODUCTIVE PROBLEMS, AUTOIMMUNE DISEASE, AND CANCER IN DOGS

Ethoxyquin is a synthetic antioxidant that is included in animal foods and some human foods as a preservative to protect fats and fat-soluble vitamins from oxidative degradation (see Section 3, pp. 180-185). Without the inclusion of antioxidants in pet foods, oxidative processes lead to rancidity of the product. Rancid fat is offensive in odor and flavor and includes compounds that are toxic when consumed. The inclusion of antioxidants in commercial pet foods ensures the safety, nutritional integrity, and flavor of the product during the time that it will be fed to companion animals.

Although ethoxyquin has been approved by the Food and Drug Administration (FDA) and used in foods for more than 30 years, this compound has been erroneously identified by some companion animal owners and breeders as a potentially dangerous agent in pet foods. Depending on the source, ethoxyquin has been identified as being responsible for reproductive problems, autoimmune disorders, behavior problems, and/or various types of cancers in dogs and cats. All of these reports are anecdotal in nature and do not provide a method of establishing an exact role of the diet or any dietary components in the onset of disease.

Ethoxyquin's safety in foods has been extensively studied in rabbits, rats, poultry, and dogs. The original studies on which the FDA based approval for the inclusion of ethoxyquin in animal feeds included a 1-year chronic toxicity study in dogs. Data from this and other studies were used when ethoxyquin was first marketed to determine a "safe tolerance level" of 150 parts per million (150 mg/kg) of food.[250] Subsequent studies failed to show any adverse health or reproductive effects of ethoxyquin when it was fed to several generations of dogs and at levels of up to 360 mg/kg of the diet (the highest concentration that was tested).[251,252] During one of these studies, the dogs mated and produced viable litters of puppies. Data from a recent study have shown that feeding high levels of ethoxyquin may result in pigment accumulation in the liver and an increase in serum levels of certain liver enzymes.[253] Although the significance of these changes must be determined, this information still does not support the contention that ethoxyquin is responsible for the variety of health problems that have been reported by pet owners to the FDA. In response to the new data, pet food manufacturers are voluntarily limiting ethoxyquin concentrations in pet foods to 75 parts per million or less. In addition, in response to consumer concerns, some pet food manufacturers have developed foods that do not contain added ethoxyquin at all. As with all additives and ingredients, ethoxyquin must be included in the list of ingredients; it is listed as a preservative.

MYTH: HIGH-FAT PET FOODS CAUSE HYPERLIPIDEMIA

Most people are aware of the relationship of dietary fat and cholesterol to the development of atherosclerosis and coronary artery disease in humans and of the importance of limiting these nutrients in their diet. In recent years, this knowledge has led some pet owners to apply these same nutritional principles to the diet of their companion animals. However, there exist some very basic differences between these species in the ways in which dietary fat is assimilated and metabolized. Unlike humans, dogs and cats are capable of consuming a wide range of dietary fat and still maintaining normal blood lipid levels. This is presumably because dogs and cats first evolved as carnivorous predators with a diet that normally contained a high proportion of animal fat. The capability to consume, digest, and assimilate a high-fat diet has remained with these species throughout the domestication process.

Both hyperlipidemia and atherosclerosis are rare conditions in dogs and cats. When cases of these conditions do occur, they are either of genetic origin or develop secondary to other disease states. For example, an inherited defect in lipoprotein lipase activity in cats causes elevated triglyceride and cholesterol levels in affected cats.[254] The disorder eventually leads to the development of severe peripheral nerve paralysis. It is proposed that an autosomal recessive mode of inheritance, similar to that of an analogous disease in humans, is responsible for this disorder. There is also some evidence for the existence of an inherited defect in lipid metabolism in Miniature Schnauzers, Beagles, and, possibly, Brittany Spaniels.[255,256,257] Abnormally elevated plasma cholesterol concentrations have also been identified in Briards, suggesting the existence of an inherited disorder of lipid metabolism in this breed (see Section 6, pp. 389-393).[258] A second cause of hyperlipidemia in companion animals is the presence of certain preexisting disorders. Diseases that may cause secondary hyperlipidemia include diabetes mellitus, hypothyroidism, pancreatitis, hypoadrenocorticism, nephrotic syndrome, and liver disease.[259] Certain medications such as glucocorticoids and immunosuppressant drugs may also result in transient increases in blood lipid levels in some pets.

When elevated triglyceride levels occur in dogs and cats, they may produce clinical signs of anorexia, lethargy, abdominal pain, seizures, vomiting, diarrhea, and lipid-laden aqueous humor. Hypercholesterolemia, on the other hand, may be related to the development of atherosclerotic lesions, lipemia retinalis, and lipid opacification of the cornea.[255,256,257,258,259] Traditionally, the dietary treatment for hyperlipidemia in dogs and cats has been a low-fat diet. Both primary and secondary hyperlipidemia appear to respond well to a strict adherence to low-fat, low-calorie diets in these species.[256,257,258,259] However, feeding a low-fat diet to healthy pets with the intention of preventing hyperlipidemia and elevated cholesterol levels is unnecessary. Balanced, low-fat diets can be used for the treatment of obesity and for weight maintenance in adult pets that lead sedentary lifestyles. However, the concerns that humans have with dietary lipids and heart disease do not apply to companion animals, except in the specific circumstances discussed above.

MYTH: COPROPHAGY IS CAUSED BY A NUTRIENT DEFICIENCY

Coprophagy (stool eating) is relatively common in dogs and is infrequently observed in cats. Contrary to popular belief, the majority of dogs who coprophagize are not consuming a diet that is deficient in one or more essential nutrients, nor do they have gastrointestinal disease.[260] Most dogs will consume the feces of ruminant or nonruminant herbivorous species such as horses, cattle, deer or rabbits. In addition, many dogs who live with cats will eat cat feces if given access to the litter box. Although less common, some dogs also consume canine feces, including their own.

The dog's evolutionary history provides a reasonable explanation for this behavior. Although the dog's ancestor, the wolf, is considered to be a social predator, this species is also an adept food scavenger. Unlike the more carnivorous feline species, most canids will eat carcasses killed by natural causes or other predators; various types of vegetation and fruits; and even garbage. Eating feces is a manifestation of scavenging behavior and is observed both in pet dogs and in captive and wild wolves. Although ingestion of herbivorous species' feces may supplement the dog's diet with certain vitamins, there is no evidence that dogs (or wolves) selectively coprophagize in an attempt to obtain nutrients that are deficient in their diet. In addition, female dogs and wolves routinely consume the feces of their puppies. It has been theorized that this behavior may continue after puppies are whelped, or that it can be socially facilitated between dogs within the same household. The best way to prevent stool eating is to limit access to fecal matter by monitoring walks, restricting the dog's access to the feces of wild animals such as rabbits and deer, and keeping the yard free of feces. In addition, there are several behavioral techniques that are available to deter dogs that coprophagize frequently.

SECTION 5

KEY POINTS

- Canine and feline couch potatoes? Unfortunately, like contemporary American humans, increasing numbers of cats and dogs are obese. Recent surveys report obesity rates from 24% to 34% among dogs and from 25% to 40% among cats. It can be theorized that a sedentary lifestyle, along with overfeeding highly palatable and energy-dense foods, may be responsible.

- It is known that health problems in humans begin to increase when a person's weight is 15% or more above their ideal. Similarly, health problems among dogs and cats probably increase with obesity. Such problems include hyperinsulinemia, glucose intolerance, diabetes mellitus, pulmonary and cardiovascular disease, exercise and heat intolerance, and orthopedic problems. Surgical risk is higher, and the incidences of postoperative morbidity and mortality increase.

- Once new fat cells are added to the body, their number cannot be decreased below a minimum level. Understandably, to avoid obesity in adulthood, it is important to provide pets with proper weight control throughout their periods of growth.

- Although the cause of obesity seemingly could be explained by simple mathematics (i.e., more energy is taken in than is expended), there are many underlying causes for such an imbalance, not all of which are completely understood.

- The notion that an individual or animal is obese because of "low metabolism" is a fallacy. In fact, research in humans has shown that the resting metabolic rate (RMR) of obese subjects is actually higher than that of normal-weight subjects.

- Although it is true that obesity is more common among neutered pets, a contributing cause is that the age of the pet at neutering (between 6 months and 1 year) corresponds with a natural decrease in the pet's growth rate and energy needs. Thus owners should decrease the amount fed during this period in the pet's development.

- External stimuli, such as diet palatability, food composition and texture, and the timing and environment of meals, appear to be important factors leading to overconsumption and obesity.

- Just like their human counterparts, animals (especially dogs) tend to eat more, regardless of their initial level of hunger, when the food is highly palatable and presented in a social setting with others present. More weight is gained when the excess calories are provided by fat than when provided by protein or carbohydrate sources.

- The benefits of exercise, which are well known to human athletes, also can have a positive effect on overweight pets. Exercise can positively affect an animal's normal physiological control of food intake, and it supports a higher proportion of lean tissue to fat tissue, which contributes to maintaining a normal RMR during weight loss.

- Most commercial pet foods formulated for weight loss or for consumption by sedentary pets have decreased levels of fat. However, some replace fat with digestible carbohydrates, such as corn and rice, and some use indigestible fiber, which results in increased fecal volume and defecation frequency.

- **Tip:** Many of the preventive and causative factors for obesity are the same for humans and animals. Lowering both your own and your pet's intake of fat and increasing the amount of exercise performed will benefit you both. People and their pets should take more walks, and people can even team up with their pets to improve health and maintain ideal weight.

- Heredity is not completely responsible for many forms of developmental skeletal disease, such as canine hip dysplasia. Environmental factors such as nutrition are also responsible. Research has shown that excess caloric intake during growth and a high calcium intake are two important nutritional factors in the development of skeletal disease. Therefore the well-intentioned efforts of some owners to maximize the growth rate of puppies by feeding excessive amounts of a balanced diet can actually lead to orthopedic problems.

- During certain periods of growth, the bones of large dogs are thinner and weaker than those of smaller dogs, and this may partially explain the predisposition for skeletal abnormalities among large and giant breeds.

- **Caution:** Although some breeders recommend routine calcium supplementation for growing puppies, this practice is unnecessary and can sometimes lead to several serious health disorders. Excess calcium has been shown to lead to many orthopedic problems, ironically the types of problems that the supplementation was supposed to help prevent.

- Calcium supplementation during pregnancy and lactation is generally contraindicated. A high-quality, commercial pet food formulated for feeding through gestation and lactation is recommended.

- Although frank deficiencies of vitamins are highly unusual in pets today, select deficiencies and toxicities can occur as a result of improper feeding practices. Feeding excessive levels of foods that contain marginal levels of vitamin E and high amounts of polyunsaturated fatty acids (PUFAs) can lead to vitamin E deficiency in cats. On the other hand, feeding cats foods that contain too much vitamin A can lead to toxicity. Thiamin deficiency can be induced by feeding

370

raw fish, and biotin deficiency can be caused by feeding raw egg whites. Both raw fish and raw egg whites contain inhibitory substances.

- Supplementing a cat's diet with liver, cod liver oil, or other fish liver oils can cause vitamin A and D toxicosis.

- **Tip:** People should resist the temptation to give a large amount of human foods to pets. Many problems can result, such as obesity, deficiencies of minerals and vitamins, parasite transmission, toxic levels of some vitamins and minerals, orthopedic deformities, digestive upsets, and diarrhea.

- **Caution:** Although small amounts of chocolate given occasionally as special treats are not likely to be harmful, death has been reported to occur when dogs ingest larger quantities of chocolate (from theobromine toxicity). Because dogs generally love the taste of chocolate, owners should be sure to keep chocolate out of a pet's reach; approximately $1\frac{1}{2}$ pounds (lbs) of milk chocolate could be lethal for a 25-lb dog.

- Contrary to popular belief, there is no evidence that adding brewer's yeast to pet foods repels fleas or mites.

- Although many hypotheses have been advanced for the cause of gastric dilatation–volvulus (GDV, or *bloat*), no nutrient causes have been identified. Development of GDV is not related to any component in pet foods or to the type of food that is fed. However, it is thought that large, deep-chested dogs might be predisposed to developing this often-fatal disorder. In addition, certain feeding practices, such as feeding one large meal per day, and exposure to stress may be precipitating factors.

SECTION 5

REFERENCES

1. Markwell PJ, Erk W, Parkin GD, and others: Obesity in the dog, *J Small Anim Pract* 31:533-537, 1990.

2. Armstrong J, Lund EM: Obesity: research update. In *Proceedings of the Petfood Forum*, Chicago, 1997, Watts Publishing.

3. Crane SE: Occurrence and management of obesity in companion animals, *J Small Anim Pract* 32:275-282, 1991.

4. Edney ATB, Smith AM: Study of obesity in dogs visiting veterinary practices in the United Kingdom, *Vet Rec* 118:391-396, 1986.

5. Glickman LT, Sonnenschein EG, Glickman NW, and others: Pattern of diet and obesity in female adult pet dogs, *Vet Clin Nutr* 2:6-13, 1995.

6. Sloth C: Practical management of obesity in dogs and cats, *J Small Anim Pract* 33:178-182, 1992.

7. Scarlett JM, Donoghue S, Siadla J, and others: Overweight cats: prevalence and risk factors, *J Obesity* 18:S22-28, 1994.

8. National Institute of Health: Health implications of obesity: National Institutes of Health consensus development conference statement, *Ann Int Med* 103:1073-1077, 1985.

9. Vasselli JR, Cleary MP, van Itallie TB: Modern concepts of obesity, *Nutr Rev* 41:361-373, 1983.

10. van Itallie TB: Morbid obesity: a hazardous disorder that resists conservative treatment, *Am J Clin Nutr* 33:358-363, 1980.

11. Mattheeuws D, Rottiers R, Kaneko JJ, and others: Diabetes mellitus in dogs: relationship of obesity to glucose tolerance and insulin response, *Am J Vet Res* 45:98-103, 1984.

12. Mattheeuws D, Rottiers R, Baeyens D, and others: Glucose tolerance and insulin response in obese dogs, *J Am Anim Hosp Assoc* 20:287-290, 1984.

13. Edney ATB: Management of obesity in the dog, *Vet Med Small Anim Clin* 69:46-49, 1974.

14. Kealy RD, Lawler DF, Ballam JM, and others: Five-year longitudinal study on limited food consumption and development of osteoarthritis in coxofemoral joints of dogs, *J Am Vet Med Assoc* 210:222-225, 1997.

15. Shofer FS, Sonnenschein EG, Goldschmidt NM, and others: Histopathologic and dietary prognostic factors for canine mammary carcinoma, *Breast Canc Res Treat* 13:49-60, 1989.

16. Scarlett JM, Donohue S: Health effects of obesity in cats, *Proc Waltham Int Symp Pet Nutr Health*, 90, 1997.

17. Knittle JL, Fellner FG, Brown RE: Adipose tissue development in man, *Am J Clin Nutr* 30:762-766, 1977.

18. Bjorntorp P: The role of adipose tissue in human obesity. In Greenwood MRC, editor: *Obesity— contemporary issues in clinical nutrition*, New York, 1983, Churchill Livingstone.

19. Lemonnier D: Effect of age, sex and site of cellularity of the adipose tissue in mice and rats rendered obese by a high fat diet, *J Clin Invest* 51:2907, 1972.

20. Faust IM, Johnson PR, Hirsch J: Long-term effects of early nutritional experience on the development of obesity in the rat, *J Nutr* 110:2027-2034, 1980.

21. Johnson PR, Stern JS, Greenwood MRC, and others: Effect of early nutrition on adipose cellularity and pancreatic insulin release in the Zucker rat, *J Nutr* 103:738-743, 1973.

22. Sibley KW: Diagnosis and management of the overweight dog, *Br Vet J* 140:124-131, 1984.

23. Kaufman E: Obesity in dogs, *Vet Tech* 7:5-8, 1986.

24. Leibowitz SF: Hypothalamic neurotransmitters in relation to normal and disturbed eating patterns. In Wurtman RJ, Wurtman JJ, editors: *Human obesity*, New York, 1987, New York Academy of Sciences.

25. Houpt KA, Hintz HF: Obesity in dogs, *Can Pract* 5:54-57, 1978.

26. Ravussin E, Burnand B, Schutz Y, and others: Twenty-four hour energy expenditure and resting metabolic rate in obese, moderately obese and control subjects, *Am J Clin Nutr* 35:566-573, 1982.

27. Halliday D, Hesp R, Stalley SF, and others: Resting metabolic rate, weight, surface area and body composition in obese women, *Int J Obes* 3:1-6, 1979.

28. Hoffmans M, Pfeifer WA, Gundlach BL, and others: Resting metabolic rate in obese and normal weight women, *Int J Obes* 3:111-118, 1979.

29. James WPT, Davies HL, Bailes J, and others: Elevated metabolic rates in obesity, *Lancet* 1:1122-1125, 1978.

30. Ashwell M: Brown adipose tissue—relevant to obesity?, *Hum Nutr App Nutr* 30:763-770, 1983.

31. Nair KS, Halliday D, Garrow JS: Thermic response to isoenergetic protein, carbohydrate or fat meals in lean and obese subjects, *Clin Sci* 65:307-312, 1983.

32. Horton ES: An overview of the assessment and regulation of energy balance in humans, *Am J Clin Nutr* 38:972-977, 1983.

33. Applegate EA, Upton DE, Stern JS: Food intake, body composition and blood lipids following treadmill exercise in male and female rats, *Physio Behav* 28:917-920, 1982.

34. Meyer DJ: Clinical manifestations associated with endocrine disorders, *Vet Clin North Am Small Anim Pract* 7:433-441, 1977.

35. Milne KL, Hayes Hm Jr: Epidemiologic features of canine hypothyroidism, *Cornell Vet* 71:3-14, 1981.

36. Panciera DL: A retrospective study of 66 cases of canine hypothyroidism, *J Am Vet Med Assoc* 204:761-767, 1994.

37. Randolph JF, Jorgensen LS: Selected feline endocrinopathies, *Vet Clin North Am Small Anim Pract* 14:1261-1270, 1984.

38. Nesbitt GH, Izzo J, Peterson L, and others: Canine hypothyroidism: a retrospective study of 108 cases, *J Am Vet Med Assoc* 177:1117-1122, 1980.

39. Panciera DL: Clinical manifestations of canine hypothyroidism, *Vet Med*, 44-49, Jan 1997.

40. Anderson RK: Canine hypothyroidism, *Small Anim Pract* 1:103-109, 1979.

41. Peterson ME: Hyperadrenocorticism, *Vet Clin North Am Small Anim Pract* 14:731-749, 1984.

42. Anderson RS: obesity in the dog and cat, *Vet Ann* 14:182-186, 1975.

43. Houpt KA, Coren B, Hintz HF, and others: Effect of sex and reproductive status on sucrose preference, food intake and body weight of dogs, *J Am Vet Med Assoc* 174:1083-1085, 1979.

44. Root M: Early spay-neuter in the cat: effect on development of obesity and metabolic rate, *Vet Clin Nutr* 2:132-134, 1995.

45. Duch DS, Chow FHC, Hamar DW, and others: The effect of castration and body weight on the occurrence of the feline urological syndrome, *Fel Pract* 8:35-40, 1978.

46. Fettman MJ, Stanton CA, Banks LL, and others: Effects of neutering on body weight, metabolic rate and glucose tolerance of domestic cats, *Res Vet Sci* 62:131-136, 1997.

47. Flynn MF, Hardie EM, Armstrong PJ: Effect of ovariohysterectomy on maintenance energy requirement in cats, *J Am Vet Med Assoc* 209:1572-1581, 1996.

48. Cleary MP, Vasselli JR, Greenwood MR: Development of obesity in Zucker (fa/fa) rat in absence of hyperphagia, *Am J Physiol* 238:E284-292, 1980.

49. Lin PY, Romsos DR, Vander Tuig JG, and others: Maintenance energy requirements, energy retention and heat production of young obese (ob/ob) and lean mice fed a high fat or high-carbohydrate diet, *J Nutr* 109:1143-1153, 1979.

50. Kleyn PW, Fat W, Kovats SG, and others: Identification and characterization of the mouse obesity gene "tubby": a member of a novel gene family, *Cell* 85:281-290, 1996.

51. Brook CGD, Huntley RMC, Slack J: Influence of heredity and environment in determination of skin fold thickness in children, *Br Med J* 2:719-721, 1975.

52. Bouchard C: Body composition in adopted and biological siblings, *Hum Biol* 57:61-75, 1985.

53. Stunkard AJ, Sorensen TIA, Hanis C, and others: An adoption study of human obesity, *N Engl J Med* 314:193-198, 1986.

54. Houpt KA, Smith SL: Taste preferences and their relation to obesity in dogs and cats, *Can Vet J* 22:77-81, 1981.

55. Scalafani A, Springer O: Dietary obesity in adult rats: similarities to hypothalamic and human obesity syndromes, *Physiol Behav* 17:461-471, 1976.

56. Slattery JM, Potter RM: Hyperphagia: a necessary precondition to obesity?, *Appetite* 6:133-142, 1985.

57. Hill SW: Eating responses of humans during meals, *J Comp Physiol Psych* 86:652-657, 1974.

58. Edelman B, Engell D, Bronstein P, and others: Environmental effects on the intake of overweight and normal-weight men, *Appetite* 7:71-83, 1986.

59. Fabry P, Tepperman J: Meal frequency—a possible factor in human pathology, *Am J Clin Nutr* 23:1059, 1970.

60. Blundell JE: Nutritional manipulation for altering food intake. In Wurtman RJ, Wurtman JJ, editors: *Human obesity*, New York, 1987, New York, Academy of Sciences.

61. Hand MS, Armstrong PJ, Allen TA: Obesity: occurrence, treatment and prevention, *Vet Clin North Am Small Anim Pract* 19:447-475, 1989.

62. Wilkinson MJA, McEwan NA: Use of ultrasound in the measurement of subcutaneous fat and prediction of total body fat in dogs, *J Nutr* 121:S47-S50, 1991.

63. Sunvold GD, Bouchard GF: Assessment of obesity and associated metabolic disorders. In Reinhart GA, Carey DP, editors: *Recent advances in canine and feline nutrition*, vol 2, Iams Nutrition Symposium Proceedings, Wilmington, Ohio, 1998, Orange Frazer Press.

64. Toll PW, Gross KL, Berryhill SA, and others DE: Usefulness of dual energy x- ray absorptiometry for body composition measurement in adult dogs, *J Nutr* 124(suppl):2601S-2603S, 1994.

65. Jensen MD: Research techniques for body composition assessment, *J Am Dietetic Assoc* 93:A22, 1993.

66. Munday HS, Booles D, Anderson P, and others: The repeatability of body composition measurements in dogs and cats using dual energy x-ray absorptiometry, *J Nutr* 124(suppl):2619S-2621S, 1994.

67. Joshua JO: The obese dog and some clinical repercussions, *Small Anim Pract* 11:601-606, 1970.

68. Iams Company: How to visually assess cat and dog body condition, *Iams Food for Thought Technical Bull*, No. 77R, 1996.

69. Laflamme D: Development and validation of a body condition score system for cats: a clinical tool, *Feline Pract* 25:13-18, 1997.

70. Laflamme D: Development and validation of a body condition score system for dogs, *Canine Pract* 22:10-15, 1997.

71. Ravussin E, Burnand B, Schutz Y, and others: Energy expenditure before and during energy restriction in obese patients, *Am J Clin Nutr* 41:753-759, 1985.

72. Weinsier RL, Wilson LJ, Lee J: Medically safe rate of weight loss for the treatment of obesity: a guideline based on risk of gallstone formation, *Am J Med* 98:115-117, 1995.

73. Mayer J, Marshall NB, Vitalle JJ: Exercise, food intake and body weight in normal rats and genetically obese adult mice, *Am J Physiol* 177:544-548, 1954.

74. Pi-Sunyer FX: Exercise effects on calorie intake. In Wurtman RJ, Wurtman JJ, editors: *Human obesity*, New York, 1987, New York Academy of Sciences.

75. Butterwick F, Markwell PJ: Changes in the body composition of cats during weight reduction by controlled dietary energy restriction, *Vet Rec* 138:354-357, 1996.

76. Burgess NS: Effect of a very-low-calorie diet on body composition and resting metabolic rate in obese men and women, *J Am Diet Assoc* 91:430-434, 1991.

77. Schultz CK, Bernauer E, Mole PA: Effects of severe caloric restriction and moderate exercise on basal metabolic rate and hormonal status in adult humans (abstract), *Fed Proc* 39:783, 1980.

78. Scheuer J, Tipton CM: Cardiovascular adaptations to physical training, *Ann Rev Physiol* 39:221-251, 1977.

79. Laflamme DP, Kuhlman G, Lawler DF: Evaluation of weight loss protocols for dogs, *J Am Anim Hosp Assoc* 33:252-259, 1997.

80. Burkholder WJ, Bauer JE: Foods and techniques for managing obesity in companion animals, *J Am Vet Med Assoc* 5:658-662, 1998.

81. Brown RC, Ambrose J: The effect of weight loss on the resting metabolic rate in the obese dog (abstract), *Fed Am Soc Exp Biol* 5:A961, 1991.

82. Center SA, Crawford MA, Guida L and others: A retrospective study of cats (n=77) with severe hepatic lipidosis: (1975-1990), *J Vet Int Med* 7:349-359, 1993.

83. Butterwick RF, Watson TDG, Markwell PJ: The effect of different levels of energy restriction on body weight and composition in obese cats, *Proc 13ᵗʰ Ann Vet Intern Med Forum,* 1029.

84. Biourge VC, Groff JM, Munn RJ and others: Experimental induction of hepatic lipidosis in cats, *Am J Vet Res* 55:1291-1302, 1994.

85. Center SA: Safe weight loss in cats. In Reinhart GA, Carey DP, editors: *Recent advances in canine and feline nutrition*, vol 2, Iams Nutrition Symposium Proceedings, Wilmington, Ohio, 1998, Orange Frazer Press.

86. Leblanc J, Diamond P: The effect of meal frequency on postprandial thermogenesis in the dog, *Fed Proc* 44:1678, 1985 (abstract).

87. Danforth E Jr: Diet and obesity, *Am J Clin Nutr* 41:1132-1145, 1985.

88. Danforth E Jr: The role of thyroid hormones and insulin in the regulation of energy metabolism, *Am J Clin Nutr* 38:1006-1017, 1983.

89. Schwartz RS, Ravussin E, Massari M, and others: The thermic effect of carbohydrate versus fat feeding in man, *Metabolism* 34:285-293, 1985.

90. Acheson KJ, Ravussin E, Wahren J, and others: Nutritional influences on lipogenesis and thermogenesis after a carbohydrate meal, *Am J Physiol* 246:E62-E70, 1984.

91. Center SA, Reynolds AP, Harte J, and others: Clinical effects of rapid weight loss in obese pet cats with and without supplemental L-carnitine, *J Vet Int Med* 11:118, 1997.

92. Bouchard GF, Sunvold GD: Dietary modification of feline obesity with a low fat, low fiber diet. In Reinhart GA, Carey DP, editors: *Recent advances in canine and feline nutrition*, vol 2, Iams Nutrition Symposium Proceedings, Wilmington, Ohio, 1998, Orange Frazer Press.

93. Porikos K, Hagamen S: Is fiber satiating? Effects of a high fiber preload on subsequent food intake of normal-weight and obese young men, *Appetite* 7:153-162, 1986.

94. Levine AS, Tallman JR, Grace MK, and others: Effect of breakfast cereals on short-term food intake, *Am J Clin Nutr* 50:1303-1307, 1989.

95. Burley VJ, Leeds AR, Blundell JE: The effect of high and low fibre breakfasts on hunger, satiety and food intake in a subsequent meal, *Int J Obes* 1(suppl):87-93, 1987.

96. Burley VJ, Blundell JE: Time course of the effects of dietary fiber on energy intake and satiety. In Southgate DAT, Waldron K, Johnson IT, and others, editors: *Dietary fiber: chemical and biological aspects*, Cambridge, UK, 1990, Royal Society of Chemistry.

97. Butterwick RF, Markwell PJ: Effect of amount and type of dietary fiber on food intake in energy-restricted dogs, *Am J Vet Res* 58:272-276, 1997.

98. Butterwick RF, Markwell PJ: Effect of level and source of dietary fibre on food intake in the dog (abstract), *Proc Waltham Int Symp Pet Nutr Health*, 1993.

99. Jackson JR, Laflamme DP, Owens SF: Effects of dietary fiber content on satiety in dogs, *Vet Clin Nutr* 4:130-134, 1997.

100. Jewell DE, Toll PW: Effects of fiber on food intake in dogs, *Vet Clin Nutr* 3:115-118, 1996.

101. Eastwood MA, Brydon WG, Tadesse K: Effect of fiber on colon function. In Spiller GM, Kay RM, editors: *Medical aspects of dietary fiber*, New York, 1980, Plenum Press.

102. Vahouny GV, Cassidy MM: Dietary fibers and absorption of nutrients (review) *Proc Soc Exp Biol Med* 180:432-446, 1985.

103. Leibetseder J: Fibre in the dog's diet. In Anderson RS, editor: *Nutrition and behavior in dogs and cats*, Oxford, England, 1984, Permagon Press.

104. Cummings JH: Nutritional implications of dietary fiber, *Am J Clin Nutr* 31:S21-S29, 1978.

105. Fernandez R. Phillips SF: Components of fiber impair iron absorption in the dog, *Am J Clin Nutr* 35:107-112, 1982.

106. Fahey GC Jr, Merchen NR, Corbin JE, and others: Dietary fiber for dogs. Part I. Effects of graded levels of dietary beet pulp on nutrient intake, digestibility, metabolizable energy and digesta mean retention time, *J Anim Sci* 68:4229-4235, 1990.

107. Sunvold GD, Fahey CG Jr, Merchen NR, and others: Dietary fiber for dogs. IV. In vitro fermentation of selected fiber sources by dog fecal inoculum and in vivo digestion and metabolism of fiber-supplemented diets, *J Anim Sci* 73:1099-1119, 1995.

108. Sunvold GD, Fahey CG Jr, Merchen NR, and others: Dietary fiber for cats: in vitro fermentation of selected fiber sources by cat fecal inoculum and in vivo utilization of diets containing selected fiber sources and their blends, *J Anim Sci* 73:2329-2339, 1995.

109. Burrows CF, Kronfeld DL, Banta CA, and others: Effects of fiber on digestibility and transit time in dogs, *J Nutr* 112:1726-1732, 1982.

110. Goggin JM, Schryver HF, Hintz HF: The effects of ad libitum feeding and caloric dilution on the domestic cat's ability to maintain energy balance, *Feline Pract* 21:7-11, 1993.

111. Rogers QR, Morris JF, Freedland RA: Lack of hepatic enzymatic adaptation to low and high levels of dietary protein in the adult cat, *Enzyme* 22:348-356, 1977.

112. Hendriks WH, Moughan PJ, Tarttelin MF: Dietary excretion of endogenous nitrogen metabolites in adult domestic cats using a protein-free diet and the regression technique, *J Nutr* 127:623-629, 1997.

113. Biourge VC, Massat B, Groff JM, and others: Effects of protein, lipid or carbohydrate supplementation on hepatic lipid accumulation during rapid weight loss in obese cats, *Am J Vet Res* 55:1406-1415, 1994.

114. Dimski DS: Feline hepatic lipidosis, *Sem Vet Med Surg (Small Anim)* 12:28-33, 1997.

115. Center SA, Reynolds AP, Harte J, and others: Clinical effects of rapid weight loss in obese pet cats with and without supplemental L-carnitine (abstract), *J Vet Int Med* 11:118, 1997.

116. Brady LJ, Armstrong MK, Muiruri KL: Influence of prolonged fasting in the dog on glucose turnover and blood metabolites, *J Nutr* 107:1053-1061, 1977.

117. Rapoport A, From GLA, Husdan H: Metabolic studies in prolonged fasting. I. Inorganic metabolism and kidney function, *Metabolism* 14:31-46, 1965.

118. Rapoport A, From GLA, Husdan H: Metabolic studies in prolonged fasting. II. Organic metabolism, *Metabolism* 14:47-64, 1965.

119. Lemieux G, Plante GE: The effect of starvation in the normal dog including the Dalmatian Coach Hound, *Metabolism* 17:620-630, 1968.

120. Bruijne JJ, De Altszuler N, Hampshire J: Fat mobilization and plasma hormone levels in fasted dogs, *Metabolism* 30:190-194, 1981.

121. Owen OE, Felig P, Morgan A: Liver and kidney metabolism during prolonged starvation, *J Clin Invest* 48:574-583, 1969.

122. Stunkard AJ: Conservative treatments for obesity, *Am J Clin Nutr* 45:1142-1154, 1987.

123. Fidanza F: Effects of starvation on body composition, *Am J Clin Nutr* 33:1562-1566, 1980.

124. Isner JM, Sours HE, Paris AL: Sudden, unexpected death in avid dieters using the liquid-protein-modified-fast diet, *Circulation* 60:1401-1412, 1979.

125. Johnson JA, Austin C, Breuer GJ: Incidence of canine appendicular musculoskeletal disorders in 16 veterinary teaching hospitals from 1980-1989, *J Vet Comp Orthop Trauma* 7:56-69, 1994.

126. Richardson DC, Zentek J: Nutrition and osteochondrosis, *Vet Clin North Am Small Anim Pract* 28:115-135, 1998.

127. Richardson DC, Toll PWL: Relationship of nutrition to developmental skeletal disease in young dogs, *Vet Clin Nutr* 4:6-13, 1997.

129. Richardson DC: The role of nutrition in canine hip dysplasia, *Vet Clin North Am Small Anim Pract* 22:529-541, 1992.

130. Kasstrom H: Nutrition, weight gain and development of hip dysplasia, *Acta Radiol* 334(suppl):135-179, 1975.

131. Slater MR, Scarlett JM, Kaderly RE, and others: Breed, gender, and age risk factors for canine osteochondritis dissecans, *J Vet Comp Orthop Trauma* 4:100-106, 1991.

132. Slater MR, Scarlett JM, Donoughue S, and others: Diet and exercise as potential risk factors for osteochondritis dissecans in dogs, *Am J Vet Res* 53:2119-2124, 1992.

133. Willis MB: Hip scoring: a review of 1985-1986, *Vet Rec* 118:461-462, 1986.

134. Corley EA, Hogan PM: Trends in hip dysplasia control: analysis of radiographs submitted to the Orthopedic Foundation for Animals: 1974 to 1984, *J Am Vet Med Assoc* 187:638-640, 1985.

135. Saville PD, Lieber CS: Increases in skeletal calcium and femur thickness produced by undernutrition, *J Nutr* 99:141-144, 1969.

136. Dluzniewska KA, Obtulowicz A, Koltek K: On the relationship between diet, rate of growth and skeletal deformities in school children, *Folia Med Craco* 7:115-126, 1965.

137. Hedhammar A, Wu F, Krook L, and others: Overnutrition and skeletal disease—an experimental study in growing Great Dane dogs, *Cornell Vet* 64(suppl 5):1-159, 1974.

138. Kealy RD, Olsson SE, Monti KL, and others: Effects of limited food consumption on the incidence of hip dysplasia in growing dogs, *J Am Vet Med Assoc* 201:857-863, 1992.

139. Lust G, Geary JC, Sheffy BE: Development of hip dysplasia in dogs, *Am J Vet Res* 34:87-91, 1973.

140. Lust G, Rendano VT, Summers BA: Canine hip dysplasia: concepts and diagnosis, *J Vet Med Assoc* 187:638-640, 1985.

141. Kealy RD, Lawler DF, Ballam JM, and others: Five-year longitudinal study on limited food consumption and development of osteoarthritis in coxofemoral joints of dogs, *J Am Vet Med Assoc* 210:222-225, 1997.

142. Olsson SE, Reiland S: The nature of osteochondrosis in animals, *Acta Radiol Scand* 358(suppl):299-306, 1978.

143. Dammrich K: Relationship between nutrition and bone growth in large and giant dogs, *J Nutr* 121:S114-S121, 1991.

144. Crenshaw TD, Budde RQ, Lauten SD, and others: Nutritional effects on bone strength in the growing canine. In Reinhart GA, Carey DP, editors: *Recent advances in canine and feline nutrition*, vol 2, Iams Nutrition Symposium Proceedings, Wilmington, Ohio, 1998, Orange Frazer Press.

145. Alexander JE, Wood LLH: *Comparative growth study* (technical report), Lewisburg, Ohio, 1990, The Iams Company.

146. Lepine AJ: Nutritional management of the large breed puppy. In Reinhart GA, Carey DP, editors: *Recent advances in canine and feline nutrition*, vol 2, Iams Nutrition Symposium Proceedings, Wilmington, Ohio, 1998, Orange Frazer Press.

147. Nap RC, Hazewinkel HAW, Vorrhout G, and others: The influence of the dietary protein content on growth in giant breed dogs, *J Vet Comp Orthop Trauma* 6:1-8, 1993.

148. Association of American Feed Control Officials: Pet food regulations. In *AAFCO official publication*, Atlanta, 1998, The Association.

149. Blum JW, Zentek J, Meyer H: Unterscuchngen einer unterschiedlichen Energiveersorgung auf die Wachstumsintensitat und Skelettentwicklung bei wachsenden Doggen, *J Vet Med* 39:568-574, 1992.

150. Hazewinkel HAW, Goedegebuure SA, Poulos PW, and others: Influences of chronic calcium excess on the skeletal development of growing Great Danes, *J Am Anim Hosp Assoc* 21:377-391, 1985.

151. Hazewinkel HA: Calcium metabolism and skeletal development of dogs. In Burger IH, Rivers JPW, editors: *Nutrition of the dog and cat*, Cambridge, England, 1989, Cambridge University Press.

152. Goedegebuure SA, Hazewinkel HAW: Morphological findings in young dogs chronically fed a diet containing excess calcium, *Vet Pathol* 23:594-605, 1986.

153. National Research Council: *Nutrient requirements of dogs*, National Academy of Sciences, Washington, DC, 1974, National Academy Press.

154. National Research Council: *Nutrient requirements of dogs*, National Academy of Sciences, Washington, DC, 1985, National Academy Press.

155. Carrig CB: Comparative radiology: dysplasia in the canine forelimb. In Potchem ET, editor: *Current concepts in radiology*, vol 3, St Louis, 1977, Mosby.

156. Stephens LC, Norrdin RW, Benjamin SA: Effects of calcium supplementation and sunlight exposure on growing Beagle dogs, *Am J Vet Res* 466:2037-2042, 1985.

157. Allen LH: Calcium bioavailability and absorption: a review, *Am J Clin Nutr* 35:783-808, 1982.

158. Hedhammer A, Krook L, Schrijver HF, and others: Calcium balance in the dog. In Anderson RS, editor: *Nutrition of the dog and cat*, Oxford, England, 1980, Pergamon Press.

159. Hazewinkel HAW, Brom WE, van den Klooster AT, and others: Calcium metabolism in Great Dane dogs fed diets with various calcium and phosphorus levels, *J Nutr* 121:S99-S106, 1991.

160. Robertson BT, Burns MJ: Zinc metabolism and zinc-deficiency syndrome in the dog, *Am J Vet Res* 24:997-1002, 1963.

161. Kunkle GA: Zinc responsive dermatoses in dogs. In Kirk RW, editor: *Current veterinary therapy VII: small animal practice*, Philadelphia, 1980, WB Saunders.

162. Hunt JR, Johnson PE, Swan PB: Dietary conditions influencing relative zinc availability from foods in the rat and correlations with in vitro measurements, *J Nutr* 117:1913-1923, 1987.

163. Pecoud A, Donzel P, Schelling JL: Effect of foodstuffs on the absorption of zinc sulfate, *Clin Pharmacol Ther* 17:469-474, 1975.

164. Lauten SD, Brawner WR, Hathcock JT: Growth and body composition of the large breed puppy as affected by diet. In Reinhart GA, Carey DP, editors: *Recent advances in canine and feline nutrition*, vol 2, Iams Nutrition Symposium Proceedings, Wilmington, Ohio, 1998, Orange Frazer Press.

165. Goodman SA, Montgomery RD, Fitch RB, and others: Serial orthopedic examinations of growing Great Dane puppies fed three diets varying in calcium and phosphorus. In Reinhart GA, Carey DP, editors: *Recent advances in canine and feline nutrition*, vol 2, Iams Nutrition Symposium Proceedings, Wilmington, Ohio, 1998, Orange Frazer Press.

166. Rumph PF: Kinetic gait analysis in developing Great Dane dogs. In Reinhart GA, Carey DP, editors: *Recent advances in canine and feline nutrition*, vol 2, Iams Nutrition Symposium Proceedings, Wilmington, Ohio, 1998, Orange Frazer Press.

167. Kuhlman G, Boourge V: Nutrition of the large and giant breed dog with emphasis on skeletal development, *Vet Clin Nutr* 4:89-95, 1997.

168. Austad R, Bjerkas E: Eclampsia in the bitch, *J Small Anim Pract* 17:793-798, 1976.

169. Boda JM, Cole HH: The influence of dietary calcium and phosphorus on the influence of milk fever in dairy cattle, *J Dairy Sci* 37:360-372, 1954.

170. Wiggers KD, Nelson DK, Jacobson NL: Prevention of parturient paresis by a low-calcium diet prepartum: a field study, *J Dairy Sci* 58:430-431, 1975.

171. Gratzl E, Pommer A: Moller-Barlow's disease in the dog, *Wien Tierarztl Mschr* 28:481-492, 513-519, 531-537, 1941.

172. Alexander JW: Selected skeletal dysplasias: craniomandibular osteopathy, multiple cartilaginous exostoses, and hypertrophic osteodystrophy, *Vet Clin North Am Small Anim Pract* 13:55-70, 1983.

173. Stogdale L: Foreleg lameness in rapidly growing dogs, *J South Afr Vet Assoc* 50:61-68, 1979.

174. Meier H, Clark ST, Schnelle GB, and others: Hypertrophic osteodystrophy associated with disturbance of vitamin C synthesis in dogs, *J Am Vet Med Assoc* 130:483-491, 1957.

175. Grondalen J: Metaphyseal osteopathy (hypertrophic osteodystrophy) in growing dogs: a clinical study, *J Small Anim Pract* 17:721-735, 1976.

176. Holmes JR: Suspected skeletal scurvy in the dog, *Vet Rec* 74:801-813, 1962.

177. Woodard JC: Canine hypertrophic osteodystrophy; a study of the spontaneous disease in litter mates, *Vet Pathol* 19:337-354, 1982.

178. Muir P, Dubielzig RR, Johnson KA, and others: Hypertrophic osteodystrophy and calvarial hyperostosis, *Comp Cont Ed Pract Vet* 18:143 151, 1996.

179. Teare JA, Krook L, Kallfelz A, and others: Ascorbic acid deficiency and hypertrophic osteodystrophy in the dog: a rebuttal, *Cornell Vet* 69:384-401, 1979.

180. Clarke RE: Hypertrophic osteodystrophy in the canine associated with a lowered resistance to infection—an unusual case history, *Aust Vet Pract* 8:39-43, 1978.

181. Schulz KS, Paynd JT, Aronson E: *Escherichia coli* bacteremia associated with hypertrophic osteodystrophy in a dog, *J Am Vet Med Assoc* 199:1170-1173, 1991.

182. National Research Council: *Nutrient requirements of cats*, National Academy of Sciences, Washington, DC, 1986, National Academy Press.

183. Cordy DR: Experimental production of steatitis (yellow fat disease) in kittens fed a commercial canned cat food and prevention of the condition by vitamin E, *Cornell Vet* 44:310-318, 1954.

184. Gaskell CJ, Leedale AH, Douglas SW: Pansteatitis in the cat: a report of five cases, *J Small Anim Pract* 16:117-121, 1975.

185. Munson TO, Holzworth J, Small E, and others: Steatitis ("yellow fat") in cats fed canned red tuna, *J Am Vet Med Assoc* 133:563-568, 1958.

186. Griffiths RC, Thornton GW, Willson JE: Pansteatitis (yellow fat) in cats, *J Am Vet Med Assoc* 137:126-128, 1960.

187. Watson ADJ, Porges WL, Huxtable CR, and others: Pansteatitis in a cat, *Aust Vet J* 49:388-392, 1973.

188. Lewis LD, Morris ML, Hand MS: Renal failure. In *Small animal clinical nutrition*, ed 3, Topeka, Kan, 1987, Mark Morris Associates.

189. English PB, Seawright AA: Deforming cervical spondylosis of the cat, *Aust Vet J* 40:376-381, 1964.

190. Cho DY, Frey RA, Guffy MM, and others: Hypervitaminosis A in the dog, *Am J Vet Res* 36:1597-1603, 1975.

191. Goldy GG, Burr JR, Longardner CN, and others: Effects of measured doses of vitamin A fed to healthy Beagle dogs for 26 weeks, *Vet Clin Nutr* 3:42-49, 1996.

192. Cline JL, Czarnecki-Maulden GL, Losonsky JM, and others: Effect of vitamin A on bone density and mucosal epithelium in dogs (abstract), *J Anim Sci* 73(suppl):192, 1995.

193. Seawright AA, English PB, Gartner RJW: Hypervitaminosis A and deforming cervical spondylosis of the cat, *J Comp Pathol* 77:29-38, 1967.

194. United States Department of Agriculture: Nutritive value of foods, *Home and Garden Bulletin*, No 72, Washington, DC, 1981, US Government Printing Office.

195. Lucke VM, Bardgett PL, Mann PGH, and others: Deforming cervical spondylosis in the cat associated with hypervitaminosis A, *Vet Rec* 82:141-142, 1968.

196. Riser WH, Brodey RS, Shirer JF: Osteodystrophy in mature cats: a nutritional disease, *J Am Radiol Soc* 9:37-46, 1968.

197. Smith DC, Proutt LM: Development of thiamine deficiency in the cat on a diet of raw fish, *Pro Soc Exp Bio Med* 56:1-5, 1944.

198. Jubb KV, Saunders LZ, Coates HV: Thiamine deficiency encephalopathy in cats, *J Comp Pathol* 66:217-227, 1956.

199. Loew FM, Martin CL, Dunlop RH, and others: Naturally occurring and experimental thiamine deficiency in cats receiving commercial cat food, *Can Vet J* 11:109-113, 1970.

200. Jarrett J: Thiaminase-induced encephalopathy, *Vet Med Small Anim Clin* 65:705-708, 1970.
201. Houston D, Hulland TJ: Thiamine deficiency in a team of sled dogs, *Can Vet J* 29:383-385, 1988.
202. Everett GM: Observations on the behavior and neurophysiology of acute thiamin deficient cats, *Am J Physiol* 141:139-149, 1944.
203. Shen CS, Overfield L, Murthy PNA, and others: Effect of feeding raw egg white on pyruvate and propionyl CoA carboxylase activities on tissues of the dog, *Fed Proc* 36:1169, 1977.
204. Greve JH: Effects of thyroid and biotin deficiencies on canine demodicosis, *Dissert Abstr* 24:1757, 1963.
205. Pastoor FJH, van Herck H, van Klooster A, and others: Biotin deficiency in cats as induced by feeding a purified diet containing egg white, *J Nutr* 121:S73-S74, 1991.
206. Carey CJ, Morris JG: Biotin deficiency in the cat and the effect on hepatic propinyl CoA carboxylase, *J Nutr* 107:330-334, 1977.
207. Baker JR, Hughes IB: A case of deforming cervical spondylosis in a cat associated with a diet rich in liver, *Vet Rec* 83:44-45, 1968.
208. Seawright AA, Hrdlicka J: Severe retardation of growth with retention and displacement of incisors in young cats fed a diet of raw sheep liver high in vitamin A, *Aust Vet J* 50:306-315, 1974.
209. Seawright AA, Steele DP, Clark L: Hypervitaminosis A of cats in Brisbane, *Aust Vet J* 44:203-206, 1968.
210. Clark L, Seawright AA, Hrdlicka J: Exostoses in hypervitaminotic A cats with optimal calcium-phosphorus intakes, *J Small Anim Pract* 11:553-561, 1970.
211. Fry PD: Cervical spondylosis in the cat, *J Small Anim Pract* 9:59-61, 1968.
212. Gans JH, Korson R, Cater MR, and others: Effects of short-term and long-term theobromine administration to male dogs, *Toxicol Appl Pharmacol* 53:481-496, 1980.
213. Welch RM, Hsu SY, DeAngelis RL: Effect of arvelor 1254, phenobarbital and polycyclic aromatic hydrocarbons on the plasma clearance of caffeine in the rat, *Clin Pharmacol Ther* 22:791-798, 1977.
214. Drouillard DD, Vesell ES, Dvorchick BN: Studies on theobromine disposition in normal subjects, *Clin Pharmacol Ther* 23:296-302, 1978.
215. Hoskam EG, Haagsma J: Chocolate poisoning terminating in the death of two Dachshunds, *Tijdschr Diergeneesk* 99:523-525, 1974.
216. Decker RA, Meyers GH: Theobromine poisoning in a dog, *J Am Vet Med Assoc* 161:198-199, 1972.
217. Glauberg A, Blumenthal PH: Chocolate poisoning in the dog, *J Am Anim Hosp Assoc* 19:246-248, 1983.
218. Zoumas BL, Kreiser WR, Martin RA: Theobromine and caffeine content of chocolate products, *J Food Sci* 45:314-316, 1980.
219. Shannon WR: Thiamine chloride: an aid in the solution of the mosquito problem, *Minn Med* 26:799-803, 1943.
220. Eder HL: Flea bites: prevention and treatment with thiamine hydrochloride, *Arch Ped* 62:300, 1945.
221. Halliwell REW: Ineffectiveness of thiamine (vitamin B_1) as a flea-repellent in dogs, *J Am Anim Hosp Assoc* 18:423-426, 1982.
222. Baker NF, Farver TB: Failure of brewer's yeast as a repellent to fleas on dogs, *J Am Vet Med Assoc* 183:212-214, 1983.
223. Farkas MC, Farkas JN: Hemolytic anemia due to ingestion of onions in a dog, *J Am Anim Hosp Assoc* 10:65-66, 1974.
224. Spice RN: Hemolytic anemia associated with ingestion of onions in a dog, *Can Vet J* 17:181-183, 1976.
225. Kay JM: Onion toxicity in a dog, *Mod Vet Prac* 64:477-478, 1983.
226. Muller GH, Kirk RW, Scott DW: *Small animal dermatology*, ed 4, Philadelphia, 1989, WB Saunders.
227. Kirk RW: Nutrition and the integument, *J Sm Anim Pract* 32:283-288, 1991.

228. The Iams Company: *Data*, Iams Technical Center, Lewisburg, Ohio, 1993.

229. Brockman DJ, Washabau RJ, Drobatz KJ: Canine gastric dilation/volvulus syndrome in a veterinary critical care unit: 2965 cases (1986-1992), *J Am Vet Med Assoc* 207:460-464, 1995.

230. Glickman LT, Glickman NW, Perez CM, and others: Analysis of risk factors for gastric dilatation and dilatation-volvulus in dogs, *J Am Vet Med Assoc* 204:1465-1471, 1994.

231. Tordoff RJ: Gastric dilatation-volvulus, *Comp Cont Ed Pract Vet* 1:142-149, 1979.

232. Bredal WP, Eggertsdottir AV, Austefjord O: Acute gastric dilatation in cats: a case series, *Acta Vet Scand* 37:445-451, 1996.

233. Glickman LT, Lantz GC, Schellenberg DB, and others: A prospective study of survival and recurrence following the acute gastric dilatation-volvulus syndrome in 136 dogs, *J Am Anim Hosp Assoc* 34:253-259, 1998.

234. Brourman JD, Schertel ER, Allen DA, and others: Factors associated with perioperative mortality in dogs with surgically managed gastric dilatation-volvulus: 137 cases (1988-1993), *J Am Vet Med Assoc* 208:1855-1858, 1996.

235. Glickman L: Epidemiology of gastric dilation-volvulus in dogs, *Proc XXI Cong World Small Anim Vet Assoc*, 9-11, 1996.

236. Eggertsdottir AV, Moe L: A retrospective study of conservative treatment of gastric dilatation-volvulus in the dog, *Acta Vet Scan* 36:175-184, 1995.

237. Glickman L, Emerick T, Glickman N, and others: Radiological assessment of the relationship between thoracic conformation and the risk of gastric dilatation-volvulus in dogs, *J Vet Rad Ultrasound* 37:174-180, 1996.

238. Schellenberg D, Yi Q, Glickman N, and others: Influence of thoracic conformation and genetics on the risk of gastric dilatation-volvulus in Irish Setter dogs, *J Am Anim Hosp Assoc* 34:64-73, 1998.

239. Schaible RH, Ziech J, Glickman NW, and others: Predisposition to gastric dilatation-volvulus in relation to genetics of thoracic conformation in Irish Setters, *J Am Anim Hosp Assoc* 33:379-383, 1997.

240. Glickman LT, Glickman NW, Schellenberg DB, and others: Multiple risk factors for the gastric dilatation-volvulus syndrome in dogs: a practitioner/owner case-control study, *J Am Anim Hosp Assoc* 33:197-204, 1997.

241. Elwood CM: Risk factors for gastric dilatation in Irish Setter dogs, *J Small Anim Pract* 39:185-190, 1998.

242. Van Kruiningen HJ, Wojan LD, Stake PE, and others: The influence of diet and feeding frequency on gastric function in the dog, *J Am Anim Hosp Assoc* 23:145-153, 1987.

243. Burrows CF, Bright RM, Spencer CP: Influence of dietary composition on gastric emptying and motility in dogs: potential involvement in acute gastric dilatation, *Am J Vet Res* 46:2609-2612, 1985.

244. Burrows CF, editor: *Bloat panel report*. In the proceedings of a meeting, June 10-11, 1987.

245. Cott B, Shelton M, DeYoung DW: Preliminary report on a GDV questionnaire, *Purebred Dogs: Am Kennel Gaz* 92:76-77, 1975.

246. Caywood D, Teague HD, Jackson DA: Gastric gas analysis in the canine gastric dilatation-volvulus syndrome, *J Am Anim Hosp Assoc* 13:459-462, 1977.

247. Rogolsky B, Van Kruiningen HJ: Short-chain fatty acids and bacterial fermentation in the normal canine stomach and in acute gastric dilatation, *J Am Anim Hosp Assoc* 14:504-515, 1978.

248. Leib MS, Wingfield WE, Twedt DC, and others: Plasma gastrin immunoreactivity in dogs with acute gastric dilatation-volvulus, *J Am Vet Med Assoc* 185:205-208, 1984.

249. Hall JA: Canine gastric dilatation volvulus update, *Sem Vet Med Surg Small Anim* 4:188-193, 1989.

250. Monsanto Chemical Company: *A five-year chronic toxicity study in dogs with santoquin*. In a report to the Food and Drug Administration, 1964.

251. Monsanto Chemical Company: *Ethoxyquin backgrounder*, December 1996.

252. Dzanis DA: Safety of ethoxyquin in dog foods, *J Nutr* 121:S163-S164, 1991.

253. Dzanis DA: Ethoxyquin, product families and more. In *Proceedings of the Petfood Forum*, Chicago, 1998, Watts Publishing.

254. Jones BR, Johnstone AC, Cahill JI, and others: Peripheral neuropathy in cats with inherited primary hyperchylomicronaemia, *Vet Rec* 119:268-22, 1986.

255. Rogers WA, Donovan EF, Kociba GJ: Idiopathic hyperlipoproteinemia in dogs, *J Am Vet Med Assoc* 166:1087-1091, 1975.

256. Hubert B, Braun JP, La Farge F, and others: Hypertriglyceridemia in two related dogs, *Comp Anim Pract* 1:33-35, 1987.

257. Whitney MS, Boon GD, Rebar AH, and others: Ultracentrifugal and electrophoretic characterization of the plasma lipoproteins of Miniature Schnauzer dogs with idiopathic hyperlipoproteincmia, *J Vet Intern Med* 7:253-260, 1993.

258. Watson P, Simpson KW, Bedford PGC: Hypercholesterolemia in Briards in the United Kingdom, *Res Vet Sci* 54:80-85, 1993.

259. Bauer JE: Evaluation and dietary considerations in idiopathic hyperlipidemia in dogs, *J Am Vet Med Assoc* 206:1684-1687, 1995.

260. Overall KL: Coprophagia, In *Clinical behavioral medicine for small animals*, St Louis, 1997. Mosby.

6

Nutritionally Responsive Disorders

Nutrition is a vital component for the health of all companion animals. Section 5 presented information about the results of feeding imbalanced diets and inappropriate food items or providing excess calories during growth and adulthood. Another way that nutrition affects the health of an animal is through inherited disorders of nutrient metabolism. There are several diseases in companion animals that are genetic in origin and affect an animal's ability to either digest, absorb, or metabolize certain nutrients. These disorders are examined in Chapter 30. Dietary management, when effective, is also discussed.

Nutrition also affects health when diet is used to either manage or treat disease. Dietary therapy plays an important role in the treatment of a number of chronic diseases in dogs and cats, even though the underlying cause of the disease may be unrelated to diet. For example, dietary therapy has been proven to be efficacious in the management of diabetes mellitus, urolithiasis, chronic kidney failure, certain skin disorders and intestinal diseases, and feline hepatic lipidosis. Although dietary intervention is occasionally used with a number of other canine and feline diseases, only those disorders for which dietary management has been proven (through controlled research) to be effective in companion animals are included in the chapters of this section.

CHAPTER

30

Inherited Disorders
of Nutrient Metabolism

 Clinical disease can occur in some companion animals as a result of the inability to absorb, assimilate, or metabolize specific nutrients. In some cases, breed predispositions can be found, and the disorder appears to have a genetic basis. Five specific examples in dogs involve lipid metabolism, purine metabolism, and the nutrients vitamin B_{12}, copper, and zinc. Although inherited disorders of metabolism are less well documented in cats, a familial hyperlipidemia has been reported in this species (Table 30-1).

TABLE **30-1**

Selected Inherited Disorders of Nutritional Metabolism

Disorder	Breeds Affected	Treatment
Malabsorption of vitamin B_{12}	Giant Schnauzer	Intramuscular injections of B_{12}
Copper-storage disease	Doberman Pinscher Bedlington Terrier West Highland White Terrier Cocker Spaniel	Copper-restricted diet, zinc acetate supplementation
Lethal acrodermatitis	Bull Terrier	None
Zinc malabsorption	Siberian Husky Alaskan Malamute Great Dane Doberman Pinscher	Zinc supplementation
Hyperlipidemia	Miniature Schnauzers, cats	Restricted-fat, restricted-calorie diet
Abnormal purine metabolism	Dalmatians	Reduced-purine diet, production of alkaline urine, adequate hydration, allopurinol

MALABSORPTION OF VITAMIN B$_{12}$ IN GIANT SCHNAUZERS

Vitamin B$_{12}$ (cobalamin) is required by the body as a coenzyme for several metabolic reactions and for normal deoxyribonucleic acid (DNA) synthesis and erythropoiesis. A deficiency results in macrocytic anemia and neurological impairment. Absorption of B$_{12}$ from the diet requires the presence of a compound called intrinsic factor (IF). In the dog, IF is produced by the gastric mucosa and the pancreas and binds to cobalamin as it passes through the gastrointestinal tract.[1] The IF-B$_{12}$ complex then attaches to specific receptor sites on cells lining the intestinal mucosa and is absorbed into the body. Without the presence of IF, cobalamin absorption is severely impaired.

Like other species, dogs require very small amounts of dietary vitamin B$_{12}$ because of the body's ability to store adequate amounts of B$_{12}$ in the liver for long periods of time. In addition, efficient reabsorption of excreted vitamin B$_{12}$ through the enterohepatic circulation results in efficient conservation of this nutrient. As a result, naturally occurring deficiencies of vitamin B$_{12}$ are not common in the canine species.

Inherited vitamin B$_{12}$ malabsorption has been recognized in Giant Schnauzers.[2] Analysis of pedigrees and a series of breeding studies have demonstrated a simple autosomal recessive mode of inheritance.[3] This disorder appears to be limited to Giant Schnauzers and has not yet been identified in other breeds. The incidence in Giant Schnauzers is not known.

Clinical signs develop when puppies are between 6 and 12 weeks of age, and include failure to thrive, lethargy, loss of appetite, neutropenia (decreased white blood cell count), and nonregenerative anemia. Diagnosis can be confirmed through analysis of serum B$_{12}$ levels, response to parenteral administration of the vitamin, and the presence of elevated levels of methylmalonic acid in the urine. Methylmalonic acid is excreted only when the normal metabolism of certain amino acids, fatty acids, and cholesterol is blocked because of the lack of a necessary B$_{12}$-containing coenzyme. Normally, dogs excrete less than 10 milligrams (mg) of methylmalonic acid per gram (g) of creatinine in the urine. Giant Schnauzers with vitamin B$_{12}$ malabsorption excrete between 4000 and 6000 mg/g of creatinine.[2]

Tests have shown that the intestinal absorption of nutrients in affected dogs is normal, with the exception of vitamin B$_{12}$. Moreover, oral administration of vitamin B$_{12}$, with or without IF, is not effective in resolving clinical signs or in raising serum B$_{12}$ levels. These results and immunoelectron microscopy studies of ileal morphology have indicated that the defect may be located at the level of the cell receptor in the small intestine. Specifically, affected dogs lack a receptor for the IF-cobalamin complex in their brush border microvilli.[3] Long-term treatment of this disorder involves the regular administration of intramuscular injections of vitamin B$_{12}$. This injection bypasses the intestine and provides tissues with the necessary vitamin. Complete resolution of clinical signs has been reported with a dosage as low as 1 mg every 4 to 5 months. In other cases, a weekly dosage of 0.5 mg has been used.[2]

COPPER-STORAGE DISEASE

Copper is needed by the body for iron absorption and transport, hemoglobin formation, and normal functioning of the cytochrome oxidase enzyme system (see Section 1, p. 47, and Section 2, pp. 126-127). The normal metabolism of copper in the body involves the passage of excess copper through the liver and its excretion in bile. Disorders that affect bile excretion often result in an accumulation of copper in the liver, sometimes to toxic levels. In these cases, copper toxicosis in the liver is a secondary disorder that develops as an effect of the primary liver disease. However, a primary, hepatic copper-storage disease exists in certain breeds of dogs. In these cases, the underlying cause of the disease is an accumulation of copper in the liver that eventually results in liver disease. This disorder has been named canine copper toxicosis or copper-storage disease and occurs most prevalently in Bedlington Terriers and West Highland White Terriers and less commonly in Doberman Pinschers and Cocker Spaniels.[4,5]

Inherited canine copper-storage disease involves the impaired removal of copper from the liver, resulting in accumulation of the mineral as the dog ages. Its development is independent of diet and eventually causes chronic, degenerative liver disease. The mode of inheritance in Bedlington Terriers is a simple, autosomal recessive gene that shows no sex predilection.[6,7] The disease in West Highland White Terriers is similar, but the mode of inheritance has not been completely established.[4]

Normal liver copper concentration in dogs ranges between 200 and 400 parts per million (ppm) of dry weight, and this level remains constant throughout life.[8] Dogs with copper-storage disease begin to accumulate the mineral shortly after birth. Biopsies of the livers of affected puppies show increased copper in the hepatocytes as early as $5\frac{1}{2}$ months of age.[9] During the first few months of life, while copper is accumulating, there is no liver damage, and serum levels of liver enzymes remain within normal range. But when hepatic copper reaches a toxic level of approximately 2000 ppm, centrolobular hepatitis with concomitant elevation of liver enzymes develops. Dogs vary significantly in the age at which toxic levels are reached. Even after toxicity occurs, levels continue to accumulate, reaching as high as 10,000 ppm.[10]

The recent identification of a DNA marker for the copper toxicosis locus in Bedlington Terriers (marker C04107) has led to the ability to reliably diagnose individual cases and to identify pedigrees and lineages in which the gene for this disorder is prevalent.[11,12] Serum chemistry profiles are useful preliminary screening tools for the onset of liver disease in young dogs. Liver biopsies should be taken if elevated levels of the liver enzyme alanine amino transaminase are observed. Clinical signs of disease are usually not manifested until the dog is between 4 and 8 years old, although some may show signs as early as 1 year or as late as 11 years of age.[4] Widespread liver necrosis and post-necrotic cirrhosis begin to cause clinical signs that are associated with liver disease. Lethargy, anorexia, vomiting, abdominal pain, and, occasionally, ascites and icterus are observed. Some dogs suffer acute tubular necrosis in the kidneys and show polyuria and polydipsia in addition to signs of liver disease.[4] Acute episodes of liver necrosis may cause sudden death in a small number of affected dogs.

Treatment involves lifelong feeding of a copper-restricted diet and the administration of medications that either decrease intestinal absorption or increase urinary excretion of copper.[4,13] Two chelating agents, penicillamine and trientine, have been used in dogs with copper-storage disease and act by increasing urinary excretion of copper.[10,14,15] However, despite the reported use of these drugs, controlled efficacy and treatment regimen studies have not been conducted in this species, and penicillamine may be toxic in some animals.[4,13]

Recent evidence shows that zinc acetate, which functions to block the intestinal absorption of copper, may be the treatment of choice for dogs with copper-storage disease.[13] Results of a study that examined the efficacy of zinc acetate in the treatment of copper-storage disease in Bedlington Terriers and West Highland White Terriers found that administration at dosages that resulted in plasma zinc concentrations of 200 to 500 micrograms (μg)/deciliter (dl) suppressed hepatic inflammatory disease and reduced hepatic copper concentrations. It appeared that hepatic function could be restored by the long-term administration of zinc acetate in affected dogs. The administration of 100 mg of zinc acetate twice daily is recommended for the first 3 months of treatment. After this period, the dosage can be reduced to 50 mg twice daily. For maximum effectiveness, the zinc should not be administered with the dog's food. Plasma zinc concentrations should be measured every 2 to 3 months to determine that the level has increased appropriately and does not exceed 1000 μg/dl. Affected dogs require lifelong therapy. Copper status must be monitored closely to guard against the potential for copper deficiency.

ZINC MALABSORPTION

Although zinc deficiency and zinc-responsive dermatosis can be caused by feeding an imbalanced diet, another potential cause involves an inherited predisposition of impaired zinc absorption. Several breeds of dogs appear to be affected by zinc malabsorption, and varying levels of severity of this disorder have been reported. The most severe zinc-related disorder is lethal acrodermatitis in Bull Terriers. This genetic disease is inherited as an autosomal recessive gene and results in an inability to absorb dietary zinc, even when high levels of the mineral are added to the diet.[16] A cell-mediated immunodeficiency also occurs in affected dogs. Growth is stunted, and severe skin lesions develop by the time the puppies are 10 weeks old.[17] The immunodeficiency results in increased susceptibility to pyoderma and multiple infections throughout the body. There is also some evidence that the behavioral disorders of tail-chasing and idiopathic aggression in this breed may be related to zinc malabsorption.[18] This disorder is invariably fatal and has a median survival age of only 7 months.[16]

A less severe zinc-responsive disorder occurs in Alaskan Malamutes, Siberian Huskies (Figure 30-1), and, occasionally, Great Danes and Doberman Pinschers.[19,20,21,22] Research has shown that Alaskan Malamutes afflicted with inherited chondrodysplastic dwarfism have an impaired ability to absorb intestinal zinc.[22] Dwarfism in this breed has a simple autosomal recessive inheritance, and zinc mal-

FIGURE 30-1

Inherited zinc malabsorption in a Siberian Husky. **A**, *Face and* **B**, *hock.*

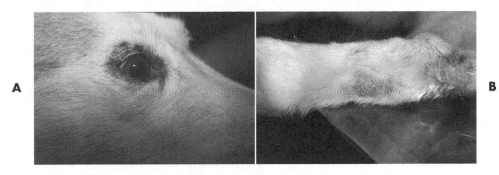

(Reprinted with permission of Candace Sousa, DVM, Animal Dermatology Clinic, Sacramento, California.)

absorption appears to be a component of this disorder. However, impaired zinc absorption has also been described in Malamutes that are not afflicted with chondrodysplasia.[20]

The onset of this syndrome usually occurs at puberty, and some dogs show signs only during times of physiological stress, such as pregnancy or exposure to weather extremes. Dermatological signs include crusting, scaling, and underlying suppuration around the face, elbows, scrotum, prepuce, and vulva. In chronic cases, hyperpigmentation of the affected skin surface is seen. The dogs are usually not pruritic until the lesions have become extensively crusted. Mild to moderate weight loss and a dull, dry coat are also observed. Histopathological examinations of skin biopsies show diffuse parakeratotic hyperkeratosis.

Oral supplementation with zinc results in rapid resolution of the skin lesions within 7 to 10 days. In most dogs, supplementation is required throughout life to prevent a recurrence of clinical signs.[14] A therapeutic dose of 100 mg of zinc sulfate administered twice daily is recommended.[14] Zinc sulfate can cause emesis in some dogs, but this can be prevented in most cases by giving the mineral with the dog's food. In a small proportion of cases, supplementation is necessary only during periods of stress. Although unusual, similar cases have also been reported in growing Great Danes.[15,17] The mode of inheritance of this disorder in all breeds is currently unknown.

HYPERLIPIDEMIA

The term *hyperlipidemia* is used interchangeably with *hyperlipoproteinemia* and refers to elevated levels of triglycerides and/or cholesterol in animals that have been fasted for at least 12 hours.[23] Most of the cases of hyperlipidemia seen in companion animals occur secondary to another underlying disorder that affects lipid metabolism. Diseases that may cause secondary hyperlipidemia include diabetes mellitus, hypothyroidism, pancreatitis, nephrotic syndrome, and liver disease.[24] In addition, certain medications such as glucocorticoids and immunosuppressant drugs may cause transient increases in blood lipid levels. Familial, or primary, hyperlipidemia refers to cases in which a heritable basis for hyperlipidemia can be found. Two well-documented inherited disorders of lipid metabolism occur in dogs and cats: hyperlipidemia in Miniature Schnauzers and lipoprotein lipase (LPL) deficiency in cats.

Lipoprotein Metabolism

A basic understanding of the mechanisms of lipid transport in the blood is necessary for an examination of hyperlipidemia. Because lipids are insoluble in water, transport in the blood requires complexing with more soluble molecules, such as proteins and phospholipids. Free fatty acids (FFAs) are carried in the bloodstream by albumin, a serum protein. Triglycerides and cholesterol esters are carried by lipoproteins, which are spherical macromolecular complexes made up of a lipid core surrounded by a thin outer membrane. Apoproteins, the proteins that are present in the lipoprotein's outer membrane, are recognition sites for target tissues and act as enzyme cofactors in lipid metabolism reactions.[25]

Lipoproteins can be categorized according to their lipid components and resultant aqueous densities. Like humans, dogs have four major classes of lipoproteins, each of which has a principal lipid component and one or more transport functions. *Chylomicrons* are synthesized in response to the absorption of fat from the intestine and function in the transport of dietary triglyceride to extrahepatic tissues and cholesterol to the liver. Chylomicrons appear in the blood approximately 2 hours postprandially, causing a transient increase in plasma triglyceride concentration. When they are delivered to tissues, the triglycerides are hydrolyzed to fatty acids and glycerol by the enzyme LPL. The second category of lipoproteins, called *very–low-density lipoproteins* (VLDLs), transport endogenous triglycerides from the liver to extrahepatic tissues for use as an energy source or for storage in adipose tissue. In contrast to chylomicrons, VLDLs are produced continuously so that in the fasting state VLDLs are the main carriers of endogenously produced triglyceride. *Low-density lipoproteins* (LDLs) transport cholesterol from the liver to extrahepatic tissues for incorporation into cell membranes and for steroid hormone synthesis. Finally, the *high-density lipoproteins* (HDLs) also transport cholesterol, but they are responsible for moving excess cholesterol out of extrahepatic cells back to the liver for excretion in bile, a process called "reverse cholesterol transport."

Postprandial hyperlipidemia is a natural occurrence that reflects a transient rise in chylomicrons; in dogs it normally resolves within 6 to 10 hours following consumption of a meal.[26,27] However, persistent hyperlipidemia in a fasted dog or cat is an abnormal response and is associated with a number of health risks. In dogs, fasting serum triglyceride concentrations greater than 150 mg/dl and/or total cholesterol concentration greater than 300 mg/dl are considered hyperlipidemic. Values for cats are fasting triglyceride and/or cholesterol values of greater than 100 mg/dl or 200 mg/dl, respectively.[28]

A number of health problems may be caused by persistent hyperlipidemia in companion animals. Hypertriglyceridemia, especially when severe, is associated with abdominal pain, vomiting, diarrhea, anorexia, seizures, hepatomegaly, and the abnormal deposition of lipid in certain tissues.[26,28,29] Like some hereditary hypertriglyceridemias in humans, elevated triglyceride levels in dogs and cats may also increase the risk for development of acute pancreatitis.[25,30] Hypercholesterolemia is not common in dogs and cats, and when it does occur it is not associated with as many health risks as is hypertriglyceridemia. Corneal lipid depositions have been reported in dogs as a result of elevated blood cholesterol.[31] In contrast to humans, dogs and cats rarely develop atherosclerosis in response to hypercholesterolemia, and when atherosclerosis is seen it is usually the result of congenital or spontaneous hypothyroidism.[32]

Hyperlipidemia in Miniature Schnauzers

Hyperlipidemia in Miniature Schnauzers is a well-documented disorder.[30,33,34] It is reported that many clinically normal dogs of this breed are found to have persistent fasting hyperlipidemia during routine veterinary examinations.[30] There is no sex predilection, and the disorder is usually first seen in Schnauzers that are more than 4 years of age. The hyperlipidemia is caused by elevated triglycerides and is typically characterized by chylomicron excess. Serum cholesterol levels are either normal or slightly increased.[25] Increased serum lipase and amylase activities have been recognized in hyperlipidemic Miniature Schnauzers that present with acute pancreatitis. In these cases, the pancreatitis is believed to be caused by the hypertriglyceridemia.

Affected dogs are either asymptomatic or have recurrent episodes of abdominal pain or distress, vomiting, and/or diarrhea. Seizures have also been associated with persistent hyperlipidemia in this breed.[33] Owners may report that episodes of abdominal distress last several days, followed by spontaneous recovery. In many cases, the clinical signs and history are similar to those of dogs with acute pancreatitis, but radiographic and laboratory evidence do not often support this diagnosis. This syndrome has been termed "pseudo pancreatitis" by one investigator.[30] Hyperlipidemia in Miniature Schnauzers is believed to be hereditary because of the high breed predisposition and because most affected Miniature Schnauzers lack evidence of diseases that cause secondary hyperlipidemia.[25]

The underlying cause of primary hyperlipidemia in Miniature Schnauzers is not known. However, it is theorized that either a familial deficiency of the enzyme LPL or the absence of an apoprotein that functions to activate LPL may be responsible. The enzyme LPL is located in capillary and endothelial tissue and hydrolyzes the triglycerides that are transported by chylomicrons and VLDLs for transport into cells. A defect in the synthesis or activity of this enzyme prevents the delivery of dietary triglycerides to tissues and leads to the retention of chylomicrons and impaired VLDL metabolism. The absence of an important apoprotein called apo C-II would have a similar effect. Apo C-II is normally a component of chylomicrons and VLDL and is a cofactor for LPL. In humans, individuals with an apo C-II deficiency have clinical symptoms similar to individuals with LPL deficiency.[35]

Feline Lipoprotein Lipase Deficiency

An inherited deficiency of LPL is the cause of a hyperchylomicronemia that is well recognized in the cat and has been shown to be inherited as an autosomal recessive trait.[36,37,38,39,40,41] The hyperlipidemia is caused by markedly elevated fasting triglyceride concentrations as a result of increased chylomicrons and, to a lesser extent, VLDLs.[42] Clinical signs may or may not be present, and the severity of clinical disease is not well correlated with the degree of hyperlipidemia. The age of onset of clinical signs varies from as young as 3 weeks to middle age.[42] When cats present with clinical disease, the most common signs include the development of subcutaneous xanthomas (lipid deposits) and lipemia retinalis. The xanthomas occur most often in areas of the body where trauma caused damage to capillaries, leading to extravasation of lipids. Variable peripheral neuropathies are seen in some cases. The signs of nerve damage develop slowly and are characterized by the loss of conscious proprioception and motor function, with retention of sensation of pain. These neuropathies are thought to be caused by compression of nerves by lipid granulomata at sites of trauma.[25]

Investigations of this disorder have shown that the plasma of affected cats has significantly reduced LPL activity after heparin administration when compared with the plasma of normal cats.[36,38,40] Heparin administration stimulates the release of active LPL and is used as a measure of LPL activity. Another study of a family of cats reported that the affected cats produced an abnormal LPL protein that failed to bind normally to vascular endothelium, rendering it inactive.[40] These results support the theory that an inherited disorder of lipid metabolism involving a deficiency of active LPL occurs in the cat.

Diagnosis of Primary Hyperlipidemia

In cases of hyperlipidemia, all causes of secondary hyperlipidemia must be ruled out before a diagnosis of primary hyperlipidemia can be made. A 16-hour fasting blood sample should be taken and cholesterol and triglyceride concentrations should be measured.[23] If there is a history of recurrent abdominal pain, vomiting, or diarrhea, serum amylase and lipase activities should be measured to monitor pancreatic pathology. The pet's breed, family lineage, age, and clinical history can be used to support a diagnosis.

Quantification of the plasma concentrations of each lipoprotein class may assist in the differential diagnosis of hyperlipidemia. An estimate of the lipoprotein pattern can be obtained through electrophoresis. An electrophoretic technique used for human lipoprotein analysis has also been adapted and validated for use in the dog.[43] However, electrophoretic separation of lipoproteins is not a disease-specific technique and cannot always differentiate between functional classes of elevated lipoproteins.[25] Laboratory techniques that can accurately identify lipoproteins not adequately differentiated by electrophoresis are not used by most diagnostic laboratories, and samples must be referred to research laboratories.[25] If a LPL deficiency is suspected in a cat, determination of plasma activity of this enzyme is suggested. LPL activity can be indirectly assayed by collecting plasma before and after the administration of heparin. However, this technique does not differentiate between hepatic lipase and LPL. Special procedures can be used to differentiate between these two enzymes for diagnostic purposes.[44]

Dietary Treatment of Primary Hyperlipidemia

The aim of treatment for primary hyperlipidemia is to reduce and maintain plasma lipid concentrations at levels that no longer predispose the dog or cat to health risks. Dietary intervention is recommended in animals that have fasting hypertriglyceridemia of greater than 500 mg/dl or hypercholesterolemia greater than 750 mg/dl.[28,29] Miniature Schnauzers that have fasting hypertriglyceridemia but no clinical signs should be treated if the hyperlipidemia persists in two consecutive samples taken several weeks apart.[30]

In both dogs and cats, a diet that is restricted in fat and calories is recommended. Feeding less fat decreases the influx of triglyceride-containing chylomicrons into the bloodstream, reduces the load on LPL, and promotes the clearance of chylomicrons and VLDLs. For successful dietary management, the diet should contain less than 20% fat, with an ideal level of between 8% and 12% (on a dry-matter basis [DMB]).[27,30] Follow-up blood samples should be taken several weeks after switching to the new diet. It is imperative that the restricted-fat diet is the animal's only source of food. All table scraps and extra treats must be discontinued. Owners should be cautioned that dogs with hyperlipidemia may be susceptible to acute pancreatitis, and that a single high-fat meal may result in the onset of this disease. If a fat-restricted diet normalizes blood triglyceride levels, dietary management should be continued for the remainder of the pet's life.

Feeding a low-fat diet to cats with LPL deficiency has been shown to normalize blood lipid levels and cause a regression of xanthomas and peripheral neuropathies within 12 weeks of lowering plasma lipid concentrations.[36,45] Similarly, clinical signs in Miniature Schnauzers usually resolve when serum triglyceride levels are normalized.[33] Most Miniature Schnauzers with hyperlipidemia can be successfully managed by diet, but more drastic fat reduction may be necessary as the pet ages. If any clinical signs of acute pancreatitis develop, periodic follow-up examinations should be conducted and veterinary care should be sought immediately.

In some cases, reducing the level of fat in the diet is not sufficient to reduce blood lipid levels. There are several lipid-lowering drugs that are approved for use in humans but not in dogs or cats. Although there are some reports of success using drugs such as clofibrate, gemfibrozil, and pharmacological doses of niacin, the efficacy of these therapies has not been proven. Marine fish oils, which contain high amounts of omega-3 fatty acids such as eicosapentaenoic acid and docosahexaenoic acid, have also been used as an adjunct therapy for hyperlipidemia in dogs.[23,36]

Studies with humans have shown that these oils reduce plasma triglyceride and cholesterol concentrations by decreasing the production of VLDLs.[46] Improved triglyceride levels have been reported in hyperlipidemic dogs receiving supplemental marine oil at doses up to 30 to 60 mg/kilogram (kg) daily, with no clinical or biochemical side effects.[23,27,47] Although not effective for all dogs, marine oil supplementation may help to normalize blood lipid levels in animals that are not responding adequately to dietary fat restriction alone.

The amelioration of clinical signs is the best indicator of long-term prognosis in pets with primary hyperlipidemia. The animal's health is invariably improved if dietary fat restriction is strictly enforced and blood lipid levels can be lowered to normal or near-normal concentrations. Naturally, the presence of any secondary, underlying disorders that could contribute further to hyperlipidemia, such as insulin-dependent diabetes mellitus (IDDM) or hypothyroidism, increase the health risks and make long-term management more difficult in these pets.

PURINE METABOLISM IN DALMATIANS

Purines are components of the nucleic acids that are found in the nucleus of plant and animal cells. All mammals are capable of synthesizing purines for tissue growth and maintenance. Purines are also obtained through the reuse of dietary or endogenous nuclear material. Nuclear material that is ingested and hydrolyzed contains purine bases that can be converted back into nucleotides to be used for growth and maintenance by the body. Normal cellular turnover and tissue maintenance, along with the digestion of excess dietary purines, results in purine catabolism. A primary end product of purine catabolism is uric acid. If the liver enzyme uricase is present, uric acid is further degraded to form the compound allantoin. Uric acid that is not converted to allantoin is present in body tissues as its salt, monosodium urate.

Most mammals, with the exception of humans, the higher apes, and Dalmatians, convert most uric acid to allantoin and as a result excrete very little urate in the urine. Dalmatians are unique in that they excrete both urate and allantoin in their urine as end products of purine metabolism.[48,49] Compared with other breeds of dogs, Dalmatians have increased levels of urate and decreased levels of allantoin in the bloodstream and urine.[50] Other breeds of dogs excrete 10 to 60 mg of urate per 24-hour period, and their serum urate concentration is approximately 0.25 mg/dl.[49,51,52] In contrast, Dalmatians excrete approximately 400 to 600 mg of urinary urate in a 24-hour period.[48,50,53] However, these values can range from less than 200 mg to greater than 1 g of uric acid. The mean serum urate concentration in Dalmatians is about 0.5 mg/dl, with a range of 0.3 to 4.0 mg/dl, approximately two-fold to four-fold the values in other dog breeds.[49,51]

There appear to be two separate underlying mechanisms that are responsible for the Dalmatian's high production of uric acid and low production of allantoin. A defective uric acid transport system in the liver results in decreased oxidation of uric acid to allantoin by the enzyme uricase.[54] The second problem involves the kidneys.

Compared with other species and other breeds of dogs, Dalmatians have reduced renal tubular reabsorption of urate.[49] In other breeds, 98% of the uric acid in the glomerular filtrate is reabsorbed in the proximal tubules and returned to the liver for further oxidation to allantoin. Dalmatians have reduced ability to reabsorb uric acid in the proximal tubules, resulting in increased urinary excretion of urate. Although few studies have examined the mode of inheritance of these defects in the Dalmatian, it has been suggested that altered purine metabolism in this breed is the result of an autosomal recessive gene.[55]

Altered purine metabolism in Dalmatians does have some medical significance. Although allantoin is highly soluble, urate has a low aqueous solubility. Its accumulation in the body can result in the precipitation of urate crystals out of the serum or urine. In humans, crystallization occurs in body tissues when serum urate values are greater than 6.5 mg/dl.[56] The presence of urate crystals causes the medical affliction that is commonly called "gout," which is characterized by inflammation, swelling, and painful joints. Interestingly, although Dalmatians do not convert uric acid to allantoin, their serum does not attain levels that are high enough to cause gout. Rather, because of the reduced reabsorption of urate in the renal tubules, Dalmatians excrete large amounts of urate in the urine, preventing buildup in the serum. Although this capability appears to protect Dalmatians from developing signs of gout, the shift of excess urate from the serum to the urine carries with it other problems.

The presence of a high concentration of urate in the urinary tract of Dalmatians appears to predispose dogs of this breed to the development of urate urolithiasis. In dogs, urate uroliths or calculi are composed primarily of ammonium urate, and a sufficiently high concentration of both urate and ammonium in the urine is necessary for the formation of these uroliths. Studies show that although urate calculi account for only 5% of calculi found in dogs, 45% to 65% of those that are seen come from Dalmatians. Furthermore, 75% to 100% of calculi found in Dalmatians are composed completely or partially of urate.[57,58,59] Urate urolithiasis is significantly more common in male Dalmatians than in females.[53,59,60] The anatomical differences between the urethras of males and females may partially explain this disparity. The small, rounded urate crystals pass readily through the wider female urethra, but they may tend to lodge in the male urethra as it enters the narrow groove in the os penis. However, others have reported that female dogs that are not Dalmatians are more likely to form urate-containing calculi than males.[53] Therefore it appears that additional factors may be responsible for the higher incidence or urate urolithiasis in male Dalmatians.

Clinical signs of urolithiasis in the dog, regardless of the type of urolith present, depend on the duration of the urolithiasis, the size of the uroliths, their location in the tract, and the presence or absence of a concomitant urinary tract infection. General signs include frequent urination and the voiding of small amounts of urine, the appearance of pain or straining during urination, and hematuria. Urethral obstruction is characterized by anuria, depression, anorexia, vomiting, and/or diarrhea. Complete obstruction always constitutes a medical emergency.

Although high urinary uric acid excretion is a major predisposing factor for the development of urate urolithiasis in Dalmatians, it is not the sole cause. Most

Dalmatians excrete urate in the urine at a concentration above its solubility limits. However, not all Dalmatians develop urate uroliths, and urate excretion is not well-correlated with the development of uroliths.[61] Other predisposing factors that may be involved include urinary ammonium concentration, urinary pH, the presence of a urinary tract infection, and dietary purine intake. The incidence of urate urolithiasis in the Dalmatian breed is not known, but it has been suggested that the majority of dogs never experience clinical signs of this disease, and that the incidence rate may be as low as 1%.[62]

Treatment for urate urolithiasis in dogs usually requires surgical removal of the calculi. Prophylactic measures for Dalmatians that are predisposed to urate urolithiasis include feeding a diet that promotes an alkaline urine and is low in purines, as well as ensuring adequate hydration.[52] A reduced-purine diet decreases the amount of urate precursors present in the urine, and the production of an alkaline urine increases the solubility of urate uroliths. The diet should provide moderate to low levels of high-quality protein. Moderate restriction of protein results in decreased ammonium ion production from the catabolism of excess protein. Ingredients that are high in protein also tend to be high in purines. The moderate restriction of protein therefore also reduces purine intake. Oral administration of sodium bicarbonate is effective in changing the alkalinity of the urine. It is hypothesized that control of any concomitant urinary tract infections may also aid in preventing recurrence.[61]

Daily administration of the drug allopurinol is often used as a prophylactic method in Dalmatians that are predisposed to urate urolithiasis.[63] Allopurinol is an inhibitor of the enzyme xanthine oxidase, which is necessary for the degradation of purines. Administration of this drug results in a decrease in uric acid production. However, this can result in increased levels of xanthine in the urine and lead to urinary calculi that contain xanthine. An increased incidence of this type of calculi has been reported in Dalmatians that have received this drug.[59,64]

CHAPTER

31

Diabetes Mellitus

 Diabetes mellitus is a chronic endocrine disorder that occurs in both dogs and cats. It is caused by the relative or absolute deficiency of the hormone insulin, which is produced by the beta cells of the pancreas. Insulin stimulates the transport of glucose and other nutrients across cell membranes for cellular use and is involved in a number of anabolic processes within the body. A lack of insulin activity leads to elevated blood glucose levels (hyperglycemia) and an inability of tissues to receive the glucose that they need (glucoprivation). Primary clinical signs include polyuria, polyphagia, polydipsia, and, in some cases, weight loss. Diagnosis is usually made using the initial signs of the disorder, which are the presence of a persistent hyperglycemia and a persistent or concurrent glycosuria.[65,66]

INCIDENCE

It is estimated that diabetes has an incidence between 0.2% and 1% in dogs and cats seen at small animal clinics.[67] A large proportion of these diabetic pets are obese at the time of diagnosis. In dogs, other factors that appear to be related to the development of diabetes are hormonal abnormalities such as hypothyroidism and Cushing's syndrome, recurrent episodes of pancreatitis, pancreatic islet-cell destruction, stress, and genetic predisposition.[68,69] In cats, the most significant risk factor for the development of diabetes is increasing age. Between 70% and 90% of diabetic cats are 7 years or older, and more than 65% are 10 years or older.[67,70] Other predisposing factors for cats include inactivity, presence of pancreatic neoplasia, long-term administration of progesterone or progestin, and, possibly, genetics.[70,71,72]

CLASSIFICATION

Diabetes mellitus is considered a heterogeneous syndrome, with its primary characteristic being a persistent and detrimental hyperglycemia. In humans, diabetes is typically classified as either type I or type II. *Type I diabetes* (also referred to as *insulin-dependent diabetes* [IDDM]) is identified by an absolute lack of endogenous insulin and a resultant dependence upon exogenous insulin for survival. This form of the disease is caused by the autoimmune destruction of the pancreatic beta cells by T cells and antibodies. Type I diabetes appears to be relatively common in dogs, as indicated by the presence of islet cell antibodies.[73] Type I diabetes is not well documented in cats, and the prevalence of islet cell antibodies in this species has not been reported. Although up to 70% of cats with diabetes require insulin therapy for survival, the proportion of these cats who have type I diabetes (i.e., an absolute lack of endogenous insulin production) is not known.[74,75]

In humans, the term *type II diabetes* is usually used interchangeably with the term *non–insulin-dependent diabetes mellitus* (NIDDM). Individuals with this form of the disease do not usually require exogenous insulin therapy for survival, although insulin or oral hypoglycemic agents may be administered to better manage blood glucose levels. Type II diabetes is characterized by impaired insulin secretion; insulin resistance; and amyloid deposition in the islets of the pancreas. The total amount of insulin secreted after a meal may be increased, normal, or decreased, and the pattern of insulin secretion is usually abnormal.[75,76] Insulin resistance occurs when an elevated concentration of circulating hormone is needed to adequately maintain blood glucose levels. Based upon glucose tolerance tests and measured levels of serum insulin, it appears that insulin resistance is a common feature of canine and feline diabetes.[77,78] The persistent hyperglycemia that results from insulin resistance and abnormal insulin secretion results in glucose toxicity. Glucose toxicity exacerbates the metabolic abnormalities of diabetes and leads to impaired insulin secretion and loss of beta cells. Although many cats and dogs are identified as having type II diabetes, more of these animals require insulin therapy than humans with type II diabetes do, probably because of a greater loss of beta cells.[79,80] Because the effects of glucose toxicity are initially reversible, some cats with NIDDM that are treated with insulin may revert to a state that does not require insulin weeks to months after the glycemia has been controlled through insulin administration.[81]

Amyloid deposition in pancreatic islets is a consistent histological finding in cats with diabetes. Amyloid is a precipitation product of a pancreatic compound called amylin. Amylin is co-secreted with insulin and helps to maintain normal blood glucose levels by stimulating the breakdown of muscle glycogen. Amyloid deposition contributes to a loss of the insulin-secreting beta cells of the pancreas, eventually causing decreased or insufficient insulin secretion. It is theorized that the extensive amyloid deposition observed in diabetic cats is at least partially responsible for the need to administer exogenous insulin therapy to many cats with type II diabetes.[74]

Insulin resistance primarily manifests itself after insulin binds to its cellular receptors, resulting in a decreased conversion of circulating glucose to glycogen or fat. In addition to being a characteristic of type II diabetes, insulin resistance also occurs as an adaptive response to low carbohydrate intake, allowing blood glucose levels to be conserved and maintained immediately after eating a low-carbohydrate meal.[82,83] It has been hypothesized that, as a species, the domestic cat is naturally

TABLE 31-1

Forms of Diabetes Mellitus

Form	Major Underlying Cause	Incidence in Dogs and Cats	Treatment
Type I	Inability of beta cells to synthesize or secrete insulin	70% to 80% of cases	Exogenous insulin and dietary management
Type II	Insensitivity of peripheral tissues to insulin; impaired insulin secretion	20% to 30% of cases	Weight loss, dietary management and/or hypoglycemic agents; insulin therapy (in some cases)

insulin resistant when compared with other more omnivorous or herbivorous species. Insulin resistance would be expected to confer an adaptive advantage for a species that evolved as an obligate carnivore, consuming a diet that was high in protein and fat but low in carbohydrate (see Section 2, pp. 71-72).[83] Therefore, peripheral resistance to insulin may represent an adaptive mechanism that allows the delivery of protein and fat to tissues while conserving blood glucose levels. If this theory is correct, it would follow that the consumption of a diet that is high in carbohydrate (such as some commercially available cat foods) would require cats to secrete much higher levels of insulin after eating than would be secreted after eating a high-protein, high-fat meal. Over time, the beta cells of the pancreas may no longer be able to meet this enhanced need, resulting in an abnormal or impaired insulin response. Although this hypothesis has also been developed and examined with humans (typically referred to as the "carnivore connection"), more study and research is needed with the cat to clarify the implications of insulin resistance in this species. Regardless, it is prudent to advise that because obesity and inactivity further contribute to insulin resistance, an elderly cat that consumes a high-carbohydrate diet, is overweight, and leads a sedentary lifestyle is expected to be at greatest risk for the development of type II diabetes (Table 31-1).

CLINICAL SIGNS

All of the clinical signs observed in pets with diabetes mellitus are associated with the short- or long-term effects of hyperglycemia. Polydipsia, polyuria, polyphagia, and/or weight loss are usually the first signs observed. The microvascular effects of diabetes contribute to the development of cataracts and renal disease. Polyneuropathy develops in some cases and can manifest as weakness, depression, or urinary and bowel incontinence. Bacterial infections are common in animals with poor glycemic control. All of these complications can be minimized or prevented through stringent control of blood glucose levels in diabetic animals.

The general therapeutic goals in diabetes management are to minimize postprandial (after-meal) hyperglycemia, prevent hypoglycemia when insulin is being administered, resolve and minimize clinical signs, prevent or delay long-term complications, and improve overall health. These goals can be achieved through exogenous insulin administration, oral hypoglycemic agents, diet, weight loss (if indicated), exercise, and the control of concurrent illness. The remainder of this chapter focuses primarily on the role of diet and weight control in managing diabetes mellitus in dogs and cats.

DIETARY TREATMENT

Dietary goals for dogs and cats with IDDM are to improve regulation of blood glucose by delivering nutrients to the body during periods when exogenous insulin is active and to minimize postprandial fluctuations in blood glucose levels. Dietary management does not eliminate the need for insulin replacement therapy, but it can be used to improve glycemic control. Dietary treatment for pets with NIDDM can be instrumental in improving glycemic control and preventing the need to institute exogenous insulin therapy. Factors that must be considered when developing an appropriate diet for a diabetic pet include the consistency and type of diet, its nutritional adequacy and nutrient composition, and the pet's caloric intake and feeding schedule.

Consistency and Type of Diet

Dogs and cats with diabetes should be fed a food that contains consistent amounts and sources of nutrients. Specifically, the type and quantity of nutrients that are delivered to the body should remain consistent from day to day, and the proportions of calories in the diet that are supplied by carbohydrate, protein, and fat should stay constant. For pets with IDDM, the provision of a consistent diet allows the insulin dosage to be adjusted to closely fit the needs of the animal. Similarly, if pets with NIDDM are being treated with oral hypoglycemic agents, the provision of a consistent diet is helpful in maintaining normal blood glucose levels. Changes in the ingredients or nutrient composition of a diet can disrupt the tight coupling of blood glucose levels with insulin activity that is needed for proper glycemic control. Therefore, only pet foods that are prepared using a fixed formulation should be selected for diabetic pets (see Section 3, pp. 194-195). Manufacturers that use fixed formulations ensure that the nutrient composition and ingredients of a food remain consistent between batches. In contrast, manufacturers that use variable formulations will change ingredients depending on the availability and market prices. If information about the formulation type is not readily available, it can be obtained by contacting the manufacturer directly. Homemade diets should also be avoided with diabetic pets because of difficulties with maintaining nutrient consistency.

The type of commercial product that is fed is also of importance. Semimoist pet foods or snacks should not be fed to diabetic pets. Postprandial blood glucose and

insulin responses have been shown to be highest when dogs are fed semimoist foods, compared with when they are fed either canned or dry pet foods.[84] This increase appears to be because of the high level of simple carbohydrate found in semimoist products. These nutrients require minimal digestion in the small intestine and are rapidly absorbed following a meal. In contrast, the digestible carbohydrates found in dry and canned foods are made up primarily of complex carbohydrates (starch). Starches require enzymatic digestion to simple sugars before they can be absorbed into the body. This process slows the rate of delivery of glucose to the bloodstream. Complex carbohydrates and certain types of fiber also affect the rate of food passage through the gastrointestinal tract and the absorption of other nutrients in the diet. Dry pet foods generally contain higher levels of both complex carbohydrates and plant fiber than semimoist or canned foods do.

Nutritional Adequacy and Nutrient Composition

The first consideration when identifying a food for a diabetic pet is the nutritional adequacy of the diet. Because long-term management is involved, the food must be nutritionally complete and balanced and must supply optimum levels of all the essential nutrients required by the pet. The methods discussed in Section 3 can be used to determine the nutritional adequacy of a commercial product. As discussed previously, the labels of over-the counter pet foods will indicate if feeding trials have been conducted or if the food has merely been formulated to meet the Association of American Feed Control Officials' (AAFCO's) *Nutrient Profiles*. A food that has been adequately tested using the AAFCO's animal feeding test protocols should be selected. If a veterinary diet is prescribed, the label will not show this information, but the veterinarian should have literature available that fully describes the selected product.

Energy-Containing Nutrients   Ideal protein, carbohydrate, and fat levels in diets for diabetic dogs and cats have not been thoroughly investigated. However, some recommendations can be made based upon studies with human diabetics and knowledge about the metabolic changes associated with diabetes in companion animals. In humans, high-protein diets are not recommended because of the incidence of diabetic nephropathy, a condition that may be exacerbated by the intake of large amounts of protein.[69] However, in dogs and cats, this complication of diabetes is rare, and protein restriction for diabetic dogs and cats is neither necessary nor recommended. Rather, diabetic dogs and cats should be fed high-quality protein in amounts that meet their daily requirements. If chronic renal failure develops as a complication of diabetes, protein must be restricted accordingly to control azotemia (see pp. 462-465).

Fat intake by diabetic dogs and cats should also be moderately restricted if the pet is overweight. Alterations in lipid metabolism can cause the development of hypercholesterolemia and hepatic lipidosis in some animals. Restricted fat intake helps to prevent or minimize these changes and facilitates weight loss or weight management. One advantage of dietary fat in the nutritional management of diabetes is its effects upon gastric motility. High levels of dietary fat delay gastric emptying and consequently may modulate the postprandial glycemic response.[85] In humans, diets containing monounsaturated fats have been shown to decrease serum total cholesterol, very–low-density lipoproteins (VLDLs), and triglycerides without increasing blood glucose levels. However, this advantage is offset by the potentiating effect of dietary fat upon insulin resistance and its potential to exacerbate blood lipid abnormalities that occur as complications of diabetes.[86] Because of these discrepant effects and because of the contribution of dietary fat to energy density, the diet for diabetic pets should be relatively low in fat while still containing adequate levels of essential fatty acids (EFAs). As a general rule (and with the exception of extremely underweight diabetic pets), the fat content of pet foods for diabetic pets should not exceed 20% of the metabolizable energy (ME) calories in the diet (Box 31-1).

The carbohydrate content of diets for diabetic pets is an important consideration because this nutrient has the greatest influence upon postprandial blood glucose levels. A diet that minimizes the glycemic response is desirable because lessening fluctuations in blood glucose contributes to better control of diabetes and its associated complications. The term *glycemic index* refers to a ranking system that categorizes foods based upon their effects on blood glucose levels. In general, complex carbohydrates (starches) have a lower glycemic index than simple carbohydrates because they are more slowly digested and absorbed.[86] Types of starch differ in glycemic effects depending upon the plant source, its physical form, and the type of cooking and processing used. For example, studies with humans have shown that whole-grain starches have a lower glycemic index than highly refined starch sources.[87] Human subjects also demonstrate higher blood glucose and insulin responses when refined forms of wheat starch are consumed, compared with the response to potato or barley starches.[88,89] Barley in particular has been identified as a starch source that may be well-suited for diabetic diets.[89,90]

Similar variations in glycemic response have been observed in dogs. In a recent study, diets containing 30% starch from either corn, wheat, barley, rice, or sorghum were fed to healthy adult dogs for a minimum of 2 weeks.[91] Feeding rice resulted in the highest postprandial glycemic and insulin responses of the five starches that

BOX **31-1**

Dietary Management of Diabetes Mellitus: Diet Characteristics

Nutritionally complete and balanced
Consistent proportion of carbohydrate, fat, and protein
Consistency of ingredients (fixed formulation)
Greater than 40% of calories supplied by complex carbohydrate
Carbohydrate includes starch sources that minimize glycemic response
Moderate fiber level
High-quality protein source
Moderately restricted in fat (≤20% of total calories)

were studied. In comparison, feeding sorghum resulted in a comparatively lower glycemic response, and feeding barley resulted in a moderate glucose response and a reduced insulin response. Wheat and corn generally resulted in intermediate glycemic and insulin responses. Several factors may be responsible for these differences. The proportion of amylose and the amount of dietary fiber that are associated with the starch source both affect glycemic responses.[92] Different types of rice contain varying amounts of amylose. Those with a high amylose content result in a higher glycemic response.[87] The relatively low glycemic index of barley has been attributed to its high amount of associated fiber and beta-glucan.[93] Because glycemic response is an important consideration when selecting diets for diabetic pets, these results indicate that both the amount and the source of the starch in the diet must be considered. While feeding rice may increase postprandial hyperglycemia, feeding barley or sorghum modulates the glucose and insulin response and therefore may be a better choice for diabetic pets. Currently, a diet that is low in simple carbohydrates and high in complex carbohydrates (starch) and that contains moderately increased fiber is recommended for diabetic pets (see the next section).[69,94,95] As a general rule, complex carbohydrate should provide 40% or more of the calories in foods for diabetic pets.

Dietary Fiber   The role of dietary fiber in the management of diabetic pets has been studied extensively in recent years. Both the amount and the type of fiber have been considered. A frequently used classification scheme divides fiber into one of two broad categories: soluble fiber or insoluble fiber. Soluble fibers include pectin, gums, mucilages, a few of the hemicelluloses, and fructooligosaccharides (FOS). These fibers have high water-holding capacities, delay gastric emptying, and are believed to slow the rate of nutrient absorption across the intestinal surface. Most soluble fibers are also highly fermentable by bacteria in the large intestine. Insoluble fibers include cellulose, lignin, and most of the hemicelluloses. These fibers have less initial water-holding capacity, cause a decrease in gastrointestinal transit time, and are less efficiently fermented by gastrointestinal bacteria.[96]

Research with human subjects indicates that a diet containing a high proportion of complex carbohydrate and soluble fiber dampens the postprandial glycemic response and aids in glycemic control.[97,98] Fiber promotes the slowed digestion and absorption of dietary carbohydrate, which results in a flattening of the glucose response curve after meals. Postprandial hyperglycemia is reduced when both soluble and insoluble fibers are fed, but soluble fibers have the most pronounced effect.[99,100,101,102] Soluble fiber also has the added benefit of causing a decrease in the low-density lipoprotein fraction of blood cholesterol in human subjects.[103] The proposed mechanism of action for soluble fiber is the ability of this type of fiber to form a gel in aqueous solutions, which results in an impairment of the convective transfer of glucose and water to the absorptive surface of the intestine.[101] These "gel-forming" fibers are referred to as viscous fibers. As fiber viscosity increases, so does the fiber's ability to slow glucose diffusion, resulting in pronounced flattening of the glycemic response curve and improved control of glycemia in diabetic subjects.[104,105,106]

Recent studies with dogs demonstrate similar effects of dietary fiber. When groups of dogs with experimentally induced diabetes mellitus were fed diets containing 15% fiber, significant reductions in 24-hour blood glucose fluctuations and urinary glucose excretion were reported.[107] Slight reductions in monthly insulin requirements and blood glycosylated hemoglobin concentration were also observed. These effects occurred when either insoluble fibers (cellulose) or soluble fibers (pectin) were included as the food's primary fiber source. However, it is important to note that the experimental diets used in this study were created by adding supplemental fiber or carbohydrate to a balanced food, resulting in dilution of calories and nutrients. These diets were compared with a high-carbohydrate, low-fat control diet that was not diluted. As a result, the control diet differed from the experimental diets not only in its fiber content, but also in fat content, caloric density, and nutrient density. As a result, dogs consuming the high-fiber diets were also consuming fewer calories per meal than dogs fed the control diet. Therefore, it cannot be determined if the dampening effects of the fiber-containing diets upon postprandial glycemia in this study were due to slowed absorption of glucose, ingestion of fewer calories, or a combination of these two factors.

In a second study, a group of dogs with naturally occurring IDDM were fed a commercial, canned diet that was diluted by the addition of either 20 grams (g) of wheat bran (insoluble fiber) or 20 g of guar (soluble fiber).[108] When the dogs consumed the canned food without added fiber, they all developed hyperglycemia within 60 minutes of eating, followed by development of a relative hypoglycemia between 90 and 240 minutes. The addition of guar to this diet abolished the postprandial hyperglycemia in four of six dogs and significantly reduced it in the remaining two dogs. The addition of wheat bran also reduced the maximal postprandial peak in blood glucose, but to a lesser extent. These effects were observed in both diabetic dogs and healthy control dogs.

While the effect upon daily postprandial fluctuations in blood glucose is an important criteria for a diabetic diet, an equally important criteria is the diet's long-term influence upon glycemic control and health. Recently, the effects of feeding increased amounts of insoluble fiber to dogs with naturally occurring IDDM were examined during two 8-month periods.[109] Canned diets containing either 23% or 11% total dietary fiber supplied primarily by insoluble fiber (cellulose) were fed to 11 dogs. Caloric intake was controlled to provide an amount of food that maintained each dog's initial body weight. The dogs accepted both diets equally and maintained body weight with only slight fluctuations. Although daily caloric intake was slightly less when dogs consumed the high-fiber diet versus the low-fiber diet, this difference was not significant. Although there were no significant differences between the two treatment groups, when evaluated individually 9 of the 11 dogs showed improved when they were consuming the high-fiber diet, compared with when they were consuming the low-fiber diet. Significant reductions in daily insulin requirements, fasting blood glucose, 24-hour mean blood glucose, urinary glucose excretion, glycosylated hemoglobin concentrations, and serum cholesterol were observed during the high-fiber period. In contrast, 2 of the 11 dogs demonstrated better glycemic control while consuming the low-fiber diet. It was noted that although there were not significant differences, daily caloric intakes were lower for the nine dogs while consuming the high-fiber diets and for the two dogs while consuming the low-fiber diets. These results suggest that caloric intake may have at least partially influenced glycemic control in the dogs in this study, despite attempts to provide consistent daily caloric intake.

These results suggest that feeding a diet containing increased amounts of insoluble fiber may improve control of glycemia in some dogs with naturally occurring diabetes mellitus, but may not be appropriate for all dogs. It is also important to note that during the course of this long-term study, 4 dogs (from an original group of 15) died or were euthanized because of diabetic complications, and 9 of the 11 remaining dogs developed concurrent disorders that are commonly associated with diabetes. These disorders developed with approximately equal frequency when dogs were fed the low- or high-fiber diets and were controlled with appropriate treatment. However, this observation raises the question of whether or not the degree of glycemic control that is reported when a high-fiber diet is fed has long-term clinical benefits to the pet. Although improved glycemic control was observed in 9 of 11 dogs, overall health and quality of life were not evaluated. Long-term studies of fiber-containing diets that include a larger number of dogs and examine the effects of fiber-containing diets on the incidence and management of associated diabetic disorders are warranted.

Feeding different types of soluble fibers and fiber blends has also been studied in dogs.[110,111,112] One group of researchers examined the effect of feeding a blend of FOS and beet fiber on diet digestibility and glycemic response in healthy adult dogs.[110] FOS are natural polymers of fructose that are found in various plants such as bananas, onions, and barley. This fiber is resistant to hydrolysis in the small intestine but is highly fermented in the large intestine (see pp. 501-503). Sugar beet fiber is a moderately fermentable fiber that is frequently included in commercial pet foods. When healthy adult dogs were fed diets containing either 0%, 5% or 10% of an FOS and beet fiber blend, the highest fiber diet caused significant decreases in postprandial glucose concentration and preprandial (fasting) serum cholesterol concentration. Increases in fiber intake were associated with increased fecal output and water content and slightly decreased protein digestibility. However, the fiber blend had no effect on fasting blood glucose concentration or postprandial insulin response. Because daily caloric intake was kept constant in this study, the glycemic and cholesterol effects were not attributable to decreased energy intake. It was postulated that the influence of soluble fiber on serum metabolites may have been due to the effects of its fermentation products on nutrient and lipid metabolism in the liver or upon secretion of gastrointestinal tract hormones that control nutrient metabolism.[112,113]

The effects of increasing soluble fiber viscosity on flattening of the postprandial glycemic response curve have also been studied in dogs.[111,114,115] Dog foods containing either 1% or 3% carboxymethylcellulose (CMC) of either high or low viscosity were fed to healthy dogs, and postprandial serum glucose and insulin concentrations were measured.[111] Dogs fed the high-CMC diets developed soft feces or diarrhea, while dogs fed the low-CMC diets had normal stools. The production of soft feces or diarrhea in dogs consuming diets containing soluble fiber has been reported previously and is considered to be a common side effect of feeding this type of fiber.[116,117] As in the case of insoluble fiber, dogs had widely divergent responses to the consumption of CMC. Because of these variations, no statistically significant effects of CMC or viscosity were found. However, dogs fed diets containing 1% high-viscosity CMC showed the lowest mean values for postprandial glucose and insulin and had the longest time for postprandial blood glucose to return to the normal fasting range. In addition, serum glucose concentrations consistently decreased below the normal fasting range by 30 minutes after eating in dogs fed CMC-containing diets. This was not observed in dogs fed the control diet. These results suggest that the CMC may delay gastric emptying or slow nutrient absorption. In contrast, dogs fed the 3% CMC diet had the highest postprandial increases, indicating enhanced glucose absorption. These inconsistent results suggest that high amounts of CMC may actually enhance glucose absorption, although a specific mechanism for this response is not known.

Recent research examining the efficacy of high-fiber diets for the management of diabetic pets may have raised more questions than it has answered. While increased amounts of insoluble fiber have been shown to dampen the postprandial glycemic curve, it is possible that this is an effect of decreased energy intake caused by dilution of the diet, rather than a direct effect of fiber. Moreover, fiber's ability to provide long-term health benefits or improved quality of life or to prevent or ameliorate diabetic complications has not been evaluated. The use of soluble fiber may have efficacy in delaying gastric emptying and slowing glucose absorption in the intestine. However, high amounts of soluble fiber are not well tolerated by dogs and can cause increased fecal water, loose stools, and diarrhea. Moreover, dogs appear to have highly variable responses to the inclusion of both types of fiber in their diets. It seems probable that the best solution will be found in creating fiber blends that function to slow gastric emptying time, modulate glucose absorption, and dampen the postprandial glycemic curve in diabetic pets. Further studies are necessary that examine different types and levels of fiber and the long-term benefits of diets containing these fibers for diabetic pets.

Chromium   The trace mineral chromium has been recognized as an essential nutrient needed for glucose metabolism since the late 1950s.[118] The biologically active form of chromium functions as a potentiator of insulin action and is called *glucose tolerance factor*. The precise composition of this factor is not known, but it appears that nicotinic acid is an essential component.[119,120] Theories for the mechanism of action of glucose tolerance factor include direct interaction with insulin, effect on the production of insulin receptors, and postreceptor metabolic interaction.[121,122,123]

Chromium deficiency in humans is associated with abnormal glucose utilization and insulin resistance and has been hypothesized to be a factor in the development of adult-onset diabetes. Although variable results are reported, improved glucose tolerance is seen in some human diabetics when their diets are supplemented with this mineral.[123,124,125] Chromium supplementation has also been shown to increase glucose uptake by tissues in swine and cattle.[126,127] These results suggest that chromium supplementation may have a role in improving glycemic control in diabetic pets.

A recent set of experiments examined the effect of chromium supplementation on glucose metabolism and insulin sensitivity in healthy adult dogs.[128] In two experiments, groups of 24 Beagles were fed diets containing either 0, 0.15, 0.3, or 0.6 parts per million (ppm) of supplemental chromium tripicolinate. Dogs that received supplemental chromium had lower plasma glucose concentrations for 30 minutes and slightly higher glucose clearance rates for between 10 and 30 minutes following intravenous glucose administration when compared with the values for dogs that did not receive supplemental chromium. Chromium supplementation was associated with lower fasting blood glucose levels, but it did not affect the serum insulin response to glucose infusion. These results are consistent with those reported in humans and other species and suggest that chromium supplementation in dogs increases tissue sensitivity to the effects of insulin. Although the effects observed in these studies were relatively small, these data indicate that increasing the level of chromium in diets formulated for diabetic pets may improve glucose tolerance and aid in glycemic control. Further studies of the effects of chromium supplementation on glucose metabolism in pets with naturally occurring diabetes and of the potential long-term benefits of supplementation are needed before specific recommendations for this nutrient can be made.

Caloric Intake and Weight Control

The relationship between obesity and NIDDM in humans is well documented. Studies with dogs and cats have shown that a similar relationship exists in these species.[129,130] Baseline plasma insulin level and insulin response to a glucose load increase linearly in dogs as a function of their degree of obesity. This effect occurs in both healthy and diabetic animals.[129] Similarly, a study with cats found that healthy but obese cats had normal fasting plasma glucose concentrations, but the study showed abnormal results on glucose tolerance tests and slightly elevated baseline serum insulin concentrations.[123] Significant delays in initial insulin response and substantially increased insulin responses at a later phase of the glucose tolerance test were found in the overweight cats. Decreased tissue sensitivity to insulin and impaired beta-cell responsiveness to stimuli are believed to be the cause of these changes. Specifically, the tissue of obese animals has decreased numbers of cellular insulin receptors, and the receptors that are present have reduced binding affinity.[131,132] In some cases, a postreceptor, intracellular defect in insulin action also occurs.[133] Ultimately these changes decrease the body's ability to respond to insulin. Over time, beta-cell hyperresponsiveness develops, and baseline insulin and insulin secretion increase in an attempt to compensate for the obesity-induced cellular resistance to insulin.

Weight reduction and control is an important aspect of the dietary management of diabetic animals that are overweight. When obesity is reduced in dogs and cats with abnormal insulin-secretory responses, glucose tolerance often improves.[129] In addition, weight loss in pets with IDDM can result in enhanced tissue sensitivity to insulin, resulting in lowered daily insulin requirements. When a diabetic pet is overweight, caloric intake should be designed for weight loss and the eventual maintenance of ideal body weight. A diet that contains a high proportion of complex carbohydrates and reduced fat provides decreased energy density. However, a diet that is low in energy density must also contain adequate levels of all nutrients in forms that are available for digestion and absorption. A commercial diet that is formulated to be complete and balanced while containing moderate fiber levels, increased complex carbohydrates, and reduced fat is recommended. Adding complex carbohydrates or fiber to a normal diet in an attempt to decrease energy density is contraindicated because this practice may cause increased stool volume, loose stools, or diarrhea and can lead to nutrient imbalances. When weight loss is instituted with pets that have IDDM, the pet's blood glucose should be carefully monitored and adjustments in insulin made as glucose tolerance improves.

Timing of Meals

The feeding schedule for pets receiving insulin should be planned so that nutrients are delivered to the body during peak periods of exogenous insulin activity. This span will be determined by the type of insulin used and the time of day it is administered. Several small meals should be provided throughout the period of insulin activity, as opposed to feeding a single large meal. Feeding several small meals helps minimize postprandial fluctuations in blood glucose levels. Other factors that affect the degree of hyperglycemia that occurs following a meal include the composition of the food and the type of insulin administered.

If insulin is administered early in the morning, the first meal should be given immediately before the insulin injection. If the pet refuses to eat on any occasion, the insulin injection can be withheld, thereby preventing the subsequent possibility of hypoglycemia. The remaining three or four meals in the day can be given at equally spaced intervals, depending on the action of the insulin used. Taking blood samples and measuring blood glucose levels every 1 to 2 hours throughout a 24-hour period will indicate if the feeding schedule coincides adequately with insulin activity. If postprandial blood glucose levels rise above 180 milligrams (mg)/deciliter (dl), the interval between feeding and insulin administration should be decreased. If hyperglycemia still occurs, the size of the meal should be decreased and/or the number of meals provided per day should be increased. Likewise, a meal should always be provided within 1 to 2 hours following the lowest blood glucose level.[117,134]

Once an appropriate pet food and feeding schedule have been selected, the management program should be strictly adhered to. Pets that have previously been fed free-choice should be gradually switched to the new regimen. Although most dogs will adapt quickly, cats can be very resistant to changes in their feeding routine and in the type of food that is fed. This resistance can make dietary management of a diabetic cat difficult for some owners. Mixing the new food into the cat's previous food and changing to a meal-feeding regimen over a period of several weeks can help decrease these problems.[135] Allowing cats to nibble over the period of insulin activity is also effective in some cases. Supplemental foods should not be given, and feeding times should vary as little as possible. Periodic monitoring of blood glucose levels can be used to adjust the diet as the pet loses weight, changes the amount of exercise it gets, or requires adjustments in insulin dosage.

C H A P T E R

32

Dietary Management of Urolithiasis in Cats and Dogs

 Lower urinary tract disease is a common disorder in dogs and cats, affecting approximately 7% of cats and 3% of dogs seen at veterinary clinics.[136] Urolithiasis is a specific type of lower urinary tract disease characterized by the presence of urinary crystals (crystalluria) or macroscopic concretions (uroliths or calculi) within the bladder or lower urinary tract, as well as associated clinical signs. Urethral plugs often contain varying proportions of mineral matter and so are classified with urolithiasis.[137] In cats, urolithiasis is now considered to be one manifestation of a collection of lower urinary tract disorders collectively referred to as *feline lower urinary tract disease* (FLUTD).

Urolithiasis is associated with a set of diverse risk factors and can be caused by several different types of mineral aggregates. Dogs reportedly show breed predilections for certain types of urolith formation and are more susceptible to infection-induced urolithiasis than cats are. In both species, identification of the mineral composition of uroliths is important because dietary treatment or management must be directed toward eliminating the specific type of urolith present. The following chapter reviews types of uroliths found in dogs and cats, risk factors for their development, and the use of diet to treat, manage, or prevent recurrence of urolithiasis.

INCIDENCE AND CLINICAL SIGNS

Urolithiasis is typically a disease of adult animals. In cats, it is rarely seen in animals younger than 1 year, and the majority of cats are first diagnosed when they are between 2 and 6 years of age.[136] In dogs, the mean age at time of diagnosis is between 6½ and 7 years.[138] In both species, age of onset is related to the type of urolith present. For example, struvite, urate, and cystine calculi are associated with dogs younger than those having either oxalate or silica calculi.[138]

409

While both male and female pets are affected, gender predispositions are reported for different types of uroliths. For example, female cats have a higher prevalence of struvite urolithiasis than male cats, but more than 70% of cases of calcium oxalate urolithiasis are seen in male cats.[139] Recent studies with dogs have shown a similar relationship between gender and mineral prevalence.[138] Struvite-, urate-, or apatite-containing calculi are more common in females, while oxalate-, cystine-, and silica-containing stones are seen more often in males.

Breed predilections for urolithiasis have been examined in both dogs and cats.[139,140,141,142,143] Early studies reported that compared with domestic short hair cats, Siamese had a decreased risk and Persians had an increased risk of developing FLUTD.[139,140] More recently, studies of the prevalence of calcium oxalate uroliths in cats found that Himalayans and Persians show a relatively higher incidence when compared with other breeds.[141] It has been speculated that breed characteristics such as low activity and a tendency toward obesity may be influential factors. Breed predilections for urolithiasis in dogs seem to be more pronounced. Calcium oxalate uroliths are most common in Miniature Schnauzers, Lhasa Apsos, and certain Terrier breeds.[142,143] In contrast, urate-containing calculi are most often seen in Dalmatians and English Bulldogs, while Dachshunds, English Bulldogs, and Chihuahuas appear to be at increased risk for the development of cystine-containing calculi.[142]

Clinical signs of urolithiasis in dogs and cats are nonspecific and depend on the location, size, and number of crystals or uroliths present within the urinary tract. Uroliths may be found in the bladder, urethra, kidneys, or, rarely, ureters. Although uroliths can be up to several millimeters (mm) in diameter, most are the size of a grain of sand or are even microscopic. Initial clinical signs include frequent urination, dribbling of urine, and urination in inappropriate places. Hematuria and a strong odor of ammonia in the urine are often observed. Pet owners may report additional signs of dysuria, such as prolonged squatting or straining following urination (often confused with constipation) and frequent licking of the urogenital region. These signs are frequently the only signs that owners report to veterinarians.

BOX 32-1

Clinical Signs of Urolithiasis in Dogs and Cats

Frequent urination
Urination in inappropriate places
Prolonged squatting or straining following urination
Hematuria
Licking of urogenital region
Dribbling of urine
Depression
Anorexia
Vomiting and diarrhea
Dehydration

In some cases, partial or total urethral obstruction may develop. When obstruction occurs, a variable mixture of mineral components and a proteinaceous colloidal matrix forms a plug that molds itself to the shape of the urethral lumen.[144] Although this can occur in any dog or cat, it is most commonly reported in male cats, presumably because of their longer and narrower urethras and the sudden narrowing at the bulbourethral glands as the urethra enters the penis.[145,146] If obstruction is complete, uremia develops rapidly and is characterized by abdominal pain, depression, anorexia, dehydration, and vomiting and diarrhea. Increased back pressure of urine can cause renal ischemia, ultimately resulting in permanent renal damage. In severe cases the distended bladder may rupture, causing a transitory relief of signs, followed rapidly by the development of peritonitis and death. Uremia alone leads to coma and death within 2 to 4 days, so partial or total obstruction always represents a medical emergency (Box 32-1).

UROLITH MINERAL TYPE

The mineral composition of uroliths in dogs and cats is most commonly either struvite (magnesium ammonium phosphate) or calcium oxalate. Other less frequently seen mineral composites include ammonium urate, xanthine, cystine, calcium phosphate, and silica. Until recently, struvite was the most commonly reported urolith in cats, followed by calcium oxalate. However, the mineral composition of uroliths retrieved from cats has changed within the past 10 years, which is reflected in a substantial increase in calcium oxalate urolithiasis.[147] A similar trend has occurred in dogs.[148] However, a major difference between struvite urolithiasis in cats and dogs is that most struvite uroliths in cats are not associated with urinary tract infection (called *sterile struvite*), while urinary tract infection is common in dogs with struvite urolithiasis.

STRUVITE UROLITHIASIS IN CATS

Early studies reported that more than 95% of uroliths in cats were composed of struvite.[149,150] However, the incidence of this type of urolith has changed significantly within the last 10 years. A study conducted in 1981 found that 78% of feline uroliths analyzed at the Minnesota Urolith Center were composed of struvite and only 1% of calcium oxalate.[147] By 1993, the incidence of struvite urolithiasis decreased to 43% of the cases, while the incidence of calcium oxalate urolithiasis increased to 43%. Although there was a significant increase in calcium oxalate uroliths during this period, the presence of calcium oxalate in urethral plugs did not change, remaining at less than 1%.

Because struvite crystals were found to be the most prevalent cause of urolithiasis in cats, research during the early 1980s focused on preventing these crystals from forming in the urine and on the development of effective dietary management for cats with struvite urolithiasis. Although it now appears that a substantial proportion of cases may have other causes, prevention of the formation of struvite crystals is still an important and effective protocol for the management of urolithiasis in many cats. Current evidence indicates that three distinct types of struvite urolithiasis occur in cats.[151,152] These are: (1) sterile struvite uroliths, (2) infection-induced struvite uroliths, and (3) urethral plugs containing a variable quantity of struvite crystals. Treatment and dietary management is directed at promoting dissolution of struvite crystals and treating urinary tract infection and inflammation if these are involved.

Struvite Formation

Several conditions are necessary for the formation of struvite crystals in the urinary tract.[152] First, a sufficient concentration of the composite minerals magnesium, ammonium, and phosphate must be present. In addition, these minerals must remain in the tract for an adequate period to allow crystallization to occur. Therefore the production of concentrated urine and small volumes of urine are thought to be contributing factors.[152] Finally, a pH that is favorable for crystal precipitation must exist within the urinary tract environment. Struvite is soluble at a pH below 6.6, and struvite crystals form at a pH of 7.0 and above.[153] Sterile struvite urolithiasis in cats is associated with the previous factors and the absence of a detectable urinary tract infection. However, while the presence of an alkaline urine is necessary for the initial formation of struvite crystals, studies of cats affected with sterile struvite urolithiasis have found that the urine of affected cats is not consistently alkaline. For example, a group of 20 cats with naturally occurring sterile struvite uroliths had a mean urine pH of 6.9 ± 0.4 at the time of diagnosis.[154] Practitioners must be cautioned that the production of a neutral or acidic urine upon presentation should not be interpreted as precluding struvite as the underlying cause of urolithiasis.

Infection-induced struvite urolithiasis is less common in cats than dogs, but it still represents an important form of disease. Infection with urease-producing bacterial species (especially *Staphylococcus*) accompanied by signs of urolithiasis and the presence of struvite in the urinary tract are necessary for diagnosis. These microbes release the enzyme *urease*. Urease hydrolyzes urea to ammonia, causing increased concentrations of ammonia and phosphate ion, two components of struvite. The increased ammonia ion further contributes to urine alkalinization. Abnormalities in local host defense mechanisms, such as a perineal urethrostomy, and the quantity of urea that is found in the cat's urine may predispose a cat to infection-induced urolithiasis.[155,156] However, because most cats are innately resistant to bacterial urinary tract infection, infection-induced struvite urolithiasis is encountered less commonly than sterile struvite.

Dietary Risk Factors

Diet and feeding practices represent important risk factors for struvite urolithiasis in cats (Box 32-2). These include the food's urine-acidifying properties, level of magnesium, digestibility, caloric density, and water content. The cat's feeding schedule may also be important. More than any of the other risk factors involved, these are

BOX 32-2

Dietary Risk Factors for Struvite Urolithiasis in Cats

Urine-acidifying properties (production of an alkaline urine)
High magnesium level
Low digestibility and caloric density
Low moisture content
Feeding regimen (meal-feeding)
Low water intake and balance

elements of a cat's life over which pet owners have some control and that can be modified during the treatment and long-term management of struvite urolithiasis.

One of the factors necessary for the formation of struvite in urine is the presence of sufficient concentrations of its three composite minerals, magnesium, ammonium, and phosphate. Feline urine always contains high amounts of ammonium because of the cat's high protein requirement and intake. Urine phosphate in healthy cats is also usually high enough for struvite formation, regardless of dietary phosphorus intake. The concentration of urine magnesium, on the other hand, is normally quite low and is directly affected by diet.[157]

Early investigations of feline struvite urolithiasis focused on dietary magnesium as a causal agent. The manipulation of dietary magnesium levels to produce or prevent phosphate urolithiasis had previously been well documented in rats and sheep.[158,159] This work was used to suggest a role of this mineral in the etiology of urolithiasis in domestic cats. One of the first studies showed that urethral obstruction and cystoliths could be induced in adult male cats when they were fed a diet containing either 0.75% or 1.0% magnesium and 1.6% phosphate.[160] The obstructing uroliths were composed primarily of magnesium and phosphate. Subsequent work showed that high levels of dietary phosphorus were not necessary for urolith development, but they did increase the risk for urolith formation when dietary magnesium was also high.[161] However, if magnesium intake was low, the incidence of urolith formation was low, regardless of the level of phosphorus. In a later study by the same group, cats were fed diets containing 0.75%, 0.38%, or 0.08% magnesium on a dry-matter basis (DMB). Seventy-six percent of the cats that were fed 0.75% magnesium and 70% of the cats that were fed 0.38% magnesium developed urolithiasis and obstructed within 1 year or less, whereas none of the cats fed 0.08% did.[157] Similarly, when random-source and specific-pathogen–free cats were fed diets containing either high magnesium or high magnesium and high phosphorus levels, urethral obstruction was induced.[162] The obstructing material was identifiable as struvite by radiographic crystallography in one of the seven affected cats.

These studies demonstrate the relationship between increasing magnesium in the diet and an increased rate of urolith formation and urethral obstruction in cats. However, the significance of these data to the role of dietary magnesium in naturally occurring feline struvite urolithiasis is questionable. The levels of dietary magnesium used in these studies were all substantially higher than those normally found in commercial cat foods. The domestic cat requires only 0.016% available magnesium for growth and maintenance.[163] The Association of American Feed Control Officials' (AAFCO's) *Nutrient Profiles* requires cat foods to contain a minimum of 0.04% magnesium.[164] Most commercial cat foods contain slightly higher than this amount but still less than 0.1%. Although the magnesium in naturally occurring ingredients is not 100% available, these levels without exception supply cats with their magnesium requirement. The amount of magnesium in cat foods is higher than the cat's minimum requirement for magnesium, but it is still substantially lower than the levels used in experimental studies to induce struvite formation (0.4% to 1.0%).

A second problem with data from early studies involved the composition of experimentally produced uroliths. The struvite found in naturally occurring cases is composed of three minerals: magnesium, ammonium, and phosphate. However, experimentally induced uroliths in some studies were actually made up of magnesium phosphate, with no detectable ammonium.[160,161] The composition of urethral plugs that caused obstruction in cats fed experimental diets was also different from the composition of urethral plugs of cats with spontaneous disease. Although the experimentally induced plugs were composed almost exclusively of struvite crystal aggregations, urethral plugs found in spontaneous disease are most often composed of a mucogelatinous protein matrix that contains varying amounts of minerals (usually struvite), sloughed tissue, blood, and inflammatory cells.[165,166,167]

The most important confounding factor of these studies involved the form of magnesium added to the experimental diets. A group of investigators examined the effects of two different forms of supplemental dietary magnesium on the urine pH of adult cats.[168] The data showed that the addition of 0.45% magnesium chloride to a basal diet resulted in a significant lowering of urine pH. In contrast, when the cats were fed the same basal diet supplemented with 0.45% magnesium oxide, a significantly higher alkaline pH was produced. In a free-choice feeding regimen, mean urine pH in cats fed the basal diet was 6.9, and urine pH values in cats fed the magnesium chloride– and magnesium oxide–supplemented diets were 5.7 and 7.7, respectively. When urine samples were examined microscopically, crystal formation was observed in cats fed the basal diet and the magnesium oxide–containing diet, but not in cats fed the magnesium chloride–containing diet. Therefore, at the same level of magnesium intake, urine pH and the formation of crystals were affected by the form of magnesium included in the diet. The observation that high levels of magnesium result in increased struvite formation may have been confounded by the effect of magnesium chloride versus magnesium oxide on urine pH. It can be concluded that similarities exist between early studies of experimentally induced struvite urolithiasis and naturally occurring disease, but the presence of significant differences and confounding factors show that magnesium intake is not singularly responsible for the natural development of struvite urolithiasis. Recent evidence indicates that dietary magnesium is less significant than urine pH, urine volume, and water balance as a dietary risk factor.

As discussed previously, struvite crystals form in feline urine with a pH of 7.0 or greater and are soluble at a pH of 6.6 or less.[160] Normal, healthy cats typically have an acid urine with a pH between 6.0 and 6.5, except after meals.[157] In all animals, the consumption of a meal results in a rise in urine pH within 4 hours. This effect, called the *postprandial alkaline tide*, is caused by renal compensation for the loss of gastric acids that are secreted during digestion of the meal. To compensate for the loss of acid and to maintain normal pH in body fluids, the kidneys excrete alkaline ions, resulting in an increased urine pH. The magnitude of the alkaline tide is directly proportional to the size of the meal and to the acidifying or alkalinizing components within the meal. Depending on the nature of the diet and the size of the meal, the postprandial alkaline tide in cats can result in a urine pH as high as 8.0.[169]

Several studies have demonstrated the importance of urine pH in the formation of struvite crystals in cats.[168,169,170,171,172] One study examined the effects of feeding a canned diet, a dry diet, or a dry diet supplemented with a urine acidifier (1.6% ammonium chloride) on urine pH and struvite formation in adult male cats.[170] Urine pH was highest in cats fed the dry diet (7.55). The addition of ammonium chloride reduced urine pH to 5.97. The canned diet produced urine with a mean pH of 5.82. The most significant findings of this study concerned urine struvite formation. Struvite crystals were present in 78% of the cats fed the dry diet but only 9% of the cats fed the dry diet plus ammonium chloride. Intakes of dry matter (DM), magnesium, and other minerals were the same for cats fed each of the dry diets. None of the cats fed the canned diet developed urinary struvite crystals. In addition, when urine samples from all cats were adjusted to a pH of 7.0 using 0.5 molar (M) sodium hydroxide, 46% of the cats fed the canned diet and all of the cats fed the ammonium chloride–supplemented dry diet showed typical struvite formation. These results show that at similar levels of energy, DM, and magnesium intake, the most important factor affecting feline struvite formation is urine pH.

Regardless of the level of magnesium intake by a cat, the dietary manipulation of urine pH consistently affects struvite formation. When a dry diet containing a high level of magnesium (0.37%) was fed to adult male cats, the addition of 1.5% ammonium chloride resulted in a urine pH of 6.0 or less.[171] Cats fed the diet without supplemental ammonium chloride produced urine with a pH of 7.3. Of the non-supplemented cats, 7 of the 12 formed struvite uroliths and obstructed on two occasions, but only 2 of the cats fed the acidifying diet obstructed on a single occasion. When the diets of the seven obstructed cats were supplemented with ammonium chloride, they experienced no further episodes of struvite urolith formation or obstruction. Radiographic examination prior to supplementation revealed visible uroliths, which dissolved after 3 months of consuming the acidifying diet. Similar results have been reported when diets containing levels of magnesium commonly found in commercial pet foods were fed. When adult cats were fed a purified diet containing only 0.045% magnesium, struvite formed, and the cats showed clinical signs of urolithiasis when the diet produced an alkaline urine.[167] However, if ammonium chloride was added as an acidifying agent, clinical signs disappeared within 4 days and did not recur while the acidifying diet was fed.

The domestic cat is a carnivorous mammal. Compared with an omnivorous or herbivorous diet, a carnivorous diet has the effect of increasing net acid excretion and decreasing urine pH.[173,174] This urine-acidifying effect is primarily a result of the high level of sulfur-containing amino acids found in meats. Oxidation of these amino acids results in the excretion of sulfate in the urine and a concomitant decrease in urine pH.[175] In addition, a diet that contains a high proportion of meat is lower in potassium salts than a diet containing high levels of cereal grains, which have been shown to produce an alkaline urine when metabolized.[176,177] Therefore the inclusion of high levels of cereal grains and low levels of meat products in some commercial cat foods may be a contributing factor to the development of struvite urolithiasis. For example, the struvite-producing, commercial dry diet that was used in one study contained 46% cereal grains, primarily in the form of wheat meal.[170] Although a certain amount of cereal is necessary for the extrusion and expansion process of dry foods, high levels of these products may contribute to the production of an alkaline urine. Conversely, the inclusion of large amounts of meat products in cat foods usually contributes to the production of a more acid urine.

As pet food manufacturers search for ingredients to include in cat foods that will naturally produce an acid urine, each ingredient must be separately evaluated for its effect on urine pH. For example, one study compared the urine-acidifying effects of corn gluten meal, poultry meal, and meat and bone meal when diets containing these ingredients were fed to cats.[178] Of the ingredients tested, corn gluten meal had the strongest acidifying effect on urine. Unlike most plant protein sources, corn gluten meal contains higher concentrations of sulfur-containing amino acids than either poultry meal or meat and bone meal. Corn gluten meal is unusual in that it is a cereal protein that produces an acid urine when fed to cats.

Water Balance and Urine Volume

Decreased urine volume may be an important risk factor for the development of urolithiasis in cats. Diets that cause a decrease in total fluid turnover can result in decreased urine volume and increased urine concentration, both of which may contribute to struvite formation. It has been suggested that dry cat foods contribute to decreased fluid intake and urine volume. An early study showed that cats fed a dry cat food had decreased total water intakes when compared with cats consuming similar energy levels from canned food.[179] Cats did increase voluntary water intake when fed the dry food but not in sufficient amounts to fully compensate for the lower moisture content of the food. In another experiment, adult cats were fed a semipurified, basal diet containing varying levels of moisture.[180] The cats consuming a diet containing 10% moisture had an average daily urine volume of 63 milliliters (ml). This volume increased to 112 ml/day when the moisture content of the diet was increased to 75%. Urine specific gravity was also slightly higher in cats that were fed the low-moisture food. In both of these studies, the differences in urine volume were attributed to lower total water intake in the cats that were consuming low-moisture foods.

However, in contrast to these studies, two other groups of investigators found no difference in water consumption between cats fed dry diets and those fed canned diets.[179,180] It appears that diet composition, especially fat content and caloric density, influences water turnover in cats fed different types of commercial diets.[181] A study examined the effects of diet type, composition, and digestibility on water-excretory patterns in cats.[181] A comparison of three canned diets showed that when cats were fed diets containing high levels of fat (34% and 28% of DM), significantly less DM was consumed than when cats were fed a canned diet containing a relatively low level of fat (14%). Fecal DM and fecal water content were lower in cats fed the high-fat diets. Because total water intake was the same for all cats, the cats consuming the high-fat diets excreted significantly higher volumes of water in their urine to achieve water balance. Further evidence supporting the importance of caloric density and fat content is demonstrated by a comparison of the low-fat canned food to three dry cat foods in the same study. Water volume in urine and feces was similar between cats fed the low-fat, canned ration and cats fed the three dry diets. Other than the large difference in water content, the nutrient content of the low-fat, canned food was very similar to that of the dry diets. Energy digestibility of the canned diet was also equivalent to that of the dry diets (79.3% and 78.7%, respectively) and was significantly lower than the mean digestibility of the high-fat, canned diets (90.3%). Statistical analysis of these data revealed that the percentage of water excreted in the urine of cats is directly related to the fat and energy content of the diet, with correlation coefficients of 0.96 and 0.94, respectively.

Some investigators have advocated feeding only canned cat food to cats with a history of urolithiasis.[182,183] The intent is to increase water intake and cause a resultant increase in urine volume and decrease in urine specific gravity. However, the water content of the diet is probably not as important as are caloric density, fat content, and digestibility. As was evident in the previously mentioned study, a poorly digestible canned diet may not contribute to increased urine volume if large amounts of water are excreted in the feces. Conversely, the consumption of a cat food (canned or dry) that is energy-dense and highly digestible will result in lower total DM intake. This decrease will be accompanied by decreased fecal volume and fecal water and increased urine volume. These effects may be beneficial in preventing urolithiasis in cats because urine will contain a lower concentration of the mineral components that lead to urolith formation. In addition, an increase in urine volume also stimulates an increased frequency of urination, thus decreasing the time available for struvite formation.

Feeding Method

The postprandial alkaline tide occurs as a result of meal ingestion and the subsequent excretion and loss of gastric acids.[184] Many factors affect its duration and magnitude. Domestic cats are nibblers by nature. When fed free-choice, most cats eat small meals every few hours throughout the day.[185,186] In general, this feeding regimen has the effect of reducing the magnitude of the alkaline tide but prolonging its duration. In contrast, depending on the alkalinizing effects of the diet, meal-feeding may cause greater fluctuations of shorter duration. The effects of a feeding regimen are further influenced by the type of diet fed, the eating patterns of the cat, and various dietary components.

In one study, cats were fed a dry, commercial food, either on a free-choice basis or once daily. The urine pH of cats fed ad libitum was maintained between 6.5 and 6.9 throughout the day. In cats fed the same diet once daily, urine pH increased 2 hours after the meal to 7.7 and then gradually decreased for the remainder of the day.[172] Another group of researchers fed cats two dry foods and three canned foods on an ad libitum basis and recorded urine pH throughout a 24-hour period.[157] One of the dry foods and two of the canned foods resulted in constant urine pH values of less than 6.3. However, the other dry and canned foods produced pH values that ranged from 6.5 to higher than 7.0. When the same foods were meal-fed once daily, all of the foods except one dry and one canned product resulted in peak urine pH values of greater than 7.0 within 4 hours after the start of the meal. These values all declined to less than 6.5 by approximately 16 hours after the meal. One dry and one canned food maintained pH values of 6.6 or less, even when meal-fed. These differences were attributed to different urine-acidifying components/ingredients present in the foods. More recently, a study that examined the long-term effects of acidifying diets found that ad libitum feeding was essential to maintain a mean urine pH of less than 6.5, even when an acidifying diet was fed.[187] The lower urine pH in cats fed ad libitum was attributed to the consumption of numerous small meals throughout the day, which minimized the amount of gastric acid secreted for each meal and subsequently decreased the postprandial alkaline tide.

In addition to urine pH, the effects of feeding regimen on urine volume and composition are important considerations. In a study that examined the relationship between method of feeding, food and water intake, urine volume, and urine composition, the period of highest urinary excretion of magnesium and phosphorus occurred preprandially and therefore did not coincide with the daily alkaline tide.[188] This study also found that ad libitum–fed cats had increased frequency of urination and greater total urine volume when compared with meal-fed cats. These effects may be beneficial in minimizing urolith formation. Although these results indicate that the highest concentration of composite minerals does not occur during the time they would be most likely to precipitate, this may not be a necessary condition for struvite formation. Research has shown that urine pH is directly related to the size of the meal, and this relationship can be described by a simple linear model.[189] In other words, as the size of the meal increases, so does postprandial urine pH. These data also showed that as postprandial urine pH increased, the presence of struvite crystals increased accordingly. Struvite did not form when urine pH was maintained at less than 6.6.

DIETARY MANAGEMENT

In clinical cases in which obstruction has occurred, immediate care involves stabilization of the cat's condition, fluid replacement therapy, and relief of bladder distention and urethral obstruction. Removal of the obstruction can usually be accomplished by either flushing the urolith or urethral plug out of the urethra or by cystocentesis. However, while cystocentesis immediately relieves the distended bladder, it usually does not remove the obstructing uroliths. Bacterial urinary tract infections, if present, should be managed by appropriate antimicrobial therapy. Long-term dietary management involves the removal or dissolution of any remaining struvite uroliths and the feeding of an appropriate diet that prevents struvite formation.

Remaining struvite uroliths that are present in the urinary tract can be removed either through surgical means or diet-induced dissolution. Surgical intervention provides immediate relief to the animal, followed by recovery within 3 to 7 days. On the other hand, dietary dissolution is a noninvasive procedure but can take several months to be effective. When dietary intervention is used, the diet should be formulated to reduce the urinary concentration of magnesium and produce an acid urine with a pH of 6.3 or less.[190] Increasing sodium chloride in the diet has been suggested as an agent to induce polydipsia and resultant polyuria with the intent of producing a more dilute urine and increasing the frequency of urination.[191] However, feeding increased amounts of sodium to cats increases renal excretion of calcium and so may contribute to the formation of calcium oxalate uroliths.[190] For this reason, increased sodium chloride is not recommended. Depending on the size and number of the uroliths present, complete dietary dissolution usually takes between 5 and 7 weeks.[192] There is also evidence suggesting that infection-induced struvite uroliths may take longer for dissolution than sterile struvite uroliths.[154] Regardless of the difference in time for dissolution, the eradication of infection caused by urease-producing bacteria is the most important factor in cats with infection-induced struvite urolithiasis.

A urine pH between 6.0 and 6.3 is desirable during the struvite dissolution phase of treatment.[153,190] Once a diet has been selected, urine pH should be monitored 4 to 8 hours after initial consumption to ensure that adequate (but not excessive) acidification is occurring. Only the prescribed diet should be fed, with no additional supplements or other cat foods. During the dissolution phase, cats should be monitored for struvite dissolution at 2- to 4-week intervals, using either palpation or radiography. Periodic evaluation of urine sediment for crystalluria may be helpful in assessing progress, but because many healthy, normal cats develop urine struvite crystals, the presence of crystalluria should not be interpreted as persistent urolithiasis.[178,193] The diet should be continued for at least 1 month following complete dissolution of struvite.[153,194,195] After this period, the diet can be changed to a maintenance product demonstrated to be effective in the management of struvite urolithiasis.

A maintenance diet that is fed to prevent the recurrence of struvite urolithiasis should produce a slightly acidified urine, be moderate in caloric density and high in digestibility, and contain a relatively low level of magnesium. A urine pH of 6.6 or less prevents the formation of struvite crystals. Therefore, a pH range between 6.0 and 6.5 is desirable for long-term maintenance. Dietary ingredients that have the effect of increasing urinary acid excretion include proteins of animal origin (because of their high sulfur–amino acid content) and compounds that result in an elevated absorption of chloride, phosphate, or sulfate.[177] Conversely, most cereal grains contain high levels of potassium salts that have the effect of producing an alkaline urine.[170] The exception is corn gluten meal, which produces an acidic urine because of its high concentration of sulfur amino acids.[178] Most commercial cat foods that contain high amounts of cereal grains should be avoided.

Diets that are moderate in caloric density and are highly digestible will be consumed in smaller amounts, thus lowering both DM and magnesium intake. The lower DM intake results in decreased fecal matter and fecal water and increased urine volume. Feeding a canned diet with these characteristics may further contribute to increased urine volume and decreased urine specific gravity.[196] Decreased magnesium intake results in lower concentrations of urine magnesium, which is necessary for struvite formation. The percentage of magnesium in the diet is not as important as the total amount of magnesium that a cat consumes. Although some researchers believe that magnesium concentration in the diet should be 0.1% or less on a DMB, others maintain that the risk of struvite formation is only increased when magnesium levels reach 0.25% or greater.[193,195,197] Because the cat's requirement for dietary magnesium is substantially lower than the amount usually found in cat food, a general rule of thumb is to select a food that contains 0.12 % magnesium or less.

There are several high-quality, nutritionally complete commercial cat foods that meet the criteria discussed. Although many grocery store brands of dry cat food may contain relatively low concentrations of magnesium, they are often low in digestibility and contain high levels of cereal grains. A commercial cat food should not be selected only on the basis of its magnesium content. The food's caloric density, digestibility, and urine-acidifying properties should all be considered when selecting a commercial cat food for the prevention of struvite urolithiasis (Box 32-3).

Risks Associated with Overacidification

Even though the maintenance of a urine pH of 6.6 or lower prevents the formation of struvite crystals, the production of urine that is too acidic can be detrimental to a cat's health. If more acid is consumed than an animal is capable of excreting, metabolic acidosis occurs. Several studies have shown that when cats are fed a

BOX 32-3

Dietary Management for Prevention of Struvite Urolithiasis

Perform surgical removal or medical dissolution of uroliths (initial treatment).
Treat and prevent recurrence of bacterial urinary tract infection (if present).
Select a food that produces an acidified urine (pH 6.0 to 6.5).
Avoid overacidification of urine.
Select a food with a reduced magnesium content (<0.12% DMB for cats).
Select a food that is highly digestible and moderate in caloric density.
Feed either a canned food or add water to a dry food to increase water intake.
Do not feed other foods, supplements, or treats.

severely acidifying diet for several months, they develop metabolic acidosis, decreased levels of serum potassium, and depletion of body potassium stores.[198,199] Other studies indicate that the long-term feeding of highly acidifying diets containing marginal levels of potassium cause hypokalemia and kidney disease in some cats.[200,201] For example, three out of nine cats fed an acidifying diet containing 40% protein and marginal levels of potassium developed chronic renal failure within 2 years.[199]

The consumption of an acidifying diet or urine-acidifying agents that cause acidosis results in increased urinary losses of potassium and calcium and may compromise electrolyte balance.[175] When acid intake is too high, the body will reestablish acid-base balance at a decreased blood bicarbonate concentration. Carbonate and phosphate are resorbed from bone to supply cations, and the calcium that is resorbed is excreted in the urine. Prolonged losses of calcium as a result of renal acidosis may eventually lead to bone demineralization and osteoporosis.[202,203] Urinary acidifying agents have been shown to have detrimental effects on bone mineralization in cats. When a diet containing 3% ammonium chloride was fed to growing kittens, urine pH was significantly decreased, but the kittens also exhibited impaired growth, decreased blood pH, increased urine calcium excretion, and bone demineralization of the caudal vertebrae.[202] Similar changes were reported when adult cats were fed a diet containing 1.5% ammonium chloride.[204]

In contrast, a 2-year study found that adult cats that were ad libitum–fed two acidifying diets maintained normal ranges for all hematological and serum biochemical profiles, as well as normal blood gas values.[187] Although cats fed the two acidifying diets had slightly lower serum phosphorus, bicarbonate, and base excess values, these values all remained within laboratory reference ranges. Measurement of bone mineral density after 2 years of feeding also showed no effect of diet. When fed ad libitum, the diet used in this study resulted in the production of urine with an average pH of 6.2. Another study using 1.7 % phosphoric acid to induce moderate acidification of urine also reported a lack of detrimental effects after 1 year of feeding.[205] An important difference between these studies and those discussed previously is that the more recent studies used diets that included corn gluten meal, animal protein, and/or phosphoric acid as urine-acidifying components. Feeding a diet that contains ingredients that promote moderate urine acidification appears to present less risk for overacidification than does supplementing a cat's diet with a urine-acidifying agent such as ammonium chloride.

Another effect of an acidified urine may be to promote the formation of another type of urolith. Although struvite is soluble in an acid urine, an acid pH may increase the likelihood of calcium oxalate formation. The prolonged feeding of a highly acidified diet leads to a loss of calcium in the urine, making this mineral available for the formation of calcium-containing uroliths. In addition, feeding a low-magnesium diet can exacerbate this problem because urine magnesium appears to inhibit calcium oxalate formation.[206] The incidence of calcium oxalate urolithiasis in cats has increased while struvite urolithiasis has decreased during the past several years.[147] It is theorized that the widespread feeding of acidifying diets that contain low levels of magnesium may be a contributing factor to this trend (see p. 424).

STRUVITE UROLITHIASIS IN DOGS

Until recently, there was very limited information available regarding the incidence of urolithiasis and the prevalence of different types of uroliths in dogs. However, analysis of data collected at the Minnesota Urolith Center and the Urinary Stone Analysis Laboratory in California has provided valuable information regarding the age, breed, and sex of affected dogs and the mineral composition and location of calculi.[207,208,209] Although dogs may develop several different types and combinations of uroliths, struvite uroliths are the most frequently diagnosed type.[148] Similar to its occurrence in cats, struvite urolithiasis is a disease of primarily adult dogs. The mean age of diagnosis is between 4 and 6 years, and female dogs are disproportionately more likely to be affected than males.[208] Certain breeds have an increased incidence of struvite urolithiasis when compared with the general population of dogs. The Bichon Frise, Dachshund, Miniature Schnauzer, Poodle, Pekingese, Pug, Welsh Corgi, Beagle, Cocker Spaniel, Springer Spaniel, and Labrador Retriever are more frequently affected.[148,207,209] Conversely a relatively lower risk for the development of struvite calculi is reported in the Dalmatian, Pomeranian, and Maltese.

Sterile vs. Infection-Induced Struvite

Similar to its production in cats, the production of sterile struvite in dogs is associated with the production of alkaline urine without a detectable urinary tract infection. However, the incidence of sterile struvite in proportion to that of infection-induced struvite urolithiasis is lower in dogs than in cats.[156] The association between urinary tract infection and struvite urolithiasis in dogs is well documented.[210,211,212] In contrast, urinary tract infections are often absent in dogs with calcium oxalate–, cystine-, urate-, or silica-containing calculi.[213] A recent study of more than 11,000 canine urinary calculi specimens found *Staphylococcus intermedius* in 30% of affected males and 54% of affected females.[214,215] There was a significant correlation between the presence of struvite calculi and a positive culture for this organism in both genders. Bacterial species most often cultured from dogs with struvite urolithiasis include *Staphylococcus, Proteus* species, and uriaplasmas.[148] It has been suggested that dogs that produce urine with a high concentration of urea may be more susceptible to this type of urolithiasis because bacterial urease converts the urea to ammonia, which is a component of struvite. However, an association between urinary urea concentration and struvite formation has not been documented in dogs.

Female dogs are more likely than males to develop struvite urolithiasis. One report found that 94% of the urocystoliths retrieved from female dogs were composed of struvite.[207] While male dogs also developed struvite, they showed a greater assortment of mineral types. In addition, female dogs show a higher incidence of infection-induced struvite when compared with males.[214] While struvite-, calcium phosphate (apatite)–, and urate-containing calculi are more common in female dogs, oxalate-, cystine-, silica-, brushite-, and xanthine-containing calculi are more common in males. One potential cause for this difference is anatomical. The shorter urethra of the female dog may facilitate the ability of opportunistic bacteria to move up the urethra into the bladder to cause infection.[214,216] It has also been suggested that dogs who are confined indoors may have longer periods of urine retention, increasing the potential for bacterial growth within the urinary tract.

Dietary Management

Surgical removal of uroliths is necessary in most cases of struvite urolithiasis in dogs, especially if the uroliths are located in the ureters or urethra. An advantage to surgical intervention is that clinical signs are quickly relieved, and treatment can then focus on eliminating urinary tract infections and preventing recurrence. An alternative, nonsurgical method for urolith removal is voiding urohydropropulsion.[217]

Medical dissolution of struvite uroliths using a calcuolytic diet has also been used in dogs. Acidifying diets that contain restricted levels of protein have been used. However, while this is often an appropriate and successful method of struvite dissolution in cats, it is not as successful in dogs.[218] Protein restriction was once used as a method of decreasing urinary urea, an important substrate for urease-positive bacteria. However, proper antimicrobial treatment is more effective at controlling bacterial populations in the urinary tract, and restricted-protein diets have been associated with low palatability and acceptance. Because most struvite calculi found in dogs contain significant amounts of non-struvite minerals, which will not dissolve in response to an acidifying diet, medical dissolution is no longer recommended for most cases of canine struvite urolithiasis.[218] In all cases, appropriate antimicrobial therapy must be instituted if urinary tract infection is present. This should be continued for 3 to 4 weeks after dissolution or removal of uroliths. Antibiotic therapy is not necessary for dogs with sterile struvite urolithiasis.

The protocol for prevention of recurrence of struvite urolithiasis includes feeding a diet that produces a moderately acidic urine and reduces the concentration of struvite components and preventing recurrence of urinary tract infection.[218,219] A diet that promotes the production of urine with a pH between 6.4 and 6.6 is recommended. Once an appropriate acidifying diet has been selected, no other foods, supplements, or treats should be fed. The diet should also contain sufficient but not excessive amounts of high-quality protein. Keeping the dog's urinary tract free of bacterial infection is the most important factor for prevention of infection-induced struvite urolithiasis. Following a complete course of full-dose antimicrobial therapy, a reduced therapeutic dose of an antimicrobial agent is often administered for up to 6 months. Periodic urine cultures should be conducted every 2 to 3 months to monitor the effectiveness of the regimen, and these should be continued for up to 2 years following the completion of antibiotic treatment.[218]

CALCIUM OXALATE UROLITHIASIS IN CATS

During the past decade, the prevalence of feline calcium oxalate uroliths has been increasing, and the prevalence of struvite uroliths has been substantially decreasing (see p. 411).[141,147] A suggested cause of this trend is the increased use of urine-acidifying diets containing low levels of magnesium. The inappropriate feeding of diets formulated to prevent struvite formation in cats that are actually at risk for calcium oxalate crystalluria may result in an increased incidence of clinical calcium oxalate urolithiasis.[220] Cats with this type of urolithiasis usually produce a concentrated urine (specific gravity of 1.04) that is slightly acidified (pH 6.3 to 6.7).[221] Mild acidemia is reported in some, but not all, cats. This results in mobilization of carbonate and phosphate from bones to buffer the excess acid. Calcium is concomitantly released and excreted in the urine, leading to a higher concentration of this mineral in the urine, which may also predispose to calcium oxalate formation. Calcium oxalate uroliths are found most often in the urinary bladder, but they also occur in various combinations in the urethra, kidneys, and ureters. Calcium oxalate uroliths are slightly more common in males and neutered animals than in females or intact cats.[220,221] Similar to struvite urolithiasis, calcium oxalate urolithiasis is a disease primarily seen in adult animals. Predispositions have been reported in the Burmese, Himalayan, and Persian breeds.[221]

Risk Factors

Several dietary components are potential contributors to the development of calcium oxalate calculi in cats.[218,221] Factors that may be important include the food's urine-acidifying properties and levels of magnesium, calcium, sodium, and vitamin B_6.[221] As with struvite, the focus has been on factors that either increase or decrease the concentration of the calculi's components in the urine (in this case, calcium and oxalate) and those that affect the solubility of calcium oxalate crystals.

A study of urine samples from cats fed a variety of diets found that reduction of urine pH and magnesium concentration significantly increased struvite solubility but concurrently decreased calcium oxalate solubility.[222] In addition, in vitro studies have shown that increased amounts of urinary magnesium reduce the formation of calcium oxalate crystals. This observation has led to the use of magnesium supplementation in humans to prevent the formation of calcium oxalate calculi. However, because increased dietary magnesium is a risk factor for struvite urolithiasis in cats, increasing dietary magnesium with the intent of preventing calcium oxalate formation is contraindicated in this species. Similarly, providing a diet that has an alkalinizing effect upon urine pH may prevent calcium oxalate urolith formation but is an important risk factor for struvite formation.

Several factors may affect the concentrations of calcium and oxalate in urine. The consumption of high amounts of sodium leads to increased renal excretion of calcium.[221] Vitamin D and ascorbic acid levels in the diet may be important because vitamin D promotes intestinal absorption of calcium, and ascorbic acid is a precursor of oxalate. Vitamin B_6 has been identified as a potentially important nutrient because experimentally induced vitamin B_6 deficiency has been associated with hyperoxaluria and the formation of renal calcium oxalate calculi in kittens.[223] However, naturally occurring hyperoxaluria has not been reported in cats. Moreover, supplementation with vitamin B_6 for cats that are not deficient does not reduce urinary oxalate excretion.[221]

A final possible risk factor is the presence of hypercalcemia. As discussed previously, some cats with calcium oxalate urolithiasis have mild acidemia. A slight but persistent acidemia promotes the mobilization of carbonate and phosphorus from bone to buffer the excess hydrogen ions. The concomitant mobility of calcium leads to increased serum calcium and hypercalciuria. It has been postulated that because hypercalcemia promotes urinary excretion of calcium, it may predispose the precipitation of calcium oxalate. While serum concentration of minerals, including calcium, are normal in most cats with calcium oxalate urolithiasis, moderate hypercalcemias (11 and 13 mg/dl) have been reported.[221] This observation warrants routine evaluation of serum calcium concentrations in affected patients, because hypercalcemia promotes urinary calcium excretion and may promote the formation and precipitation of calcium oxalate crystals (Box 32-4).

Dietary Management

Unlike struvite uroliths, calcium oxalate uroliths in cats cannot be dissolved using a calcuolytic diet. Therefore, this type of urolith must be removed from the urinary tract using surgical intervention or urohydropropulsion.[217,220] In some cases, very small urocystoliths may be retrieved through catheterization. If hypercalcemia is present, appropriate treatment to correct the underlying cause must be instituted. Following removal of uroliths and recovery from surgery, emphasis is placed on preventing recurrence though the use of an appropriate diet.

Goals of dietary management include reducing urinary concentrations of calcium and oxalate and maintaining a dilute urine with a pH between 6.3 and 6.9.[224] The food that is selected should contain ingredients that are highly digestible and include optimal levels of calcium and magnesium. Restriction of dietary calcium is not recommended unless absorptive hypercalcemia exists. In those cases, moderate restriction is advocated to prevent negative calcium balance. Although increased urine magnesium concentration reduces the formation of calcium oxalate crystals, this is also a risk factor for struvite urolith formation. Therefore magnesium levels in the diet should be adequate but not high. Because the consumption of excess levels of sodium may induce increased renal excretion of calcium, moderate restriction of dietary sodium has been recommended.[190]

BOX 32-4

Dietary Risk Factors for Calcium Oxalate Urolithiasis in Cats
Urine-acidifying properties (production of an acidified urine)
Reduced magnesium content (possibly)
Excess sodium consumption
Excess vitamin D and ascorbic acid intake
Low water intake and balance
Any factor that may contribute to hypercalciuria or hypercalcemia

The production of a dilute urine can be achieved by feeding a diet that is high in digestibility and moisture. Feeding a canned ration or adding water to a high-quality, highly digestible dry food is recommended. Potassium citrate is often included in diets that are formulated to prevent recurrence of calcium oxalate urolithiasis. Potassium citrate has an alkalinizing effect on urine pH, and when excreted in the urine, citrate forms a soluble salt with calcium (Box 32-5).[221,225]

CALCIUM OXALATE UROLITHIASIS IN DOGS

Uroliths composed of calcium oxalate are the second most common type found in dogs.[226,227] Like struvite uroliths, calcium oxalate uroliths can develop in dogs of any age, but it is primarily a disease of adult animals. More than half of the cases occur in dogs between the ages of 5 and 12 years.[226] In contrast to struvite urolithiasis, male dogs are more likely than females to be affected.[218] The incidence of calcium oxalate urolithiasis in both genders has increased dramatically in the past 15 years, possibly in response to the increased use and availability of dog foods that promote the production of an acidified urine.[218]

Risk Factors

Risk factors are similar to those for cats and include mild acidemia, decreased urine pH, hypercalciuria, production of a concentrated urine, and possibly consumption of an acidifying diet or excessive amounts of vitamin C. Miniature Schnauzers are most commonly affected, accounting for about 25% of cases of calcium oxalate urolithiasis in dogs.[226] Other breeds that are more frequently affected include the Lhasa Apso, Yorkshire Terrier, Miniature Poodle, Shih Tzu, and Bichon Frise. Hypercalcemia is not common, but it is seen in some cases. This is associated with increased urine calcium excretion, normal serum calcium values, and normal or low serum parathyroid hormone concentration.[228] There is also recent evidence that the presence of hyperadrenocorticism increases a dog's risk for developing calcium oxalate urolithiasis.[229]

Dietary Management

As it is for cats, the only effective treatment for dogs with clinically active calcium oxalate uroliths is removal, through either surgery, catheterization, or urohydropropulsion. If hypercalciuria is present, the underlying cause, if known, should be addressed. If an acidifying food or supplemental vitamin C is being fed, the dog should be switched to a food that promotes a neutral urine pH and contains ingredients that are high in quality and digestibility. All supplements should be discontinued. Increased water intake is recommended to promote the production of a dilute urine. This can usually be accomplished through either feeding a canned diet or adding water to a dry food immediately before feeding (Box 32-5). As with cats, potassium citrate is often included in diets that are formulated to prevent recurrence of calcium oxalate urolithiasis in dogs because of its urine-alkalinizing effect.[225]

BOX 32-5

Dietary Management for Prevention of Calcium Oxalate Urolithiasis

Perform removal of uroliths through surgery, urohydropropulsion, or catheterization (initial treatment).

Treat hypercalcemia (if present).

Select a food that produces a neutral or slightly acidified urine (pH 6.3 to 6.9).

Select a food with optimal calcium and magnesium levels.

Select a food that is highly digestible and moderate in caloric density.

Select a food with normal (not excess) sodium and supplemental potassium citrate.

Feed either a canned food or add water to a dry food to increase water intake.

Do not feed other foods, supplements, or treats.

OTHER TYPES OF UROLITHS FOUND IN CATS

Other mineral types found in feline uroliths include purine (ammonium urate or xanthine), cystine, and calcium phosphate.[136,147] Purine uroliths make up a relatively small fraction of uroliths seen in cats and are most commonly located in the urinary bladder. Although the underlying cause is usually not known, the production of an acidic, highly concentrated urine and the consumption of a food high in purine precursors (such as liver) may be risk factors for this type of urolith. Calcium phosphate (apatite) is found in 1% or less of naturally occurring feline uroliths.[147] A primary risk factor for this type of urolith in other species is the presence of primary hyperparathyroidism. However, this association has not been reported in cats.[147,230] Cats with cystine uroliths have increased urine concentration of the amino acids cystine, arginine, lysine, and ornithine.[190] Although medical protocols for the dissolution of this type of urolith have not been developed, cystine is soluble in alkaline urine and precipitates in acidified urine. Therefore urine-acidifying foods should not be fed to cats with this type of urolith.

Recently, it has been theorized that a substantial proportion of cats diagnosed with nonobstructive lower urinary tract disease may be affected by a disease that is similar to interstitial cystitis in humans.[196] In cats, the disorder has been called *idiopathic cystitis* to reflect its unknown etiology.[231] A diagnosis is made based upon clinical signs of lower urinary tract disease, abnormalities of urinalysis, and urinary tract lesions identified by imaging studies. Clinically, a diagnosis of idiopathic cystitis is made in cats with signs of lower urinary tract disease and urinalysis abnormalities for which no obvious cause can be found. Most cats diagnosed with idiopathic cystitis produce an acidic urine and are fed a dry cat food. Although little is known about its underlying cause, the currently recommended dietary management of idiopathic cystitis is to change the cat's diet to promote production of a more dilute urine. This can be accomplished by adding water to a dry food or switching to a canned ration. Potential benefits of producing less concentrated urine include the dilution of any noxious substances that may contribute to the disorder, more frequent urination patterns that decrease bladder contact time with urine, and removal of any excess crystals (if they exist).

OTHER TYPES OF UROLITHS FOUND IN DOGS

Other mineral types found in the urinary calculi of dogs include urate (usually in Dalmatians; see p. 394), calcium phosphate, silica, and cystine. Calcium phosphate is the third most common type of mineral found in canine uroliths; this type occurs more often in females than males.[138] In most cases, calcium phosphate is found as a component of mixed-mineral uroliths with either struvite or calcium oxalate. Because calcium phosphate is typically considered to be a secondary component, dietary management is usually directed toward preventing the recurrence of the primary mineral.

Silica crystals are also often found in association with other types of minerals, but these are seen more often in males than females.[232] Certain breeds of dog appear to have an increased risk for silica urolithiasis. These include the German Shepherd, Old English Sheepdog, Miniature Schnauzer, Shih Tzu, Lhasa Apso, Yorkshire Terrier, and Golden Retriever.[218,232] Surgical removal is the conventional treatment. A measure used to prevent recurrence is increasing water consumption to produce a more dilute urine.

Cystine urolithiasis is relatively rare in dogs, but when it occurs it is almost always in males.[138,233] Certain breeds are at increased risk, and it is associated with reduced renal tubular reabsorption of several basic amino acids such as lysine, arginine, ornithine, and citrulline. Following surgical removal, preventive measures include feeding a urine-alkalinizing diet and increasing water consumption to promote the production of a less concentrated urine.

C H A P T E R

33

Nutritionally Responsive
Dermatoses

The skin (integument) is a metabolically active organ system that provides sensory input, protects the body from physical and infectious injury, functions in temperature control and immunoregulation, and serves as a reservoir for some nutrients.[234] The health of a pet's skin and hair coat can be affected by nutrient imbalances that involve protein, vitamin A, vitamin E, the essential fatty acids (EFAs), and zinc. Dogs and cats that are consuming high-quality, complete, balanced pet foods are unlikely to suffer from a serious deficiency or excess of any of these nutrients. However, feeding a poorly formulated or stored commercial food or preparing a homemade diet that is not correctly balanced can lead to skin disorders. In addition, any metabolic or functional disorder that affects a pet's ability to digest, absorb, or use nutrients can cause secondary nutrient imbalances that may manifest as dermatoses. A third way nutrition can affect the health of the skin is through the development of a food allergy or hypersensitivity. The development of a hypersensitivity to one or more components in the diet can be the cause of inflammatory dermatoses in dogs and cats. Dermatoses caused by both nutrient imbalances and food hypersensitivities are discussed in this chapter.

PROTEIN AND SKIN HEALTH

The importance of protein for the maintenance and development of skin tissues is well documented. A deficiency of protein in dogs and cats causes changes to the skin and hair coat. Signs include abnormal keratinization of skin and hair, depigmentation of hair shafts, and changes in sebaceous and epidermal lipids. Hairs become brittle and break off easily, and coat growth slows or stops. The lipid layer of the epidermis also becomes abnormal and loses its function as a protective barrier. The skin becomes scaly, greasy, and susceptible to secondary bacterial infections. Today, dermatoses that are induced by protein deficiency are very rare in dogs and cats. Cases of extreme protein/calorie malnutrition or starvation can result in dermatological signs, but other clinical signs of malnutrition will also be observed. When healthy pets are fed balanced, complete pet foods, signs of protein deficiency are highly unlikely.

Dietary protein may also affect skin health in terms of hypersensitivity response and effect upon subcutaneous lipid metabolism. The importance of dietary protein for pets with food-induced allergies is discussed later in this chapter. It has also been theorized that feeding different types of proteins may affect skin and serum lipid concentrations in dogs. For example, when fed to monkeys and rabbits, plant proteins are hypocholesterolemic when compared with animal proteins.[235,236]

In a study with dogs, six different protein sources (chicken, pork, lamb, fish, beef, and soy) were sequentially fed to a group of 12 dogs.[237] No differences were observed between protein treatment groups in skin histology, signs of inflammation or pruritus, or skin fatty acid levels. However, several of the dogs fed pork had increased production of scale and decreased hair regrowth following skin biopsies. These results may suggest that pork should be avoided as a protein source in dogs with seborrhea. However, additional research is needed to confirm these findings and to further investigate the role of pork in skin health.

Another study compared the effects of feeding soy protein versus a meat-based protein source and soy oil versus poultry fat on serum cholesterol, serum lipids, and cutaneous fatty acid concentrations in dogs.[238] Dietary protein had no effect upon serum cholesterol concentration and only marginal effects upon serum and skin fatty acid concentrations. However, dogs fed soy oil–containing diets had higher linoleic acid and lower oleic acid concentrations in skin and serum when compared with dogs fed diets containing poultry fat. Dogs fed diets containing poultry fat also had higher concentrations of serum arachidonic acid. While the type of fat significantly influenced serum and skin fatty acid and cholesterol concentrations in this study, these effects were not related to the type of protein that was fed.

The results of these two studies indicate that protein source does not significantly affect changes in fatty acid values or skin architecture in the dog. The effects of dietary protein on inflammatory skin disease in dogs may be related more to allergenicity and frequency of exposure rather than effects upon fatty acid metabolism or homeostasis. It is also possible that fat content in various protein sources may affect cutaneous and plasma fatty acid concentrations. Such effects are associated with the protein's fatty acid profiles and not with protein characteristics per se.

VITAMIN A–RESPONSIVE DERMATOSES

Vitamin A is necessary for normal epithelial cell differentiation and maintenance and for the process of keratinization (see Section 1, pp. 29-31, and Section 2, pp. 117-119). Both deficiencies and excesses of this vitamin cause skin lesions in dogs and cats. Signs include hair loss and poor coat condition, hyperkeratinization of the epidermis and hair follicles, scaling of the skin, and an increased susceptibility to secondary bacterial infections of the skin.[234] Vitamin A toxicity is most commonly caused by feeding an all-liver diet or by oversupplementation with cod liver oil.

More common than deficiencies or excesses, however, are certain types of skin disorders that are responsive to treatment with supplemental vitamin A. The administration of vitamin A and the retinoids (natural and synthetic analogues of vitamin A) appear to have both physiological and pharmacological effects. These compounds have been used successfully in humans and animals to treat cases of idiopathic seborrhea that are not caused by a vitamin A deficiency.[239,240] *Seborrhea* is a general term that describes the overproduction of oils and other protective secretions by the sebaceous glands in the skin. The skin usually becomes flaky, greasy, or both. Because the epidermal lipid layer is abnormal, the animal becomes prone to secondary bacterial skin infections that can cause pruritus and further damage to the skin. Treatment of seborrhea in companion animals is usually directed toward determining the underlying cause and correcting it. However, in a substantial number of cases, an underlying cause cannot be identified and treatment is directed primarily toward the relief of clinical signs.

Certain types of seborrhea in dogs and cats respond favorably to vitamin A. Idiopathic seborrhea in Cocker Spaniels can often be kept in complete remission with vitamin A therapy.[241,242,243] Similar results have been reported in Labrador Retrievers and Miniature Schnauzers.[242,244] Vitamin A–responsive seborrhea is characterized by dry and scaly skin that progresses to oily changes. Affected dogs eventually develop large, hyperkeratotic plaques (composed of sebum and keratin) and marked follicular plugging. Lesions are most prominent on the underside of the thorax and abdomen. Hair loss and skin changes are accompanied by secondary bacterial folliculitis. Pruritus and inflammation may or may not be present.[241,244] Almost all reported cases also show moderate to severe otitis externa.

Cases of vitamin A–responsive seborrhea usually do not respond to the traditional treatments for seborrhea, which include medicated shampoos, antibiotic therapy, and glucocorticoid therapy. Although clinical signs can be used in support of a diagnosis, the diagnosis of vitamin A–responsive seborrhea can only be confirmed through favorable response to supplementation. A dose of 10,000 international units (IUs) per day is suggested, although levels as high as 50,000 IUs/day have been used.[241,242,243,244] A decrease in clinical signs is usually seen within 4 weeks, with complete remission within 2 to 6 months.[241,244] Attempts to reduce the level of vitamin A or to withdraw therapy result in a relapse of clinical signs, indicating that lifelong therapy is necessary. The dosages used represent 6 to 10 times the dog's normal requirement for vitamin A. However, no signs of vitamin A toxicity have been observed in the reported cases, even after several years of therapy. Other studies have indicated that much higher levels of vitamin A are necessary to induce clinical signs of toxicity in dogs.[245,246]

A second skin disorder that has been shown to be responsive to vitamin A supplementation is sebaceous adenitis. This chronic skin disease is characterized by the development of lymphocytic, granulomatous, or pyogranulomatous inflammation of the sebaceous glands, resulting in scaling, skin lesions, and hair loss. Over time, sebaceous glands are progressively destroyed, and inflammation diminishes. Standard

Poodles, Akitas, Chow Chows, and Vizslas are more frequently affected with this disorder than the general population of dogs.[247,248] In Poodles, the disease is believed to be transmitted by an autosomal recessive gene.[249] Some of the treatments used to manage sebaceous adenitis include antiseborrheic shampoos, topical application of propylene glycol or EFAs, and systemic administration of cyclosporine or synthetic retinoids (vitamin A derivatives).

A recent study of 30 dogs examined the efficacy of using two synthetic retinoids, isotretinoin and etretinate, to treat the clinical signs of sebaceous adenitis.[250] Dogs that had been diagnosed with the disorder were treated for a minimum of 2 months with one of the two retinoids. Forty-seven percent of the dogs given isotretinoin and fifty-three percent given etretinate were successfully treated and were maintained on retinoid therapy indefinitely. Although it was previously thought that Akitas respond poorly to synthetic retinoids, this study reported successful treatment in 10 of the 11 Akitas included.[248,251] These results suggest that retinoids may be an effective treatment for some dogs with sebaceous adenitis. An initial dosage of 1 milligram (mg)/kilogram (kg) of body weight per day of either isotretinoin or etretinate is recommended.[250]

It is important to note that these skin conditions are not caused by a vitamin A deficiency. In all reported cases, the dogs were being fed a high-quality, complete and balanced, commercial dog food. Moreover, serum levels of vitamin A were normal, and no other signs of vitamin A deficiency were observed. One group of investigators also reported that the skin changes seen in cases of vitamin A–responsive dermatosis differed significantly from those seen with a true vitamin A deficiency.[241] It is likely that the effect of vitamin A is the result of a pharmacological action of the vitamin on epithelial cells, rather than a result of the vitamin's role as an essential nutrient.[239]

VITAMIN E–RESPONSIVE DERMATOSES

It has been suggested that vitamin E may play a role in certain skin disorders in dogs. The occurrence of demodicosis (skin lesions caused by the demodectic mange mite *Demodex canis*) has been associated with decreased blood levels of vitamin E. It has been theorized that a subclinical vitamin E deficiency causes suppression of the immune system, which in turn increases a dog's susceptibility to the *Demodex* mite. In one study, a group of dogs with demodicosis were treated with supplemental vitamin E, and significant improvement was observed.[252] However, other studies have reported that vitamin E supplementation had no effect on demodicosis.[17] More controlled research is necessary before definitive conclusions can be made concerning the role of vitamin E in the control of this disorder in dogs.

Supplementation with large amounts of vitamin E has been shown to control primary acanthosis nigricans in Dachshunds. This disorder is characterized by hair loss and extreme hyperpigmentation (blackening) and thickening of the skin. As the disease progresses, varying degrees of greasiness, crusting, rancid odor, and secondary bacterial infections develop. Pruritus is usually absent or mild during the

per day is recommended by some authors.[19,257] Others suggest an initial dosage that provides 1 mg of elemental zinc/day.[261] The initial dose should be administered for at least a 30-day period to determine the response to treatment. A response should be seen within 6 weeks of initiation of supplementation and, in most cases, skin lesions show a rapid response, with complete healing within 2 weeks.

Zinc supplementation confirms a diagnosis of zinc-responsive dermatosis and aids in rapid recovery. However, providing a complete and balanced food that supplies adequate levels of zinc and does not include inhibitory substances is recommended in all cases. Continued supplementation with zinc after correction of the diet is necessary when an inherited problem with zinc metabolism exists.

ESSENTIAL FATTY ACIDS AND SKIN DISEASE

As components of cell-membrane phospholipids and precursors for a variety of regulatory compounds, the EFAs maintain the health and integrity of epithelial tissue in the body. Because of its high cell turnover rate, the skin is especially susceptible to EFA deficiencies.[262] The omega-6 fatty acids that are considered to be essential nutrients include linoleic acid in dogs and linoleic and arachidonic acid in cats (see Section 2, pp. 94-95). Although the essential nature of omega-3 fatty acids has been controversial, alpha-linolenic acid is considered to be essential for vertebrate species by most fatty acids researchers today.[263]

In dogs, an EFA deficiency results in a dry, dull coat; hair loss; and the eventual development of skin lesions. Over time, the skin becomes pruritic, greasy, and susceptible to infection. A change in the surface lipids in the skin alters the normal bacterial flora and predisposes the animal to secondary bacterial infections.[19,260] Epidermal peeling, interdigital exudation, and otitis externa have also been reported in EFA-deficient dogs. Linoleic acid deficiency in cats results in similar signs.

Naturally occurring skin disease as a result of EFA deficiency is rare in companion animals today. Healthy companion animals that are fed high-quality foods are not at risk of developing an EFA deficiency. When a deficiency does occur, it is usually the result of feeding a diet that is either poorly formulated or has been stored improperly. If the food has been stored at high temperatures or beyond the stated expiration date, there is a risk of EFA loss as a result of oxidative changes to the food. When an EFA deficiency is suspected, it is better to change the diet to one that is well formulated and has been stored properly, rather than to attempt to correct a deficiency by adding supplemental fatty acids.

Omega-6 and Omega-3 Fatty Acids

EFA supplementation and dietary manipulation of EFA metabolism appear to have some efficacy in the treatment of certain skin disorders that are not the result of a dietary deficiency of EFAs. The polyunsaturated fatty acids (PUFAs) are divided into several series based on the position of the first double bond in the carbon chain. Of greatest interest are the omega-3 and omega-6 series of fatty acids. The omega-3 (or n-3) fatty acids have the first double bond located at the third carbon atom from the terminal methyl group. The omega-6 fatty acids have the first double bond at the sixth carbon atom (see Section 1, p. 21). The incorporation of both types of fatty acids into cell membranes and their availability for synthesis of new compounds are affected by the molecule's chain length, the degree of saturation, and the position of the first double bond.

Algae synthesize large amounts of omega-3 fatty acids. As a result, most marine animal tissues contain high concentrations of these fatty acids. Sources of omega-3 fatty acids in pet foods include cold-water fish oils as well as whole-fat flax (flax oil is an enriched source of alpha-linolenic acid). Land animals, in contrast, have higher concentrations of the omega-6 fatty acids in their tissues because most plants consumed by these animals contain greater amounts of omega-6 than omega-3 fatty acids.[47] Enriched sources of omega-6 fatty acids in pet foods include corn, safflower, sunflower, and cottonseed oils. Soy and canola oils contain high levels of omega-6 fatty acids, as well as some alpha-linolenic acid. An omega-6 fatty acid that is of particular interest, gamma-linolenic acid (18:3n-6), is found in borage, black current, and evening primrose oil.[264] Oils containing a large proportion of monounsaturated fatty acids, such as olive oil, and saturated animal fats are not considered enriched in either omega-3 or omega-6 fatty acids (Table 33-2).

Fatty Acids as Eicosanoid Precursors

In addition to providing structural integrity to cell membranes, membrane fatty acids also have specific roles in the regulation of cell functions. Arachidonic acid, gamma-linolenic acid, eicosapentaenoic acid (EPA), and docosahexaenoic acid (DHA) are all precursors for the synthesis of eicosanoids. Eicosanoids are immunoregulatory molecules that have local and short-lived hormone-like effects and include the prostaglandins, leukotrienes, prostacyclins, and thromboxanes.[263] Eicosanoids are involved in inflammatory reactions, immunoregulation, and epidermal cell prolifer-

TABLE 33-2

Sources of Omega-3 and Omega-6 Fatty Acids in Pet Foods

Omega-6 Fatty Acid Sources	Omega-3 Fatty Acid Sources
Corn oil (70% linoleic acid)	Coldwater fish oils (12% to 15% EPA*)
Safflower oil (78% linoleic acid)	Flaxseed (57% alpha-linolenic acid)
Sunflower oil (69% linoleic acid)	Canola oil (8% alpha-linolenic acid)
Cottonseed oil (54% linoleic acid)	Soybean oil (7% alpha-linolenic acid)
Soybean oil (54% linoleic acid)	

Note: The following fats and oils are poor sources of omega-6 and omega-3 fatty acids: lard, mutton fat, coconut oil, and olive oil.
*EPA = Eicosapentaenoic acid (20:5n-3)

ation. When cellular injury occurs, membranes release their component fatty acids, which are then metabolized to eicosanoids. The amount and type of eicosanoid synthesized is determined by the availability and type of fatty acid precursor and by the activities of the two metabolic enzyme systems, cyclooxygenase and lipozygenase.[265] In addition to producing different families of eicosanoids, omega-3 and omega-6 fatty acids compete for these two metabolic pathways for conversion.[260,266]

Eicosanoids are one of several mediators of inflammation in the skin of dogs and cats. During an inflammatory response, the release and metabolism of omega-6 fatty acids produces the 2-series prostaglandins, the 4-series leukotrienes, hydroxyeicosatetraenoic acid, and thromboxane A_2 (Figure 33-2). These agents are immunosuppressive at high levels, proinflammatory, promote platelet aggregation, and act as potent mediators of inflammation in type-I hypersensitivity reactions.[267,268] In contrast, the release and metabolism of omega-3 fatty acids produces mediators with much less inflammatory activity. Those compounds are antiaggregatory, not immunosuppressive at levels normally found in the body, and vasodilatory. They include the 3-series prostaglandins, the 5-series leukotrienes, hydroxyeicosapentaenoic acid, and thromboxane A_3.

FIGURE **33-2**

Metabolism of omega-3 and omega-6 series fatty acids.

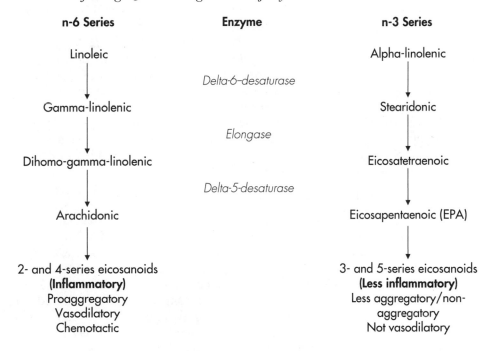

Influence of Omega-6 and Omega-3 Fatty Acids on Eicosanoid Production

In recent years, research with humans, laboratory animals, and companion animals has shown that the ratio of omega-6 to omega-3 fatty acids in tissues can be manipulated by diet, and that these manipulations influence the inflammatory response. Increasing the amount of omega-3 fatty acids in skin and other tissues leads to decreased production and activity of the proinflammatory eicosanoids and increased synthesis of the less inflammatory metabolites.[269] Several factors are responsible for this effect. First, omega-6 and omega-3 fatty acids compete directly for the same enzyme systems. As a result, increasing the proportion of omega-3 fatty acids competitively inhibits the metabolism of omega-6 fatty acids when fatty acids are released from membranes during an inflammatory reaction. Second, the compounds produced from the metabolism of omega-3 fatty acids are less inflammatory than those produced from arachidonic acid.[270] Finally, two end products of EPA metabolism are leukotriene B_5 (LTB$_5$) and 15-hydroxyeicosapentaenoic acid. There is evidence that these compounds inhibit the potent proinflammatory action of leukotriene B_4 (LTB$_4$) and may diminish LTB$_4$-mediated allergic or inflammatory conditions.[271]

It appears that the amount and type of omega-3 fatty acids and the ratio of omega-6 to omega-3 fatty acids in the diet must be considered when determining effects on eicosanoid synthesis.[272-274] A study with healthy dogs showed that feeding a diet containing an omega-6:omega-3 ratio between 5:1 and 10:1 resulted in the production of significantly lower levels of LTB$_4$ and significantly higher levels of the less inflammatory metabolite LTB$_5$ in the skin, compared with the levels that were produced when the dogs were fed a diet with ratios of 28:1 or higher.[275] The neutrophils of dogs fed diets containing the lowest omega-6:omega-3 ratios (5:1 and 10:1) also had decreased LTB$_4$ and increased LTB$_5$ concentrations. Cells from lipopolysaccharide-stimulated skin biopsy samples synthesized 48% to 62% less LTB$_4$ and 48% to 79% more LTB$_5$ when compared with samples obtained before the experimental diets were fed. Similar changes were observed in neutrophils. These responses were considered to be clinically significant because decreases in tissue LTB$_4$ concentrations of 50% or more are typically large enough to attenuate an inflammatory response.[276,277]

Dietary Fatty Acids and Allergic Skin Disease

Allergic skin diseases are common in companion animals and are characterized by extreme pruritus, self-trauma to the skin, and secondary bacterial infection. Flea-bite hypersensitivity has accounted for the largest number of reported cases, with atopic disease (allergic inhalant dermatitis) ranking second and food hypersensitivity third.[278,279] It has been estimated that approximately 10% to 15% of the canine population is affected by one or more types of allergic skin disease.[280,281] In addition, many pets with atopy are sensitive to more than one allergen, which may include house dust mites or dust, molds, weeds, grasses, and trees.[278] Observations of breed and family predilections, along with results of limited breeding trials, indicate that some dogs are genetically predisposed to develop atopy.[281,282] Breeds that are at increased risk include Chinese Shar Peis, Dalmatians, Irish Setters, Golden Retrievers, Boxers, Labrador Retrievers, Belgian Tervurens, and several Terrier and toy breeds.[283,284] In cats, allergic skin disease most commonly manifests as miliary dermatitis, symmetrical truncal alopecia, eosinophilic plaques and granuloma, and facial pruritus.[278,279]

Clinical signs of allergic skin disease develop when the animal is exposed to the offending antigen and sensitized mast cells in the skin degranulate and release inflammatory agents. These compounds include histamine, heparin, proteolytic enzymes, chemotactic factors, and various types of eicosanoids. As discussed previously, the types of fatty acids present in the cell membranes and the activity of the cyclooxygenase and lipoxygenase enzyme systems determine the specific type of eicosanoids produced during an inflammatory response.

Various fatty acid supplements have been used to manage signs of inflammatory skin disease in companion animals. Most recently, the importance of the omega-6 and omega-3 fatty acids has been recognized. Studies have shown than many dogs and cats with inflammatory skin disease have favorable responses to the addition of omega-3 fatty acids to the diet or to adjustments in the ratio of omega-6 to omega-3 fatty acids. While early studies examined the use of omega-3 fatty acid supplements, more recent experiments have revealed enhanced effectiveness when dietary levels of both omega-3 and omega-6 fatty acids are adjusted, thus affecting the ratio of omega-6 to omega-3 fatty acids that are fed.

Fatty Acid Supplements

The use of supplements that are enriched with omega-3 fatty acids has become popular in the management of canine inflammatory skin disease. Omega-3 fatty acids that are commonly supplemented are EPA (20:5n-3) and DHA (22:6n-3), which are found in certain types of fish oil. Alpha-linolenic acid (18:3n-3), found in flax, has also been used. However, supplementation of the pet's regular diet with fatty acids has met with variable success. A review of five separate clinical tests of a commercial supplement (DVM Derm Caps) showed that fatty acid supplementation was effective in controlling pruritus in 11% to 27% of dogs with inflammatory skin disease.[285,286,287,288,289] In one study, 93 dogs with a diagnosis of atopic dermatitis were treated with a commercial fatty acid supplement containing 15 mg of EPA per capsule.[285] A dose of one capsule per 9 kg (20 pounds [lbs]) of body weight was given. One third of the dogs showed a good or excellent response to the supplement, but only 17 dogs (18%) required no additional therapy. A second study using the same supplement reported that 11% of dogs with atopy, food allergy, or flea bite allergy were adequately controlled by the supplement alone with no other treatment necessary.[286]

An omega-6 fatty acid that has been used in the treatment of inflammatory skin disease is gamma-linolenic acid (18:3n-6). Once consumed, gamma-linolenic acid is readily converted to dihomo-gamma-linolenic acid in the liver, where it is then further metabolized to either the monoenoic prostaglandins and thromboxanes or to arachidonic acid (Figure 33-3). The more active pathway is toward the production of the monoenoic prostaglandins (PGE_1) because the rate-limiting delta-5-desaturase step for arachidonic acid production is quite slow in animals.[266] Like the eicosanoids that are produced from EPA, PGE_1 is less inflammatory than the dienoic prostaglandins produced from arachidonic acid. Therefore it is expected that providing gamma-linolenic acid in the diet will promote the formation of dihomo-gamma-linolenic acid and the monoenoic prostaglandins, rather than the formation of arachidonic acid and its more inflammatory metabolites.

When dogs' diets are supplemented with evening primrose oil, plasma levels of dihomo-gamma-linolenic acid increase.[290] Similarly, when dogs with atopy that had been controlled by feeding a supplement containing omega-3 fatty acids and gamma-linolenic acid were switched to a supplement containing only olive oil (a poor source of both omega-3 and omega-6 fatty acids), plasma levels of dihomo-gamma-linolenic acid subsequently decreased.[291] A return of clinical signs in these dogs paralleled the reduction in dihomo-gamma-linolenic acid. It has been postulated that atopic disease in some dogs may be a manifestation of a deficiency of the enzyme delta-6-desaturase, the rate-limiting step between conversion of linoleic acid to gamma-linolenic acid.[292,293] Providing gamma-linolenic acid would be expected to bypass this step of fatty acid metabolism and provide substrate for the production of the monoenoic prostaglandins. However, the effectiveness of providing gamma-linolenic acid to pruritic dogs with the intent of increasing production of dihomo-gamma-linolenic acid is still controversial. A recent study comparing pruritic and healthy dogs found that unmedicated dogs with signs of atopy naturally have higher concentrations of dihomo-gamma-linolenic acid in subcutaneous fat when compared with levels in dogs with healthy skin.[294] These results

FIGURE **33-3**

Production of gamma-linolenic acid metabolites.

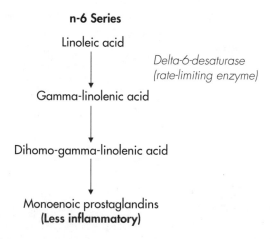

n-6 Series

Linoleic acid

Delta-6-desaturase (rate-limiting enzyme)

Gamma-linolenic acid

Dihomo-gamma-linolenic acid

Monoenoic prostaglandins
(Less inflammatory)

suggest that dogs with atopy may instead possess an abnormality in dihomo-gamma-linolenic metabolism caused by a deficiency in delta-5-desaturase. These conflicting data indicate that there may be several underlying causes of atopy in dogs. While some atopic animals show abnormal fat absorption and clearance, others may have deficiencies of delta-6- and/or delta-5-desaturase activities.[295,296]

Supplements containing combinations of evening primrose oil and fish oil (source of the omega-3 fatty acids EPA and DHA) are effective in the long-term control of atopy in some dogs and cats.[262,287,291,297,298,299] When 33 dogs were treated with this type of supplement, 18% needed no other treatment, and 7% showed a significant reduction in clinical signs.[262] Similar results have been reported in cats. When the diets of 14 cats that had a diagnosis of miliary dermatosis were supplemented with various combinations of evening primrose oil and fish oil, improvements in clinical signs were observed with either evening primrose oil alone or a combination of evening primrose oil and fish oil.[298] In contrast, supplementation with fish oil alone was not effective. After 12 weeks of treatment, 11 of 14 cats showed a favorable response to the combination of 80% evening primrose oil and 20% fish oil. A second study with cats found that 40% of cats with nonlesional pruritus and 67% of cats with eosinophilic granuloma complex responded favorably to dietary supplementation with a product containing EPA, gamma-linolenic acid, decahexaenoic acid, safflower oil, natural glycerin, and vitamin E.[299] It has been speculated that cats may differ from dogs in their response to omega-3 fatty acids because cats have been shown to lack omega-3 fatty acid activity in the skin and because they have a lower activity of the enzyme delta-6-desaturase (see Section 2, pp. 94-95).

While a small number of allergic pets have been shown to require no additional therapy when provided with a dietary fatty acid supplement, most that respond still require concurrent administration of antihistamines or low doses of corticosteroids to control pruritus.[289,300,301] In addition, a substantial proportion of dogs and cats show no response at all to fatty acid supplementation. There are several possible reasons for the variable responses that have been observed. First, there are a number of different agents that mediate inflammation and pruritus in dogs and cats with allergic dermatitis. Therefore, the manipulation of fatty acids would not be expected to work in all cases. A second factor may involve the manner in which fatty acid therapy is administered. Supplementing a companion animal's diet with a fatty acid-containing capsule does not account for the levels or proportions of fatty acids present in the regular diet. The exact quantities and ratio of fatty acids in the regular diet are usually not known. It is therefore extremely difficult to achieve an effective fatty acid profile through supplementation. The effectiveness of fatty acid therapy relies upon competitive inhibition between omega-6 and omega-3 fatty acids and their metabolites. If the pet's regular diet already contains high levels of omega-6 fatty acids, providing an omega-3 fatty acid supplement may not effectively change the proportion of these types of fatty acids present in the tissues.

Several studies have shown that allergic pruritus is not controlled in dogs using the recommended doses of omega-3 fatty acid supplements.[300,302] Other studies have reported that 2 to 10 times the recommended dose may be necessary to achieve clinical results in pruritic dogs.[291,292] High doses of supplements increase the risk of causing an imbalanced fatty acid ratio in the diet and can become cost-prohibitive for some clients. Fatty acid supplements have also been associated with undesirable side effects such as lethargy, vomiting, diarrhea, and urticaria in some dogs and cats.[299,303] An added risk with use of omega-3 fatty acids is oversupplementation, which may lead to decreased platelet aggregation and increased blood clotting time.[303,304]

Altering the Dietary Omega-6:Omega-3 Fatty Acid Ratio

When modifying dietary fatty acid levels to manage inflammatory disease, the goal is to supply optimal amounts of linoleic acid to meet a dog's essential dietary requirement and at the same time produce a potentially less inflammatory fatty acid metabolic profile. Recent research indicates that using a total dietary approach in which both the quantity and the ratio of omega-6 and omega-3 fatty acids are controlled may be an effective means of altering tissue eicosanoid profiles and reducing pruritus in allergic pets. Recent results of an experiment with healthy adult dogs showed that feeding a diet that contains an omega-6:omega-3 ratio between 5:1 and 10:1 results in changes in skin leukotriene concentrations that are considered to be clinically significant.[275] Omega-3 fatty acid–enriched diets have also been shown to modify the biochemical components of the inflammatory stage of wound healing in the skin of dogs.[305] Specifically the concentration of antiinflammatory fatty acids and eicosanoids in 4-day-old skin wounds increased, and the concentration of proinflammatory fatty acids and eicosanoids decreased as the proportion of omega-3 fatty acids in the diet increased. Moreover, the omega-3 concentrations that were fed in these studies did not negatively impact platelet reactivity, coagulation assays, fibrinogen concentration, or antithrombin III activity.[306]

Clinical studies have examined the effectiveness of varying the dietary omega 6:omega-3 fatty acid ratio in managing inflammatory skin disease. In one study, 31 pruritic dogs were fed a veterinary-exclusive commercial diet containing an adjusted fatty acid ratio of 5:1 for a period of 8 weeks.[207] All of the dogs had been diagnosed with atopy, adverse reactions to food, or a combination of these two conditions. Twenty-eight dogs completed the trial, and fourteen dogs (45%) showed a good to excellent response to the dietary change. Another feeding trial was conducted with 18 non–food-allergic, atopic dogs fed a lamb-and-rice diet containing an omega-6:omega-3 fatty acid ratio of 5.3:1.[296] The dogs' clinical responses were evaluated by both a veterinarian and the owner. In this study, 44% of the dogs (8 of 18) had a good or excellent response to the test diet within 7 to 21 days of feeding. Upon refeeding the original diet, all showed a return of clinical signs. Pruritus was again alleviated by reintroduction of the test diet in all eight dogs. An important result of this study was the positive response in dogs that had previously been unresponsive to a dietary fatty acid supplement containing omega-3 and omega-6 fatty acids. Of 11 dogs that had been previously treated unsuccessfully with the supplement, 7 (65%) had a good or excellent response to the test diet.

Recommended Doses and Ratios

Documentation of appropriate doses of supplements and ratios of fatty acids to include in pet foods is lacking. Experimental data show that changes in skin concentrations of fatty acids are maximized after 3 to 12 weeks of supplementation or feeding a new diet. However, great variability is seen with the type and ratio of fatty acids that are used.[188,201] One problem is that there are currently no canine or feline recommended daily allowances for omega-3 fatty acids.[264] The American Association of Feed Control Officials' (AAFCO's) linoleic acid minimum requirement is 1% dry matter (DM) for dogs and 0.5% for cats. In many commercial pet foods, omega-6 fatty acids contribute more than 4% of the food's energy. It is therefore possible that excessive levels of omega-6 fatty acids may obfuscate an effective dose of omega-3 fatty acids, even when high levels are supplemented.

A review of several therapeutic diets commonly recommended for pets with skin or gastrointestinal inflammation found that the omega-3 fatty acid concentration typically provided between 0.6% and 2% of the daily energy intake, with one food containing as high as 4%.[264] It was suggested that a daily dietary omega-3 intake of between 2% and 4% of energy effectively increases membrane and plasma omega-3 concentrations. Likewise, a reasonable starting dose for a fatty acid supplement is one that supplies 175 mg of omega-3 fatty acids per kg of body weight per day. This recommended dose is substantially higher than those recommended on the labels of most commercial fatty acid supplements.

As discussed previously, the ratio of dietary omega-6 to omega-3 fatty acids appears to be as important as the total amount of omega-3 fatty acids. The easiest and most effective way to modulate this ratio is by incorporating it directly into the pet's normal diet. Based on current studies, a ratio between 5:1 and 10:1 seems to be the most effective in altering tissue lipid and eicosanoid concentrations and modifying the inflammatory response. The omega-6 fatty acid content should meet the EFA requirements of dogs and cats, but it should not exceed 4% of the metabolizable energy (ME) calories. Several additional benefits of a total dietary approach include improved client compliance, achievement of a specifically targeted omega-6:omega-3 ratio, and safety (no danger of oversupplementation).

FOOD HYPERSENSITIVITY (ALLERGY)

Dogs and cats can have adverse reactions to dietary ingredients for a number of reasons (Table 33-3). Dietary hypersensitivity occurs when an animal develops a specific immunological reactivity (allergy) to one or more components in the diet. Hypersensitivities differ significantly from food intolerances, in which the animal responds adversely to its diet but displays no evidence of an immune-mediated response. Intolerances include problems such as a lack of the intestinal enzyme lactase, food toxicities, and pharmacological reactions to dietary ingredients.[308,309] In contrast, true food hypersensitivity is a result of antibody–, immune complex–, or cell-mediated–immune reactions.[310] Because dietary hypersensitivity usually manifests

TABLE 33-3

Causes of Adverse Reactions to Food in Dogs and Cats

Food allergy (hypersensitivity)	Immune-mediated adverse reaction to a food component
Food intolerance	Nonimmunological adverse reaction of a metabolic, idiosyncratic, toxic, or pharmacological nature to a food component
Metabolic adverse reaction	Abnormal metabolic response to a food component, usually due to an inborn error of metabolism
Food idiosyncracy	Abnormal response to a food substance; resembles a hypersensitivity response but does not have an immunological basis
Food toxicity (poisoning)	Adverse reaction to a contaminating organism or toxin present in a food
Pharmacological reaction	Due to pharmacological or druglike effect of a food component (e.g., histamine in poorly preserved fish)

as a dermatosis, the discussion included in this section is limited to this type of dietary problem.

Description and Incidence

Compared with other types of dermatitis, food hypersensitivity is considered to be relatively rare in dogs and cats.[311,312] It has been estimated that food-induced allergic dermatitis constitutes 1% of all dermatoses seen by small-animal veterinarians and 10% of the inflammatory dermatoses diagnosed.[313,314] However, other researchers report that dietary hypersensitivities account for between 23% and 62% of all nonseasonal allergic dermatoses.[311,315] Although the estimated incidence rates vary considerably, it has been generally accepted that dietary hypersensitivity ranks third in incidence to inhalant allergies and flea bite allergies as a cause of pruritic skin disease in dogs and cats.[316]

Dietary hypersensitivity can develop at any age. Unlike inhalant allergies (atopy) and flea-bite dermatitis, which often take several years to develop, signs of food hypersensitivity often first occur in pets that are less than 1 year of age. In two reports, 19% and 33% of the cases developed initial clinical signs when they were less than 1 year of age.[317,318] Similarly, a study of 25 dogs diagnosed with a food allergy found that more than 50% were less than 1 year old at the onset of clinical signs.[319] These data suggest that food allergy should always be considered when an immature pet exhibits a nonseasonal allergic dermatitis.

The onset of dietary allergy can be seen at any time of the year and is not typically associated with a recent dietary change. In one study, 68% of the dogs had been fed the offending diet for 2 years or more before clinical signs developed.[313] No significant sex or age predilections have been observed. Although the presence of a genetic component has not been proven, one study did find that among purebred dogs, German Shepherds and Golden Retrievers appeared to be overrepresented when compared with a general hospital population.[319] This difference was not significant but suggests the possibility of a genetic predilection in these breeds. Other breeds that appear to be at increased risk include the Soft-Coated Wheaton Terrier, Dalmatian, West Highland White Terrier, Collie, Chinese Shar Pei, Lhasa Apso, Cocker Spaniel, English Springer Spaniel, Miniature Schnauzer, and Labrador Retriever.[320]

Some investigators have reported that, unlike atopy and flea-bite allergy, dietary hypersensitivity does not respond well to corticosteroid treatment.[234,321] However, other studies have found that a significant number of cases show a decrease in clinical signs when treated with systemic glucocorticoids.[317,319] In one study, 72% of the dogs with a diagnosis of food allergy had either a partial or complete response to corticosteroid therapy.[319] A favorable response to the systemic administration of glucocorticoids therefore does not reliably exclude food allergy as an underlying cause of clinical signs.

Etiology

The immunological mechanisms that cause food hypersensitivity are incompletely understood. The disorder is currently considered to be the result of type-I and/or type-III immediate hypersensitivity responses. A type-I response is responsible for the severe pruritus that is seen after ingesting the offending dietary antigen. A type-III response, on the other hand, is thought to be responsible for the acute intestinal signs (diarrhea) that are seen in a small number of animals.[316,322] Delayed (type-IV) hypersensitivities, which occur several hours to days after ingesting the offending antigen, may also be involved.[322]

Food antigens are generally proteins, lipoproteins, glycoproteins, or polypeptides. It is possible that some of the processing procedures used to produce commercial pet foods increase the antigenicity of certain dietary components.[309,321,323] This would be one explanation for the observation that some allergic pets tolerate homemade diets but develop an allergic response to commercial diets that contain the same ingredients.[318] Beef, soy, and dairy products are the most common causes of food allergies in dogs and cats.[316,319,323,324] Other dietary ingredients to which dogs and cats have developed allergies include wheat, pork, chicken, corn, horse meat, egg, and fish.[309] It appears that these ingredients are common allergens because they are often used in pet foods, thus increasing the likelihood of exposure, as opposed to any characteristics that confer unique antigenicity.[325,326]

A single animal may be allergic to one specific ingredient in the diet, or it may exhibit multiple hypersensitivities. There are conflicting reports regarding the frequency at which multiple hypersensitivities are observed in dogs and cats. While some researchers have reported finding many instances of multiple hypersensitivities, others report that these are rare.[311,313,315,325] A recent study of 25 dogs with signs consistent with food hypersensitivity reported that the mean number of allergens per dog was 2.4, and 64% of the dogs reacted adversely to two or more dietary ingredients.[326] These results indicate that multiple hypersensitivities should always be considered when diagnosing and treating food allergies.

It has been proposed that early weaning of puppies or kittens may predispose some pets to the development of food allergies later in life.[324] In healthy animals, the small intestine possesses a protective barrier that limits the absorption of macromolecules. In young puppies and kittens, this protective barrier is not completely functional. When foreign food proteins are introduced to the immature gut, some may pass across the intestinal barrier, penetrate the lymphoid tissue, and trigger an immunological response. Disease states that disrupt the small intestine's immunological barrier may have a similar effect. This theory is speculative at this time, but it may explain the early onset of food allergies in some pets. Further research must be conducted to determine the exact role that early weaning or the disruption of the intestine's protective barrier may play in the development of dietary hypersensitivities.

Clinical Signs

In most dogs and cats, dietary hypersensitivities manifest as allergic dermatoses. Studies have shown that 97% of allergic companion animals show dermatological signs alone, and 10% to 15% develop gastrointestinal disease with or without skin disease.[318,321,327] The most common dermatological sign in dogs and cats is an intense pruritus.[310,327] Initially, this usually occurs between 4 and 24 hours after ingesting the offending antigen. Over time, chronic cases show constant pruritus with no evident association between eating and an exacerbation of signs.[316] The onset of pruritus is not accompanied by other skin changes. However, the pet's intense scratching, biting, and self-trauma quickly lead to secondary lesions. In dogs, the areas of the body most often affected are the feet, axillae, and inguinal area.[316,328] Cats are affected most intensely around the head, neck, and ears.[324,329] In severe cases in both species, generalized pruritus over the entire body is seen.[308] Excessive scratching and licking leads to hair loss and reddening of the skin. Papular eruptions occur in approximately 40% of reported cases, and secondary bacterial infections are seen in about 20%.[308] Other secondary changes may include chronic inflammation, crusting, seborrhea, and hyperpigmentation.

Persistent otitis externa, with or without infection, is often seen in both dogs and cats, and in some cases it is the only presenting sign. A small number of cases have also been reported that showed only a recurrent pyoderma not associated with pruritus. The pyoderma subsided with antibacterial therapy but continued to recur until the diet was changed.[319] Skin disease caused by dietary hypersensitivity is usually nonseasonal. However, if multiple sensitivities are present (e.g., dietary allergy plus atopy or flea-bite allergy), the dietary sensitivity may not manifest clinically until another sensitivity is also triggered and the dog or cat reaches its pruritic threshold. This situation can cause the signs to appear to be seasonal in nature (Table 33-4).[308,324]

Diagnosis and Treatment

Diagnosis of food hypersensitivity involves first ruling out other potential causes of the allergic dermatosis. These causes include atopy, flea-bite dermatitis, and drug hypersensitivities. Obtaining a full diet history is equally important. When a food allergy is suspected, the standard method of diagnosis includes three phases: (1) feed-

TABLE 33-4

Signs of Dietary Hypersensitivity in Dogs and Cats

Dogs	Cats
Intense pruritus (on the feet, axillae, and inguinal area)	Intense pruritus (on the head and neck)
Self-induced skin trauma	Self-induced trauma
Chronic inflammation of skin	Ulcerative dermatitis
Papular eruptions	Miliary dermatitis
Hair loss	Hair loss
Hyperpigmentation/scaling	Cutaneous hyperesthesia
Otitis externa	Seborrhea
Secondary bacterial infections (e.g., recurrent pyoderma)	Vomiting/diarrhea (common)
Vomiting/diarrhea (in 10% to 15% of cases)	

ing an elimination diet and demonstrating an amelioration of clinical signs, (2) challenging the pet with the original diet and observing a return of clinical signs, and (3) feeding selected ingredients to identify the specific offending dietary antigens (Box 33-1). Intradermal skin testing and serological testing have been shown to be unreliable in diagnosing food allergies in dogs and cats.[323,330]

By definition, an elimination diet contains protein and carbohydrate sources to which the pet has not previously been exposed. In most cases, this means selecting a food that contains ingredients not typically included in commercial pet foods. A recent survey of 123 pet foods available in grocery stores reported that the most commonly used ingredients include chicken, beef, egg, soy, milk, corn, rice, and wheat.[326] Less commonly used ingredients were lamb, fish, turkey, oat, kelp, barley, flax, alfalfa, and potatoes. Ingredients that were rarely seen in grocery store pet foods were sorghum, rabbit, venison, rye, and quinoa. Suggested elimination diets are those that include lamb, rabbit, venison, or fish as a protein source, and rice, potatoes, or barley as a carbohydrate source.[310,323] However, because lamb and rice have become relatively common ingredients in all types of commercial pet foods in recent years, these foods may have lost their suitability as an elimination diet for many pets.

A homemade pet food is often recommended for the elimination phase of diagnosis because some pets with food hypersensitivity will still react to commercial diets and because few commercial diets contain only one carbohydrate and one protein source. For example, 20% of dogs that were asymptomatic when fed a homemade diet of lamb and rice became pruritic again when fed a commercial preparation containing the same ingredients.[318] Another controlled study showed that 16% of dogs with diagnosed food hypersensitivity developed allergic reactions to a commercial diet that was manufactured as an elimination diet for the diagnosis of dietary hypersensitivity.[325] These differences may provide evidence that the

BOX 33-1

Three Phases of Food Hypersensitivity Diagnosis

1. **Feeding the elimination diet.** The diet should consist of a single protein and a single carbohydrate source to which the animal has not been previously exposed. The diet should be introduced gradually over a 4-day period. Improvement in clinical signs is usually observed within 3 weeks but may take up to 10 weeks.
2. **Feeding a challenge diet to confirm.** The pet's original diet or a diet that is known to cause an allergic reaction in the animal should be fed. If pruritus occurs within 4 hours to 14 days, a diagnosis of dietary hypersensitivity is confirmed.
3. **Identifying the offending dietary ingredients.** One suspected offending ingredient should be added to the elimination diet. The animal should be monitored for signs of allergic response. This process should be repeated for all suspected ingredients. Common pet food ingredients are most likely to be the cause of food hypersensitivity (e.g., beef, soy, chicken, egg, dairy, wheat, corn).

processing of some commercial pet foods may enhance the antigenicity of some food components. It is thought that the inclusion of poor-quality ingredients that are partially resistant to heat treatment or digestion may also increase the antigenicity of proteins in commercial foods.[309] For these reasons, a commercial food selected as an elimination diet should contain high-quality raw ingredients. Commercially prepared elimination diets have the benefits of economy, convenience, and assurance of consistency and nutritional adequacy.

If a homemade elimination diet is selected, a ratio of 1:2 to 1:4 parts protein source to carbohydrate source can be used. The pet's diet should be gradually changed to this food over a period of 3 to 4 days. The elimination diet should then be fed exclusively, with no additional treats or table scraps. In addition, all chew toys that are made of animal products must be removed, and chewable vitamins or heartworm medication must be replaced with pure forms of medication. Some dogs and cats will show improvement after eating the elimination diet for only 3 weeks, but an 8- to 10-week trial period may be needed to establish a diagnosis.[308] A study of 51 dogs with a food allergy reported that only 25% responded to an elimination diet after 3 weeks of feeding, but more than 90% responded by 10 weeks.[320] In general, a 50% or greater reduction of pruritus and skin disease is accepted as diagnostic for dietary hypersensitivity.[314] Some pets may have a dietary hypersensitivity occurring concomitantly with other pruritic dermatoses, such as flea-bite allergy or atopy. When this occurs, feeding an elimination diet often causes a decrease in pruritus and skin disease but does not result in the complete resolution of signs. If pruritus is not diminished during the elimination phase, then either food allergy is not the diagnosis or the elimination diet being used still contains an ingredient to which the pet is allergic.

A conclusive diagnosis can be made if the pet's former diet is reintroduced as a challenge diet and pruritus returns within 4 hours to 14 days.[316,319] The final phase of diagnosis, identification of specific antigens, is accomplished by adding single food items to the elimination diet and assessing for a return of clinical signs. Because beef, soy, and dairy products account for the majority of dietary hypersensitivities in dogs and cats, these ingredients should be tested first. It is generally accepted that only a very small amount of allergen is necessary to evoke a hypersensitivity response.[324,331] Adding powdered milk at a level of $\frac{1}{2}$ to 2 tablespoons (tbsp) per meal provides exposure to the antigens found in dairy products.[328] If no return of signs is seen after 10 to 14 days, the next ingredient can be tested.[319] Food items that are readily available to pet owners can be easily tested. Cooked beef, wheat flour, and soy meal can each be tested by adding $1\frac{1}{2}$ to 2 tbsp per meal. Only one new substance should be added and tested at a time, and if a food causes an allergic reaction, the elimination diet should be fed until all signs are resolved before proceeding to another item. If no clinical signs are observed within 14 days of adding a test ingredient, the pet is probably not allergic to that food. Because a substantial number of animals are allergic to more than one food component, testing should include as many common pet food proteins as possible.[326]

The identification phase of diagnosis can be very tedious and time-consuming for many pet owners. In addition, some owners are reluctant to risk the recurrence of clinical signs in their pet. After completing the elimination and challenge phases and arriving at a diagnosis of food allergy, some pet owners choose to simply find a diet that their pet tolerates without attempting to identify the specific ingredients to which the pet reacts. Simply changing to a new, commercial pet food is rarely effective because most commercial foods contain similar ingredients. Diets should be selected that contain single protein and carbohydrate sources to which the pet has not been exposed and that are not expected to cause a reaction. Feeding the elimination diet as a long-term maintenance diet is acceptable if this diet has been determined to be complete and balanced.

The lifetime nutritional management of pets with dietary hypersensitivity requires feeding a diet that is palatable, complete and balanced, and does not contain the offending antigen or antigens. The protein included in the diet should be of very high quality and highly digestible. Poorly digested proteins retain their inherent antigenicity during heat processing of the product. In addition, incomplete digestion within the gastrointestinal tract may result in increased antigenicity in some poor-quality proteins.[309] The inclusion of a reduced omega-6:omega-3 fatty acid ratio may also help manage inflammation and pruritus. Although a homemade diet may be used safely for the elimination phase of diagnosis, these are not recommended for long-term maintenance because they are expensive and inconvenient and may not be complete and balanced. Commercial products offer economy and convenience, and unlike most homemade diets, they are guaranteed to be nutritionally complete and balanced.

Some pets with diagnosed food hypersensitivities eventually develop additional sensitivities to ingredients in the new diet.[308] In these cases, the identification phase must be repeated, and another suitable diet must be found. Similarly, it is possible for the original sensitivity to become diminished and allow the pet to once again consume a diet containing that ingredient.[308] Because dietary hypersensitivity is not always responsive to corticosteroid therapy and because of the long-term side effects of corticosteroids, emphasis is placed on strict adherence to dietary management rather than on drug therapy. But with either treatment, the therapeutic objective is management of the disorder because dietary hypersensitivity can never be cured. Any small dietary indiscretion on the part of the owner or the pet does not cause direct harm but may lead to damage from pruritus and self-induced trauma. In some cases, repeated failures to adhere to the new diet decrease the chance of obtaining relief when fed an elimination diet. It is therefore very important that pet owners are aware of the need for strict compliance in order to control clinical signs.

CHAPTER
34

Chronic Renal Failure

DESCRIPTION AND CLINICAL SIGNS

Chronic renal failure in dogs and cats is characterized by an irreversible and progressive loss of kidney function and the development of clinical signs that reflect the kidneys' decreasing ability to perform normal regulatory and excretory functions. There are many potential causes for the initial kidney damage that leads to chronic disease. These causes include, but are not limited to, trauma, infection, immunological disease, neoplasms, renal ischemia (decreased blood flow to the kidneys), genetic anomalies, and exposure to toxins. Although renal disease can develop at any age, chronic renal disease is most commonly seen in older pets.[332] In most cases the initial underlying cause is no longer present when the pet develops chronic renal failure. This is due to the ability of the kidney to compensate for large proportions of functional tissue loss. However, over time these compensatory mechanisms may break down, leading to progressive loss of kidney function and signs of chronic disease.

Nephrons are the functional units of the kidneys. Each nephron consists of a glomerulus and a system of tubules within which reabsorption and excretion occur. The glomerulus is a tuft of capillaries where water, waste products, and electrolytes from the blood are filtered. The tubules originate at the base of the glomerulus and selectively reabsorb many of the blood components present in the filtrate. When the filtrate reaches the final portion of the tubule, it contains only those compounds that are going to be excreted as waste in the urine. The healthy kidney contains thousands of nephrons and has a substantial functional reserve.

Blood flow through the kidneys is very high, with approximately one fourth of cardiac output filtered through the kidneys each minute. The waste products of protein catabolism, such as urea, creatinine, uric acid, and ammonia, are removed and excreted in the urine. In addition, electrolytes and trace minerals are filtered, reabsorbed, and selectively excreted. The kidneys are also important in the normal regulation of fluid balance, pH, and blood pressure and for the production of the hormone erythropoietin and the active form of vitamin D. The progressive loss of these functions leads to functional loss and eventual clinical signs of chronic renal disease.

The compensatory mechanisms of the healthy nephrons that remain after initial renal injury allow the kidneys to function normally even after the loss of a large proportion of tissue. A loss of at least 70% to 85% of functional capacity usually occurs before a pet begins to show clinical signs of renal failure.[332,333] One of the first signs that most pet owners notice is increased water consumption and increased urination. This effect is caused by a reduced capacity to concentrate urine, resulting in an increased volume of urine and increased frequency of urination. Some dogs may appear to regress in their housebreaking or may involuntarily empty their bladder while sleeping. Polydipsia accompanies the increased urination because the dog compensates to maintain fluid balance. Polyuria and polydipsia are less commonly observed in cats because cats usually become uremic before they lose the ability to concentrate urine.[334] In addition, owners of indoor cats that use litter boxes are less likely to notice increased urination even when it does occur.

Many of the clinical signs seen in dogs and cats with advanced renal failure are associated with the degree of azotemia or uremia that is present. This is commonly referred to as *uremic syndrome*.[335] *Azotemia* refers to the accumulation of nitrogenous waste products in the blood, waste products composed primarily of urea nitrogen and/or creatinine. The term *uremia* technically means elevated concentrations of urea in the blood, but it commonly refers to the collection of clinical signs associated with renal failure. Although urea is singularly only a minor uremic toxin, serum urea levels are associated with the adverse clinical signs that reduce quality of life and contribute to morbidity in patients with chronic renal failure.[336] These signs include decreased appetite or anorexia, vomiting, depression, electrolyte and pH disturbances, mucosal ulcers, and weight loss. Some pets also develop chronic diarrhea and neurological signs. Aberrations in phosphorus and calcium metabolism lead to secondary renal hyperparathyroidism, which causes renal osteodystrophy (bone demineralization) and deposition of calcium phosphate in soft tissues. In many cases of chronic renal failure, the inability of the kidneys to produce erythropoietin and a reduced lifespan of red blood cells lead to the development of a normocytic, normochromic anemia (Box 34-1).[337]

Diagnosis of chronic renal disease in dogs and cats is based on medical history, clinical signs, serum chemistry, and urinalysis. Pets with chronic renal failure develop elevated blood urea nitrogen (BUN) and plasma creatinine levels as a result of reduced glomerular function. Although BUN and creatinine measurements have been used for many years as the primary indicator of renal health in dogs and cats, they are relatively insensitive tests and do not accurately reflect the magnitude of renal functional loss.[338,339] The relationship between glomerular filtration rate (GFR) and serum urea and creatinine concentrations is not linear, and up to 75% of renal function must be lost before BUN and creatinine values increase above the normal range.[338] Subsequently, values rise rapidly in response to small additional losses of renal function. Despite these deficiencies, BUN and serum creatinine still provide practitioners with a rapid screening test for assessing glomerular function in clinically affected patients. Plasma creatinine levels of between 2.0 and 3.5 milligrams (mg)/

BOX 34-1

Clinical Signs of Chronic Renal Failure

Polyuria
Increased frequency of urination
Polydipsia
Depression
Diarrhea
Vomiting
Anorexia
Renal osteodystrophy
Anemia
Neurological impairment

deciliter (dl) are indicative of mild to moderate renal disease. Levels higher than 3.5 mg/dl usually indicate advanced failure or end-stage renal disease.[337,340] Plasma creatinine is a sensitive indicator of renal dysfunction and is not affected by dietary protein intake. In contrast, BUN is strongly affected by the consumption of a protein-containing meal. Therefore all samples should be taken 12 hours postprandial. A fasting BUN of greater than 35 mg/dl may be an indication of some level of kidney dysfunction. A loss of concentrating ability and elevated serum phosphorus (greater than 5 mg/dl) also provides supportive evidence for a diagnosis of chronic renal failure.[337] Laboratory test results may also show a normocytic, normochromic anemia; lymphopenia; hypercholesterolemia; or metabolic acidosis.[335] Both lipase and amylase may be increased in the absence of pancreatitis due to decreased renal filtration.

With chronic renal disease, the gradual decline in GFR is responsible for the inability of the kidneys to filter and excrete waste products efficiently. However, early detection of kidney dysfunction is difficult in dogs and cats because clinical signs of uremia only develop after 60% to 70% of renal function has been lost. The most accurate and sensitive method for detecting early changes in renal function and for monitoring disease progression is to measure GFR. This test requires 24-hour urine collection by a veterinarian and measures the rates at which blood is filtered through the kidneys and waste products are removed and excreted.[337] An estimate of GFR can also be obtained by measuring the renal clearance of exogenous creatine.[341,342] Unfortunately, these tests usually require expensive equipment and are very time-consuming and tedious to perform, so they are not available in most clinical settings. Recently, efforts to produce a simpler and less expensive method for measuring GFR have reported success with using iohexol, an iodine-based radiographic contrast compound.[343,344] These test may be especially important because early detection of a decreasing GFR can be the signal for nutritional interventions that can actually slow the progression of renal failure. Waiting for the appearance of azotemia or a loss of concentrating ability delays the use of these measures.

PROGRESSIVE NATURE

The occurrence of chronic renal failure is preceded by some type of renal insult or injury that causes a loss of nephrons. Following this initial episode, the kidneys undergo structural and functional compensatory adaptations. Specifically, these changes include increased glomerular capillary hypertension, increased single nephron glomerular filtration rate (SNGFR), and renal hypertrophy (growth of remnant nephrons).[345,346,347,348,349] The increase in GFR in the surviving nephrons causes the kidneys' total GFR to be higher than the level that would be predicted following the reduction in renal mass. These changes enable a damaged kidney to compensate and function for variable and extended periods of time at normal or near-normal capacity. During this compensatory phase, clinical signs of renal disease are not evident.

Depending on the extent of the damage to the kidneys and on other factors that can influence the progression of disease, renal function may eventually begin to decline. When this occurs, the progressive and irreversible loss of functioning nephrons causes a gradual reduction in total GFR and in the kidneys' ability to excrete waste products from the body. The inability to excrete waste products and the compromised regulatory functioning of the kidneys leads to clinical signs of renal failure. Renal failure can progress to end-stage disease even after the initial cause of injury has been resolved and in the absence of active renal disease. It appears that the loss of a certain critical mass of nephrons can result in self-perpetuating, progressive renal disease. Studies in dogs have indicated that between $3/4$ and $15/16$ of renal mass must be destroyed before progression occurs.[350] However, great variability is seen among individuals. Some dogs and cats never develop progressive disease, even when an extremely high proportion of renal mass has been destroyed.[351]

Many factors may contribute to the progression of renal disease in dogs and cats. Evidence from early studies with rats suggested that the alterations that compensate for the initial loss of active tissue may eventually contribute to progressive deterioration of the remaining tissue.[348,352] These studies led to the hypothesis that hyperfiltration and hypertension of surviving nephrons ultimately would cause cellular injury, resulting in progressive glomerulosclerosis and a loss of nephron function. This postulation has been termed the *hyperfiltration theory* and appears to explain the progressive nature of renal disease in several strains of laboratory rat.[353,354,355] While glomerular hypertrophy and hypertension occur in dogs and cats with decreased renal function, the role of these changes in disease progression is still unclear.[343,356,357] Several studies with dogs indicate that the adaptive changes that occur following a loss of renal tissue do not lead to the progressive glomerulosclerosis that has been reported in rats.[342,358,359] In contrast, therapies that reduce glomerular hypertension have been shown to protect the kidneys from further damage in dogs with experimentally induced diabetic nephropathy.[360,361] These results indicate that a reduction in glomerular hypertension may be beneficial to dogs with chronic renal disease.

ROLE OF DIET IN PROGRESSION

Other factors that may contribute to spontaneous progression of renal disease in dogs and cats include systemic hypertension, hyperparathyroidism, intrarenal inflammation, hyperlipidemia, renal mineralization, and renal ammoniagenesis. Each of these factors is influenced to some degree by the pet's diet and nutritional status. Chronically elevated serum phosphate levels can contribute to hyperparathyroidism and renal mineralization; dietary fatty acids affect serum lipid levels, intrarenal blood pressure, and inflammation; dietary sodium may influence the development of systemic hypertension; and metabolic acidosis affects ammonia production in the kidneys.

The goals of dietary management of chronic renal failure are to ameliorate clinical signs of uremia (see p. 462) and, if possible, slow or stop the progression of the disease. Until recently, dietary protein was the major nutrient identified as important in slowing disease progression. However, recent evidence indicates that protein may not be a factor in disease progression in dogs and cats, while other nutrients may play significant roles. Dietary components that may influence the rate of progression of chronic renal failure in dogs and cats include phosphorus, the type of fatty acids included in the diet, and nutritional factors that affect the body's acid-base status.

Protein

Feeding a high-protein diet results in increased renal blood flow and increased postprandial GFR in all species that have been studied, including the dog.[353,362] This effect is seen in both healthy animals and animals with compromised kidney function. Studies have shown that the restriction of dietary protein reduces these effects and slows the progression of chronic renal disease in a susceptible strain of male rats with experimentally reduced renal mass.[348,353] Restricting dietary protein also slows the development of progressive disease in healthy Fischer 344 rats that are genetically predisposed to develop chronic renal disease as they age.[363,364]

These effects have not been observed in dogs. In contrast to rats, feeding elevated protein levels has not been shown to cause a progression of renal disease in dogs with either experimentally induced or naturally occurring renal disease.[358,359,365,366,367] In one long-term study, diets containing either 19%, 27% or 56% protein were fed to dogs with a ¾ reduction in renal mass for a period of 4 years.[365] The dogs that were fed the high-protein diet (56% protein) had higher GFR and renal plasma flow rates than the dogs that were fed the low-protein diet (19% protein). However, significant morphological or functional deterioration in the remaining nephrons of the kidneys was not observed in any dogs. The investigators were unable to establish a cause and effect relationship between protein feeding and the progression of renal disease in the dogs that were studied. Feeding the high-protein (56%) and the low-protein (19%) diets was associated with slight proteinuria, but the 27%-protein diet did not cause this effect. In contrast to the rats that were studied, none of the dogs in this study developed elevated BUN levels or clinical signs of chronic renal disease in response to consuming moderate- or high-protein diets.

In another study, three groups of dogs with induced renal failure were fed three diets varying in protein, fat, carbohydrate, and mineral content.[367] Over a 40-week period, dogs that were fed the high-protein, high-phosphorus diet (44.4% protein, 2.05% phosphorus) showed the highest mortality rate. However, mortality was associated with uremia caused by the increased protein, rather than uremia caused by the development of progressive nephron destruction. There was no evidence of a decline in GFR (an indication of progressive renal disease) in the dogs fed the high-protein diet. These results indicate that the increased mortality was caused by the extrarenal, clinical effects of feeding high amounts of protein to dogs with renal failure and not to an enhanced progression of renal disease caused by the diet.

Although the previous studies do not support the hypothesis that protein affects the progression of chronic renal failure in dogs, other studies have also failed to show that restricting dietary protein inhibits the initial development or progression of renal disease. Early studies with rats reported that feeding low-protein diets prolonged life and delayed the development of chronic renal disease.[353,368,369] However, subsequent studies have shown that the benefits that had been attributed to low protein were actually a result of the low intakes of these diets and the subsequent low energy consumption of the rats throughout life. The low energy intake significantly slowed growth (which continues throughout life in rats) and retarded the progression of chronic renal disease.[364,370] Unfortunately, the belief that feeding a low-protein diet prevents the development and the progression of renal disease had already been applied to several other species, including companion animals. However, this theory is without supportive scientific evidence in either dogs or cats.

In dogs, the moderate restriction of dietary protein is not effective in modifying glomerular hypertrophy after a loss of kidney function. When dogs with a $^{15}/_{16}$ loss of kidney function were fed a moderately restricted diet containing 16% protein, the adaptive changes of hyperfiltration, capillary hypertension, and glomerular hypertrophy still occurred.[345] A second study of dogs with a $^{7}/_{8}$ loss of functional kidney tissue reported that renal lesions were indistinguishable between dogs that were fed a diet containing 15% protein and those that were fed a diet containing 31% protein over a 14-month period.[347]

Recent studies with cats have shown similar results. When cats with experimentally-induced renal failure were fed either a high-protein diet (51.7%) or a low-protein diet (27.6%), cats consuming the low-protein diet showed fewer and less severe glomerular lesions in the remnant kidney.[371,372] However, the low-protein diet was less palatable, and cats consuming this diet had significantly lower caloric intakes than those consuming the high-protein diet, leading to weight loss and signs of protein deficiency. Because of this confounding effect, the authors of the study concluded that restriction of calories and protein led to less glomerular injury in cats with induced renal failure when compared with cats fed a diet replete in calories and protein.

A subsequent study was undertaken to elucidate the separate effects of protein and calorie intake on the progression of renal disease in cats.[373] A group of 28 adult female cats with experimentally induced renal failure was divided into four groups according to initial GFR. Each group received one of four diets for a 12-month period: low protein/low calorie, low protein/high calorie, high protein/low calorie, or high protein/high calorie. GFR did not decrease in any of the groups during the 12-month study period. Mild to moderate renal glomerular lesions were observed in all groups, but their development was not affected by either protein level or caloric intake. On the other hand, nonglomerular lesions in the kidneys were reported in cats fed the high-caloric diets but not in those fed the high-protein diets. The cat appears to be similar to the dog in that feeding a diet containing adequate protein does not exacerbate chronic renal disease. Long-term studies with the cat are still necessary to evaluate the effects of dietary protein over periods of more than 1 year.

The severe restriction of dietary protein in both dogs and cats may be associated with several inherent dangers. Protein deficiency results in impaired immunological response and resistance to infection, reduced hemoglobin production and anemia, decreased plasma protein levels, and muscle wasting.[374,375] Because it has been hypothesized that elderly pets experience losses of renal function as a normal process of aging, it has become popular to advocate feeding low-protein diets to older animals, with the intent of slowing the rate of renal deterioration. However, no research has shown that there is an obligatory loss of kidney function with aging in either dogs or cats.[376,377,378] It is known, however, that elderly pets require adequate levels of high-quality protein to help to minimize losses of protein reserves and satisfy their maintenance needs (see Section 4, pp. 282-284). Restricting protein in older pets when it is not necessary can lead to further loss of protein reserves, malnutrition, and clinical signs associated with protein or amino acid deficiency. Diets with severely reduced protein are low in palatability, causing reduced intake that can further exacerbate protein deficiency. For example, when a diet containing 27.6% protein was fed to cats with ⅚ renal ablation, the cats consumed significantly less food when compared with cats fed 51.7% protein.[371] The cats fed the low-protein diet lost weight and developed hypoalbuminemia, a clinical sign of protein malnutrition. In contrast, cats fed the high-protein diet gained weight and did not develop protein deficiency. Consideration of the detrimental effects of protein restriction is particularly important in cats because this species does not readily adapt to reduced-protein diets (see Section 2, pp. 105-111).

Current evidence suggests that mechanisms that can alter the progression of renal disease in the rat do not have the same effect in the dog and cat. Dogs appear to be resistant to the glomerulosclerosis and loss of renal function associated with aging and adaptive changes in nephrons and protein-feeding in the rat.[376] Studies indicate that although high-protein feeding can exacerbate clinical signs by leading to azotemia in dogs with advanced renal failure, there is no evidence that dietary protein causes a progressive destruction of nephron functioning in the remaining normal tissue. It is hypothesized that the absence of systemic hypertension in dogs with renal disease and the fact that dogs do not normally develop the same type of renal disease as rats explain the differences between dogs and rats.[234,249] In addition, unlike the rat, the dog does not continue to grow throughout its life and typically consumes only one to two meals per day, compared with the nibbling regimen of the rat. In dogs, hyperfiltration following the consumption of a meal that contains protein lasts for a short time, as opposed to continuously throughout a 24-hour period in the rat.[223] Preliminary studies with cats indicate that the cat is similar to the dog, and that routine restriction of protein in cats with chronic renal disease with the intent of slowing disease progression is not supported.

Phosphorus

Another dietary factor that may be involved in the progression of renal disease in companion animals is the level of phosphorus in the diet. As chronic renal failure progresses, GFR declines and leads to a decreased ability to excrete phosphorus. In addition, declining kidney function leads to an inability to produce calcitriol (active vitamin D) and to degrade parathyroid hormone (PTH). Together, these changes result in aberrations in phosphorus and calcium metabolism and can ultimately result in hyperphosphatemia, bone demineralization (osteodystrophy), and the deposition of calcium phosphate crystals in soft tissues. The deposition of calcium and phosphorus in renal tissue causes inflammation, scarring, and subsequent loss of nephrons.[379] It has been hypothesized that the restriction of dietary phosphorus will help to control renal secondary hyperparathyroidism, resulting in decreased mineralization and less damage to functioning nephrons, ultimately slowing the progression of renal disease.

Studies with rats have shown that phosphorus restriction is effective in minimizing or preventing proteinuria and in slowing the structural and functional changes that occur in the remaining healthy nephrons.[380] Similar studies with dogs have found that the dietary restriction of phosphorus can slow the progression of clinical disease and prolong survival in azotemic dogs with induced chronic renal failure.[381] In addition, when diets containing 32% protein and varying levels of phosphorus were fed to dogs with induced renal failure, the dogs that were fed the low-phosphorus diets had significantly higher GFR values when compared with dogs fed the high-phosphorus diets.[382] However, over time, renal lesions developed that were not influenced by the level of phosphorus in the diet, indicating that other factors were involved in the progression of the disease. Beneficial effects of phosphorus restriction that are independent of the level of protein in the diet were found in a study comparing the effects of high and low dietary protein and phosphorus in dogs with a $^{15}/_{16}$ reduction in renal mass.[383] Survival time and GFR stability were enhanced in dogs fed reduced phosphorus (0.4%) but were not affected by the level of protein fed. There is also evidence that normal phosphorus intake in cats with induced renal disease causes increased mineralization of renal tissue, and that dietary restriction can prevent these changes.[384] Current evidence suggests that dietary phosphorus may affect the progression of renal disease in dogs and cats, but progression of disease can still occur even with restricted dietary phosphorus.

Dietary Lipids

The amount and type of fat in a pet's diet may affect the progression of renal disease. Hyperlipidemia has been identified as a causal factor in uremic renal failure in some species.[385,386] Like rats and humans, dogs and cats with renal dysfunction often exhibit elevated serum cholesterol and triglycerides. In addition, the degree of hyperlipidemia has been shown to be directly related to further losses of renal function in dogs with experimentally induced renal disease.[381] When dogs with induced renal failure were fed a diet enriched in polyunsaturated fatty acids (PUFAs) (safflower oil or menhaden fish oil) they had lower blood lipid levels, compared with dogs fed a diet containing saturated fat.[387] These results indicate that replacing a proportion of saturated fat with polyunsaturated fat may be helpful in ameliorating the hyperlipidemia seen in pets with chronic renal disease.

A second factor affecting the progression of renal disease is the presence of increased vascular pressure in the kidneys, specifically within the glomerular capillaries. In rats, manipulations that increase glomerular pressure contribute to the progression of chronic renal failure, and factors that reduce glomerular hypertension are renoprotective.[353,388] Modifications of the level of omega-3 fatty acids in the diet affects glomerular pressure and the progression of renal disease in rats. However, while some researchers report benefits of feeding omega-3 fatty acids, others found that feeding this class of fatty acid was associated with a worsening of disease in rats.[389,390,391] Similarly, while some human patients with immune-mediated forms of renal disease have benefited from supplementation with omega-3 fatty acids, others have showed no change in condition.[392,393]

Like rats and humans, dogs and cats with chronic renal disease develop glomerular hypertension.[346,356] A recent study of diabetic dogs demonstrated that therapies aimed at reducing glomerular hypertension significantly slowed the progression of kidney disease.[360,361] It is speculated that lowering glomerular pressure may also be of benefit to dogs and cats with other forms of chronic renal failure.[389] Dietary lipids influence intrarenal pressure through the effects of renal eicosanoid metabolism.[389] Eicosanoids, produced from fatty acids, are one of several mediators of inflammation in many different tissues of the body (see pp. 436-437). During an inflammatory response, the release and metabolism of omega-6 fatty acids produces the 2-series prostaglandins, the 4-series leukotrienes, hydroxyeicosatetraenoic acid, and thromboxane A_2 (TXA_2). Two omega-6 derived eicosanoids, prostaglandin E_2 (PGE_2) and prostacyclin, are vasodilatory and proinflammatory and function in the kidney to increase renal blood flow and GFR. In contrast, TXA_2 causes vasoconstriction and has variable effects on GFR. Omega-3 fatty acid–derived eicosanoids are less potent inflammatory agents, and omega-3–derived thromboxanes have less vasoconstrictive and platelet aggregating effects. Because omega-6 and omega-3 fatty acids compete for the same enzyme systems, increasing tissue concentrations of omega-3 fatty acids causes a diminution of the 2-series eicosanoids derived from the omega-6 fatty acid arachidonic acid, thus down-regulating intrarenal inflammatory responses.

A link between production of the 2-series of prostaglandins and thromboxanes and progressive renal disease has been proposed. This theory is based on studies that suggest glomerular hypertension is affected by renal eicosanoids, and that supplementation with omega-3 fatty acids (marine fish oil) can reduce renal hypertension and may slow the progression of chronic renal disease.[353] A recent study measured the effects of three different types of fat on GFR in dogs with induced renal failure.[395] Dogs were fed a low-fat diet supplemented with either menhaden fish oil (a source of omega-3 fatty acids), safflower oil (a source of unsaturated omega-6 fatty acids) or beef tallow (a source of saturated omega-6 fatty acids) for a period of 20 months. Dogs fed the menhaden fish oil–supplemented diet had reduced proteinuria and lower serum creatinine, cholesterol, and triglyceride values when compared with dogs fed either safflower oil or beef tallow. While six out of seven dogs fed the diet enriched with omega-6 fatty acids showed progressive loss of renal function over the 20-week period, dogs fed the diet supplemented with omega-3 fatty acids did not exhibit signs of progression and actually had GFR test values indicating a slight increase in renal function at the end of the trial (Figure 34-1). These results indicate that omega-3 fatty acids may be renoprotective, while supplementation with omega-6 fatty acids may contribute to disease progression.

FIGURE **34-1**

Change in GFR (%) in dogs supplemented with menhaden fish oil, beef tallow, or safflower oil. *P < 0.05.*

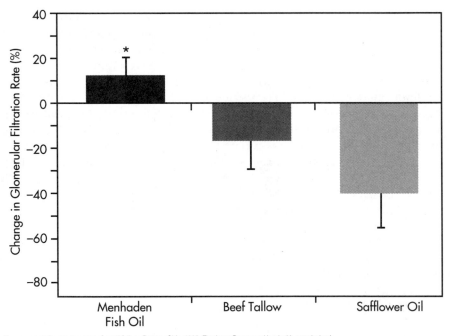

(From *New concepts in management of renal failure*, Dayton, Ohio, 1998, The Iams Company. Used with permission.)

A second study examined the effects of fatty acid supplementation in dogs with spontaneous chronic renal failure.[396] Dogs were fed fatty acid supplements containing either safflower oil or menhaden fish oil for a 6-week period. Dogs fed the omega-3 supplement maintained GFR for the entire 6-week period and exhibited decreased levels of urinary PGE_2. The dogs supplemented with safflower oil had increased GFR and increased urinary PGE_2 concentrations. Although dogs fed safflower oil had higher GFR values, it is theorized that this was a short-lived effect caused by increased renal blood flow. The rise in PGE_2 is indicative of increased intrarenal pressure, which over time may contribute to the progression of disease.[335] The somewhat conflicting results of these two studies indicate the need to fully elucidate the role of omega-6 and omega-3 fatty acids in the progression of chronic renal disease in dogs and cats over greater periods. Such studies are especially important for the cat, given the paucity of studies in this species and the cat's special fatty acid needs.

Other Contributing Nutrients

High levels of sodium in the diet have been said to exacerbate the progression of chronic renal failure through enhancement of systemic hypertension.[335] There is also limited evidence in rats that sodium restriction may slow the progression of chronic renal disease.[397] For this reason, moderate sodium restriction has been recommended for pets with chronic renal failure. However, sodium restriction is not universally accepted because systemic hypertension is not a consistent finding in dogs and cats with renal failure. Moreover, unnecessarily decreasing dietary sodium may exacerbate compromised renal concentrating ability due to reduced intrarenal sodium content, and it may cause increased production of angiotensin in response to lowered systemic levels of sodium. Currently, there are no published studies showing a benefit of sodium restriction in pets with renal failure.

Metabolic acidosis occurs commonly in pets with chronic renal failure and is caused by the reduced ability of the kidneys to excrete acids. For example, a retrospective study of cats with naturally occurring renal failure reported that approximately 80% of cats were diagnosed with metabolic acidosis.[398] The development of acidosis in cats may be exacerbated by the acidifying nature of many commercial maintenance diets. Acidosis contributes to renal injury and uremia and to excessive renal tubular generation of ammonia. These changes all are believed to contribute to a progressive loss of renal function. In addition, there is an apparent association between metabolic acidosis and negative potassium balance in cats, which may further contribute to disease progression.[205,399] Supplementation with alkalinizing agents is used to limit the requirement for renal excretion of acid and to normalize body acid-base balance. Oral sodium bicarbonate and potassium citrate are recommended for dogs. Because cats with chronic renal disease are often hypokalemic, potassium citrate should be used with this species.

DIETARY MANAGEMENT

When chronic renal disease has been diagnosed in a dog or cat, dietary management can be implemented with the goals of minimizing the clinical, biochemical, and physiological consequences of the loss of kidney function. Alterations in the kidneys' ability to excrete waste products and to regulate metabolism of certain nutrients and hormones are the cause of the clinical signs that the animal experiences. Although dietary therapy does not "cure" chronic renal disease, it can minimize clinical signs and contribute to a pet's health, well-being, and longevity. Recent evidence also indicates that modifying certain nutrients in the diet may slow the progression of disease. A major goal of dietary management is to minimize the accumulation of protein catabolites in the blood while still providing adequate protein for the pet's maintenance needs. In addition, adequate calories from nonprotein sources must be provided to minimize the use of either body tissues or dietary protein for energy. Other nutrients of concern include dietary fat, fiber, phosphorus, sodium, potassium, and water-soluble vitamins (Box 34-2).

Protein

A distinction must be made between restricting protein with the proposed purpose of slowing or stopping the progression of renal disease and restricting protein with the purpose of managing clinical signs. Although studies with rats indicate that protein restriction is beneficial in slowing the progression of chronic renal disease, research does not support this finding in dogs and cats (see pp. 455-458). In contrast, when chronic renal disease has been definitively diagnosed in a dog or cat through the appearance of clinical signs, diminished GFR, and changes in blood chemistry data, restriction of dietary protein may be beneficial and is recommended for the management of clinical signs.

The accumulation of the nitrogenous end products of protein and amino acid metabolism causes many of the clinical and metabolic signs of chronic renal failure. Urea is the most abundant of these metabolites and can be readily measured in the blood. Although urea is only a mild uremic toxin, its concentration parallels the levels of other, more potent nitrogenous toxins and can be used as an index to mon-

BOX 34-2

Goals of Dietary Management of Chronic Renal Disease

Maintain nitrogen balance by providing optimal protein nutrition.
Provide adequate nonprotein calories.
Minimize azotemia and associated clinical signs.
Normalize serum phosphorus.
Normalize blood pH.
Normalize electrolyte balance.

itor the extent of disease and clinical signs. Together these components produce nausea, vomiting, osmotic diuresis, and a decreased lifespan of red blood cells.[337] Normalizing the levels of urea and other nitrogenous waste products in the blood through the restriction of dietary protein contributes to a return of appetite; weight gain; and a lessening of other clinical signs.[340,374]

The generation of urea is directly proportional to the daily turnover of dietary and body protein. Protein that is ingested in excess of the animal's requirement is metabolized for energy, producing urea and other end products that must then be excreted by the kidneys. Similarly, when inadequate calories are ingested or when an animal is in a catabolic state, body protein is used for energy, also resulting in the synthesis of urea. A reduction in the excretory capacity of the kidneys results in an elevation of urea and other components in the blood, because they are retained by the body. A primary goal of dietary therapy is to provide an optimal amount of protein and adequate nonprotein calories to prevent the breakdown of body tissue for energy. These changes minimize the amount of urea and other nitrogenous end products that are produced. In most cases, this necessitates a moderate restriction of dietary protein and a change in the type of protein included in the diet.

Minimum protein and amino acid requirements for pets with chronic renal failure have not been established. Therefore the decision to control protein intake is determined by the patient's clinical signs and degree of impairment of renal function. Protein restriction is suggested only when a pet's BUN is greater than 65 to 80 mg/dl and when serum creatinine is greater than 2.5 mg per 100 milliliters (ml).[374,400,401] Although the normal range for fasting BUN is between 10 and 24 mg/dl, most dogs do not show clinical signs of renal disease until BUN exceeds 60 to 80 mg/dl and there is a loss of 75% or more of renal function.[374,401] Pets that have only slightly elevated BUN values (30 to 60 mg/dl) and are not showing clinical signs do not benefit from protein restriction.[402]

The goal of dietary protein restriction is to maintain the animal's BUN below a level of 60 mg/dl. In dogs and cats, as in other animals, a direct relationship exists between the BUN/serum creatinine ratio and dietary protein. The minimum daily protein requirement for dogs has been determined to be between 1.25 and 1.50 grams (g) of protein per kilogram (kg) of body weight.[403] This recommendation assumes that the protein is of very high biological value. Early recommendations for the level of protein to feed to uremic dogs varied from 0.66 g/kg to 2.2 g/kg per day.[404,405,406] However, a study of dogs with induced renal disease found that feeding a diet containing 1.6 g/kg of protein or less caused signs of protein deficiency.[407] This is equivalent to feeding a diet containing 8.2% protein on a dry-matter basis (DMB).[408] Increasing the protein level to 2 g/kg still aided in the control of BUN levels and clinical signs of renal disease but did not cause protein malnutrition. The potential to induce protein deficiency necessitates conservative restriction of dietary protein in dogs with renal disease. Because uremic animals tend to be in a catabolic state, their minimum protein requirement may be even slightly higher than that of a normal dog.[335] In addition, dogs with proteinuria may require more dietary protein than dogs without proteinuria. Considering this, dogs with chronic renal failure should not be fed diets containing less than 2.2 g of protein/kg of body weight per day.[335] In all cases, the highest level of protein that results in an amelioration of clinical signs and controls BUN levels without compromising protein and amino acid nutrition should be fed.

In dogs with mild to moderate renal disease, a diet containing between 12% and 28% protein on a DMB is recommended, with the exact level dependent on the animal's clinical and biochemical response.[340,409] In cases of severe renal disease, when GFR has deteriorated to only 10% to 20% of normal, protein must be progressively restricted to approach a level that is close to the pet's minimum daily requirement. Depending on the degree of clinical signs and the energy level of the diet, a pet food containing between 10% and 15% protein may be needed, provided that the protein is of high biological value.[340,408] At this level of dysfunction, a balancing act occurs between providing a diet that will ameliorate clinical signs yet will still provide adequate amounts of nutrients. Once a modified diet has been selected and found to be acceptable to the pet, progressive improvement of clinical signs such as a reduction in vomiting, improved appetite, weight gain, and improved physical activity is generally seen within 2 to 4 weeks. Weekly monitoring of BUN and serum creatinine and evaluation of clinical response should be used to determine the need for either increasing or decreasing dietary protein level.

Modification of dietary protein for cats with chronic renal failure must account for the cat's naturally higher protein requirement and its inability to adapt to low-protein diets (see Section 2, pp. 105-111). The effectiveness of restricted protein intake in managing clinical signs of chronic renal disease in cats is not well studied. When cats with naturally occurring renal failure were fed a diet containing either normal or reduced levels of protein and phosphorus, the group fed lower protein and phosphorus exhibited decreasing BUN and serum phosphorus levels over the 6-week study period.[410] However, the health of cats fed both high and low protein and phosphorus deteriorated during the study. Subjective changes in health were assessed as being less severe in the cats fed the restricted diet, but long-term survival and the rate of disease progression were not reported. Moreover, the design of this study did not allow separation of the effects of low protein from those of reduced phosphorus.

Because cats have significantly higher protein requirements than dogs, reduced protein diets formulated for dogs should not be fed to cats. It is currently recommended that cats with chronic renal failure be fed the maximum level of protein that will control uremia and its associated clinical signs.[374] One method of accomplishing this is to determine a cat's current protein intake as a percentage of calories and to slowly decrease dietary protein until clinical signs are managed. For example, if a cat is currently eating a diet that contains 38% protein calories, the proportion of protein in the diet should be reduced to 30% of metabolizable energy (ME). Serum biochemistries and clinical signs should be measured after 1 to 3 weeks and, if necessary, the diet can be adjusted further. This method allows precise control over the protein content of a cat's diet without the risk of unnecessarily restricting protein. It is especially important to monitor cats that are consuming reduced protein diets for signs of protein malnutrition.[411] Signs of protein deficiency include hypoalbuminemia, anemia, weight loss, and loss of lean body mass. If these

signs occur, dietary protein should be gradually increased until these abr.
are corrected.

In dogs and cats, it is important to adjust the protein level of the diet t
the needs of an individual animal. If protein restriction is adequate, a 50% or g
reduction in BUN should occur.[337] Improvement in clinical signs is generally .
within 3 to 4 weeks. Most dogs and cats will show a reduction in vomiting, r
proved appetite, weight gain, and improved physical activity. Consistent monito.
ing of BUN values and clinical response to the diet can be used to indicate the need
to either increase or decrease the protein level. If progressive deterioration of renal
function occurs, adjustments in the diet to maintain an acceptable BUN may be necessary. Chemistry profiles and complete blood counts should also be measured periodically to monitor the pet for anemia, acidemia, or electrolyte imbalances.

The type of protein included in the restricted protein diet is very important.
Only protein sources that are highly digestible and of high biological value should
be used. These sources include eggs, dairy products, soy protein isolates, and some
lean muscle meats. Poor-quality proteins and ingredients that are not highly digestible should be avoided. The therapeutic diet can be either a commercially prepared product or a homemade diet. Advantages of using a commercially prepared
diet include convenience and the assurance of consistency in the formulation. However, preparing a homemade diet may allow greater flexibility in the level of protein and other nutrients that are included, thus providing a diet that is specifically
formulated to meet a pet's individual needs. Homemade diets may also be more
palatable for some pets than some commercially prepared products. Because of
their tendency to develop anorexia, cats with renal disease should be fed diets that
are highly palatable and acceptable. Commercial feline maintenance diets should be
avoided because many are formulated to be acidifying and so may contribute to an
exacerbation of metabolic acidosis.[411] Decisions regarding the type of diet to use
can be made based on the pet's response to treatment and the capabilities and preferences of the owner.

Fat

It is important that diets formulated for pets with chronic renal disease contain
enough nonprotein calories to spare protein from being used as an energy source.
Fat is an excellent energy source for dogs and cats and also promotes diet palatability. The type of fat included in the diet is also very important. Hyperlipidemia has
been shown to be causally linked to the progression of chronic renal disease in
dogs and other species.[381,385,412] Additionally, hyperlipidemia in dogs with induced
renal failure can be ameliorated by feeding a diet enriched in PUFAs that are supplied as either safflower oil or menhaden fish oil.[413] Unsaturated fatty acids in the
omega-3 family (e.g., certain marine fish oils, flax oil) may be the preferred source
because of the beneficial effects that this class of fatty acids have on intrarenal hemodynamics and inflammation. Preliminary studies indicate that diets rich in
omega-3 fatty acids may offer a novel approach to slowing the progression of this
disease in dogs (see pp. 459-461).

urrently recommended that fatty acid supplements containing omega-6
ds not be administered to pets with chronic renal failure. Conversely, in-
g omega-3 fatty acids in the diet may be beneficial. While one method of in-
ng omega-3 fatty acids is to add a supplement to the diet, the ratio of omega-6
mega-3 fatty acids can be better controlled by feeding a diet that contains ad-
ted amounts of these fatty acids. Although an ideal ratio for dogs with renal dis-
ase has not been identified, current evidence suggests that feeding a diet containing a ratio of 5:1 is beneficial.[413] Studies of the effects of modifying dietary fatty acids
in cats with renal disease have not been published. Because of the cat's unique fatty
acid needs, no recommendations for this species can yet be made.

Phosphorus

The decrease in GFR that occurs during renal failure results in a decreased ability
to excrete phosphorus. This decreased ability leads to phosphorus retention, hyperphosphatemia, and renal secondary hyperparathyroidism. These factors are believed to promote the formation of calcium phosphate crystals and the deposition
of these crystals in the kidneys and other soft tissues, which may lead to further loss
of nephrons and progression of disease (see p. 458).[379,380] Additionally, the chronic
elevation of PTH that is caused by retention of phosphorus results in excessive
demineralization of bone and pathological changes that are associated with bone
loss.

A goal of dietary therapy is to normalize serum phosphorus concentrations and
prevent bone demineralization and deposition of calcium phosphate crystals in soft
tissues. In moderate cases of renal disease, when serum phosphorus is slightly elevated, a decrease in the level of phosphorus in the diet may be sufficient to achieve
normalization of serum phosphorus. Because dietary protein is a principal source
of phosphorus, restriction of protein and the use of reduced phosphorus protein
sources contribute to this dietary modification. However, as the disease progresses,
dietary restriction does not always control blood phosphorus levels and may not be
sufficient to control the long-term effects of hyperparathyroidism and bone disease.
Intestinal phosphate-binding agents must then be used in conjunction with reduced
dietary phosphorus to normalize the serum phosphorus concentration.[400,405] These
agents are administered with a meal and limit the gastrointestinal absorption of
phosphorus. The compounds most commonly used are aluminum hydroxide and
aluminum carbonate.[340]

Blood phosphorus concentration should be monitored regularly, and the diet
and the binding agents should be adjusted until normalization of serum phosphorus is achieved. Calcium supplementation and vitamin D supplementation should
be avoided until serum phosphorus levels are under control. Providing additional
calcium in the presence of hyperphosphatemia may further contribute to soft tissue
mineralization. Once serum phosphorus concentration has been normalized, calcium and/or vitamin D can be supplemented to aid in the control of renal hyperparathyroidism and bone disease. Calcium carbonate at a dosage of 100 mg/kg of
body weight is recommended.[337]

Although some studies with dogs showed that restriction of dietary phosphorus prevented or reversed renal secondary hyperparathyroidism, most research indicates that dietary restriction alone does not consistently reduce serum PTH levels.[402,414] Moreover, serum phosphorus does not appear to be a sensitive predictor of renal secondary hyperparathyroidism.[402] It has been hypothesized that chronically elevated PTH may be more affected by decreased levels of active vitamin D (calcitriol) than by elevated phosphorus. As kidney function declines, the ability to produce calcitriol is compromised. Subsequently, low calcitriol levels stimulate the release of PTH. It therefore appears that restriction of dietary phosphorus alone may not be sufficient to prevent hyperparathyroidism in some dogs with chronic renal failure. Phosphate-binding agents, calcium supplementation, and administration of calcitriol may be necessary to treat the hyperparathyroidism of renal disease in these animals.[415]

Dietary Fiber

The reduced ability of the kidneys to excrete nitrogenous end products of protein catabolism is a major cause of the uremic signs and laboratory abnormalities seen in animals with chronic renal failure. As discussed previously, providing a reduced level of dietary protein that is of very high quality can decrease the body's need to oxidize dietary amino acids and excrete the nitrogenous end products. A second approach to managing nitrogen excretion is to alter the route of excretion. Recent studies have shown that the amount and type of fiber included in the diet influences nitrogen excretion and urea concentrations in the blood. Specifically, feeding fermentable fiber alters the flux of urea and ammonia in the large intestine and cecum, resulting in a shift of urea excretion from the kidneys via urine to the large intestine via feces. Because an alternate route of urea excretion is available, BUN values decrease. Feeding fermentable fibers has been shown to cause a repartitioning of nitrogen into the feces in humans, rats, and dogs.[416,417,418,419,420]

The underlying mechanism involves the effects of dietary fiber on bacterial growth in the gastrointestinal tract. Feeding fermentable fiber results in increases in bacterial growth and activity in the large intestine. This is accompanied by increased colonic blood flow, tissue weights, surface area, and nitrogen excretion.[420,421,422,423] The increased fecal nitrogen is due primarily to excretion of a greater proportion of bacterial mass. The intestinal bacterial that proliferate synthesize the enzyme urease, which converts urea to ammonia and carbon dioxide. The ammonia is subsequently used by bacteria as a source of nitrogen for protein synthesis. This process functions to remove urea nitrogen from circulation and incorporate it into bacterial protein, which is ultimately excreted via the feces (Figure 34-2).

The effect of fermentable fiber on patterns of nitrogen excretion has recently been studied in dogs. When healthy adult dogs were fed a diet containing a blend of fermentable fibers (beet pulp, fructooligosaccharides [FOS], and gum arabic), apparent digestibility of dry matter (DM) and organic matter decreased slightly due to excretion of nonfermentable fiber components and increased bacterial mass.[336] This was accompanied by a slight decrease in apparent protein digestibility (91.3% vs.

FIGURE 34-2

Effect of fermentable fiber on patterns of nitrogen excretion.

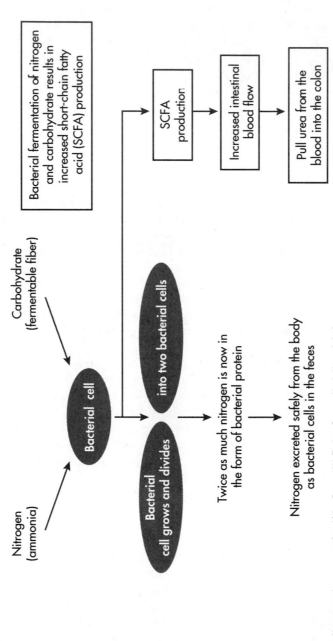

Bacterial fermentation of nitrogen and carbohydrate results in increased short-chain fatty acid (SCFA) production

SCFA production

Increased intestinal blood flow

Pull urea from the blood into the colon

Carbohydrate (fermentable fiber)

Nitrogen (ammonia)

Bacterial cell

Bacterial cell grows and divides

into two bacterial cells

Twice as much nitrogen is now in the form of bacterial protein

Nitrogen excreted safely from the body as bacterial cells in the feces

88.2%). Dogs fed the fiber-containing diet had excellent stool scores, with no adverse effects such as diarrhea or formation of soft stools. Changes in protein digestibility due to feeding fermentable fibers to dogs has been shown to be caused by the increased excretion of bacterial nitrogen as opposed to a decreased digestibility of dietary protein within the small intestine.[420,424] These results support the theory that fermentable fiber can be used to repartition nitrogen excretion through intestinal bacterial protein in dogs.

The efficacy of repartitioning nitrogen excretion using fermentable fiber in the diet for dogs with chronic renal disease has also been examined. Because fermentable fiber is capable of repartitioning nitrogen excretory patterns away from the kidneys and toward the large intestine, it is possible that more dietary protein can be fed without negatively impacting azotemia and its associated signs. When dogs with experimentally induced renal insufficiency were fed either a control diet or a diet supplemented with a fermentable fiber blend, GFR was unchanged, while BUN values and urinary excretion of urea nitrogen decreased (Figures 34-3 and 34-4).[425] Because there was no change in renal function, this indicates that the reduced concentration of urea in the blood was a result of enhanced fecal nitrogen excretion.

Preliminary results of the use of fermentable fiber in the diets of dogs with naturally occurring renal disease are encouraging as well. The clinical response to feeding a low- or moderate-protein diet containing a fermentable fiber blend to dogs in various stages of chronic renal failure was studied.[426] All of the dogs in the study had previously been fed a conventional renal diet that was severely restricted in protein (14% DM). At the start of the study, the dogs were switched to either a moderate-protein (21.1%) or low-protein (17.5%) renal diet, based upon initial BUN and creatinine values. In addition to fiber content and higher protein level, the two experimental diets also had an adjusted omega-6 to omega-3 fatty acid ratio of approximately 5:1, compared with a ratio of 22:1 in the conventional renal diet. All of the diets contained reduced levels of phosphorus. Blood chemistries, hematocrit and hemoglobin counts, and overall health were monitored for a 10-week period and compared with values collected at the start of the study.

Results indicated that the inclusion of dietary fiber in the two experimental renal diets successfully partitioned nitrogen excretion away from the kidneys. For example, none of the dogs fed the moderate protein had increased BUN values, and two showed reduced blood ammonia values, even though the diet contained approximately 50% more protein than the conventional renal diet that had previously been fed. It appears that adequate protein to meet the nutritional recommendation for adult maintenance was provided to these dogs without the side effect of exacerbating azotemia. The dogs also showed a trend toward lower serum triglyceride values as a result of the lower percentage of calories provided by fat and the adjusted omega-6 to omega-3 fatty acid ratio. Owners reported an overall improvement in the quality of their dog's coat in all of the reported cases, again reflecting better protein nutrition in these dogs. The dogs with more advanced renal disease were fed the second experimental renal diet, which contained approximately 25% more protein than the conventional renal diet. Similar to the first group of dogs, these dogs either maintained or lowered BUN and creatinine values over the 10-week period.

FIGURE 34-3

*Effect of feeding fermentable fiber on percent nitrogen in urine. *P < 0.05.
**Expressed as a percent of no-fiber value.*

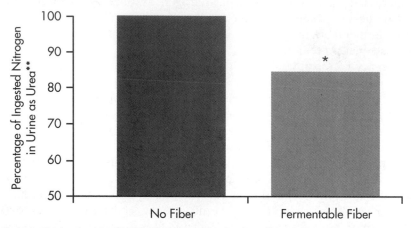

(From World Small Animal Veterinary Association: *Clinical Nutrition Symposium proceedings,* Dayton, Ohio, 1998, The Iams Company. Used with permission.)

FIGURE 34-4

*Effect of feeding fermentable fiber on BUN. *P < 0.05.
**Expressed as a percent of no-fiber value.*

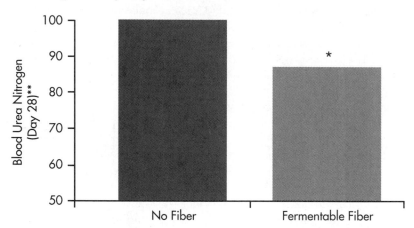

(From World Small Animal Veterinary Association: *Clinical Nutrition Symposium proceedings,* Dayton, Ohio, 1998, The Iams Company. Used with permission.)

Preliminary results indicate that including a blend of fermentable fiber sources in the diet of dogs with chronic renal failure is efficacious because it allows higher levels of protein to be fed to uremic dogs, thus providing optimal protein nutrition and preventing the development of protein deficiency. Dogs tolerate a blend of fermentable fibers with no adverse effects on gastrointestinal function or fecal score. Despite the lack of side effects in dogs, previous work with cats has shown that cats are less tolerant of fermentable fiber in the diet.[427] Feeding cats highly fermentable fiber causes significant reductions in protein and lipid digestibility. For this reason, high levels of fermentable fiber in the diets of cats are not currently recommended. It is possible that the inclusion of certain types of fiber blends may be efficacious in this species, but more studies are needed before recommendations can be made.

Other Nutrients

Additional nutrients that are of concern in the diets of dogs and cats with renal disease include sodium, potassium, the water-soluble vitamins, and, possibly, bicarbonate. The major route of sodium excretion in dogs is through the urine.[428] In humans and other species, sodium retention and systemic hypertension is a common sequela of chronic renal disease. However, hypertension is not a common occurrence in dogs and cats.[429] In addition, dogs and cats with renal disease demonstrate limited renal responsiveness and decreased tolerance to sudden changes of sodium content in the diet.[337] Diets for pets with renal disease should also contain adequate levels of potassium to prevent the hypokalemia that occurs in some cases, most often in cats.[405] When polyuria is present, supplementation with water-soluble vitamins is advisable because of excessive losses of these vitamins in the urine.

Reduced renal mass is associated with an increase in the production of ammonia by the renal tubules. This results in a rise in renal tissue ammonia concentration, which can cause local toxic and inflammatory effects and further contribute to renal damage.[405] In severe cases, systemic metabolic acidosis may occur as a result of compromised capacity to regulate acid-base balance. Supplementation with sodium bicarbonate or potassium citrate may ameliorate some of the damage as a result of increased ammonia production in the kidneys and will aid in the treatment of metabolic acidosis. A dosage of 5 to 10 grains of sodium bicarbonate, given orally every 10 to 12 hours, is recommended (Box 34-3).[405]

BOX 34-3

Practical Feeding Tips: Dietary Management of Chronic Kidney Disease

Provide the highest dietary protein that will maintain a BUN of less than 60.

Provide a highly digestible, high–biological value protein source.

Provide an adequate amount of nonprotein calories.

Restrict dietary phosphorus and regularly monitor serum phosphorus level.

Feed a diet that has an adjusted omega-6 to omega-3 fatty acid ratio of 5:1.

Feed a diet containing a moderate level of fermentable fiber to aid in the control of azotemia (dogs only).

Provide intestinal phosphate binding agents, if necessary.

When necessary, provide supplemental calcium and vitamin D once serum phosphorus is normalized.

Monitor intake of sodium bicarbonate, potassium, and water-soluble vitamins closely. Adjust diet as necessary.

CHAPTER

35

Feline Hepatic Lipidosis

Feline hepatic lipidosis is an acquired disorder caused by the excessive accumulation of triglycerides in the cells of the liver, which ultimately interferes with the liver's ability to function.[430] It is one of the most common hepatobiliary disorders of cats and in the past has been associated with a very high mortality rate.[431,432] But in recent years, the long-term prognosis of cats with hepatic lipidosis has dramatically improved. This is due in large part to the use of early and aggressive tube feeding, which successfully reverses the condition in many cats.[433,434] However, despite progress in treatment, the underlying cause of hepatic lipidosis remains poorly understood. In the majority of cats, hepatic lipidosis is the only detectable underlying abnormality, and for this reason, the syndrome is referred to as *idiopathic hepatic lipidosis* (IHL).[435] Less commonly, hepatic lipidosis occurs secondarily to other pathological conditions such as inflammatory bowel disease, renal disease, or diabetes mellitus.

INCIDENCE AND CAUSE

In healthy animals, a dynamic relationship exists among the fatty acids that are located in adipose tissue, traveling in the blood, and stored in the liver. Circulating fatty acids are taken up by the liver, where they are either metabolized for energy or converted to triglycerides and secreted back into the circulation. If the supply of fatty acids to the liver exceeds the liver's capacity to oxidize or secrete them, lipidosis occurs.[436] Hepatic lipidosis may also occur as a result of impaired oxidation of fatty acids in hepatocytes or due to an inability of the liver to secrete the very–low-density lipoproteins (VLDLs) that carry triglycerides in the bloodstream. Recent studies support the theory that the origin of excess hepatic triglycerides in cats with IHL is from fatty acids mobilized from adipose tissue.[437,438] Most researchers agree that the pathogenesis of IHL is probably multifactorial, involving factors that affect fatty-acid mobilization to the liver as well as the oxidation of fatty acids or synthesis and secretion of VLDLs.[432]

IHL is fairly common and is usually is seen in middle-aged cats with a history of obesity. Females are reported to be twice as likely to be affected as males, but this may reflect a higher incidence of obesity in the females that were studied, rather than a true gender difference.[435] In the majority of cases, a cat will have experienced a period of stress followed by partial or complete anorexia. Although obesity in cats is not typically associated with hepatic accumulation of lipids, the metabolic changes caused by prolonged fasting lead to rapid and severe hepatic fat accumulation and the clinical signs associated with liver disease. For example, when five healthy but obese cats were fasted for a period of 4 to 6 weeks, three of the cats remained healthy and two developed overt clinical and laboratory signs of IHL.[439] Subsequent studies by the same group reported that voluntary fasting could be induced by changing the diets of obese cats from a highly palatable commercial diet to a less palatable purified diet.[440] All of the cats refused to eat the new diet and developed histological signs of hepatic lipidosis over a period of 4 to 7 weeks.

Although prolonged fasting appears to be a consistent finding in cats that develop IHL, the exact metabolic changes responsible for the rapid accumulation of lipid in the liver are not fully understood. Cats diagnosed with IHL typically show signs of protein malnutrition such as muscle wasting, anemia, and hypoalbuminemia. It has been hypothesized that deficiencies of arginine and methionine, secondary to anorexia and protein malnutrition, are involved in the onset of IHL. The cat requires a dietary source of the amino acid arginine for the production of urea in the liver. When the cat stops eating, prolonged anorexia leads to a deficiency of arginine. Urea cycle activity is depressed, and ammonia begins to accumulate in the blood. Byproducts of this disruption in the urea cycle also interfere with lipoprotein synthesis in the liver.[441] Moreover, a deficiency of one or more essential amino acids may limit the synthesis of the proteins needed for production of lipoproteins by the liver, leading to the accumulation of triglycerides.[442] Supportive research for the role of protein has shown that the administration of small amounts of protein to obese cats during fasting helps to prevent the accumulation of hepatic lipids.[4343]

Carnitine is a compound that is synthesized primarily in the liver and is necessary for the transport of long-chain fatty acids into cellular mitochondria for oxidation. Human subjects with carnitine deficiency show severe fat accumulation in the liver and other organs and develop signs of liver disease.[444] Because of this association in humans, it had been theorized that a deficiency of carnitine may be the cause of IHL in cats. However, carnitine concentrations in the plasma, liver, and skeletal muscle of cats with hepatic lipidosis are normal.[445,446] In addition, the plasma concentration of ketone bodies is elevated in cats with IHL, which indicates that there is no impairment of fatty acid oxidation in cats with this disorder.[447]

CLINICAL SIGNS AND DIAGNOSIS

Clinical signs of IHL include complete or partial anorexia with a duration of 7 days or longer; depression; jaundice; weight loss; and muscle wasting.[435,448,449,450,451] Vomiting and/or diarrhea are occasionally reported. Owners usually report that the cat suddenly stopped eating following a period of lifestyle change or stress. Commonly reported stresses include a move to a new house, the arrival of new pets into the household, or a sudden change in diet.[447] Laboratory findings show increased serum activities of liver-associated enzymes, increased serum bilirubin and bile acid concentrations, and, in some cases, increased blood urea nitrogen (BUN) and plasma ammonia concentration.[440,449] A nonregenerative anemia characterized by irregularly shaped erythrocytes is typically seen.[435,449] The initial diagnosis of IHL is made using medical history, clinical signs, and the results of laboratory tests. The diagnosis is confirmed by a liver biopsy or fine-needle aspirate showing excessive lipid accumulation in the sampled hepatocytes.

TREATMENT

Regardless of the metabolic cause of IHL, it is essential for the cat's recovery that an early diagnosis is made and that supportive fluid and nutritional therapy is started as soon as possible. Aggressive tube feeding is the treatment of choice because afflicted cats will not eat voluntarily. Force-feeding is not recommended because it can further stress the cat and does not provide an accurate measure of the pet's caloric intake. For these reasons, tube feeding with a nasogastric tube or gastrostomy is preferred by most veterinarians.[452,453] The use of a gastrostomy tube involves direct surgical entry into the cat's stomach. This procedure allows accurate and consistent delivery of nutrients and does not interfere with the cat's ability to swallow.[451,452] Although surgical complications are a risk, most cats tolerate gastrostomy tubes better than pharyngostomy tubes.

The composition of an ideal therapeutic diet for cats recovering from IHL has not been determined. A variety of diets have been recommended, including blenderized high-protein cat diets, human enteral products, and veterinary enteral products.[453,454] Because it is generally accepted that the provision of optimal levels of dietary protein is essential, a product that provides 30% to 50% of metabolizable energy (ME) calories as protein, 30% to 40% as fat, and 20% to 30% as digestible carbohydrate is recommended.[447] Cats that show clinical signs of hepatoencephalopathy initially need to be fed a reduced-protein diet. Protein content can be gradually increased as neurological signs resolve.

The initial tube feeding should provide $\frac{1}{4}$ to $\frac{1}{2}$ of the cat's calculated ME requirement. This is gradually increased over a 1-week period to the cat's ME requirement. A minimum of four feedings should be provided per day. Signs of hepatic dysfunction begin to resolve as soon as the cat is receiving adequate protein and energy intake. However, most cats require 3 to 6 weeks of intense dietary therapy before laboratory values normalize, clinical improvement occurs, and the cat's appetite returns. Because it appears that acquired food aversion is a component of the anorexia seen in many cats with IHL, oral feeding should not be introduced until tube feeding is well established and the cat voluntarily shows a strong interest in food when it is presented.[449]

The cat's owner must be willing to assist with the nursing care of the pet because cats with hepatic lipidosis may not eat well for several months. As the cat's appetite returns, the frequency of tube feedings should be slowly decreased until the cat is consuming adequate calories voluntarily. When vomiting can be controlled and long-term adequate protein and calorie intake is ensured, treatment is usually successful. However, because many cats refuse to eat voluntarily for a period of weeks to several months, management can be difficult for pet owners and prognosis will be guarded until the cat begins to eat voluntarily. Supportive treatment involves minimizing any stress that the animal may experience and, in some cases, administering appetite stimulants.[455] Although some investigators advocate supplying supplemental carnitine during tube feeding, recent evidence indicates that this is probably unnecessary.[430,446] Throughout the treatment period, frequent monitoring of liver-associated enzymes in serum can be used as an indicator of hepatic recovery.[439]

Because most cats with IHL have a history of obesity, it is prudent to prevent weight regain following recovery. If the cat is still overweight, a weight loss protocol that allows a slow rate of weight loss and includes a diet containing optimal levels of protein should be followed (see Section 5, pp. 322-326). Veterinary supervision is warranted to ensure a slow rate of weight loss and prevent the recurrence of IHL. Most importantly, the cat's lifestyle and living conditions should be managed to minimize or prevent stressful events that may lead to subsequent episodes of anorexia.

36

Dental Health and Diet

 Periodontal disease and inflammation of the gingivae are common disorders in dogs and cats.[456,457] Gingivitis is caused by the formation and persistence of dental plaque on the surface of the teeth. If untreated, this can progress to periodontal disease, which affects the gingivae, periodontal ligament, cementum, and alveolar bone. Periodontal disease is associated with oral pain, malodorous breath, ulceration, and the loss of alveolar bone and teeth. The bacteremia that often accompanies periodontitis may also lead to damage of other organs in the body. Although a direct causal relationship has not been proven, periodontal disease has been implicated as contributing to diseases involving the kidneys, cardiovascular system, lungs, and immune system.[458,459] Because periodontal disease is a common and serious disorder in dogs and cats, recent studies have focused on nutrition and diet as risk factors for its development and as potential means for reducing gingivitis and preventing its progression to periodontal disease.

DESCRIPTION AND INCIDENCE

The types of dental health problems that occur in dogs and cats differ somewhat from those typically seen in humans. Because of the sharp inclined planes of their dentition, dogs and cats are not susceptible to the formation of tooth caries (i.e., cavities). In dogs, demineralization of teeth is not common because of the alkaline nature of their saliva. Cats, in comparison, can produce saliva with a more acidic pH, making tooth demineralization possible in this species. Overall, the three primary dental problems that are seen in dogs and cats are oral malodor, gingivitis, and periodontal disease. Odontoclastic resorptive lesions in cats also have been associated with gingival inflammation and, possibly, periodontal disease.[460,461]

Periodontal disease is one of the most common diseases observed by small-animal practitioners, and it is the most prevalent type of oral disorder. It has been reported in domestic pets for at least 70 years and is currently considered a worldwide problem.[462] For example, gingival inflammation and heavy calculus deposits were found in 95% of research colony dogs, 2 years old or older, in a study conducted more than 30 years ago.[463] Another early study reported moderate to severe periodontal disease in 75% of necropsied pet dogs that were between 4 and 8 years of age.[464] More recently, a study of 63 pet dogs aged 1 year or older reported that almost all of the dogs had gingivitis, and 53% had evidence of periodontitis.[465]

Periodontal disease in dogs is strongly associated with increasing age and appears to be most prevalent in small and toy breeds.[462,466] It is thought that the drastically reduced jaw size and crowding of teeth of small dogs may be predisposing factors. The progressive nature of periodontal disease and the likelihood that supragingival changes may go unnoticed by owners until there is significant damage to the periodontium explain the increased incidence in older animals.

Although there are relatively little epidemiological data relating to cats, it is speculated that the incidence of gingivitis and periodontal disease is similar in cats and dogs. A study conducted with cats in England found evidence of periodontal disease in 60% of cats older than 3 years.[456] Odontoclastic resorptive lesions are also a commonly diagnosed dental disorder of cats. A recent study of 145 adult cats found evidence of these lesions in 48% of the animals studied.[467] Other groups have found incidence values between 23% and 67%.[467,468]

Oral Malodor

Oral malodor (halitosis) is commonly reported in pets and is perceived by many owners to be a significant problem.[469] Moreover, malodor is considered to be a precursor or manifestation of more serious dental disease and may be the first clinical sign that owners report to their veterinarians. As in humans, oral malodor in dogs and cats can be caused by oral or non-oral factors. Non-oral etiologies include gastrointestinal, lung, and systemic disease.

In the majority of cases, the predominant source of halitosis is within the oral cavity. Microbial metabolism of protein-containing substances such as food debris, exfoliated epithelium, saliva, and blood result in the production of volatile sulfur compounds (VSCs).[470,471] These compounds, particularly mercaptyl sulfide and hydrogen sulfide, produce breath malodor when exhaled.[472,473] In addition to the microbial flora in the mouth, two other factors that influence the production of malodor are saliva pH and glucose concentration. Specifically, saliva with a low pH and relatively high glucose concentration suppresses odor formation, while the production of saliva with an alkaline pH and low glucose concentration is associated with increased production of odor.[474,475]

Breath malodor is associated with gingivitis and periodontitis. A recent study with dogs demonstrated significant correlations between the production of VSCs in the mouth, the amount of plaque and calculus accumulation on the tooth surface, and the severity of gingivitis.[476] Another study found that dogs with a high degree of oral malodor were more likely to have moderate to severe periodontal disease when compared with dogs with less malodor.[477] This association is further demonstrated by evidence that veterinary periodontal therapy causes a significant reduction in previously established oral malodor.[478] One explanation for this is that chronic inflammation and tissue damage provides increased protein substrate for microorganisms in the mouth, enhancing the production of VSCs.[479] The heavier plaque that occurs with dental disease may also provide a favorable anaerobic environment and additional substrate for the formation of VSCs.[480] The VSCs may also have detrimental effects on the structural integrity of epithelial tissue in the mouth, further contributing to the pathogenesis and progression of periodontal disease.[481]

Gingivitis and Periodontal Disease

Gingivitis is a nonspecific term referring to inflammation of the gingivae (gums). Periodontal disease is a plaque-induced, progressive inflammatory disease affecting the gingiva, periodontal ligaments (connective tissue between the tooth root and socket), and alveolar bone.[464]

The presence and proliferation of certain species of anaerobic bacteria and the inflammatory responses of the host contribute to the progressive destruction of the periodontium.[462] As the supporting connective tissues and adjacent bone are weakened, teeth become loose and may be lost. Periodontal disease itself causes discomfort and pain and, if left untreated, can lead to bacteremia. In a study of 39 dogs with periodontal disease, 15% had bacteremia on presentation.[482] This increased to 67% after veterinary dental manipulation. Cats with periodontitis are similarly susceptible to bacteremia.[483] As stated previously, the bacteremia associated with periodontal disease is thought to be a risk factor for kidney disease, bacterial endocarditis, and pulmonary disease, especially in older animals.[484,485,486]

Initial stages of gingivitis are caused by the persistence of dental plaque and calculus. When a clean tooth surface is exposed to saliva, a pellicle, composed of a thin layer of glycoprotein, forms within minutes. Plaque-forming bacteria, which are part of the normal oral flora, adhere to the pellicle and proliferate. Within 24 hours, a smooth layer of plaque covers the entire tooth surface. Plaque is a soft, gelatinous material composed of bacteria and their metabolic byproducts, oral debris, and salivary components. Mature plaque is not removed by normal actions of the tongue or by rinsing of the mouth. Rather, mechanical abrasion from chewing or tooth brushing is necessary for plaque removal.

Left undisturbed, aerobic and facultative anaerobic bacteria proliferate as the plaque thickens and matures. Over time, salivary calcium salts are deposited on the plaque, producing calculus. Calculus is a hard deposit that provides a rough surface, promoting accumulation of more plaque and also contributing to tissue damage as it extends into the gingival sulcus. Gingivitis occurs when plaque and calculus form at the neck of the tooth, leading to inflammation and tissue damage. As the gingival sulcus enlarges into a periodontal pocket, the area provides an oxygen-depleted environment that allows proliferation of anaerobic bacteria. Periodontal disease becomes established when the periodontal ligament is exposed to plaque, bacteria, and bacterial byproducts.

In some animals, gingivitis persists without progressing into periodontitis. However, in most, untreated gingivitis eventually progresses to periodontal disease. Clinical signs of gingivitis and periodontal disease include oral malodor, gingival sensitivity and bleeding, tooth loss, and difficulty eating.

Feline Odontoclastic Resorptive Lesions

Although rare in dogs, odontoclastic resorptive lesions are one of the most common dental problems reported in the domestic cat.[468,487] These lesions are commonly referred to as neck lesions or cervical line lesions because the dental defect is often found at the neck area of the tooth. They are characterized by odontoclastic resorption of the tooth's enamel, dentin, or cementum.[488]

Mandibular premolars and molars are the most frequently affected teeth, although canine teeth and incisors may also develop these lesions. As with periodontal disease, the incidence of resorptive lesions is strongly correlated with increasing age. Although the underlying etiology of odontoclastic lesions in cats is not known, it is clear that these lesions are not dental caries. It is theorized that they may develop in response to localized inflammatory responses associated with gingivitis and periodontal disease.[489] For this reason odontoclastic resorptive lesions are usually classified as a form of periodontal disease in the cat.[490]

Because resorptive lesions are very painful to the cat, difficulties in eating and refusal to eat are often the first signs reported by owners. Other signs include oral malodor, gingivitis, and excessive salivation. Gingival inflammation and proliferation are commonly observed in cats with dental lesions, but it is not known if this is a result of the resorptive lesion or an underlying cause. The inflammation associated with odontoclastic lesions may provide a favorable environment for plaque formation and bacterial proliferation, which lead to gingivitis and possible periodontitis. Alternatively, resorptive lesions may develop in response to the localized and chronic inflammation of gingivae that is associated with periodontal disease. It is known that activity of odontoclasts, the cells responsible for demineralization, is stimulated by chronic inflammation.[491] Moreover, bacterial populations associated with chronic inflammatory disease in the cat's mouth may provide the acidic microenvironment necessary for the tooth decalcification that occurs with resorptive lesions.[492]

Initial physical evaluation of a cat's mouth may not reveal damage to the tooth because of the progressive nature of the disorder. Over time, there is eventual loss of the tooth crown and root. Diagnosis usually requires dental examination and radiographs.[493] Feline resorptive lesions are typically categorized into four stages, with treatment and management procedures dependent upon the stage of the disease at the time of diagnosis.[494,495] While dental prophylaxis and application of a fluoride cavity varnish may stop or slow progression of the early stages, extraction of the tooth is usually necessary in more advanced stages of the disease.

ROLE OF DIET IN THE DEVELOPMENT OF DENTAL DISEASE

The most important factor that influences the development of gingivitis and periodontal disease in dogs and cats is the presence and persistence of undisturbed plaque on tooth surfaces. Therefore management and feeding practices that minimize plaque and calculus formation or aid in their removal are important in the prevention of periodontal disease. Factors that are important include the frequency of tooth brushing, the type of diet that is fed, whether or not table scraps or noncommercial foods are fed, and the frequency of access to chew toys, rawhide chews, and biscuits.

Once plaque has been deposited on the surface of the tooth, it must be removed mechanically through abrasion provided by diet, tooth brushing, or chewing on supplemental chew toys or foods. Use of the antimicrobial agent chlorhexidine digluconate is effective for the reduction of breath malodor, plaque accumulation, and gingivitis in dogs.[496,497] However, the success of chlorhexidine and other agents is greatly enhanced when they are used in conjunction with brushing, and the use of a chemical mouthwash alone is not effective in removing the hardened calculus that forms when plaque is allowed to accumulate. For this reason, an approach that provides frequent and consistent mechanical removal of plaque and calculus is desirable (see pp. 486-488).

Hard vs. Soft Diet

The type of diet that is fed has been implicated as a potential risk factor for the development of dental disease in dogs and cats. Early studies reported that dogs fed a soft diet developed clinical and histological signs of periodontal disease earlier in life than those fed a dry diet.[498,499] The severity of disease in dogs fed a soft diet was also greater than that observed in dogs fed a dry biscuit diet. In another study, dogs fed a diet that required mastication did not develop gingivitis during the 1-month trial period.[500] In contrast, dogs fed the same diet in a minced, soft form developed gingivitis and had signs associated with developing periodontal disease.

Recently, survey studies have been used to identify dietary risk factors associated with periodontal disease in dogs. Data from a group of 63 pet dogs in the United States showed that gingivitis and calculus were less common in dogs fed dry dog food as the major portion of their diet, compared with those fed canned food.[465] However, indicators of tooth mobility, tooth loss, and periodontal disease did not differ significantly with the type of diet fed. Another study conducted by the Japanese Small Animal Veterinary Association collected data from more than 2600 dogs.[501] Analysis showed that dental calculus was found in 34% of dogs fed primarily dry food and 42% of dogs fed primarily canned or home-cooked food. Results from both of these studies indicate that while feeding a dry-type dog food may help decrease the severity or slow the progression of dental disease, dogs still accumulate plaque and develop gingivitis and periodontal disease when fed a dry diet.

A similar relationship between wet and dry diet and the development of dental disease has been reported in cats.[502] The gingivae of growing kittens fed a dry cat food remained healthy, showing little inflammation or accumulation of calculus. In contrast, a group of kittens fed a canned food for the same period developed oral malodor, gingivitis, and calculus. Another study reported that cats had greater plaque accumulation when fed a canned diet, compared with the accumulation in cats fed a dry commercial food for a period of only 2 weeks.[503] The Japanese survey discussed previously also included 745 cats. As with dogs, dental calculus was significantly less common when dry food was fed. It was concluded that feeding dry food is less likely to be associated with calculus formation than feeding a canned or homemade diet.

Current indications are that soft foods such as canned commercial diets or home-prepared foods are less effective than hard, dry foods in providing the abrasion needed to remove plaque that normally forms on teeth. However, it is important to realize that dry pet foods do not effectively prevent the development of gingivitis and periodontal disease, since in most studies a substantial proportion of animals fed dry diets still developed signs associated with progressive dental disease.

Opportunities for Chewing

It appears that the dental benefits afforded by feeding a dry pet food are directly associated with opportunity and frequency of chewing. A study of 1350 dogs in North America examined the relationship between the occurrence and severity of calculus and periodontal disease and the type of diet and chew toys that dogs received.[504] A significant linear relationship was found between decreasing calculus score and access to an increasing number of chewing materials. Although less significant, this trend was also observed for gingivitis.

When the type of food alone was considered, there was no significant association between feeding a diet made up exclusively of dry pet food and the degree of calculus, gingivitis, or tooth attachment loss. However, in dogs that were fed dry food, access to rawhide chews and other types of chewing materials was significantly associated with a reduced accumulation of calculus and less gingival inflammation and attachment loss. Rawhide chew materials were the most effective in preventing dental disease, followed by various types of hard bones. In this study, feeding hard biscuits as a supplement to the dry diet did not provide any additional dental benefit. In contrast, dogs that were not exclusively fed dry food obtained little or no dental benefit from additional chew materials. The authors concluded that there was a consistent (if not always significant) trend towards a widespread protective effect of access to supplemental chewing materials in dogs that were fed dry pet food, compared with dogs fed primarily soft food or a mixture of food types.

Another study with 67 dogs showed similar results.[505] Providing dogs with rawhide chews as a supplement to their normal dry diet led to significant removal of preexisting supragingival calculus over a period of 3 weeks. Providing cereal biscuits instead of rawhide was somewhat helpful, but less so than providing rawhide.

Two recent studies examined the dental effects of feeding a rawhide chew that was formulated to promote dental hygiene.[506,507] In the first study, dogs were fed a dry maintenance diet and provided with tooth brushing every other day.[506] Half of the dogs also received one rawhide chew once a day. Dental health was assessed over a period of 3 weeks. While plaque accumulation and gingivitis occurred in all of the dogs, significantly less gingivitis developed when the chew was added to the regimen. After the study period, deposits of calculus and stain were greater with tooth brushing only, compared with that when the teeth were brushed and the chew was provided. In the second study, the effects of the chew on dental health were measured in the absence of regular tooth brushing.[507] Similar results were reported. While gingivitis developed in both groups of dogs, the daily provision of chewing materials significantly decreased the severity. These results indicate that chewing materials are helpful in reducing the degree of gingivitis through direct mechanical cleaning of the tooth surfaces. However, because dogs given the dental chews still showed some level of plaque accumulation and gingivitis, it appears unlikely that this level of reduction can completely prevent the development of periodontitis.

The variable results associated with specific types of chewing toys and different effects on mandibular and maxillary teeth suggest that owners should provide a variety of different types of chewing materials to their dogs. It appears that a cumulative effect is afforded by feeding a dry food and providing additional and varied chew toys. This may occur because dogs fed a dry pet food have at least one and possibly two or more opportunities for extended chewing each day. It is possible that the additive effect of consuming a dry diet plus having frequent access to chew toys surpasses a relative "chewing threshold" that affords some level of protective effect that is not reached when a canned or soft food is fed. It is also possible that dogs fed dry pet foods may by nature or through learning be more frequent or vigorous "chewers". This theory is supported by data from a study showing that dogs given rawhide chews varied significantly in their level of interest and in the speed with which they chewed and consumed the rawhide.[508] Videotaping chewing episodes allowed the authors to divide dogs into categories of slow and fast chewers. Dogs classified as slow chewers had less calculus accumulation at the end of the 12-month test period when compared with fast chewers, indicating that the amount of time a dog spends chewing each day is an important factor.

While providing chewing materials is beneficial for dental health in dogs, this is generally not an approach that can be used for cats. Although individual cats that enjoy chewing on hard bones or rawhide may exist, most pet cats do not engage in frequent or prolonged bouts of chewing. An examination of the cats' evolutionary history provides a possible explanation for this difference. Unlike dogs, which evolved from a species that hunted large ungulates and spent a great deal of time chewing bones and tough connective tissue, the cat evolved from the small African wild cat (*Felis libyca*), which hunted primarily small rodents, such as mice. The cat's prey was rapidly consumed, with minimal chewing, and numerous mice were caught and eaten each day. As a result, our domestic cat (*Felis catus*) has neither the dentition nor (it appears) the desire to spend large amounts of time chewing on bones or other types of chew toys.

Special Diets and Biscuits

While it is generally accepted that persistence of plaque and subsequent development of gingivitis and periodontal disease are facilitated by feeding soft diets and impeded by hard foods, it is not known to what extent diet can replace or enhance regular prophylactic dental care. In recent years, efforts have been made to formulate biscuits and complete commercial diets that effectively prevent or slow the accumulation of plaque and calculus when fed to dogs. For example, a study with Beagles tested the ability of feeding specially formulated "tartar control" biscuits to reduce plaque formation.[509] When groups of 20 dogs were fed canned food as their primary diet and given either 10 regular dog biscuits, 10 experimental "tartar control" biscuits, or no biscuits each day, dogs fed both biscuit types had less plaque accumulation, but the experimental control biscuits were slightly more effective. However, the implications of these differences are difficult to determine since neither calculus formation nor gingivitis were reported in this study.

Other studies have examined the effect of incorporating the compound sodium hexametaphosphate (HMP) into coatings for snack biscuits.[510,511] Sodium HMP is a chemical sequestrant that forms soluble complexes with several cations, including calcium. It is theorized that when small amounts of HMP are included in food, chewing allows the HMP to adhere to plaque, form soluble complexes with calcium, and then be washed away. Because the inorganic portion of tooth calculus in dogs contains predominantly calcium carbonate and small amounts of calcium phosphate, inclusion of HMP was expected to prevent or decrease calculus formation.[512]

A series of studies compared the dental effects of daily supplementation with HMP-coated biscuits to dogs fed either dry dog food or dry dog food moistened with water.[510,511] After pretreatment with dental prophylaxis (scaling and polishing), dogs were supplemented daily with either conventional biscuits, experimental biscuits coated with HMP, or no biscuits. In both types of feeding regimens (dry and moistened diet), the daily ingestion of HMP-coated biscuits reduced but did not completely prevent the formation of calculus. A more pronounced reduction of calculus occurred in dogs fed the moistened diet than in those fed a dry maintenance diet. Overall, reductions in calculus formation varied between 30% and 63%. However, the degree of gingivitis was not measured, nor was it possible to predict the clinical significance of the reported reductions in calculus. While feeding hard biscuits formulated for calculus control reduced the development of deposits on teeth, it did not completely prevent it. The degree to which the biscuits could slow or prevent the development of gingivitis or periodontal disease was not studied and is not currently known.

In addition to biscuits, some manufacturers have produced pet foods that are promoted as "oral care" diets. The effects of feeding an adult maintenance food that was purportedly formulated to reduce plaque, stain, and calculus formation were compared with the effects of feeding a conventional dry adult maintenance diet.

Dogs were fed each diet for a period of 3 weeks. At the end of the test period, dogs fed the specially formulated diet had 19% less plaque, 44% less stain, and 32% less calculus accumulation.[513] Signs of gingivitis and periodontitis were not reported. A previous study by the same group found that dogs fed the oral care diet developed less oral malodor after a 1-week feeding period.[514] The authors concluded that the type of processing and ingredients used in the test food helped to reduce the accumulation of plaque, stain, and calculus but did not completely prevent their occurrence. However, the clinical significance of these results is not known, because the effect of this level of reduction on the development of gingivitis or periodontal disease has not been studied.

Because of the documented importance of providing chewing materials for promoting dental health, a second study was conducted to compare the aforementioned oral care diet with feeding a conventional dry dog food plus an oral hygiene rawhide chew.[515] Plaque and calculus formation and development of gingivitis were studied over a 3-week test period. Results showed that plaque, calculus, and gingivitis increased similarly in all of the dogs, regardless of feeding regimen. Because a control group of dogs was not included in this study, no comparison could be made between dental changes in dogs fed these two regimens and dogs fed only a conventional maintenance diet. An additional finding was that dogs fed the oral care diet lost significant amounts of body weight during the treatment period. This effect was associated with poor acceptance of the diet and a failure to eat the entire ration each day. As in the previous study, these data showed that neither regimen effectively maintained clinically healthy gingivae over a 3-week period, again suggesting that dietary approaches to oral hygiene, while helpful, cannot replace other methods of dental care such as tooth brushing and veterinary dental prophylaxis.

Overall, there are limited data available on the efficacy of feeding commercial dog foods that are specifically formulated for dental health. One group of investigators identified several dietary factors that may be important influences on dental health.[513] These included the size, shape, and density of the food's pieces; the diet's moisture level; and the inclusion of certain ingredients.[513] However, none of these factors has been studied in controlled experiments. Moreover, neither the nutrient composition nor the processing method of the diets and chews that have been studied have been described in published studies. These limitations should be taken into consideration when evaluating the true efficacy of specially formulated diets or making recommendations regarding diet components that might affect dental health. At this time, available research indicates that simply feeding a dry pet food of any type cannot replace other forms of prophylactic dental care in dogs and cats.

Diet and Feline Odontoclastic Resorptive Lesions

Although limited data are available, there is some evidence that an association exists between dental resorptive lesions and certain aspects of a cat's diet. A recent study examined risk factors for the development of odontoclastic lesions in 145 adult cats.[467] The two most important factors associated with resorptive lesions were increasing age and feeding a diet that contained low levels of magnesium. In addition, cats that had their teeth cleaned at least twice a week and were fed diets containing higher levels of magnesium, calcium, phosphorus, and potassium were less likely to develop oral lesions. Contrary to common belief, neither the type of diet fed (soft vs. hard) nor the number of feedings provided per day was associated with the development of dental lesions. Although limited data are available, a positive association has been reported between resorptive lesions and feeding noncommercial (homemade) diets, cat treats, table foods, and diets containing low amounts of calcium.[516,517]

The increased use of acid sprays as a coating on dry cat foods has led to speculation that these coatings may reduce the pH of the surface of teeth during chewing and promote an environment favorable for tooth demineralization. A study was conducted to determine whether the pH of a cat food and that of a cat's tooth surfaces after eating are correlated.[492] Cats with resorptive lesions were found to have lower tooth surface pH values than cats without lesions (7.93 vs. 8.65). However, no relationship was found between the pH of the food that was fed and the incidence or severity of dental lesions. Although the surface pH values for the commercial diets studied were all acidic (pH range between 4.9 and 6.3), ingestion caused only a very slight and transient decrease in tooth surface pH.

It appears that a cat's saliva is capable of quickly neutralizing the acidic coating of the food, resulting in only very slight alterations in tooth surface pH. Moreover, even the transient change in tooth surface pH that was observed cannot be considered clinically significant because physiological decalcification of bone and teeth occur only at a pH between 4 and 5.[518,519] Although these data did not provide further clarification of the pathogenesis of resorptive lesions, they do indicate that commercially produced dry foods that have an acid coating do not influence the development of feline neck lesions. The authors agreed with other researchers that neck lesions are probably of multifactorial origin, with chronic gingivitis and periodontitis playing a significant role. While some studies have shown certain dietary components to increase a cat's risk of developing odontoclastic lesions, more data and the completion of controlled studies are necessary before recommendations can be made regarding dietary approaches for the prevention of these lesions.

PREVENTION OF DENTAL DISEASE AND MAINTENANCE CARE

Current evidence supports a supplemental role of diet in the maintenance of dental health. However, simply feeding a dry pet food or a food promoted as an oral care diet cannot replace regular and consistent prophylactic care. The primary approach for preventing the development of gingivitis and periodontal disease includes a program of regular home care, periodic veterinary dental prophylaxis, and provision of carefully chosen and varied types of chewing materials (for dogs). Feeding a dry diet is considered to be adjunctive to these procedures.

Veterinary dental prophylaxis is conducted under general anesthesia and includes supragingival and subgingival scaling and polishing.[520] The scaling removes calculus and plaque that has formed above and below the gingival interface, and polishing removes micropitting on the tooth that provides a favorable surface for plaque deposition. The frequency of treatment depends upon the pet's rate of plaque accumulation, the degree of established gingivitis or periodontal disease, and the pet's age. Because moderate to severe dental disease is most commonly seen in older dogs and cats, the risk of frequent anesthesia administration must always be considered.[521] Generally, veterinary dental cleaning every 12 to 18 months is recommended for pets with healthy gingiva. Pets with chronic gingivitis or periodontitis will benefit from more frequent cleaning, usually every 6 to 12 months.[520] It is important for pet owners to be informed that when established dental disease is present, frequent veterinary cleaning is still necessary even in the face of optimal home care. Although daily tooth brushing can effectively remove plaque, it cannot affect the degree of subgingival disease and may even mask the progression of disease below the gingival surface.[522] Therefore regular and continued professional therapy is essential for dogs and cats diagnosed with periodontal disease.

The most effective method of home dental care is regular tooth brushing. Brushing prevents plaque accumulation and the development of gingivitis.[523] Current evidence shows that the frequency of brushing necessary to maintain clinically healthy gingivae depends on the initial condition of the tissue. For example, in studies of dogs with established gingivitis, brushing daily was effective in returning the gums to health, but brushing three times per week was not sufficient.[523,524,525] Conversely, brushing three times per week can successfully maintain dental health in dogs with no signs of gingivitis or periodontal disease.[523,526] As discussed previously, providing various types of chew materials such as rawhides, dental devices, and, possibly, some types of hard biscuits can augment, but not replace, the effectiveness of brushing.

Dental care products that contain chlorhexidine gluconate or chlorhexidine acetate have been shown to effectively reduce breath malodor and plaque formation in dogs.[496,514, 527,528] In addition, long-term use of chlorhexidine can effectively reduce gingivitis and slow the progression of periodontal disease.[527] Although several other antimicrobial agents are available, chlorhexidine is reported to be the most effective agent for long-term dental care in pets.[497,529] Its effectiveness is maximized when it is applied once or twice a day as a tooth-brushing solution, as this allows mechanical removal of plaque. However, studies with dogs have also shown that applying a chlorhexidine-containing spray or gel prevents plaque accumulation, improves breath, and helps prevent gingivitis and periodontal disease, even when not accompanied by brushing.[530] This is a distinct advantage for pet owners whose dog or cat will not tolerate frequent sessions of tooth brushing. The only reported side effects of chlorhexidine-containing dental products are an unpleasant taste and brown staining of the teeth in some animals. The staining occurs after long-term use and, though it may be aesthetically displeasing to some owners, is not harmful or pathogenic.

BOX 36-1

Practical Tips: Long-Term Preventive Dental Care of Pets

Regular veterinary dental examinations and prophylaxis (scaling and polishing) should be scheduled.

Home dental care should include regular tooth brushing (minimum of one to three times per week).

A pet dental solution or toothpaste containing chlorhexidine (or another antimicrobial agent) should be applied topically or used during tooth brushing.

Hard biscuits and chewing materials such as hard bones, rawhides, and rope toys should be provided to pets who enjoy them.

A dry pet food should be fed as the dog's or cat's primary diet.

Regardless of the type of dental agent used, all pet owners should receive instructions on home dental care and should be strongly encouraged to maintain a consistent preventive program throughout a pet's life. Although meticulous home care does not preclude the need for regular professional prophylaxis, it can reduce the accumulation of plaque, the deposition of calculus, and the development of gingivitis. This may effectively prevent periodontitis and allows a reduced frequency of veterinary dental prophylaxis. Additional care involves providing a variety of chew toys and products for dogs and feeding a dry diet. Diets consisting primarily of soft foods with no opportunities for chewing hard kibble or biscuits should be avoided unless another health condition requires their use or the pet will not accept a dry pet food. If a soft or canned food provides the primary basis of a pet's diet, frequent tooth brushing, the provision of chewing items, and veterinary prophylaxis are doubly important (Box 36-1).

C H A P T E R

37

Nutritional Management
of Gastrointestinal Disease

Gastrointestinal disease in dogs and cats is composed of a group of disorders with varying and often unrelated underlying causes. Regardless of the cause, most intestinal disorders manifest as acute or chronic diarrhea and, in some cases, vomiting or anorexia. Nutritional support is an important component of treatment because of the gastrointestinal tract's essential role in nutrient digestion and absorption. A primary goal of dietary therapy is to maintain delivery of nutrients and prevent nutrient deficiencies and malnutrition. In addition, long-term dietary management can help to repair the damaged intestinal lining, restore normal populations of intestinal microflora, promote normal gastrointestinal motility and function, and reduce gastrointestinal inflammation.[531,532] While dietary management will not always cure the underlying disease, it can have a profound influence on the ability of the intestine to recover and is an important component of veterinary treatment for the control of many types of intestinal disease.

NUTRITION-RESPONSIVE GASTROINTESTINAL DISEASES

Intestinal disorders in companion animals that have been shown to be responsive to dietary management include small intestinal bacterial overgrowth (SIBO), pathogen overgrowth, pancreatic disease, several types of inflammatory disorders, and nonspecific acute diarrhea.

Small Intestinal Bacterial Overgrowth

SIBO occurs when there are quantitative and qualitative changes to bacterial populations in the lumen of the proximal part of the small intestine.[533] While some dogs with SIBO do not have clinical signs, most develop chronic episodes of intermittent diarrhea that may be accompanied by vomiting or anorexia. A number of factors may lead to bacterial overgrowth or changes in intestinal bacterial populations. These include impaired gut motility, prolonged or excessive use of oral antibiotics, exocrine pancreatic insufficiency, and achlorhydria. A genetic predilection may occur in some breeds. German Shepherds have been reported to have an unusually high incidence of SIBO, and this has been associated with a breed-specific deficiency of secretory immunoglobulin A.[534] SIBO may also develop as a sequela to other forms of intestinal disease such as lymphocytic-plasmacytic enteritis and exocrine pancreatic insufficiency.[534,535]

Diagnosis of SIBO is confirmed through microbiological culture of duodenal fluid obtained endoscopically or during a laparotomy. In addition, elevated serum folate and deconjugated bile acids or reduced serum cobalamin provide indirect evidence for bacterial overgrowth in the proximal small intestine.[536,537] Currently, there is some dispute regarding normal and abnormal numbers of bacteria in the intestines of dogs and cats.[538,539] Traditionally, SIBO has been diagnosed using the same criteria that have been established for humans. In human subjects, SIBO is diagnosed when greater than 10^5 total or 10^4 anaerobic colony-forming units of bacteria per ml (CFU/ml) are cultured from endoscopically obtained duodenal fluid.[540] However, recent studies with dogs and cats have shown that the number of bacteria found in the small intestine of these species varies greatly and can typically be much higher than values reported in humans.[535,538] For this reason, a total bacterial count in excess of 10^7 to 10^8 CFU/ml has recently been suggested as the standard for diagnosis of SIBO in dogs and cats.[538] Even assuming this change in diagnostic criteria, it is still generally accepted that SIBO is an important primary cause of chronic diarrhea in dogs, as well as a concomitant finding in several other forms of intestinal disease.[541]

Qualitative changes in the bacterial flora are as important in SIBO as increased numbers, and these changes should always be assessed. Species of bacteria that typically increase in dogs with SIBO include coliforms, staphylococci, and enterococci, with *Clostridium* and *Bacteroides* species predominating. While clinical SIBO is less common in cats, subclinical cases have been reported based upon earlier diagnostic criteria.[542] The most common species of bacteria found in cats with SIBO were *Bacteroides* species, eubacteria, fusobacteria, and *Pasteurella* species. In addition, the cat appears to be unique in the relatively high number of clostridia found in the intestine, as compared with other carnivorous species.[539]

Pathogen Overgrowth

In all animals, genera and species of intestinal bacteria can be categorized into beneficial and harmful/pathogenic species.[543,544,545] Beneficial bacteria in the intestine have several important functions. Normal populations of these microbes inhibit the proliferation of harmful bacterial species, stimulate immune function, aid in the digestion or absorption of food, and synthesize essential vitamins. These effects are achieved through competition for oxygen, luminal substrates, and living space within intestinal niches.[538] In addition, some indigenous flora produce substances that directly inhibit the growth of other bacterial species. For example, certain species of intestinal microbes produce short-chain fatty acids (SCFAs) during the metabolism of fiber. In turn these SCFAs inhibit the growth of some pathogenic species of bacteria.[546]

Pathogen overgrowth occurs when one or more species of harmful bacteria proliferate. This may manifest as a single problem or can occur as a component of SIBO or another form of intestinal disease. An important intestinal pathogen in companion animals is *Clostridium perfringens*.[545,547] The proliferation of pathogenic species of bacteria cause harm to the host animal by producing toxins, carcinogens, or putrefactive compounds. These compounds may directly affect the intestinal mucosa, cause systemic disease, or inhibit the growth of beneficial bacteria. Signs of pathogen overgrowth include vomiting, diarrhea, weight loss, and, in some cases, systemic illness caused by the production of toxins.

Exocrine Pancreatic Insufficiency

Exocrine pancreatic insufficiency (EPI) is a well-defined gastrointestinal disorder in dogs and cats. The reduction or loss of pancreatic enzymes impairs nutrient digestion and absorption and negatively affects functioning of the small intestine.[548,549,550] EPI is reported to be the most common cause of fat malabsorption in dogs.[551] Although EPI has been less frequently reported in cats, recent evidence indicates that it is more common in this species than was previously believed.[552] The most common underlying cause of EPI in dogs is idiopathic pancreatic acinar atrophy, followed by pancreatic hypoplasia and chronic pancreatitis.[553,554] In contrast, chronic pancreatitis is the most common cause of EPI in cats.[555] Other causes in cats include adenocarcinoma and infection with the pancreatic parasite *Eurytrema procynosis*.[555,556]

Because the exocrine pancreas has a significant functional reserve, deficiencies of the proteolytic enzymes alpha-amylase and lipase result only after 85% to 90% of pancreatic tissue is lost. When this threshold is reached, severe impairment of nutrient digestion and absorption leads to malabsorption. Other intestinal effects include a decrease in protein synthesis within enterocytes, malabsorption of some vitamins, and development of SIBO or pathogen overgrowth. Recent studies indicate that SIBO is found in more than 70% of dogs with a diagnosis of EPI.[557]

Clinical signs of EPI include loose or semiformed voluminous stools or diarrhea, weight loss, and (in dogs) polyphagia. The diarrhea caused by EPI is typically osmotic due to the passage of malabsorbed dietary components along the intestinal tract. However, secretory diarrhea of the lower small intestine and colon may also be present, resulting from bacterial deconjugation of bile acids and the metabolism of unabsorbed fat to hydroxy fatty acids.[558,559] While clinical signs and history are helpful in diagnosing EPI, definitive diagnosis is made using results of the serum trypsin–like immunoreactivity assay.[560,561]

Inflammatory Bowel Disorders

Inflammatory diseases of the intestine are generally categorized according to the type of inflammatory cell that predominates in the intestinal mucosa, the area of the intestine affected, or the underlying cause, if known. *Colitis* is a general term for a condition that describes irritation or inflammation of the large intestine, and it is considered the most frequently diagnosed disorder of the large intestine in dogs and cats.[562] Colitis is classified into several forms, which include lymphocytic-plasmacytic, eosinophilic, histocytic, and granulomatous. Lymphocytic-plasmacytic enterocolitis is the most common form of inflammatory bowel disorder (IBD) in dogs.[563] Boxers and German Shepherds are at increased risk, while Basenjis are susceptible to a specific form of disease called immunoproliferative enteropathy.[563,564,565] Several forms of IBD also occur in the domestic cat, including lymphocytic-plasmacytic enteritis and eosinophilic enteritis.[566,567,568] No breed-specific predilections have been reported in cats.

Clinical signs of colitis are caused by dysfunction of the large intestine and include increased defecation frequency, tenesmus, and production of bloody or mucoid diarrhea. When IBD affects the small intestine, signs include production of large quantities of soft, bulky stools or diarrhea, with occasional steatorrhea. Contrary to large intestinal disease, weight loss and vomiting are common with small intestinal IBD. It is currently believed that IBD is a multifactorial disorder. Predisposing factors include genetics, exposure to luminal antigens and loss of immune tolerance, compromised colonocyte health, increased mucosal permeability, and impairment or insufficiency of the intestine's normal protective mechanisms.[569,570] Infection with an intestinal parasite or bacterial pathogen, bacterial overgrowth, or presence of a food antigen may all trigger an initial inflammatory response, which can persist even after the initial cause has been resolved.[571,572] Once an immune response has been initiated in the small or large intestine, production of inflammatory eicosanoids and tissue ischemia may perpetuate the inflammatory response, resulting in a cycle of chronic illness.

Treatment of IBD is directed toward eliminating the underlying cause (if one can be found), reducing inflammation, and achieving long-term remission. Traditional therapy has involved the extended use of antiinflammatory drugs such as sulfasalazine or prednisolone. However, these drugs are associated with undesirable and deleterious health effects when used for long periods.[573,574] In recent years, new regimens have been developed that focus on dietary management.[531,562] While drug therapy is still often used in the initial treatment phase to reduce inflammation and allow healing of the intestinal tract, dietary management can often maintain remission and prevent relapse. Drug therapy is then only reinstated if clinical signs return.

Nonspecific Acute Diarrhea

Nonspecific acute diarrhea refers to short episodes of diarrhea for which a cause cannot be found. In most cases, the pet remains active, there is no evidence of systemic disease, and the clinical signs are self-limiting. In dogs, this condition is commonly caused by consuming garbage, animal feces, or carrion. Overeating or a sudden change in the type or brand of food that is fed can cause acute diarrhea in both dogs and cats. Feeding a poorly formulated or inadequately prepared homemade diet or excessive amounts of table scraps can also lead to small or large intestinal diarrhea. In these cases, the diarrhea can be treated symptomatically until the animal recovers or an underlying cause can be found and treated.

INITIAL MANAGEMENT OF INTESTINAL DISEASE: FASTING VS. FEEDING

Traditionally, acute gastrointestinal disease has been nutritionally managed by instituting short-term fasting or severely reduced food intake with the intent of providing "gut rest." This approach is based upon the belief that slowing gastrointestinal tract function by withholding food allows normal gastric and peristaltic contractions to subside and promotes healing of the intestinal lining.[531] According to this approach, after a fasting period of 12 to 48 hours, a bland diet consisting of highly digestible ingredients should be fed for several days.

In recent years, the approach of fasting followed by refeeding with a bland diet has been questioned, specifically because this approach appears to be based more on convention than on evidence of efficacy.[532] Moreover, while use of the term *bland* to describe the refeeding diet enjoys ubiquitous usage, the definition of this term and the specific diet characteristics are vague and poorly defined. While a short-term fasting period to allow gut rest may be helpful in the initial treatment stage of some intestinal disorders, recent studies of intestinal disease in dogs and cats have indicated that the type of diet is very important and that diet characteristics other than "blandness" must be considered.

DIET COMPOSITION

A diet used to manage gastrointestinal disease should be selected in accordance with the specific disease being treated, the area of the gastrointestinal tract affected, and the ability of the diet to promote healing and maintain remission. Specific diet characteristics that should be considered include protein and carbohydrate sources, level and type of fat, level and type of dietary fiber, and diet digestibility.

Protein Source

Diseases that affect the small intestine, such as EPI and SIBO, can impair protein digestion and absorption. Prolonged malabsorption of dietary protein can lead to protein malnutrition, which further exacerbates existing intestinal disease through impairment of mucosal cell protein synthesis and turnover and local immune function.[575] Most seriously, a syndrome called *protein-losing enteropathy* (PLE) occurs when there is rapid and severe loss of protein from the small intestine.[534] Although

PLE is most commonly associated with idiopathic lymphangiectasia, it is believed to represent the end stage of several intestinal disorders.[576] Therefore the diet should provide a protein source that is easily digested and assimilated and contains all of the essential amino acids in their correct proportions to minimize the risk of protein malnutrition.

Any dietary protein that is not completely digested and assimilated in the small intestine travels to the large intestine, where it can be metabolized by gut microbes, causing changes in gut microflora and producing excessive amounts of ammonia and gas.[577] This can lead to large intestinal diarrhea, further exacerbating intestinal disease. In at least some pets, the development of colitis appears to be an immune-mediated response to food antigens that gain access to the colonic lamina propria and submucosa.[577,578] Once an immune response is triggered, the continuous exposure of the local immune system of the large intestine to an offending antigen results in persistent inflammation and disruption of intestinal function.

Proteins included in diets for dogs and cats with intestinal disease should be highly digestible. When hypersensitivity is suspected, a single-source protein should be fed, preferably one to which the dog or cat has not previously been exposed. Highly digestible protein sources have reduced antigenicity because less intact dietary protein is absorbed into the mucosa of the small intestine and less arrives intact or partially digested in the large intestine. Providing a single protein source also minimizes the chance of feeding a protein to which the pet has been previously sensitized. Because of a possible connection between food antigens and colitis, some authors have recommend feeding an elimination diet to treat colitis and other forms of inflammatory intestinal disease.[531,562] Elimination diets and their use in the diagnosis and management of dietary hypersensitivity are described in detail in Chapter 33 (see pp. 446-450).

Several studies of dogs and cats with colitis have shown positive results when the animals are fed an elimination diet containing a single, novel protein source.[570,579,580] Although response rates vary among studies, between 30% and 85% of dogs with idiopathic colitis respond favorably to this type of regimen. Differences in response rates may reflect variations in the diets used with respect to protein source and digestibility. Animals that did not respond with complete remission to a novel protein source often showed some degree of improvement and required lower levels of antiinflammatory medications to achieve and maintain remission.[579] A number of suitable commercially prepared veterinary diets are available. Most are formulated to provide complete and balanced nutrition and include single-source, highly digestible protein. Examples of potentially acceptable protein sources include rabbit, duck, lamb, venison, and fish.[562]

It has recently been suggested that animals with IBD are at increased risk of immunological sensitization to food proteins during the initial phase of treatment.[577] Chronic inflammation of the intestinal mucosa can lead to impaired protein digestion and damage to the intestinal lining. As a result, intact food proteins may have a greater chance of gaining access to the lamina propria and stimulating an immune response during periods of active disease.[562,577] Therefore the novel protein that is fed during the initial phase of therapy may have only short-term benefit. This theory has led to the concept of using an initial "sacrificial protein source" for the first 4 to 6 weeks of diet therapy.[577] The protein source is then changed again to a second novel and highly available source. The intent of this procedure is to introduce the second protein only after mucosal inflammation and permeability has decreased, thus minimizing the risk of the second protein resulting in hypersensitivity. Although this theory requires further investigation and substantiation, the need to change protein sources after an initial phase of treatment should be considered when selecting a diet for the management of dogs and cats with certain types of IBD.[501]

Carbohydrate

Similar to protein, a single carbohydrate source that can be easily digested and assimilated should be included in the diets of pets with gastrointestinal disease. Because gluten-induced enteropathy is the cause of intestinal disease in some dogs, particularly Irish Setters, it is prudent to include only gluten-free carbohydrates in diets formulated for intestinal disease.[584,585] Rice is ideal for most pets because cooked and blended white rice is highly digestible, does not contain gluten, and has low antigenicity in dogs and cats.[577,582,583] In contrast, wheat, oats, and barley contain gluten and so should be avoided. Other gluten-free carbohydrate sources include potato, tapioca, and corn. Potato and tapioca starches are less digestible than rice, while corn may be contraindicated in dogs with hypersensitivity to this ingredient.[309]

Level and Type of Fat

Dogs and cats with gastrointestinal disease should be fed a reduced-fat diet. High fat intake is specifically contraindicated in animals with EPI, postacute pancreatitis, and lymphangiectasia because these diseases all involve severe impairment of fat digestion and assimilation. A low-fat diet is also indicated whenever there is SIBO or reduced surface area in the small intestine. Malabsorption of dietary fat allows bacterial metabolism of unabsorbed fat to hydroxy fatty acids, while bacterial overgrowth contributes to deconjugation of bile salts, both of which stimulate secretory diarrhea in the distal small intestine and colon.[558] Although it has been suggested that cats with small bowel diarrhea tolerate high-fat diets better than dogs do, there are no published data that support this claim.[531,586] A general recommendation is to select a diet that contains 11% or 15% or less total fat (on a dry-matter basis [DMB]) for dogs and cats, respectively, with gastrointestinal disease.[587]

The recently documented antiinflammatory benefits of omega-3 fatty acids suggest that there may be a role for this class of fatty acids in the management of inflammatory intestinal disease. In addition to demonstrated benefits for pets with inflammatory skin disease (see pp. 438-439), there is also evidence that altering the omega-6:omega-3 fatty acid ratio to favor production of omega-3 metabolites alters eicosanoid profiles in the intestinal mucosa (Figures 37-1 and 37-2).[587] When dogs were fed diets containing omega fatty acid ratios of 10:1 and 5:1, intestinal and colonic mucosa eicosapentaenoic acid (EPA) (20:5n-3) and docosapentaenoic acid

FIGURE **37-1**

Effect of dietary omega-6:omega-3 fatty acid ratio on 12-week EPA concentrations in canine intestinal mucosa.

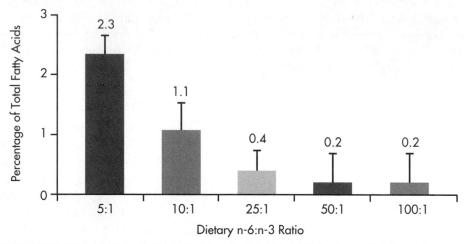

(From World Small Animal Veterinary Association: *Gastrointestinal Health Symposium*, Dayton, Ohio, 1997, The Iams Company. Used with permission.)

FIGURE **37-2**

Effect of dietary omega-6:omega-3 fatty acid ratio on 12-week EPA concentrations in canine colonic mucosa.

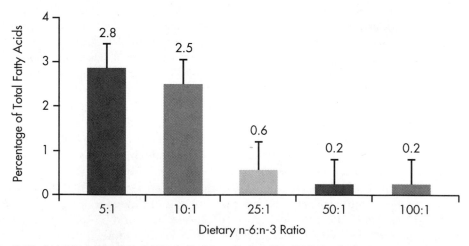

(From World Small Animal Veterinary Association: *Gastrointestinal Health Symposium*, Dayton, Ohio, 1997, The Iams Company. Used with permission.)

(22:6n-3) concentrations increased and arachidonic acid levels decreased over an 8-week period.[304,587] Regional differences were seen, with small-intestinal mucosa having a greater concentration of stearic acid (18:0) and linoleic acid (18:2n-6) than colonic mucosa and colonic mucosa having greater concentrations of eicosatrienoic (20:3n-3) and arachidonic (20:4n-6) acids.

Recent studies with humans and laboratory animals have indicated that increasing dietary omega-3 fatty acids in the diet significantly affects clinical disease.[588,589,590] When the diets of human patients with ulcerative colitis were supplemented with fish oil, they showed a 56% reduction in colitis symptoms and a 30% reduction in colonic leukotriene B_4 (LTB_4) production.[591] Another study revealed that inclusion of fish oil in the diet of patients with IBD resulted in increased concentrations of EPA and docosahexaenoic acid (DHA) and decreased arachidonic acid in intestinal mucosa lipid membranes.[592] Similarly, when human subjects consumed a fish oil supplement containing 3.2 grams (g) of EPA and 2.1 g of docosapentaenoic acid per day, significant changes occurred in intestinal eicosanoids, and improvements in histological findings and body weight were reported.[593] Of particular interest in this study was the finding that the degree of reduction of intestinal LTB_4 was similar in magnitude to that observed in patients treated with prednisolone. This effect allowed a reduction in drug dosages in patients who were receiving the fish oil supplement.

While canine colonic lipid and eicosanoid production are demonstrably altered by increasing the proportion of dietary omega-3 fatty acids, the efficacy of this class of fatty acids in the treatment of intestinal disease has not been well studied in dogs or cats. However, positive results in humans and rats, as well as the responses of canine intestinal mucosa to dietary omega-3 fatty acids, support the use of diets containing optimized omega-6 to omega-3 fatty acid ratios as an aid in managing the inflammation associated with intestinal disease. Clinical studies of dogs and cats with naturally occurring intestinal disease are necessary to further define the role of omega-3 fatty acids in the management of these disorders.

Fiber

Dietary fiber is composed of a group of structural carbohydrates and lignin that are resistant to digestion by mammalian enzymes. The major components of fiber include cellulose, hemicellulose, lignin, pectin, gums, and mucilages. Additionally, unique substances such as fructooligosaccharides (FOS) are classified as fiber because they behave similarly in the gastrointestinal tract (i.e., are not digested by mammalian enzymes). FOSs are found in a variety of fruits, vegetables, and grains. They are also produced commercially through fermentation by *Aspergillus niger* (Figure 37-3).[594]

The benefits of dietary fiber for gastrointestinal health and in the treatment and management of gastrointestinal disease in dogs and cats are now well recognized. In the past, the perceived benefits of fiber were limited to its physical effects, and distinctions were not made between different fiber types. However, in recent years, in vitro and in vivo studies have shown that different types of fiber have different effects on the function and health of the intestine.[421,427] Therefore, the type of fiber

FIGURE 37-3

Common FOS. **A,** *1-Kestose (GF₂);* **B,** *Nystose (GF₃);*
C, *1ᶠ-Beta-fructofuranosylnystose (GF₄).*

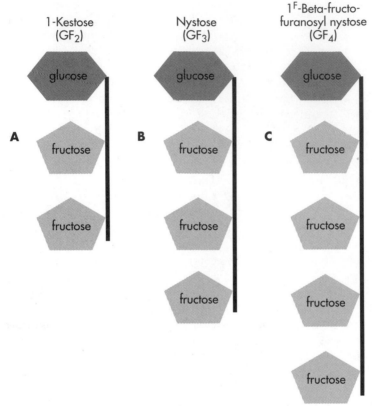

(From NAVC: *New discoveries in canine gastrointestinal disease,* Dayton, Ohio, 1996. The Iams Company.)

included in diets for pets with gastrointestinal disease is as important as the level of fiber. The classification, characteristics, and functions of dietary fiber are discussed extensively in Chapters 2 and 10 (p. 16 and p. 92).

With respect to intestinal disease, the most important considerations are the degree to which a fiber is fermented by intestinal bacteria and the amount and type of byproducts that are produced.[595,596,597] Both dogs and cats have active colonic bacteria and are capable of fermenting dietary fiber.[421,427,598] The amount of fermentation depends upon the amount of time the fiber is present in the tract, the composition of the diet, and the type of fiber that is present. For example, cellulose, gum karaya, and xanthan gum are almost nonfermentable in the intestine of the dog and cat.[421,598] Pectin and guar gum are rapidly fermented by canine and feline colonic microbes while beet pulp and rice bran are moderately fermentable sources of fiber (Tables 37-1 and 37-2).

TABLE 37-1

Fermentation Index of Fiber Sources for Dogs

Fiber Source	Fermentation Index*
Cellulose	0.2
Oat fiber	0.4
Gum karaya	0.6
Peanut hulls	0.9
Xanthan gum	1.0
Gum arabic	1.0
Gum talha	1.3
Psyllium gum	1.4
Soy hulls	1.4
Rice bran	1.8
Beet pulp	2.5
Carob bean gum	3.4
Citrus pulp	3.4
Locust bean gum	5.3
FOS	5.7
Citrus pectin	5.9
Guar gum	7.3
Lactulose	8.3

Adapted from Sunvold GD, Fahey GC Jr, Merchen NR, and others: Dietary fiber for dogs. IV. In vitro fermentation of selected fiber sources by dog fecal inoculum and in vivo digestion and metabolism of fiber-supplemented diets, *J Anim Sci* 73:1099-1109, 1995.

*Total 24-hour SCFA production (millimole [mmol]/g of substrate organic matter)

The most important end products of fiber fermentation are SCFAs. These compounds, primarily acetic, butyric, and propionic acids, comprise a preferred energy source for colonocytes, which derive more than 70% of their energy requirement from SCFAs.[599,600] Colonic cell proliferation is enhanced in the presence of SCFAs, probably as a result of increased availability of this energy source.[601] Dogs that consumed diets containing fermentable fiber had increased colon weights, mucosal surface area, and mucosal hypertrophy when compared with dogs fed a diet containing nonfermentable fiber.[602,603,604] These changes appear to be due to a greater ratio of mucosal surface area to colonic mass and are indicative of increased absorptive potential.[605,606]

The presence of SCFAs in the gastrointestinal tract has several other beneficial effects. SCFAs affect gut motility by increasing peristaltic contractions in the distal portion of the small intestine while possibly inhibiting colonic contractions.[607,608] It is postulated that the cumulative results of these two effects may prevent excessive fermentation in the small intestine while potentiating the absorption of SCFAs in the large intestine. Colonic blood flow increases in the presence of SCFAs.[609] This may

TABLE 37-2

Fermentation Index of Fiber Sources for Cats

Fiber Source	Fermentation Index*
Cellulose	0.1
Xanthan gum	0.5
Gum karaya	0.9
Gum arabic	1.3
Gum talha	1.8
Beet pulp	2.0
Rice bran	2.1
Carob bean gum	3.3
Sugar cane residue	3.4
FOS	4.3
Locust bean gum	4.8
Guar gum	5.1
Citrus pectin	5.5

Adapted from Sunvold GD, Fahey Jr GC, Merchen NR, and others: Dietary fiber for cats: in vitro fermentation of selected fiber sources by cat fecal inoculum and in vivo utilization of diets containing selected fiber sources and their blends, *J Anim Sci* 73:2329-2339, 1995

*Total 24-hour SCFA production (millimole [mmol/g] of substrate organic matter)

occur due to a relaxation of resistance arteries in the colon or simply in response to increased metabolic activity of the colonocytes. Lastly, the presence of SCFAs aids in the prevention of diarrhea by enhancing sodium absorption, promoting the growth of beneficial indigenous microflora, and inhibiting the proliferation of pathogenic microbes.[610,611,612]

In addition to positive benefits for intestinal mucosal cells, SCFAs also affect bacterial populations in the distal small intestine. When treating intestinal disease, this is an important consideration because bacterial and pathogen overgrowth is frequently seen as a primary disease or as a consequence of other forms of intestinal disease (see pp. 489-491). An important function of indigenous bacterial populations in the intestine is to help prevent overgrowth of pathogenic bacteria. They exert this effect by their patterns of SCFA production and direct inhibition of the growth of other species.[613,614,615] Beneficial bacteria also aid in the digestion and absorption of food, provide a source of vitamins to the host animal, and stimulate immune function. Conversely, proliferation of harmful bacterial species cause or exacerbate intestinal disease through the production of toxins, carcinogens, or putrefactive substances. Recent studies indicate that both the relative abilities of beneficial and pathogenic bacteria to use fiber as a substrate, as well as the amount and pattern of SCFAs that are produced, should be considered in the selection of a fiber source.[615]

There is also evidence suggesting that IBDs and intestinal healing after surgery may be positively influenced by fermentable fiber and SCFA status. The provision of specific bowel nutrients, including SCFAs, has been shown to protect intestinal tissue and promote restoration of normal intestinal function. For example, ulcerative colitis in humans is characterized by diminished rates of oxidation of butyrate in the large intestine.[616] Providing a supplemental source of butyrate to the colon has been shown to reduce the inflammatory response.[617] A study with rats examined the effects of feeding diets with or without fermentable fiber after colonic anastomoses.[618] During healing, the fiber-containing diet conferred a trophic effect on the surgical site, improving both wound strength and rate of healing.

While some SCFA production is desirable because of the beneficial effects of these compounds, more is not necessarily better. While minimal production of SCFAs occurs when cellulose is fed, maximal production occurs when fiber mixtures containing pectin are fed.[421,598] By comparison, beet pulp is moderately fermentable in the dog and cat intestine. Excessive fermentation and the production of large amounts of SCFAs in the intestinal tract of both dogs and cats can cause the production of loose stools or diarrhea and excess gas and may interfere with nutrient digestion and absorption.[420,421,427] Benefits are maximized when moderately fermentable fiber sources are selected that can provide optimal levels of SCFAs and at the same time have a nonfermentable component to provide bulk and contribute to normal peristalsis.

Fructooligosaccharides

In recent years, the use of oligosaccharides, specifically FOS, has been shown to support gastrointestinal health. One of the reasons is that FOS are selectively utilized by certain beneficial bacterial species in the gastrointestinal tract.[614,619,620] For example, most *Bifidobacterium* species, *Lactobacillus* species, and *Bacteroides* species utilize FOS as well as they do glucose, while *Eubacterium* species, *Salmonella* species, and *Clostridium* species either do not metabolize FOS or metabolize them less well than glucose.[532,621] Studies with human subjects have shown that the consumption of dietary FOS aids in preventing infection with *Clostridium* species and *Escherichia coli* and supports the growth of *Bifidobacteria* populations.[621,622] Similarly, recent in vitro and in vivo studies have shown that FOS and lactosucrose (another highly fermentable fiber) are effective in altering intestinal microbe populations in dogs and cats (Figures 37-4 and 37-5).[544,623,624,625]

Although a limited number of studies have been conducted, FOS appear to have efficacy in the treatment of SIBO in dogs. When dogs with SIBO were fed a diet containing 1% FOS for 45 days, significantly fewer aerobic and facultative anaerobic bacteria were found in both intestinal fluid and mucosal samples when compared with the samples of control dogs.[626] A recent study found that Beagles fed diets containing either cellulose (nonfermentable fiber) or a combination of beet pulp and FOS had similar fecal bacteria densities, but those fed the FOS-containing diet had lower numbers of *Enterobacteriaceae* and clostridia and higher numbers of lactobacilli and streptococci, compared with those in dogs fed the

FIGURE 37-4

Effect of dietary FOS on the concentration of lactobacilli in the feline large intestine. *P<0.05.

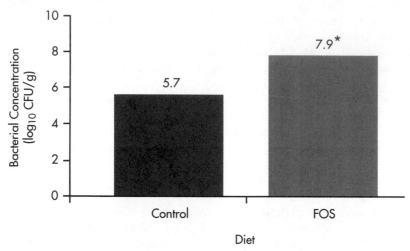

(From Sparkes AH, Papasouliotis K, Sunvold G, and others: The effect of dietary supplementation with fructo-oligosaccharides on the fecal flora of healthy cats, *Am J Vet Res* 59:436-440, 1998.)

FIGURE 37-5

Effect of dietary FOS on the concentration of Clostridium perfringens *in the feline large intestine.* *P<0.10.

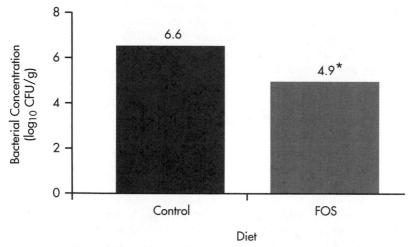

(From Sparkes AH, Papasouliotis K, Sunvold G, and others: The effect of dietary supplementation with fructo-oligosaccharides on the fecal flora of healthy cats, *Am J Vet Res* 59:436-440, 1998.)

nonfermentable fiber.[615,627] The dogs fed the FOS-containing diet also had increased small-intestinal mucosa weight and absorptive surface area and higher nutrient transport rates per unit of intestine. These results indicate that providing a fermentable fiber such as FOS may affect small intestinal bacterial populations in dogs with SIBO, while also promoting increased absorptive capacity.

When SIBO or pathogen overgrowth occur, the bacterial populations in the small intestine can be altered either by using antimicrobial drugs or by changing the diet to increase beneficial bacteria and inhibit the growth of undesirable species. While antibiotics are often effective in the treatment and management of SIBO, the risk of selectively killing the wrong populations exists, and this may result in exacerbation of SIBO. In addition, long-term use is usually required and may be associated with adverse side effects. Therefore dietary treatment, if effective, is more appealing to most pet owners. Current data indicate that including FOS and moderately fermentable fibers in diets for pets with SIBO or pathogen overgrowth aids in promoting the growth of beneficial bacterial populations and inhibits the growth of pathogenic bacteria.

Fiber Recommendations

Current data suggest that appropriate levels of moderately fermentable fiber should be included in the elimination diet that is typically used to treat IBD in dogs and cats (see p. 494). Although highly digestible diets that are very low in fiber have traditionally been used, it now appears that diets formulated to manage intestinal disease should contain between 3% and 7%, but not more than 10%, fiber (on a DMB).[532,628] A balance of fermentable and nonfermentable fiber sources should be fed to supply SCFAs and promote motility, respectively.[532] Both beet pulp and rice bran are moderately fermentable fibers and are appropriate for inclusion in gastrointestinal diets for dogs and cats. In addition, FOS are an important fermentable fiber that can provide SCFAs and be used to alter bacterial populations and numbers in pets with SIBO and pathogen overgrowth. The nutritional objective when selecting dietary fibers should be to select those that predispose to the colonization of beneficial indigenous microflora and promote sufficient SCFA production for intestinal epithelial health.

Diet Digestibility

A final consideration when selecting a diet for pets with gastrointestinal disease is digestibility. Diets formulated for the management of gastrointestinal disease should be highly digestible. When nutrients are efficiently digested and absorbed in the proximal small intestine, the remainder of the bowel is allowed to rest and the delivery of undigested nutrients to the large intestine is minimized.[577] This limits the risk of gaseousness and osmotic diarrhea in the large intestine due to malabsorption.[562] Highly digestible protein sources are less antigenic because little dietary protein is absorbed intact into the mucosa (see pp. 493-495). Diets that

BOX 37-1

Dietary Recommendations for Dogs and Cats with Gastrointestinal Disease

Highly digestible (DM digestibility coefficient greater than 90%)
Single-source, high-quality protein (rabbit, duck, lamb, venison, chicken, or fish)
Single-source, gluten-free carbohydrate (rice, potato, tapioca, or corn)
Reduced fat (less than 10%)
Adjusted fatty acid ratio (omega-6 to omega-3 ratio of 5 : 1 to 10 : 1)
Moderate fiber content (3% to 7% total dietary fiber)
Moderately fermentable fiber (fermentable and nonfermentable components)
FOS for control of intestinal microflora

require minimal digestion also reduce gastric, pancreatic, biliary, and intestinal secretions and contribute to reduced total bacterial counts in the intestine.[531] While a moderate amount of fiber should be included in the diet, excess fiber, especially nonfermentable fiber, should be avoided. Feeding excessive amounts of dietary fiber can impair protein, fat, and energy digestibility. Gastrointestinal diets should have digestibility coefficients of 90% or greater (dry-matter [DM] digestibility).[532]

GENERAL RECOMMENDATIONS

Current research and clinical studies suggest that diets formulated for dogs and cats with gastrointestinal disease should be highly digestible; contain single protein and carbohydrate sources, reduced fat, and an adjusted omega-6 to omega-3 fatty acid ratio; and include a moderate amount of fiber that has both a fermentable and nonfermentable component. Preferably the protein source should be novel, and the carbohydrate source should be gluten-free (Box 37-1).

38

Nutritional Care of Cancer Patients

Because of increased knowledge and improvements in pet health care and nutrition in recent years, many companion animals are now living well into old age. As a result, cancer has become a relatively common disease in dogs and cats, occurring most frequently in pets who are older than 5 years.[629] In addition, because of improved methods of treatment, many pets with neoplastic disease achieve full remission and experience improved quality of life and survival times. Providing dogs and cats with optimal nutrition during the early stages of the disease and throughout treatment and remission is an important component of care. Most cancer patients experience significant alterations in food intake, nutrient metabolism, and energy requirements. The underlying cause of many of these changes is a paraneoplastic syndrome called *cancer cachexia*. Research in recent years has shown that nutritional therapy is a key component in the amelioration of cancer cachexia and may also be helpful in controlling malignant disease. The following chapter reviews the metabolic and physical changes associated with cancer cachexia, the nutrient and energy needs of pets with cancer, and nutritional approaches to managing these patients. Regardless of the type of malignant disease, the ultimate goal of nutritional therapy is to provide an appropriate food that is palatable, contains available nutrients, prevents or limits the effects of cancer cachexia, and improves a pet's quality of life.

CANCER CACHEXIA

Up to 80% of human cancer patients are affected by cancer cachexia.[630] Although the incidence has not been reported for dogs and cats, clinical signs of weight loss and anorexia, along with cachexia's characteristic metabolic abnormalities, are seen in pets with a wide variety of malignancies and in varying stages of disease.[631,632] The underlying cause of cancer cachexia is a pronounced alteration in the body's metabolism of carbohydrate, protein, and fat. Over time, these metabolic changes lead to anorexia, fatigue, weight loss, impaired immune function, and malnutrition. Cancer cachexia significantly affects a patient's quality of life, ability to withstand chemotherapy or radiation treatment, and survival time.[630,633] Furthermore, recent evidence shows that the metabolic changes of cachexia occur before any clinical signs are observed.[634] This underscores the importance of early nutritional intervention when treating dogs and cats with cancer.

While cachexia is an important paraneoplastic syndrome, it is not the only cause of decreased food intake and loss of body condition in pets with cancer. Tumor-bearing animals may lose weight because of the presence or treatment of the tumor or as a result of treatment-induced side effects. In some cases, such as oropharyngeal, gastric, or small-bowel tumors, the physical presence of a tumor can interfere with nutrient intake or assimilation. Surgical procedures, chemotherapy, and radiation therapy may also negatively affect nutrient intake and metabolism. Certain chemotherapies may alter smell and taste perceptions, resulting in decreased food intake or changes in food preferences.[635,636] Anorexia, vomiting, and diarrhea are also potential side effects of chemotherapy and radiation therapy.[637] All of these effects must be addressed when assessing nutritional status and developing a dietary management protocol for pets with cancer.

Phases

Cancer cachexia has significant and persistent effects on body condition and health in many animals with cancer. Three stages of cachexia have been identified. During the first phase, the patient does not exhibit clinical signs, but biochemical changes are evident. These include elevated blood lactate and insulin levels and alterations in amino acid and lipid profiles.[638] Dogs with lymphoma have significantly higher serum lactate and insulin concentrations following intravenous dextrose infusion, compared with levels in healthy dogs.[639] These changes occur even in dogs that are not showing clinical signs of cachexia. Clinical signs develop during the second stage. The patient begins to show anorexia, weight loss, and depression and has an increased risk of experiencing detrimental side effects of cancer therapy. The third and final stage is characterized by marked losses of body fat and protein stores, severe debilitation, weakness, and biochemical evidence of negative nitrogen balance. If left untreated, cancer cachexia can be the ultimate cause of death. Indirect calorimetry studies with rats have found that the three phases usually coincide with normal, increased, and decreased energy requirements, respectively.[640]

Alterations in Carbohydrate Metabolism

The biochemical alterations of cancer cachexia involve the metabolism of carbohydrate, protein, and lipids, which in turn affects basal metabolic rate. Together, this collection of biochemical changes leads to inefficient energy utilization by the host animal and enhanced energy use by the tumor. Alterations in carbohydrate metabolism are dramatic and are at least partially related to the metabolic needs of the tumor. Tumor cells preferentially obtain energy through anaerobic glycolysis and are incapable of obtaining significant amounts of energy from either aerobic glycolysis or fat oxidation.[641,642] As a result, as a tumor grows it uses the host's supply of glucose for energy, generating large amounts of lactate, the end product of anaerobic glycolysis. The host's hepatocytes convert this excess lactate to glucose via the Cori cycle, resulting in a shift in glucose metabolism from energy-producing oxidative pathways to energy-requiring gluconeogenic pathways. The end result is a gain of energy by the tumor and a net energy loss for the host. This alteration in carbohydrate metabolism occurs as early as the preclinical stage of cancer cachexia. Therefore nutritional intervention that is aimed at shifting metabolism to benefit the host over the tumor should begin as soon as a diagnosis is made.

Biochemical abnormalities that occur in response to changes in carbohydrate use include elevated serum lactate concentrations, altered serum insulin and glucagon secretion patterns, increased rate of gluconeogenesis and glucose turnover, and insulin resistance.[643,644,645,646] Although the majority of studies have been conducted with human cancer patients or laboratory animal models, there is evidence that these changes also occur in dogs (and presumably cats). Dogs with lymphoma, a common form of cancer in many breeds, show altered responses to glucose tolerance tests, and many develop insulin resistance.[639,647] These changes occur before and after the development of clinical signs and continue after remission is achieved.[647] It is hypothesized that insulin resistance in dogs with lymphoma is due to a postreceptor defect resulting in glucose intolerance. Regardless of the underlying cause, the prevalence of glucose intolerance and insulin insensitivity mandate the need to limit and carefully select the type of carbohydrate included in foods for pets with cancer.

Alterations in Protein Metabolism

Because both the tumor and the host have obligatory protein requirements, negative nitrogen balance is common in cancer patients.[648] Growing tumors require amino acids for protein synthesis and will also use host gluconeogenic amino acids for the production of glucose. Because tumors often have a high metabolic rate, this significantly affects host protein stores and can result in abnormal serum amino acid profiles.[649] The host experiences an increased rate of whole body protein turnover, characterized by a decreased rate of protein synthesis in skeletal muscle and an increased rate of synthesis in the liver.[650,651] This imbalance eventually leads to muscle wasting, hypoalbuminemia, compromised immunity, impaired gastrointestinal function, and delayed wound healing.

Studies of human cancer patients have shown that serum levels of the gluconeogenic amino acids alanine, glutamic acid, aspartic acid, and glycine generally decrease, while concentrations of branch-chain amino acids are normal or increased.[649,652] The liver responds to this imbalance by increasing protein synthesis in an attempt to overcome tumor-induced protein and amino acid catabolism.[652] Studies of dogs with cancer have also found changes in serum amino acid profiles. A group of 32 dogs with a variety of cancers had decreased serum levels of glycine, glutamine, valine, cystine, and arginine and elevated levels of isoleucine and phenylalanine, compared with values seen in healthy control dogs.[653,654] Similar to changes in serum lactate and insulin, these alterations did not resolve when remission was achieved.

Alterations in Lipid Metabolism

A loss of body fat accounts for the majority of the weight lost by humans and animals with cancer cachexia.[655] While reduced food intake is a significant cause of this loss, humans and animals with cancer also experience decreased lipogenesis and increased lipolysis.[656] This shift results in elevated concentrations of serum free fatty acids (FFAs), very–low-density lipoproteins (VLDLs), triglycerides, acetoacetate, and beta-hydroxy butyrate.[657,658,659] In human patients with cancer, altered lipid profiles have been associated with immunosuppression and decreased survival time.[660] Similarly, dogs with untreated lymphoma had significantly elevated concentrations of serum triglycerides, FFAs, and VLDLs when compared with healthy controls.[653,661] Although serum cholesterol concentration increased in response to chemotherapy, other lipid parameters did not normalize during treatment or when the dogs attained remission.

In recent years, the importance of omega-3 fatty acids for human cancer patients and the effects of this class of fatty acids on tumor development and metastasis have been studied. (A complete review of these fatty acids and their present use in pet foods is included on pp. 435-436). The antiinflammatory effects of omega-3 fatty acids on multiple systems of the body suggest a role in treating cancer patients. In addition, there is an increasing body of evidence showing that this family of fatty acids, particularly eicosapentaenoic acid (EPA) and docosahexaenoic acid (DHA), limits tumor growth.[662,663,664,665] Studies in animal models have shown that supplementation with EPA and DHA prevents cachexia and metastatic disease.[666] Although the underlying mechanism is not completely understood, the effect appears to be related to the incorporation of long-chain omega-3 fatty acids into tumor cell membranes. This alters membrane fluidity and permeability, making tumor cells more susceptible to both chemotherapeutic agents and the host's own immune system. There is also indirect evidence that omega-3 fatty acids may be helpful in preventing the recurrence of cancer after remission has been achieved.[667]

Results of trials with human cancer patients have shown clinical benefits of omega-3 fatty acid supplementation. When 85 subjects with upper gastrointestinal cancers were fed either an omega-3 fatty acid and arginine supplement or a placebo, those receiving the supplement had improved nitrogen intake and balance, an increased rate of wound healing, reduced incidence of complications, and shortened hospitalization time when compared with patients receiving the placebo.[662] While the design of this study confounded fatty acid and arginine effects, the results suggest a benefit of omega-3 fatty acids for human cancer patients. Similar results were reported when cancer patients were supplemented with omega-3 fatty acids, arginine, and ribonucleic acid (RNA).[668]

Although available data are limited, initial research indicates that companion animals with cancer may also benefit from omega-3 fatty acids. When dogs with lymphoma were fed a food supplemented with omega-3 fatty acids (EPA and DHA) and arginine, supplemented dogs had lower plasma lactate responses to glucose tolerance tests and increased disease-free intervals and survival times when compared with affected dogs that were not supplemented.[638] Similar to studies with humans, the design of this study prevented any conclusions about a singular effect of omega-3 fatty acids because arginine was included in the supplement.

It is important to note that the majority of nutritional studies in dogs with cancer have almost exclusively examined patients with lymphoma. Although lymphoma is a common form of neoplastic disease and is seen in many different breeds of dogs, cachexia is not always observed in pets with this type of cancer.[669] Additional studies of different types of cancer in dogs and cats and their associated metabolic changes are needed. Recently, the effects of feeding increased levels of omega-3 fatty acids and arginine on irradiated skin and oral mucosa in dogs with nasal tumors were examined.[670] Feeding a food that contained increased amounts of DHA, EPA, and arginine normalized blood lactate, decreased histological evidence of radiation damage to the skin and mucosa, and improved the quality of life in dogs with these tumors.

Changes in Energy Requirements

As discussed previously, tumors obtain energy primarily through anaerobic metabolism of glucose, resulting in the production of lactate. The host must then recycle the lactate that is produced through the Cori cycle, leading to a net loss of energy. Additional energy costs to animals with cancer may include cytokine-induced increases in glucose recycling, protein degradation, and energy expenditure.[671,672,673] Therefore, at least theoretically, energy expenditure in cancer patients is expected to increase. However, studies using indirect calorimetry to measure energy expenditure in tumor-bearing subjects have reported varying results.[640, 674,675,676,677] Some investigators have reported increased energy expenditure in humans and animals with neoplastic disease. Conversely, others have found normal or reduced energy needs. These discrepancies are probably a result of several factors. Because cancer cachexia develops in stages and biochemical alterations typically precede clinical signs, animals that are in the preclinical stage of cachexia are expected to have normal energy requirements. Conversely, individuals with active, untreated cachexia may have elevated energy expenditure, while those in the final stages may be hypometabolic. Additional factors that significantly affect energy needs include the type and size of tumor and the patient's phase of treatment, severity of clinical signs, and level of activity.

Several studies using indirect calorimetry have been conducted to determine whether there are significant changes in resting energy expenditure (REE) in dogs with cancer.[678,679,680] In one study, 22 dogs with naturally occurring lymphoblastic lymphoma were fed isocaloric amounts of either a high-carbohydrate or a high-fat diet before and during chemotherapy.[679] The initial REE values in dogs with lymphoma before treatment were significantly lower than those of healthy control dogs. After 6 weeks of chemotherapy, REE values decreased further in the dogs with lymphoma, even after remission was achieved in the majority of dogs. Although there were no significant differences in mean REE between the two diet groups, the dogs fed the high-fat diet maintained slightly higher energy expenditures than those fed the high-carbohydrate diet.[678] An important consideration in this study is the fact that the healthy control animals were slightly younger than the dogs with cancer (mean ages of 5.4 versus 7 years, respectively). Although slight, this age difference may account for the lower initial mean REE in dogs with lymphoma. However, it would not account for the further decreases seen during treatment and remission. A possible explanation for these decreases may be that the dogs with lymphoma were in the first silent phase of cancer cachexia at the start of the study. This was followed by a reduction in metastatically active tumor tissue in response to treatment or possibly in response to a decrease in host metabolism caused by a loss of lean body tissue. A common side effect of chemotherapy is decreased energy intake, which could lead to a loss of lean body tissue and a decreased metabolic rate.

A second study examined the effects of surgical excision of various types of tumors on energy expenditure in dogs.[680] Removal of tumors did not significantly affect REE, regardless of tumor type. In addition, the energy expenditure of tumor-bearing dogs prior to surgery was not significantly greater or less than that of a control group of healthy dogs. In contrast to the previously described study of dogs with lymphoma, this study indicated that REE and energy needs of dogs with other types of cancer are not significantly different from healthy dogs of the same age.

Although studies of the energy requirements of dogs with cancer are limited (no studies have been published for cats), results thus far indicate that the energy needs of cancer patients do not significantly increase, and they may decrease slightly with some types of cancer. In addition, removal of the cancer through surgery or chemotherapy does not appear to appreciably affect energy needs. These data do not support the standard tenet that patients with neoplastic disease have increased energy requirements. Rather, it seems that the energy needs of dogs and cats with cancer must be addressed on an individual basis and may vary with the type of cancer, stage of the disease, and method of treatment.[669]

DIETARY MANAGEMENT OF CANCER PATIENTS

The metabolic changes associated with cancer occur before clinical signs are seen, emphasizing the importance of early nutritional intervention. Because many dogs and cats with cancer have decreased food intakes, a major goal of nutritional therapy is to select a food that is highly palatable and energy dense. The food's nutrient profile should be tailored to address the metabolic alterations of cancer cachexia, maintain normal body condition, and prevent weight loss. Provision of an appropriate diet may reverse some of the deleterious effects of neoplastic disease, improve the pet's ability to tolerate chemotherapy or radiation treatment, and enhance overall quality of life. Specific dietary recommendations should consider the stage of disease, energy needs, current and past nutritional status, and ability or willingness to eat.

Diet Characteristics

Current data indicate that food selected for cancer patients should take advantage of the differences in metabolic needs between the host animal and the tumor. The food's caloric distribution should emphasize calories originating from fat and protein, rather than from carbohydrate, because fatty acids and amino acids are not the preferred fuel source for most tumors. A diet that contains reduced carbohydrate and elevated fat and protein may supply a readily available source of energy, meet the host's protein needs, and limit the supply of carbohydrate to tumor cells.[655,681] Human cancer patients with cachexia have shown improvements in body weight, adipose stores, energy and nitrogen balance, and ability to metabolize glucose when dietary fat is increased.[682,683] Similarly, dogs with lymphoma fed a high-fat diet had lower mean lactate and insulin levels after remission when compared with dogs fed isocaloric amounts of a high-carbohydrate diet.[679] A food that contains 50% to 60% of total calories from fat, 30% to 50% of calories from protein, and the remaining proportion of calories from carbohydrate is recommended for dogs and cats with cancer.[669] In addition to shifting metabolism away from carbohydrate and toward fat, another benefit of feeding a high-fat diet to cancer patients is the increased energy density and palatability of these foods.

The type of fat included in foods for pets with cancer is also an important consideration. Documented benefits of omega-3 fatty acids, particularly the long-chain fatty acids EPA and DHA, support the inclusion of increased levels of these fatty acids and a modified omega-6 to omega-3 fatty acid ratio for pets with cancer. Although additional studies are needed, preliminary data indicate that increased dietary omega-3 fatty acids can improve alterations in metabolism associated with cancer, may affect the occurrence of metastatic disease and cachexia, and may improve the response to chemotherapy or radiation therapy. Studies of inflammatory diseases in dogs have shown that benefits are optimized when dietary omega-3 fatty acids are increased and the food contains an adjusted omega-6 to omega-3 ratio between 5:1 and 10:1 (see Section 6, p. 442).

Foods for cancer patients should contain slightly higher concentrations of protein than the levels needed for adult maintenance. Providing optimal levels of high-quality protein contributes to a positive nitrogen balance in the face of potentially increased requirements during active neoplastic disease. Losses of lean body tissue can occur during cancer cachexia and as a result of anorexia or decreased food intake. The food should contain between 30% and 50% of calories from protein, with the higher end of this range appropriate for cats.[684] Because tumor cells preferentially use gluconeogenic amino acids for energy, a food that is specifically enriched with certain amino acids may be beneficial. For example, supplemental arginine has been shown to inhibit tumor growth and metastasis, while glycine may reduce cisplatin-induced nephrotoxicity.[685,686,687] Because most of these studies have been conducted with laboratory animal models, specific recommendations for companion animals cannot be made at this time. More research is necessary to determine if there is a role for specific amino acid therapy in dogs and cats with neoplastic disease.

Calculating Energy Needs

The energy needs of companion animals with cancer can be affected by the type of tumor and the animal's stage of disease, willingness to eat, and activity level. Because ill animals are often kept in thermoneutral environments, have decreased food intakes, and are inactive, the formulas used to determine normal maintenance energy requirements for dogs and cats will not usually provide accurate estimates for pets with cancer. Conversely, an animal's resting energy requirement (RER) reflects the energy needed during a resting, postabsorptive state in a thermoneutral environment. Formulas for RER may therefore provide a better estimate of energy needs in cancer patients. An additional "illness factor" can be added to this estimate based upon the pet's degree of illness and metabolic state. For dogs, an estimate of RER can be made using the formula RER (kilocalories [kcal]/day) = 70 × (body weight$_{kilograms [kg]}$)$^{0.75}$.[669,688,689] An estimate for cats can be calculated using the formula: RER (kcal/day) = 40 × (body weight$_{kg}$). The RER estimates may need to be adjusted to account for additional energy needs for the demands of underlying disease. For dogs with cancer, a factor of 1.25 to 2 has been recommended, while 1.25 to 1.5 has been suggested for cats.[669,688]

METHODS OF FEEDING

Feeding ill patients can be achieved through delivery of nutrients enterally (into the intestinal tract) or parenterally (intravenously). Enteral feeding should be always be the delivery method of choice, provided the pet has a functional gastrointestinal tract. Compared with parenteral methods, enteral feeding prevents mucosal atrophy and bacterial overgrowth, presents less risk to the patient, and is more convenient and affordable for clients. Parenteral nutrition is only suggested when the gastrointestinal tract cannot be used and when there is an anticipated need for long-term intravenous feeding.

Oral feeding of a canned or dry ration should be the first choice for cancer patients. Many dogs and cats with cancer are capable of consuming, digesting, and assimilating food but are reluctant to eat an adequate volume of food. Decreased intake or anorexia occurs as a result of the metabolic or physiological effects of disease or in response to surgery, chemotherapy, or radiation therapy. Some pets can be encouraged to eat by offering small meals or hand-feeding, warming the food to body temperature, adding warm water to enhance the aroma and texture, or changing the type of food that is offered. Metoclopramide is often given to ameliorate nausea associated with chemotherapy, and it may stimulate eating.[638] Similarly, chemical appetite stimulants such as benzodiazepine derivatives or antiserotonin agents may be helpful in getting reluctant pets to eat. However, these drugs can have variable responses and may not be appropriate for some cancer patients because of physiological contraindications and potential side effects.[688]

When a patient is unwilling or unable to consume food orally, a feeding tube can be used. Nasoesophageal tubes provide short-term feeding to patients with normal gastrointestinal function, but they are not appropriate for animals with severe esophageal or gastric disease. Two other types of enteral feeding routes are gastrostomy tubes and jejunostomy tubes. A gastrostomy tube delivers nutrients directly into the stomach, while a jejunostomy tube bypasses the entire upper gastrointestinal tract and delivers nutrients to the small intestine. Both gastrostomy and jejunostomy tubes require surgical placement and can be left in position for extended periods of time. However, while bolus (meal) feeding can be used with nasoesophageal and gastrostomy tubes, a constant rate of infusion must be used with a jejunostomy tube. More complete discussions of the use, placement, and management of enteral feeding tubes are found in other publications.[655,689,690]

The formula selected for tube feeding should have the same characteristics as the food that would be used for oral feeding. An energy- and nutrient-dense formula minimizes the volume that must be fed. Providing a high proportion (50% or more) of calories as fat also helps delay gastric emptying and prevent diarrhea. The formula should include a soluble and insoluble fiber source that helps slow gastric emptying and supports normal gastrointestinal tract function.[638] A formula that is too nutrient-dense may induce vomiting or osmotic diarrhea, especially if a large volume is administered at one time. Therefore a balancing act between providing adequate nutrients, calories, and fluid and preventing nausea or diarrhea is often required when tube-feeding cancer patients. A blenderized canned cat or dog food works well with gastrostomy tubes, while liquid commercial veterinary products for dogs and cats can be used with nasogastric and jejunostomy tubes. The pet's total daily requirements should be administered in at least five to eight small bolus feeding per day, except when jejunostomy feeding is used. If diarrhea occurs, reduction of the rate of feeding, feeding smaller increments, or decreasing the total amount of formula administered may help the intestinal tract to adapt.

Parenteral nutrition is the only option for nutritional support in cancer patients that cannot tolerate enteral feeding, usually because of a nonfunctional or severely diseased gastrointestinal tract.[689,691,692] Regardless of the underlying disease being treated, parenteral nutrition is generally not considered for veterinary patients unless the patient is expected to require support for several days and the gastrointestinal tract is expected to heal given a sufficient period of rest. The long-term benefits of parenteral nutrition are often questionable because this route of delivery is associated with mucosal atrophy and increased medical risks such as sepsis and metabolic anomalies. Parenteral nutrition may also be cost prohibitive for many clients. When it is used, a parenteral formula for dog and cats with cancer should contain a limited amount of dextrose and 60% to 70% of calories as fat. Avoiding glucose- or lactate-containing solutions is especially important, given the metabolic changes associated with cancer.[693] As with enteral feeding, the goal is to provide the host with a readily available energy source while limiting the energy available to the tumor.

CONCLUSION

The primary challenge when feeding cancer patients is to provide adequate calories, essential nutrients, and fluids in the face of the decreased food intake and metabolic alterations that are often associated with neoplastic disease. Although more clinical trials are needed with dogs and cats with different types of cancer, current research supports the use of foods that contain increased amounts of fat and protein, reduced carbohydrate, and elevated levels of omega-3 fatty acids.

S E C T I O N 6

KEY POINTS

- Some breeds of dogs are affected by inherited disorders of nutritional metabolism. Owners should be aware of inherited disorders that are known to affect certain breeds and of testing methods that are diagnostic. In many cases, treatments are available and effective.

- Although inherited metabolic disorders are less well documented in cats than in dogs, feline lipoprotein lipase (LPL) deficiency is well recognized. Feeding a low-fat diet often results in normal blood lipid levels and a regression of symptoms.

- **Caution:** Treatment of primary hyperlipidemia in both dogs and cats entails feeding a diet restricted in fat and calories. The starting diet should contain between 8% and 12% fat on a dry-matter basis (DMB). Such a diet must be followed strictly for the remainder of the pet's lifetime. All snacks and table scraps must be eliminated. Dogs with hyperlipidemia may be susceptible to acute pancreatitis that could be brought on by a single high-fat meal.

- Dalmatians are the only breed of dog that excretes both urate and allantoin in their urine as end products of purine metabolism. They have higher levels of urate in their blood and urine than other breeds of dogs, as well as reduced renal tubular reabsorption of urate. Higher serum urate values in humans lead to a condition commonly known as "gout." The Dalmatian excretes excess urate in the urine, leading to the development of urate urolithiasis or urinary tract "stones." Although approximately half of the dogs seen with urinary calculi are of the Dalmatian breed, the overall incidence in the Dalmatian breed has been estimated to be as low as 1%.

- A large proportion of diabetic dogs and cats are obese at the time of diagnosis. Other risk factors for diabetes include hypothyroidism, Cushing's syndrome, and pancreatic disease. In cats, the risk of developing diabetes also increases greatly with age.

- The diet selected for a pet with diabetes should contain 40% or more of its calories supplied as complex carbohydrate; a moderate level of fiber; and high-quality protein; it should be moderately restricted in fat.

- **Tip:** Pets with diabetes should be fed several small meals instead of one large meal during the period of insulin activity. For example, if insulin is given early in the morning, the first meal should be provided immediately before the insulin injection. Once an appropriate feeding schedule and diet have been established, changes should be avoided. Snacks should not be given, and feeding times should be consistent.

- Urolithiasis is caused by the presence of urinary calculi in the bladder and/or lower urinary tract. In dogs and cats, the two most common types of uroliths are struvite (magnesium ammonium phosphate) and calcium oxalate.

- Owners should be aware of the clinical signs of urolithiasis in dogs and cats. Initial signs include frequent urination, urine dribbling, and urination in inappropriate places. A pet may also show prolonged squatting or straining during urination or frequent licking of the urogenital region. If obstruction occurs, uremia develops rapidly and is characterized by severe pain, anorexia, vomiting, dehydration, and depression. This is a medical emergency that can cause permanent kidney damage, bladder rupture, and death.

- Dietary risk factors for the development of struvite urolithiasis include production of an alkaline urine, meal-feeding (for cats), low water consumption, and feeding a diet that is low in digestibility, caloric density, and moisture, and high in magnesium. Dietary risk factors for the development of calcium oxalate urolithiasis include production of an acidic urine, low water consumption, and feeding a diet that contains excess sodium, vitamin D, or ascorbic acid.

- Some cutaneous disorders that respond to vitamin A therapy are not actually caused by a vitamin A deficiency. In these cases vitamin A therapy is required throughout the pet's life, but therapeutic dosages have not been found to be toxic. It is believed that there is a genetic basis for the disease in some breeds (the Cocker Spaniel in particular).

- Interestingly, a pet can develop food hypersensitivity to a food it has been consuming on a regular basis for years without problems. In most cases, food hypersensitivity manifests as dermatological problems, usually intense pruritus, although gastrointestinal problems can also occur.

- By the time an animal shows clinical signs of renal failure the kidneys may be functioning at only 15% to 30% of their original capacity. Increased water consumption and increased urination may be the first signs an owner notices. A tentative diagnosis can be inferred by medical history and clinical signs and confirmed by blood testing and urinalysis. Determination of an animal's glomerular filtration rate (GFR) is the most accurate diagnostic test.

- **Caution:** Feline idiopathic hepatic lipidosis is fairly common among middle-aged, obese cats. It most often occurs after a period of partial or complete anorexia, usually brought on by stress. Early diagnosis is critical, and owners should take note of signs of developing anorexia.

- Lifelong dental care for dogs and cats should include yearly veterinary cleaning (scaling and polishing), regular home dental care (brushing one to three times per week), and the provision of a variety of chew toys and hard biscuits to pets who enjoy them. Although it cannot replace regular dental care, feeding a dry pet food contributes to healthy gums and teeth.

- Providing moderate levels of fiber in diets for pets with gastrointestinal disease promotes the growth of beneficial microflora and contributes to proper gastrointestinal function. A fiber that contains both a fermentable and a nonfermentable component should be selected.

- Diets for pets with cancer should be formulated to account for the metabolic changes associated with neoplastic disease. A diet that is nutrient-dense, highly digestible, high in fat, and low in carbohydrate is appropriate in many cases. The diet should also contain a high quality source of protein and an adjusted omega-6 to omega-3 fatty acid ratio of 10:1 to 5:1.

- **Tip:** Pay close attention to your pet's eating habits. A change may signal an illness, and if an owner is not observant, nutritional deficiencies may develop and affect the pet's ability to cope with illness. Like humans, pets often do not want to eat when they are ill. However, proper nutrition during illness is essential for recovery. Pets' energy requirements increase in response to stress induced by illness, and the metabolic rate increases if fever is present. If the pet's appetite has decreased, owners should feed a well-balanced, nutrient-dense diet in order to ensure that nutritional needs are met even if the pet can only eat a small amount of food.

SECTION 6

REFERENCES

1. Batt RM, Horadagoda NU, Simpson KW: Role of the pancreas in the absorption and malabsorption of cobalamin (vitamin B_{12}) in dogs, *J Nutr* 121:S75-S76, 1991.

2. Fyfe JC, Jexyk PF, Giger U, and others: Inherited selective malabsorption of vitamin B_{12} in Giant Schnauzers, *J Am Anim Hosp Assoc* 25:533-539, 1989.

3. Fyfe JC, Giger U, Hall CA, and others: Inherited selective intestinal cobalamin malabsorption and cobalamin deficiency in dogs, *Pediatr Res* 29:24-31, 1991.

4. Thornburg LP, Polley D, Dimmitt R: The diagnosis and treatment of copper toxicosis in dogs, *Can Pract* 11:36-39, 1984.

5. Ubbink GH, van de Broek J, Hazewinkel HA, and others: Cluster analysis of the genetic heterogeneity and disease distributions in purebred dog populations, *Vet Rec* 142:209-213, 1998.

6. Johnson GF: Inheritance of copper toxicosis in Bedlington Terriers, *Am J Vet Res* 41:1865-1866, 1980.

7. Brewer GJ: Wilson disease and canine copper toxicosis, *Am J Clin Nutr* 67:1087S-1090S, 1998.

8. Keen CR, Lonnerdal B, Fisher GL: Age-related variations in hepatic iron, copper, zinc and selenium concentrations in Beagles, *Am J Vet Res* 42:1884-1887, 1981.

9. Thornburg LP, McAllister D, Ebinger WL, and others: Copper toxicosis in dogs. I. Copper-associated liver disease in Bedlington Terriers. II: The pathogenesis of copper-associated liver disease in dogs, *Can Pract* 12:33-38, 41-45, 1985.

10. Twedt DC, Sternlieb I, Gilbertson SR: Clinical, morphologic and chemical studies on copper toxicosis of Bedlington Terriers, *J Am Vet Assoc* 175:269-275, 1979.

11. Yuzbasiyan-Gurkan V, Blanton SH, Cao Y, and others: Linkage of a microsatellite marker to the canine copper toxicosis locus in Bedlington Terriers, *Am J Vet Res* 58:23-27, 1997.

12. Holmes NG, Herrtage ME, Ryder EJ, and others: DNA marker C04107 for copper toxicosis in a population of Bedlington Terriers in the United Kingdom, *Vet Rec* 142:351-352, 1998.

13. Brewer GJ, Dick RD, Schall W, and others: Use of zinc acetate to treat copper toxicosis in dogs, *J Am Vet Med Assoc* 201:564-568, 1992.

14. Herrtage ME, Seymout CA, Jefferies AR: Inherited copper toxicosis in the Bedlington Terrier: a report of two clinical cases, *J Small Anim Pract* 28:1127-1140, 1987.

15. Twedt DC, Whitney EL: Management of hepatic copper toxicosis in dogs. In Kirk RW, editor: *Current veterinary therapy X*, Philadelphia, 1989, WB Saunders.

16. Jezyk PF, Haskins ME, McKay-Smith WE, and others: Lethal acrodermatitis in Bull Terriers, *J Am Vet Med Assoc* 188:833-839, 1986.

17. Miller WH Jr: Nutritional considerations in small animal dermatology, *Vet Clin North Am Small Anim Pract* 19:497-511, 1989.

18. Tail chasing in a Bull Terrier, *J Am Vet Med Assoc* 202:758-760, 1993.

19. Codner EC, Thatcher CD: The role of nutrition in the management of dermatoses, *Semin Vet Med Surg Small Anim* 5:167-177, 1990.

20. Kunkle GA: Zinc responsive dermatoses in dogs. In Kirk RW, editor: *Current veterinary therapy VII*, Philadelphia, 1980, WB Saunders.

21. Fadok VA: Zinc responsive dermatosis in a Great Dane: a case report, *J Am Anim Hosp Assoc* 18:409-414, 1982.

22. Brown RG, Hoag GN, Smart ME, and others: Alaskan Malamute chondrodysplasia. V. Decreased gut zinc absorption, *Growth* 42:1-6, 1978.

23. Watson TDG, Barrie J: Lipoprotein metabolism and hyperlipoproteinemia in the dog and cat: a review, *J Small Anim Pract* 34:479-487, 1993.

24. Barrie J, Watson TDG, Stear MJ, and others: Plasma cholesterol and lipoprotein concentrations in the dog: the effects of age, breed, gender and endocrine disease, *J Small Anim Pract* 34:507-512, 1993.

25. Whitney MS: Evaluation of hyperlipidemias in dogs and cats, *Semin Vet Med Surg Small Anim* 7:292-300, 1992.

26. Watson TDG, Mackenzie JA, Stewart JP, and others: Use of oral and intravenous fat tolerance tests to assess plasma chylomicron clearance in dogs, *Res Vet Sci* 58:256-262, 1995.

27. Downs LG, Crispin SM, LeGrande-Defretin V, and others: The effect of dietary changes on plasma lipids and lipoproteins of six Labrador Retrievers, *Res Vet Sci* 63:175-181, 1997.

28. Armstrong PJ, Ford RB: Hyperlipidemia. In Kirk RW, editor: *Current veterinary therapy X: small animal practice*, Philadelphia, 1989, WB Saunders.

29. Johnson RK: Canine hyperlipidemia. In Ettinger SJ, editor: *Textbook of veterinary internal medicine*, vol 1, ed 3, Philadelphia, 1989, WB Saunders.

30. Ford RB: Idiopathic hyperchylomicronemia in Miniature Schnauzers, *J Small Anim Pract* 34:488-492, 1993.

31. Crispin SM: Ocular manifestations of hyperlipoproteinemia, *J Small Anim Pract* 34:500-506, 1993.

32. Liu SK, Tilley LP, Tappe JP, and others: Clinical and pathological findings in dogs with atherosclerosis: 21 cases (1970-1983), *J Am Vet Med Assoc* 189:227-232, 1986.

33. Bodkin, K: Seizures associated with hyperlipoproteinemia in a Miniature Schnauzer, *Can Pract* 17:11-15, 1992.

34. DeBowes LJ: Lipid metabolism and hyperlipoproteinemia in dogs, *Comp Cont Ed Pract Vet* 9:727-736, 1987.

35. Connelly PW, Maguire GF, Little JA: Familial apolipoprotein C-II deficiency associated with premature vascular disease, *J Clin Invest* 80:1597-1606, 1987.

36. Jones BR, Johnstone AC, Cahill JI, and others: Peripheral neuropathy in cats with inherited primary hyperchylomicronaemia, *Vet Rec* 119:268-272, 1986.

37. Watson TDG, Gaffrey D, Mooney CT, and others: Inherited hyperchylomicronaemia in the cat: lipoprotein lipase function and gene structure, *J Small Anim Pract* 33:207-212, 1992.

38. Bauer JE, Verlander JW: Congenital lipoprotein lipase deficiency in hyperlipemic kitten siblings, *Vet Clin Pathol* 13:7-11, 1984.

39. Johnstone AC, Jones BR, Thompson JC, and others: The pathology of an inherited hyperlipoproteinaemia of cats, *J Comp Pathol* 102:125-137, 1990.

40. Peritz LN, Brunzell JD, Harvey-Clarke C, and others: Characterization of a lipoprotein lipase class III type defect in hypertriglyceridemic cats, *Clin Invest Med* 13:259-263, 1990.

41. Smerdon T: Hyperchylomicronaemia in a litter of Siamese kittens, *Bull Fel Advis Bur*, 51-53, Autumn 1990.

42. Jones BR: Inherited hyperchylomicronaemia in the cat, *J Small Anim Pract* 34:493-499, 1993.

43. Barrie J, Nash AS, Watson TDG: A method for the quantification of the canine plasma lipoproteins, *J Small Anim Pract* 34:226-231, 1993.

44. Brunzell JD, Iverius PH, Scheibel MS, and others: Primary lipoprotein lipase deficiency in lipoprotein deficiency syndromes, *Adv Exp Med Biol* 201:227-239, 1986.

45. Grieshaber TL, McKeever PJ, Conroy, JD: Spontaneous cutaneous (eruptive) xanthomatosis in two cats, *J Am Anim Hosp Assoc* 27:509-512, 1991.

46. Harris WS: Omega-3 fatty acids: effects on lipid metabolism, *Curr Opin Lipidol* 1:5-11, 1990.

47. Logas D, Beale KM, Bauer JE: Potential clinical benefits of dietary supplementation with marine-life oil, *J Am Vet Med Assoc* 199:1631-1636, 1991.

48. Kuster G, Shorter RG, Dawson B: Uric acid metabolism in Dalmatians and other dogs, *Arch Int Med* 129:492-496, 1972.

49. Duncan H, Curtiss AS: Observations on uric acid transport in man, the Dalmatian and the non-Dalmatian dog, *Henry Ford Hosp Med J* 19:105-114, 1971.

50. Sorenson JL, Ling GV: Metabolic and genetic aspects of urate urolithiasis in Dalmatians, *J Am Vet Med Assoc* 203:857-862, 1993.

51. Briggs OM, Harley EH: Serum urate concentrations in the Dalmatian coach hound, *J Comp Pathol* 95:301-304, 1985.

52. Duncan H, Wakim KG, Ward LE: The effects of intravenous administration of uric acid on its concentration in plasma and urine of Dalmatian and non-Dalmatian dogs, *J Lab Clin Med* 58:876-883, 1961.

53. Case LC, Lind GV, Ruby AL, and others: Urolithiasis in Dalmatians: 275 cases (1981-1990), *J Am Vet Med Assoc* 203:96-100, 1993.

54. Giesecke D, Tiemeyer W: Defect of uric acid uptake in Dalmatian dog liver, *Experentia* 40:1415-1416, 1984.

55. Trimble HC, Keeler CE: The inheritance of "high uric acid excretion" in dogs, *J Hered* 29:280-289, 1938.

56. Yu TF, Gutman AB, Berger L: Low uricase activity in the Dalmatian dog simulated in mongrels given oxonic acid, *Am J Physiol* 220:973-979, 1971.

57. White EG: Symposium on urolithiasis in the dog. I. Introduction and incidence, *J Small Anim Pract* 7:529-535, 1966.

58. Brown NO, Parks JL, Greene RW: Canine urolithiasis: respective analysis of 438 cases, *J Am Vet Med Assoc* 170:414-418, 1977.

59. Osborne CA, Clinton CW, Banman LK: Prevalence of canine uroliths, Minnesota Urolith center, *Vet Clin North Am Sm Anim Pract* 16:27-44, 1986.

60. White EG, Treacher RJ, Porter P: Urinary calculi in the god. I. Incidence and chemical composition, *J Comp Pathol* 71:201-216, 1961.

61. Porter P: Urinary calculi in the dog. I. Urate stones and purine metabolism, *J Comp Pathol* 73:119-135, 1963.

62. Fetner PJ: Uric acid dermatitis, *Dalmatian Quart*, 11-13, Spring 1991.

63. Ling GV, Case LC, Nelson H, and others: Pharmokinetics of allopurinal in Dalmatian dogs, *J Vet Pharmacol Ther* 20:134-138, 1997.

64. Lind GV, Ruby AL, Harrold DR: Xanthine-containing urinary calculi in dogs given allopurinol, *J Am Vet Med Assoc* 198:1935-1940, 1991.

65. Cornelius LM: Update on management of diabetes mellitus in dogs and cats, *Mod Vet Pract* 66:251-255, 1985.

66. Williams L: Canine diabetes mellitus, *Vet Tech* 9:168-170, 1988.

67. Panciera DL, Thomas CB, Eicker SW, and others: Epizootiologic patterns of diabetes mellitus in cats: 333 cases (1980-1986), *J Am Vet Med Assoc* 197:1504-1508, 1990.

68. Stogdale L: Definition of diabetes mellitus, *Cornell Vet* 76:156-174, 1985.

69. Ihle SL: Nutritional therapy for diabetes mellitus, *Vet Clin North Am Small Anim Pract* 25:585-597, 1995.

70. Rand JS, Bobbermein LM, Hendrikz JK: Over-representation of Burmese in cats with diabetes mellitus in Queensland, *Aust Vet J* 75:402-405, 1997.

71. Goossens J, Nelson R, Feldman E: Response to therapy and survival in diabetic cats, *J Vet Int Med* 9:181, 1995.

72. Rand JS: Understanding feline diabetes, *Aust Vet Pract* 27:17-26, 1997.

73. Hoenig M: Pathophysiology of canine diabetes, *Vet Clin North Am Small Anim Pract* 25:253-256, 1995.

74. Rand JS: Pathogenesis of feline diabetes. In Reinhart GA, Carey DP, editors: *Recent advances in canine and feline nutrition*, vol 2, Iams Nutrition Symposium Proceedings, Wilmington, Ohio, 1998, Orange Frazer Press.

75. Struble AL, Nelson RW: Non–insulin-dependent diabetes mellitus in cats and humans, *Compend Contin Ed Pract Vet* 19:935-945, 1997.

76. Lutz TA, Rand JS: Plasma inulin and insulin concentrations in normo- and hyperglycemic cats, *Can Vet J* 37:27-34, 1996.

77. O'Brien TD, Hayden DW, Johnson EH, and others: High dose intravenous glucose tolerance test and serum insulin and glucagon levels in diabetic and non-diabetic cats: relationships to insular amyloidosis, *Vet Pathol* 22:250-261, 1985.

78. Mattheeuws D, Rottiers R, Kaneko JJ, and others: Diabetes mellitus in dogs: relationship of obesity to glucose tolerance and insulin response, *Am J Vet Res* 45:98-103, 1984.

79. Link KRJ, Rand JS: Glucose toxicity in cats, *J Vet Int Med* 10:185, 1996.

80. Imamura T, Koffler M, Helderman JF and others: Severe diabetes induced in subtotally depancreatized dogs by sustained hyperglycemia, *Diabetes* 37:600-609, 1988.

81. Nelson RW, Feldman EC, Ford SL, and others: Transient diabetes mellitus in the cat, *Proc Ann Conf Vet Intern Med Forum*, 794, 1992.

82. Rossetti L, Rothman DL, DeFronzo RA, and others: The effect of dietary protein on in vivo insulin action and liver glycogen repletion, *Am J Physiol* 257:E212-E219, 1989.

83. Brand Miller JC, Colagiuri S: The carnivore connection: dietary carbohydrate in the evolution of NIDDM, *Diabetologia* 37:1280-1286, 1994.

84. Holste LC, Nelson RW, Feldman EC, and others: Effect of dry, soft moist, and canned dog foods on postprandial blood glucose and insulin concentrations in healthy dogs, *Am J Vet Res* 50:984-989, 1989.

85. El-Berheri Burgess BRB: Rationale for changes in the dietary management of diabetes, *J Am Diet Assoc* 81:258-270, 1982.

86. Jenkins DJA, Wolever TMS, Taylor RH, and others: Glycemic index of foods: a physiological basis for carbohydrate exchange, *Am J Clin Nutr* 34:362-366, 1981.

87. Jarvi AE, Karlstrom YE, Garnfeldt YE, and others: The influence of food structure on postprandial metabolism in patients with non–insulin-dependent diabetes mellitus, *Am J Clin Nutr* 61:837-842, 1995.

88. Bantle JP, Laine DC, Castle GW, and others: Postprandial glucose and insulin responses to meals containing different carbohydrate in normal and diabetic subjects, *N Engl J Med* 309:7-12, 1983.

89. Wolever TMS, Bolonesi C: Source and amount of carbohydrate affect postprandial glucose and insulin in normal subjects, *J Nutr* 126:2798-2806, 1996.

90. Liljeberg HGM, Garnfeldt YE, Bjorck IME: Products based on a high fiber barley genotype, but not on common barley or oats, lower postprandial glucose and insulin responses in healthy humans, *J Nutr* 126:458-466, 1996.

91. Sunvold GD, Bouchard GF: The glycemic response to dietary starch. In Reinhart GA, Carey DP, editors: *Recent advances in canine and feline nutrition*, vol 2, Iams Nutrition Symposium Proceedings, Wilmington, Ohio, 1998, Orange Frazer Press.

92. Goddard MS, Young G, Marcus R: The effect of amylose content on insulin and glucose responses to ingested rice, *Am J Clin Nutr* 39:388-392, 1984.

93. Liljeberg HGM, Granfeldt YE, Bjorck IME: Products based on a high fiber barley genotype, but not on common barley or oats, lower postprandial glucose and insulin responses in healthy humans, *J Nutr* 126:458-466, 1996.

94. Graham PA, Maskell IE, Nash AS: Canned high fiber diet and postprandial glycemia in dogs with naturally occurring diabetes mellitus, *J Nutr* 124:2712S-2715S, 1994.

95. Nelson RW: Dietary therapy for canine diabetes mellitus. In Kirk RW, editor: *Current veterinary therapy X*, Philadelphia, 1989, WB Saunders.

96. Anderson JW: Physiological and metabolic effects of dietary fiber, *Fed Proc* 44:2902-2906, 1985.

97. Crapo PA: Carbohydrate in the diabetic diet, *J Am Coll Nutr* 5:31-43, 1986.

98. Riccardi G, Rivellese A, Pacioni D, and others: Separate influence of dietary carbohydrate and fiber on the metabolic control of diabetes, *Diabetologia* 26:116-121, 1984.

99. Jenkins JA: Dietary fiber and carbohydrate metabolism. In Spiller GA, Kay RM, editors: *Medical aspects of dietary fiber*, New York, 1980, Plenum Press.

100. Anderson JW: Dietary fiber and diabetes. In Vahouny GV, Kritchevsky D, editors: *Dietary fiber in health and disease*, New York, 1982, Plenum Press.

101. Nuttal FQ: Dietary fiber in the management of diabetes, *Diabetes* 42:503-508, 1993.

102. Vaaler S. Diabetic control is improved by guar gum and wheat bran supplementation, *Diabetic Med* 3:230-233, 1986.

103. Kay RM, Truswell AS: Effect of citrus pectin on blood lipids and fecal steroid excretion in man, *Am J Clin Nutr* 30:171-175, 1977.

104. O'Connor N, Tredger J, Morgan L: Viscosity differences between various guar gums, *Diabetologia* 20:612-615, 1981.

105. Holt S, Heading RC, Carter DC, and others: Effect of gel fiber on gastric emptying and absorption of glucose and paracetamol, *Lancet* 1:636-639, 1979.

106. Anderson JW, Akanji AO: Dietary fiber: an overview, *Diabetes Care* 14:1126-1131, 1991.

107. Nelson RW, Ihle SL, Lewis LD, and others: Effects of dietary fiber supplementation on glycemic control in dogs with alloxan-induced diabetes mellitus, *Am J Vet Res* 52:2060-2066, 1991.

108. Blaxter AC, Cripps RJ, Gruffyd-Jones TJ: Dietary fibre and postprandial hyperglycemia in normal and diabetic dogs, *J Small Anim Pract* 31:229-233, 1990.

109. Nelson RW, Duesberg CA, Ford SL, and others: Effect of dietary insoluble fiber on control of glycemia in dogs with naturally acquired diabetes mellitus, *J Am Vet Med Assoc* 212:380-386, 1998.

110. Diez M, Hornick JL, Baldwin P, and others: Influence of a blend of fructo-oligosaccharides and sugar beet fiber on nutrient digestibility and plasma metabolite concentrations in healthy Beagles, *Am J Vet Res* 58:1238-42, 1997.

111. Nelson RW, Sunvold GD: Effect of carboxymethylcellulose on postprandial glycemic response in healthy dogs. In Reinhart GA, Carey DP, editors: *Recent advances in canine and feline nutrition*, vol 2, Iams Nutrition Symposium Proceedings, Wilmington, Ohio, 1998, Orange Frazer Press.

112. Burney MI, Massimino SF, Field CJ, and others: Modulation of intestinal function and glucose homeostasis in dogs by the ingestion of fermentable dietary fibers. In Reinhart GA, Carey DP, editors: *Recent advances in canine and feline nutrition*, vol 2, Iams Nutrition Symposium Proceedings, Wilmington, Ohio, 1998, Orange Frazer Press.

113. Chen WJ, Anderson JW, Jennings D: Propionate may mediate the hypocholesterolemic effects of certain soluble plant fibers in cholesterol-fed rats, *Proc Soc Exp Bio Med* 175:215-218, 1984.

114. Reppas C, Meyer JH, Sirois J, Dressman JB: Effect of hydroxyproplymethylcellulose on gastrointestinal transit and luminal viscosity in dogs, *Gastroenterology* 100:1217-1223, 1991.

115. Reppas C, Dressman JB: Viscosity modulates blood glucose response to nutrient solutions in dogs, *Diabetes Res Clin Pract* 17:81-88, 1992.

116. Nelson RW: Dietary management of diabetes mellitus, *J Small Anim Pract* 33:213-217, 1992.

117. Nelson RW: Nutritional management of diabetes mellitus, *Semin Vet Med Surg Small Anim* 5:178-186, 1990.

118. Schwarz K, Mertz W: Chromium (III) and the glucose tolerance factor, *Arch Biochem Biophys* 85:292-295, 1959.

119. Urberg M, Zemel MB: Evidence for synergism between chromium and nicotinic acid in the control of glucose tolerance in elderly humans, *Metabolism* 36:896-899, 1987.

120. Olin KL, Stearns DM, Armstrong WH, and others: Comparative retention/absorption of [51]chromium from [51]chromium chloride, [51]chromium nicotinate and [51]chromium picolinate in a rat model, *Trace Elements Electrolytes* 11:182-186, 1994.

121. Evans GW: The effect of chromium picolinate on insulin controlled parameters in humans, *Int J Biosoc Med Res* 11:163-180, 1989.

122. Mertz W: Chromium occurrence and function in biological systems, *Physio Rev* 49:163-238, 1969.

123. Anderson RA, Polansky MM, Bryden NA, and others: Effects of supplemental chromium on patients with symptoms of reactive hypoglycemia, *Metabolism* 36:351-355, 1987.

124. Mossop RT: Effects of chromium (III) on fasting glucose, cholesterol, and cholesterol HDL levels in diabetics, *Cent Afr J Med* 29:80-82, 1983.

125. Glinsmann WH, Mertz W: Effect of trivalent chromium on glucose tolerance, *Metabolism* 15:510-520, 1966.

126. Bunting LD, Fernandez JM, Thompson DL, and others: Influence of chromium picolinate on glucose usage and metabolic criteria in growing Holstein calves, *J Anim Sci* 72:1591-1599, 1994.

127. Amoikon EF, Fernandez JM, Southern LL, and others: Effect of chromium tripicolinate on growth, glucose tolerance, insulin sensitivity, plasma metabolites and growth hormone in pigs, *J Anim Sci* 73:1123-1130, 1995.

128. Spears JW, Brown TT, Sunvold GD, and others: Influence of chromium on glucose metabolism and insulin sensitivity. In Reinhart GA, Carey DP, editors: *Recent advances in canine and feline nutrition*, vol 2, Iams Nutrition Symposium Proceedings, Wilmington, Ohio, 1998, Orange Frazer Press.

129. Mattheeuws D, Rottiers R, Baeyens D, and others: Glucose tolerance and insulin response in obese dogs, *J Am Anim Hosp Assoc* 20:287-290, 1984.

130. Nelson RW, Himsel CA, Feldman EC, and others: Glucose tolerance and insulin response in normal-weight and obese cats, *Am J Vet Res* 51:1357-1362, 1990.

131. Bar RS, Gordon P, Roth J, and others: Fluctuations in the affinity and concentration of insulin receptors on circulating monocytes of obese patients: effects of starvation, refeeding and dieting, *J Clin Invest* 58:1123-1135, 1976.

132. Lockwood DH, Hamilton CL, Livingston JN: The influence of obesity and diabetes in the monkey on insulin and glucagon binding to liver membranes, *Endocrinology* 104:76-81, 1979.

133. Olefsky JM, Ciaraldi TP, Kolterman OG: Mechanisms of insulin resistance in noninsulin-dependent (type II) diabetes, *Am J Med* 79:12-21, 1985.

134. Ferguson D, Hoenig M, Cornelius L: Diabetes mellitus in dogs and cats. In Lorenz MD, Cornelius LM, Ferguson DC, editors: *Small animal medical therapeutics*, Philadelphia, 1992, JP Lippincott.

135. Norswothy G: The difficulties in regulating diabetic cats, *Vet Med*, 342-348, Apr 1993.

136. Bartges JW: Lower urinary tract disease in older cats: what's common, what's not, *Vet Clin Nutr* 3:57-62, 1996.

137. Osborne CA, Kruger JM, Lulich JP: Feline lower urinary tract disorders: definition of terms and concepts, *Vet Clin North Am Small Anim Pract* 26:169-179, 1996.

138. Ling GV, Franti CE, Ruby AL, and others: Urolithiasis in dogs. I. Mineral prevalence and interrelations of mineral composition, age, and sex, *Am J Vet Res* 59:624-629, 1998.

139. Willeberg P: A case-control study of some fundamental determinants in the epidemiology of the feline urological syndrome, *Nord Vet Med* 27:1-14, 1975.

140. Willeberg P, Priester WA: Feline urological syndrome: associations with some time, space and individual patient factors, *Am J Vet Res* 37:975-978, 1976.

141. Osborne CA, Thumchai R, Lulich JP, and others: Etiopathogenesis and therapy of feline calcium oxalate uroliths, *Proc Ann Conf Vet Intern Med Forum*, 487-489, 1995.

142. Ling GV, Franti CE, Ruby AL, and others: Urolithiasis in dogs. II. Breed prevalence, and interrelations of breed, sex, age and mineral composition, *Am J Vet Res* 59:630-642, 1998.

143. Lulich J, Osborne CA, Thumchai R, and others: Epidemiology of canine calcium oxalate urolithiasis: Case study, *Proc Ann Conf Vet Intern Med Forum*, 490-492, 1995.

144. Gaskell CJ: Feline urological syndrome (FUS)—theory and practice, *J Small Anim Pract* 31:519-522, 1990.

145. Osborne CA, Johnston GR, Polzin DJ, and others: Feline urologic syndrome: a heterogenous phenomenon?, *J Am Anim Hosp Assoc* 20:17-32, 1984.

146. Bovee KC, Reif JS, Maguire TG, and others: Recurrence of feline urethral obstruction, *J Am Vet Med Assoc* 174:93-96, 1979.

147. Osborne CA, Thumchai R, Lulich JP, and others: Epidemiology of feline urolithiasis, *Proc Ann Conf Vet Intern Med Forum*, 482-483, 1994.

148. Kruger JM, Osborne CA, Lulich JP and others: Canine struvite urolithiasis: contrasts, changes and challenges, *Vet Clin Nutr* 5:18-21, 1998.

149. Jackson OF: The treatment and subsequent prevention of struvite uroliths in cats, *J Small Anim Pract* 12:555-568, 1971.

150. Bohonowych RO, Parks JL, Greene RW: Features of cystic calculi in cats in a hospital population, *J Am Vet Med Assoc* 173:301-303, 1978.

151. Osborne CA: Feline lower urinary tract disease: state of the science, *Proc Kal Kan Symp Treatment Dog and Cat Dis*, Vernon, California, 1992, Kal Kan Foods.

152. Osborne Ca, Lulich JP, Thumchai R, and others: Feline urolithiasis: etiology and pathophysiology, *Vet Clin North Am Small Anim Pract* 26:217-233, 1996.

153. Buffington CA, Rogers QR, Morris JF: Effect of diet on struvite activity product in feline urine, *Am J Vet Res* 51:2025-2030, 1990.

154. Osborne Ca, Lulich JP, Kruger JM, and others: Medical dissolution of feline struvite urocystoliths, *J Am Vet Med Assoc* 196:1053-1059, 1990.

155. Osborne CA, Kruger Jm, Lulich JP, and others: Disorders of the feline lower urinary tract. In CA Osborne, DR Finco, editors: *Canine and feline nephrology and urology*, Baltimore, 1995, Williams and Wilkins.

156. Osborne CA, Polzin DJ, Abdullahi SU, and others: Struvite urolithiasis in animals and man: formation, detection, and dissolution, *Adv Vet Sci Comp Med* 29:1-54, 1985.

157. Lewis LD, Morris ML: Diet as a causative factor of feline urolithiasis, *Vet Clin North Am Small Anim Pract* 14:513-527, 1984.

158. Bushman DH, Emerick RJ, Embry LB: Experimentally induced ovine phosphatic urolithiasis: relationships involving dietary calcium, phosphorus and magnesium, *J Nutr* 87:499-503, 1965.

159. Chow FHC, Brase JL, Hamar DW, and others: Effect of dietary supplements and methylene blue on urinary calculi, *J Urol* 104:315-319, 1970.

160. Rich LJ, Dysart I, Chow FHC, and others: Urethral obstruction in male cats: experimental production by addition of magnesium and phosphate to diet, *Fel Pract* 4:44-47, 1974.

161. Lewis LD, Chow HC, Taton GS, and others: Effect of various dietary mineral concentrations on the occurrence of feline urolithiasis, *J Am Vet Med Assoc* 172:559-563, 1978.

162. Kallfelz FA, Bressett JD, Wallace RJ: Urethral obstruction in random source and SPF male cats induced by high levels of dietary magnesium or magnesium and phosphorus, *Fel Pract* 10:25-35, 1980.

163. National Research Council: *Nutrient requirements of cats,* Washington, DC, 1986, National Academy of Sciences.

164. Association of American Feed Control Officials: Pet food regulations. In *AAFCO official publication,* Atlanta, 1998, The Association of American Feed Control Officials.

165. Finco DR, Barsanti JA, Crowell WA: Characterization of magnesium-induced urinary disease in the cat and comparison with feline urologic syndrome, *Am J Vet Res* 46:391-400, 1985.

166. Ross LA: Feline urologic syndrome: understanding and diagnosing this enigmatic disease, *Vet Med* 85:1194-1203, 1990.

167. Osborne CA, Kruger JP, Lulich JP, and others: Feline matrix crystalline urethral plugs: a unifying hypothesis of causes, *J Small Anim Pract* 33:172-177, 1992.

168. Buffington CA, Rogers QR, Morris JG, and others: Feline struvite urolithiasis: magnesium effect depends upon urinary pH, *Fel Pract* 15:29-33, 1985.

169. Cook NE: The importance of urinary pH in the prevention of feline urologic syndrome, *Pet Food Ind* 27:24-31, 1985.

170. Tarttelin MF: Feline struvite urolithiasis: factors affecting urine pH may be more important than magnesium levels in food, *Vet Rec* 121:227-230, 1987.

171. Taton GF, Hamar DW, Lewis LD: Evaluation of ammonium chloride as a urinary acidifier in the cat, *J Am Vet Med Assoc* 184:433-436, 1984.

172. Taton GF, Hamar DW, Lewis LD: Urinary acidification in the prevention and treatment of feline struvite urolithiasis, *J Am Vet Med Assoc* 184:437-443, 1984.

173. Chan JCM: Nutrition and acid-base metabolism, *Fed Proc* 40:2423-2428, 1981.

174. Klahr SD: Disorders of acid-base metabolism. In Chan JCM, Gill JR, editors: *Disorders of mineral, water, and acid-base metabolism*, New York, 1982, Wiley and Sons

175. Kane E, Douglass GM: The effects of feeding a dry commercial cat food on the urine and blood acid-base balance of the cat, *Fel Pract* 16:9-13, 1986.

176. Holsworth J: Nutrition and nutritional disorders. In *Diseases of the cat: medicine and surgery*, vol 1, Philadelphia, 1987, WB Saunders.

177. Harrington JT, Lemann J: The metabolic production and disposal of acid and alkali, *Med Clin North Am* 54:1543-1554, 1970.

178. Skoch ER, Chandler EA, Douglas GM, and others: Influence of diet or urine pH and the feline urological syndrome, *J Small Anim Pract* 32:413-419, 1991.

179. Anderson RS: Water balance in the dog and cat, *J Small Anim Pract* 23:588-598, 1982.

180. Gaskell CJ: Nutrition in diseases of the urinary tract in the dog and cat, *Vet Ann* 25:383-390, 1985.

181. Thrall BE, Miller LG: Water turnover in cats fed dry rations, *Fel Pract* 6:10-17, 1976.

182. Seefeldt SL, Chapman TE: Body water content and turnover in cats fed dry and canned rations, *Am J Vet Res* 40:183-185, 1979.

183. Sauer LS, Hamar D, Lewis LD: Effect of diet composition on water intake and excretion by the cat, *Fel Pract* 15:16-21, 1985.

184. Allen TA: Measurement of the influence of diet on feline urinary pH, *Vet Clin North Am Small Anim Pract* 26:363-369, 1996.

185. Kane E, Rogers QR, Morris JG, and others: Feeding behavior of the cat fed laboratory and commercial diets, *Nutr Res* 1:499-507, 1981.

186. Hart BL: Feline behavior, *Fel Pract* 9:10-12, 1979.

187. Jackson JR, Kealy RD, Lawler DF, and others: Long-term safety of urine acidifying diets for cats, *Vet Clin Nutr* 2:100-107, 1995.

188. Finco DR, Adams DD, Crowell WA, and others: Food and water intake and urine composition in cats: influence of continuous versus periodic feeding, *Am J Vet Res* 47:1638-1642, 1986.

189. Finke MD, Litzenberger BA: Effect of food intake on urine pH in cats, *J Small Anim Pract* 33:261-265, 1992.

190. Osborne CA: Diagnosis, medical treatment, and prognosis of feline urolithiasis, *Vet Clin North Am Small Anim Pract* 26:604-627, 1996.

191. Hamar DW, Chow FHC, Dysart MI, and others: Effect of sodium chloride in prevention of experimentally produced phosphate uroliths in male cats, *J Am Anim Hosp Assoc* 12:514-517, 1976.

192. Osborne CA, Polzin DJ: Prospective clinical evaluation of feline struvite urolith dissolution, *Proc Am Coll Vet Int Med* 1:4-11 to 4-16, 1986.

193. Buffington CA: Acid questions: potential dangers associated with cat food acidification, *Pet Food Ind*, 4-8, Sep-Oct 1993.

194. Osborne CAN, Polzin DJ, Kruger JM, and others: Relationship of nutritional factors to the cause, dissolution and prevention of feline uroliths and urethral plugs, *Vet Clin North Am Small Anim Pract* 19:561-581, 1989.

195. Osborne CA, Kruger JM, Polzin DJ, and others: Medical dissolution of feline struvite uroliths, *Minn Vet* 24:22-32, 1984.

196. Buffington CAT, Chew DJ: Lower urinary tract diseases in cats: the Ohio State experience, *Proc Ann Conf Vet Intern Med Forum*, 343-339, 1997.

197. Burger IH: Nutritional aspects of the feline urological syndrome (FUS), *J Small Anim Pract* 28:447-452, 1987.

198. Dow SW, Fettman MJ, Roger QR: Taurine depletion induced by experimental dietary potassium depletion and acidification of cats (abstract), *J Vet Intern Med*, 1040. 1989.

199. Dibartola SP, Buffington CA, Chow DJ: Development of chronic renal disease in cats fed a commercial diet, *J Am Vet Med Assoc* 202:744-750, 1993.

200. Dow SW, Fettman MJ, LeCouteur RS, and others: Potassium depletion in cats: renal and dietary influences, *J Am Vet Med Assoc* 191:1569, 1987.

201. Fettman MJ: Feline kaliopenic polymyopathy/nephropathy syndrome, *Vet Clin North Am Sm Anim Pract* 19:415-419, 1989.

202. Buffington CA: Feline struvite urolithiasis: effect of diet. In *Proceedings of the European Society of Veterinary Nephrology and Urology Annual Symposium*, Barcelona, Spain, 1988, Intercongress

203. Kurtz I, Maher T, Hutter HT: Effect of diet on plasma acid-base composition in normal humans, *Kidney Int* 24:670-680, 1983.

204. Ching SV, Fettman MJ, Hamar DW: The effect of chronic dietary acidification using ammonium chloride on acid-base and mineral metabolism in the adult cat, *J Nutr* 119:902-915, 1989.

205. Fettman MJ, Coble JM, Hamar DW, and others: Effect of dietary phosphoric acid supplementation on acid-base balance and mineral and bone metabolism in adult cats, *Am J Vet Res* 53:2125-2135, 1992.

206. Schwille PO, Hermann U: Environmental factors in the pathophysiology of recurrent idiopathic calcium urolithiasis (RCU) with emphasis on nutrition, *Urol Res* 20:72-76, 1992.

207. Weichselbaum RC, Feeney DA, Jessen CR, and others: Evaluation of the morphologic characteristics and prevalence of canine urocystoliths from a regional urolith center, *Am J Vet Res* 59:379-387, 1998.

208. Ling GV, Franti CE, Roy AL, and others: Urolithiasis in dogs. I. Mineral prevalence and interrelations of mineral composition, age and sex, *Am J Vet Res* 59:624-629, 1998.

209. Ling GV, Franti CE, Ruby AL, and others: Urolithiasis in dogs. II. Breed prevalence, and interrelations of breed, sex, age, and mineral composition, *Am J Vet Res* 59:630-642, 1998.

210. Osborne CA, Klausner JS, Polzin DJ, and others: Etiopathogenesis of canine struvite urolithiasis, *Vet Clin North Am Small Anim Pract* 16:67-86, 1986.

211. Weaver AD, Pillinger R: Relationship of bacterial infection in urine and calculi to canine urolithiasis, *Vet Rec* 97:48-50, 1975.

212. Clark WE: Staphylococcal infection of the urinary tract and its relations to urolithiasis in dogs, *Vet Rec* 95:204-206, 1974.

213. Osborne CA, Lulich JP, Bartges JW, and others: Canine and feline urolithiasis: relationship to etiopathogenesis to treatment and prevention. In Osborne CA, Finco DR, editors: *Canine and feline nephrology and urology*, Baltimore, 1995, Williams and Wilkins.

214. Ling GV, Franti CE, Johnson DL and Ruby AL: Urolithiasis in dogs. III. Prevalence of urinary tract infection and interrelations of infection, age, sex, and mineral composition, *Am J Vet Res* 59:643-649, 1998.

215. Ling GV, Franti CE, Johnson DL, and others: Urolithiasis in dogs. IV. Survey of interrelations among breed, mineral composition, and anatomic location of calculi, and presence of urinary tract infection, *Am J Vet Res* 59:650-660, 1998.

216. Escolar E: Structure and composition of canine urinary calculi, *Res Vet Sci* 49:327-333, 1990.

217. Lulich JP, Osborne CA, Carlson M, and others: Nonsurgical removal or urocystoliths in dogs and cats by voiding urohydropropulsion, *J Am Vet Med Assoc* 203:660-663, 1993.

218. Ling, GV: Urinary stone disease. In Ling GV: *Lower urinary tract disease of dogs and cats*, St Louis, 1995, Mosby.

219. Osborne CA, Klausner JS, Abdullahi S, and others: Medical dissolution and prevention of canine struvite uroliths. In RW Kirk, editor: *Current veterinary therapy IX*, Philadelphia, 1986, WB Saunders.

220. Osborne C: Feline calcium oxalate urolithiasis: perspectives from the Minnesota Urolith Center. In *Proceedings of the Petfood Forum*, Chicago, 1997, Watts Publishing.

221. Osborne C, Lulich J, Thumchai R, and others: Feline calcium oxalate uroliths: pathophysiology, clinical findings, diagnosis, treatment, and prevention, *Vet Clin Nutr* 1:105-114, 1994.

222. Buffington CAT: *Nutritional diseases and nutritional therapy in the cat*, ed 2, New York, 1995, Churchill Livingstone.

223. Bai SC, Sampson DA, Morris JF, and others: Vitamin B-6 requirement of growing kittens, *J Nutr* 119:1020-1027, 1989.

224. The Iams Company: *Eukanuba veterinary diets: product reference guide*, Lewisburg, Ohio, 1998, The Iams Company.

225. Marone CC: Effects of metabolic alkalosis on calcium excretion in the conscious dog, *J Lab Clin Med* 101:264-270, 1983.

226. Lulich J, Osborne C, Thumchai R, and others: Epidemiology of canine calcium oxalate urolithiasis: case study, *Proc Ann Conf Vet Intern Med Forum*, 490-492, 1995.

227. Bovee KC, McGuire T: Qualitative and quantitative analysis of uroliths in dogs: definitive determination of chemical type, *J Am Vet Med Assoc* 185:983-987, 1984.

228. Lulich JP, Osborne CA, Smith CL: Canine calcium oxalate urolithiasis: risk factor management. In Kirk RW, Bonagura JD, editors: *Current veterinary therapy XI*, Philadelphia, 1992, WB Saunders.

229. Hess RS, Kass PH, Ward CR: Association between hyperadrenocorticism and development of calcium-containing uroliths in dogs with urolithiasis, *J Am Vet Med Assoc* 212:1889-1891, 1998.

230. Klausner JS, Osborne CA: Canine calcium phosphate uroliths, *Vet Clin North Am Small Anim Pract* 16:171-180, 1986.

231. Buffington CA, Chew DJ: Lower urinary tract disease in cats: new directions, *Vet Clin Nut* 1:53-56, 1994.

232. Aldrich J, Ling GV, Ruby AL, and others: Silica-containing urinary calculi in dogs (1981-1993), *J Vet Int Med* 11:288-295, 1997.

233. Bovee KC, Thier SO, Rea C, and others: Renal clearance of amino acids in canine cystinuria, *Metabolism* 23:51-58, 1974.

234. Kirk RW: Nutrition and the integument, *J Small Anim Pract* 32:283-288, 1991.

235. Terpstra AHM, West CE, Fennis JTCM: Hypocholesterolemic effect of dietary soy protein versus casein in rhesus monkeys, *Am J Clin Nutr* 39:1-7, 1984.

236. Bauer JE, Covert SJ: The influence of protein and carbohydrate type on serum and liver lipids and lipoprotein cholesterol in rabbits, *Lipids* 19: 844-850, 1984.

237. White SD, Rosychuk RAW, Scott KV, and others: Effects of various proteins in the diet on fatty acid concentrations in the skin, cutaneous histology, clinicopathology and thyroid function in dogs. In Carey DP, Norton SA, Bolser SM, editors: *Recent advances in canine and feline nutritional research*, Proceedings of the Iams International Nutrition Symposium, Wilmington, Ohio, 1996, Orange Frazer Press.

238. Campbell KL, Czarnecki-Maulden GL, Schaeffer DJ: Effects of animal and soy fats and proteins in the diet on fatty acid concentrations in the serum and skin of dogs, *Am J Vet Res* 56:1465-1469, 1995.

239. Fadok VA: Treatment of canine idiopathic seborrhea with isotretinin, *Am J Vet Res* 47:1730-1733, 1986.

240. Strauss JS, Stranieri AM: Changes in long-term sebum production from isotretinin therapy, *J Am Acad Dermatol* 6:751-755, 1982.

241. Scott DW: Vitamin A-responsive dermatosis in the Cocker Spaniel, *J Am Anim Hosp Assoc* 22:125-129, 1986.

242. Ihrke PJ, Goldschmidt MH: Vitamin A-responsive dermatosis in the dog, *J Am Vet Med Assoc* 182:687-690, 1983.

243. Power HT, Ihrke PJ, Stannard AA, and others: Use of etretinate for treatment of primary keratinization disorders (idiopathic seborrhea) in Cocker Spaniels, West Highland White Terriers, and Basset Hounds, *J Am Vet Med Assoc* 201:419-429, 1992.

244. Parker W, Yager-Johnson JA, Hardy MH: Vitamin A responsive seborrheic dermatosis in the dog: a case report, *J Am Anim Hosp Assoc* 19:548-554, 1983.

245. Cho DY, Frey RA, Guffy MM, and others: Hypervitaminosis A in the dog, *Am J Vet Res* 36:1597-1603, 1975.

246. Kamm JJ: Toxicology, carcinogenicity, and teratogenicity of some orally administered retinoids, *J Am Acad Derm* 6:652-660, 1982.

247. Stewart LJ, White SD, Carpenter JL: Isotretinoin in the treatment of sebaceous adenitis in two Vizslas, *J Am Anim Hosp Assoc* 27:65-71, 1991.

248. Rosser EJ Jr: Sebaceous adenitis. In Kirk RW, Bonagura JD, editors: *Current veterinary therapy XI*, Philadelphia, 1992, WB Saunders.

249. Rosser EJ Jr, Dunston RW, Breen PT, and others: Sebaceous adenitis with hyperkeratosis in the Standard Poodle: a discussion of 10 cases, *J Am Anim Hosp Assoc* 23:341-345, 1986.

250. White SD, Rosychuk AS, Scott KV, and others: Sebaceous adenitis in dogs and results of treatment with isotretinoin and etretinate: 30 cases (1990-1994), *J Am Vet Med Assoc* 207:197-200, 1995.

251. Power HT, Ihrke PJ: Synthetic retinoids in veterinary dermatology, *Vet Clin North Am Small Anim Pract* 20:1525-1539, 1990.

252. Fiqueriredo C: Vitamin E serum contents, erythrocyte and lymphocyte count, PCV, and hemoglobin determinations in normal dog, dogs with scabies, and dogs with demodicosis. In *Proceedings of the Annual American Academy of Veterinary Dermatology and American College of Veterinary Dermatology*, 8, 1985.

253. Scott DW, Walton DK: Clinical evaluation of oral vitamin E for the treatment of primary canine acanthosis nigricans, *J Am Anim Hosp Assoc* 21:345-356, 1985.

254. National Research Council: *Nutrient requirements of dogs*, Washington, DC, 1985, National Academy of Sciences.

255. Ayres S, Mihan R: Is vitamin E involved in the autoimmune mechanism? *Cutis* 21:321-325, 1978.

256. Miller WH; Nonsteroidal antiinflammatory agents in the management of canine and feline pruritus. In Kirk RW, editor: *Current veterinary therapy*, Philadelphia, 1989, WB Saunders.

257. Van den Broek AHM, Thoday KL: Skin disease in dogs associated with zinc deficiency: a report of five cases, *J Small Anim Pract* 27:313-323, 1986.

258. Sousa CA, Stannard AA, Ihrke PJ: Dermatosis associated with feeding generic dog food: 13 cases (1981-1982), *J Am Vet Med Assoc* 192:676-680, 1988.

259. Robertson BT, Burns MJ: Zinc metabolism and zinc-deficiency syndrome in the dog, *Am J Vet Res* 24:997-1002, 1963.

260. Codner EC, Thatcher CD: Nutritional management of skin diseases, *Comp Cont Ed Pract Vet* 15:411-424, 1993.

261. Colombini S, Dunstan RW: Zinc-responsive dermatosis in northern-breed dogs: 17 cases (1990-1996), *J Am Vet Med Assoc* 211:451-453, 1997.

262. Lloyd DH: Essential fatty acids and skin disease, *J Small Anim Pract* 30:207-212, 1989.

263. Lands WEM: Omega-3 advances. In *Proceedings of the Petfood Forum*, Chicago, 1998, Watts Publishing.

264. Remillard RL: Omega 3 fatty acids in canine and feline diets: a clinical success or failure? *Vet Clin Nutr* 5:6-11, 1998

265. Sumida C, Graber R, Ninez E: Role of fatty acids in signal transduction: modulators and messengers, *Prost, Leuko and Essent Fatty Acids* 48:117-122, 1993.

266. Schoenherr WD, Jewell DE: Nutritional modification of inflammatory diseases, *Sem Vet Med Surg Small Anim* 12:212-222, 1997.

267. Bibus DM: Dietary control of eicosanoids. In *Proceedings of the Petfood Forum*, Chicago, 1997, Watts Publishing.

268. Yammamoto S, Hayashi Y, Takahashi Y: Reactions of mammalian lipoxygenases and cycloxygenases with various polyunsaturated fatty acids. In Sinclair A, Gibson R, editors: *Essential fatty acids and eicosanoids*, 1992, AOCS Press.

269. Lands WEM: Control of eicosanoid response intensity. In Vanderhoek J, editor: *Frontiers in bioactive lipids*, New York, 1996, Plenum Press.

270. Lands WEM, LeTellier RP, Rome LH, and others: Inhibition of prostaglandin biosynthesis, *Adv Biosci* 9:15-27, 1973.

271. Logas D, Beale KM, Bauer JE: Potential clinical benefits of dietary supplementation with marine-life oil, *J Am Vet Med Assoc* 199:1631-1636, 1991.

272. Boudreau MD, Chanmugam PS, Hart SB, and others: Lack of dose response by dietary n-3 fatty acids at a constant ratio of n-3 to n-6 fatty acids in suppressing eicosanoid biosynthesis from arachidonic acid, *Am J Clin Nutr* 54:111-117, 1991.

273. Waldron MK, Bauer JE, Hannah SS: Dietary PUFAs effects on neutrophil functions, *Proc Ann Conf Vet Intern Med Forum,* 753, 1996.

274. Bauer JE, McAlister K, Harte J: Differential metabolism of dietary omega-3 fatty acids by LCAT in polyunsaturated fat-supplemented dogs, *J Vet Int Med* 9:213, 1995.

275. Vaughn DM, Reinhart GA, Swaim SF, and others: Evaluation of dietary n-6 to n-3 fatty acid rations on leukotriene B synthesis in dog skin and neutrophils, *Vet Dermatol* 5:163-173, 1994.

276. Aked D, Foster SJ, Howarth A, and others: The inflammatory response of rabbit skin to topical arachidonic acid and its pharmacological modulation, *Brit J Pharmacol* 89:431-438, 1986.

277. Aked D, Foster, SJ: Leukotriene B4 and prostaglandin E2 mediate the inflammatory response of rabbit skin to intradermal arachidonic acid, *Brit J Pharmacol* 92:545-552, 1987.

278. Scott DW, Miller WH Jr, Griffin CE: Allergic skin disease in dogs and cats. In *Muller and Kirk's small animal dermatology*, Philadelphia, 1995, WB Saunders.

279. Chalmers S, Medleau L: Feline allergic dermatoses: diagnosis and treatment, *Vet Med* 84:399-403, 1989.

280. Chalmers SA, Medleau L: An update on atopic dermatitis in dogs, *Vet Med* 89:326-340, 1994.

281. Scott DW, Paradis M: A survey of canine and feline skin disorders seen in a university practice (1987-1988), *Can Vet J* 31:830-835, 1990.

282. Schwartzman RM: Immunologic studies of progeny of atopic dogs, *Am J Vet Res* 45:375-379, 1984.

283. Scott DW: Observations on canine atopy, *J Am Anim Hosp Assoc* 17:91-100, 1981.

284. Reedy LM, Miller WH Jr: *Allergic skin diseases of dogs and cats*, Philadelphia, 1989, WB Saunders.

285. Miller WH, Griffin GE, Scott DW, and others: Clinical trial of DVM derm caps in the treatment of allergic disease in dog: a nonblinded study, *J Am Anim Hosp Assoc* 25:163-168, 1989.

286. Scott DW, Buerger RG: Nonsteroidal anti-inflammatory agents in the management of canine pruritus, *J Am Anim Hosp Assoc* 24:425-428, 1988.

287. Miller WH, Scott DW, Wellington JR: Investigation on the antipruritic effects of ascorbic acid given alone and in combination with a fatty acid supplement to dogs with allergic skin disease, *Can Pract* 17:11-13, 1992.

288. Scott DW, Miller WH, Decker GA, and others: Comparison of the clinical efficacy of two commercial fatty acid supplements (EfaVet and DVM Derm Caps), evening primrose oil, and cold water marine fish oil in the management of allergic pruritus in dogs: a double-blinded study, *Cornell Vet* 82:319-329, 1992.

289. Paradis M, Lemay S, Scott DW: The efficacy of clemastine (Tavist), a fatty acid-containing product (DVM Derm Caps) and the combination of both products in the management of canine pruritus, *Vet Dermatol* 2:17-20, 1991.

290. Lloyd DH, Thomsett LR: Essential fatty acid supplementation in the treatment of canine atopy, *Vet Dermatol* 1:41-44, 1989.

291. Bond R, Lloyd DH: A double-blind comparison of olive oil and a combination of evening primrose oil and fish oil in the management of canine atopy, *Vet Rec* 131:558-560, 1992.

292. Campbell KL: Fatty acid supplementation and skin disease, *Vet Clin North Am Small Anim Pract* 20:1475-1486, 1990.

293. White PD: Essential fatty acids: use in management of canine atopy, *Comp Cont Ed Pract Vet* 15:451-457, 1993.

294. Taugbol O, Baddaky-Taugbol B, Saarem K: The fatty acid profile of subcutaneous fat and blood plasma in pruritic dogs and dogs without skin problems, *Can J Vet Res* 62:275-278, 1998.

295. Van den Broek AHM, Simpson JW: Fat absorption in dogs with atopic dermatitis, In Von Tscharner C, Halliwell REW, editors: *Advances in veterinary dermatology,* Philadelphia, 1990, Im Bailliere-Tindall.

296. Scott DW, Miller JR, Reinhart GA, and others: Effect of an omega-3/omega-6 fatty acid-containing commercial lamb and rice diet on pruritus in atopic dogs: results of a single-blinded study, *Can J Vet Res* 61:145-153, 1997.

297. Harvey RG: Effect of varying proportions of evening primrose oil and fish oil on cats with crusting dermatosis (miliary dermatitis), *Vet Rec* 133:208-211, 1993.

298. Harvey RG: Management of feline miliary dermatitis by supplementing the diet with essential fatty acids, *Vet Rec* 128:326-329, 1991.

299. Miller WH Jr, Scott DW, Wellington JR: Efficacy of DVM Derm Caps Liquid in the management of allergic and inflammatory dermatoses of the cat, *J Am Anim Hosp Assoc* 29:37-40, 1993.

300. Scott DW, Miller WH: Nonsteroidal management of canine pruritus: chlorpheniramine and a fatty acid supplement (DVM Derm Caps) in combination, and the fatty acid supplement at twice the manufacturers' recommended dosage, *Cornell Vet* 80:381-387, 1991.

301. Paradis M, Scott DW: Further investigations on the use of nonsteroidal and steroidal anti-inflammatory agents in the management of canine pruritus, *J Am Anim Hosp Assoc* 27:44-48, 1991.

302. Lloyd DH, Thomsett LR: Essential fatty acid supplementation in the treatment of canine atopy. A preliminary study, *Vet Dermatol* 1:41-44, 1989.

303. Scott DW, Buerger RG: Nonsteroidal anti-inflammatory agents in the management of canine pruritus, *J Am Anim Hosp Assoc* 24:425-428, 1988.

304. Vaughn DM, Reinhart GA: Dietary fatty acid ratios and eicosanoid production, *Proc Ann Conf Vet Intern Med Forum*, 1995.

305. Mooney MA, Vaughn DM, Reinhart GA, and others: Evaluation of the effects of omega-3 fatty acid-containing diets on the inflammatory stage of wound healing in dogs, *Am J Vet Res* 59:859-863, 1998.

306. Boureaux MK, Reinhart GA, Vaughn D, and others: The effects of varying dietary n-6 to n-3 fatty acid ratios on platelet reactivity, coagulation screening assays, and antithrombin III activity in dogs, *J Am Anim Hosp Assoc* 33:235-243, 1997.

307. Schick MP, Schick RP, Reinhart GA: The role of polyunsaturated fatty acids in the canine epidermis: normal structural and functional components, inflammatory disease state components, and as therapeutic dietary components. In *Recent advances in canine and feline nutritional research*, Proceedings of the Iams International Nutrition Symposium, Wilmington, Ohio, 1996, Orange Frazer Press.

308. Halliwell REW: Management of dietary hypersensitivity in the dog, *J Small Anim Nutr* 33:156-160, 1992.

309. Reinhart GA: New concepts in managing common pet allergies, *Proc Conv Can Vet Med Assoc*, 9-14, 1995.

310. Wills J, Harvey R: Diagnosis and management of food allergy and intolerance in dogs and cats, *Aus Vet J* 71:322-326, 1994.

311. Reedy LM, Miller WH: Food hypersensitivity. In *Allergic skin diseases in dogs and cats*, Philadelphia, 1989, WB Saunders.

312. Muller GH, Kirk RW, Scott DW: *Small animal dermatology*, ed 4, Philadelphia, 1989, WB Saunders.

313. Walton GS: Skin responses in the dog and cat due to ingested allergens: observations on one hundred confirmed cases, *Vet Rec* 81:709-713, 1967.

314. Scott DW: Immunologic skin disorders in the dog and cat, *Vet Clin North Am Small Anim Pract* 8:641-664, 1978.

315. Baker E: Food allergy, *Vet Clin North Am Small Anim Pract* 4:79-89, 1974.

316. August JR: Dietary hypersensitivity in dogs: cutaneous manifestations, diagnosis and management, *Comp Cont Ed Pract Vet* 7:469-477, 1985.

317. Rosser EJ: *Proceedings of the Annual Meeting of the American College of Veterinary Dermatology*, San Francisco, 47, 1990.

318. White SD: Food hypersensitivity in 30 dogs, *J Am Vet Med Assoc* 188:695-698, 1986.

319. Harvey RG: Food allergy and dietary intolerance in dogs: a report of 25 cases, *J Small Anim Pract* 34:175-179, 1993.

320. Rosser EJ: Diagnosis of food allergy in dogs, *J Am Vet Med Assoc* 203:259-262, 1993.

321. Doering GG: Food allergy: where does it fit as a cause of canine pruritus? *Pet Vet,* 10-16, May/June 1991.

322. Halliwell REW, Gorman NT: *Veterinary clinical immunology*, Philadelphia, 1989, WB Saunders.

323. Jeffers JG, Shanley KJ, Meyer EK: Diagnostic testing of dogs for food hypersensitivity, *J Am Vet Med Assoc* 198:245-250, 1991.

324. Hodgkins E: Food allergy in cats: considerations, diagnosis and management, *Pet Vet,* 24-28, Nov/Dec 1991.

325. Carlotti DN, Remy I, Prots C: Food allergy in dogs and cats: a review and report of 43 cases, *Vet Dermatol* 1:55-62, 1990.

326. Jeffers JG, Meyer EK, Sosis EJ: Responses of dogs with food allergies to single-ingredient dietary provocation, *J Am Vet Med Assoc* 209:608-611, 1996.

327. Leib MS, August JR: Food hypersensitivity. In Ettinger SJ, editor: *Textbook of veterinary internal medicine*, ed 3, Philadelphia, 1989, WB Saunders.

328. Johnson LW: Food allergy in a dog: diagnosis by dietary management, *Mod Vet Pract* 68:236-239, 1987.

329. Scott DW: Feline dermatology 1983-1985, *J Am Anim Hosp Assoc* 23:255-274, 1987.

330. Kunkle G, Horner S: Validity of skin testing for diagnosis of food allergy in dogs, *J Am Vet Med Assoc* 200:677-680, 1992.

331. Walton GS: Skin diseases of domestic animals: skin manifestations of allergic response in domestic animals, *Vet Rec* 82:204-207, 1968.

332. Polzin DJ, Osborne CA, Bartges JW, and others: Chronic renal failure. In Ettinger SJ, Feldman EC, editors: *Textbook of veterinary internal medicine*, ed 4, Philadelphia, 1995, WB Saunders.

333. Squires RA: Uraemia, In Bainbridge J, Elliott J, editors: *BSVAV manual of canine and feline nephrology and urology*, Ames, Iowa, 1996, Iowa State University Press.

334. Ross LA, Finco DR: Relationship of selected clinical renal function tests to glomerular filtration rate and renal blood flow in cats, *Am J Vet Res* 42:1023-1026, 1981.

335. Senior DF: Chronic renal failure in dogs, *Proc Cong World Small Anim Vet Assoc*, 40-45, 1998.

336. Reinhart GA, Sunvold GD: New methods for managing canine chronic renal failure, *Proc Cong World Small Anim Vet Assoc*, 46-51, 1998.

337. Bovee KC: The uremic syndrome: patient evaluation and treatment, *Comp Cont Ed Pract Vet* 1:279-283, 1979.

338. Krawiec DR: Quantitative renal function tests in cats, *Comp Cont Educ Vet Pract* 16:1279-1284, 1994.

339. Carey, DP: Clinical assessment of chronic renal failure. In Reinhart GA, Carey DP, editors: *Recent advances in canine and feline nutrition*, vol 2, Iams Nutrition Symposium Proceedings, Wilmington, Ohio, 1998, Orange Frazer Press.

340. Cowgill LD, Spangler WL: Renal insufficiency in geriatric dogs, *Vet Clin North Am Sm Anim Med* 11:727-749, 1981.

341. Finco DR, Coulter DB, Barsanti JA: Simple, accurate method for clinical estimation of glomerular filtration rate in the dog, *Am J Vet Res* 42:1874-1877, 1981.

342. Finco DR, Brown SC, Crowell WA, and others: Exogenous creatinine clearance as a measure of glomerular filtration rate in dogs with reduced renal mass, *Am J Vet Res* 52:1029-1032, 1991.

343. Watson ADJ, Lefebre HP, Laroute V, and others: Comparison of clearance tests to assess glomerular filtration rate in dogs, *Proc Ann Conf Vet Intern Med Forum*, 711, 1998.

344. Brown SA, Finco DR, Boudinot FD: Evaluation of a single injection method, using inoxol, for estimating glomerular filtration rate in cats and dogs, *Am J Vet Res* 57:105-110, 1996.

345. Brown SA, Finco DR, Crowell WA, and others: Dietary protein intake and the glomerular adaptations to partial nephrectomy in dogs, *J Nutr* 121:S125-S127, 1991.

346. Brown SA, Finco D, Crowell WA: Single-nephron adaptations to partial renal ablation in the dog, *Am J Physiol* 258:F495-F503, 1990.

347. White JV, Finco DR, Brown SA, and others: Effect of dietary protein on kidney function, morphology, and histopathology during compensatory renal growth in dogs, *Am J Vet Res* 52:1357-1365, 1990.

348. Hostetter TH, Olson JL, Rennke HG: Hyperfiltration in remnant nephrons: a potentially adverse response to renal ablation, *Am J Physiol* 241:F85-F92, 1981.

349. Olivetti GP, Anversa P, Rigamonti W, and others: Morphometry of the renal corpuscle during normal postnatal growth and compensatory hypertrophy, *J Cell Biol* 75:573-585, 1977.

350. Churchill J, Polzin D, Osborne C, and others: The influence of dietary protein intake on progression of chronic renal failure in dogs, *Semin Vet Med Surg Sm Anim* 7:244-250, 1992.

351. Brown SA: Dietary protein restriction: some unanswered questions, *Semin Vet Med Surg Sm Anim* 7:237-243, 1992.

352. Anderson S, Brenner BM: The role of intraglomerular pressure in the initiation and progression of renal disease, *J Hypertens* 4(suppl 5):S236-S238, 1986.

353. Brenner BM, Meyer TW, Hostetter TH: Dietary protein intake and the progressive nature of renal disease: the role of hemodynamically mediated glomerular injury in the pathogenesis of progressive glomerular sclerosis in aging, renal ablation and intrinsic renal disease, *N Engl J Med* 307:652-659, 1982.

354. Shimamura T, Morrison AB: A progressive glomerulosclerosis occurring in partial five-sixths nephrectomized rats, *Am J Pathol* 79:95-106, 1975.

355. Remuzzi G: Glomerular hypertrophy and progression: summary and concluding remarks, *Kidney Int* 45:S30-S31, 1994.

356. Brown SA, Brown CA: Single-nephron adaptations to partial renal ablation in cats, *Am J Physiol* 269:R1002-R1008, 1995.

357. Gonin-Jmaa D, Senior DF: The hyperfiltration theory: progression of chronic renal failure and the effects of diet in dogs, *J Am Vet Med Assoc* 207:1411-1415, 1995.

358. Finco DR, Crowell WA, Barsanti JA: Effects of three diets on dogs with induced chronic renal failure, *Am J Vet Res* 46:646-653, 1985.

359. Polzin DJ, Leininger JR, Osborne CA, and others: Development of renal lesions in dogs after $^{11}/_{12}$ reduction in renal mass, *Lab Invest* 58:172-183, 1988.

360. Brown SA, Walton C, Crawfod P, and others: Long-term effects of anti-hypertensive regimens on renal hemodynamics and proteinuria in diabetic dogs, *Kidney Int* 43:1210-1218, 1993.

361. Gaber L, Walton C, Brown S, and others: Effects of antihypertensive agents on the morphologic progression of diabetic nephropathy in dogs, *Kidney Int* 46:161-169, 1994.

362. Bourgoignie JJ, Gavellas G, Martinex E, and others: Glomerular function and morphology after renal mass reduction in dogs, *Lab Clin Med* 109:380-388, 1987.

363. Maeda H, Gleiser CA, Masoro EJ, and others: Nutritional influences on aging of Fischer 344 rats. II. Pathology, *J Gerontol* 40:671-688, 1985.

364. Masoro EJ, Iwasaki K, Gleiser CA, and others: Dietary modulation of the progression of nephropathy in aging rats: an evaluation of the importance of protein, *Am J Clin Nutr* 49:1217-1227, 1989.

365. Bovee KC, Kronfeld DS, Ramberg CF, and others: Long term measurement of renal function in partially nephrectomized dogs fed 56, 27 or 19% protein, *Invest Nephrol* 16:378-385, 1979.

366. Robertson JL, Goldschmidt M, Kronfeld DS, and others: Long term renal responses to high dietary protein in dogs with 75% nephrectomy, *Kidney Int* 29:511-519, 1986.

367. Polzin DJ, Osborne CA, Hayden DW: Influence of reduced protein diets on morbidity, mortality, and renal function in dogs with induced chronic renal failure, *Am J Vet Res* 45:506-517, 1984.

368. Tucker SM, Mason RL, Beauchene RE: Influence of diet and feed restriction on kidney function of aging male rats, *J Gerontol* 31:264-270, 1976.

369. Berg BN, Simms HS: Nutrition and longevity in the rat. II. Longevity and onset of disease with different levels of food intake, *J Nutr* 71:255-263, 1960.

370. Tapp DC, Kobayoshu S, Fernandes S: Protein restriction or calorie restriction? A critical assessment of the influence of selective calorie restriction on the progression of experimental renal disease, *Semin Nephrol* 9:343-353, 1989.

371. Adams LG, Polzin DJ, Osborne CA, and others: Effects of dietary protein and calorie restriction in clinically normal cats and in cats with surgically induced chronic renal failure, *Am J Vet Res* 54:1653-1662, 1993.

372. Adams LG, Polzin DJ, Osborne CA, and others: Influence of dietary protein/calorie intake on renal morphology and function in cats with 5.6 nephrectomy, *Lab Invest* 70:347-357, 1994.

373. Finco DR, Brown SC, Brown CA, and others: Protein and calorie effects on progression of induced chronic renal failure in cats, *Am J Vet Res* 59:575-582, 1998.

374. Osborne CA, Polzin DJ, Abdullahi S, and others: Role of diet in management of feline chronic polyuric renal failure: current status, *J Am Anim Hosp Assoc* 18:11-20, 1982.

375. Reinhart GA, Sunvold GD: New methods for managing chronic renal failure, *Proc North Am Vet Conf*, Orlando, Fla, 17-20, 1998.

376. Finco DR: Renal function in geriatric dogs—are there dietary protein effects?, *Vet Clin Nutr* 1:66-68, 1994.

377. Sheffy BE, Williams AJ, Zimmer JF, and others: Nutrition and metabolism of the geriatric dog, *Cornell Vet* 75:324-347, 1985.

378. Finco DR, Brown SA, Crowell WA, and others: Effects of aging and dietary protein intake on uninephrectomized geriatric dogs, *Am J Vet Res* 55:1282-1290, 1994.

379. Polzin DJ, Osborne CA, Lulich JP: Effects of dietary protein/phosphate restriction in normal dogs and dogs with chronic renal failure, *J Small Anim Pract* 32:289-295, 1991.

380. Lau K: Phosphate excess and progressive renal failure: the precipitation-calcification hypothesis, *Kidney Int* 36:918-937, 1989.

381. Brown SA, Crowell WA, Barsanti JA: Beneficial effects of dietary mineral restriction in dogs with marked reduction of functional renal mass, *J Am Soc Nephrol* 1:1169-1179, 1991.

382. Finco DR, Brown SA, Crowell WA, and others: Effect of phosphorus/calcium-restricted and phosphorus/calcium-replete 32% protein diets in dogs with chronic renal failure, *Am J Vet Res* 53:157-163, 1992.

383. Finco DR, Brown SC, Crowell WA, and others: Effects of dietary phosphorus and protein in dogs with chronic renal failure, *Am J Vet Res* 153:2264-2271, 1992.

384. Ross LA, Finco DR, Crowell WA: Effect of dietary phosphorus restriction on the kidneys of cats with reduced renal mass, *Am J Vet Res* 43:1023-1026, 1982.

385. French SW, Yamanaka W, Ostred R: Dietary induced glomerularsclerosis in the guinea pig, *Arch Pathol* 83:204-210, 1967.

386. Heifets M, Morrissey JJ, Parkerson ML, and others: Effect of dietary lipids on renal function in rats with subtotal nephrectomy, *Kidney Int* 32:335-341, 1987.

387. Brown SA: Managing chronic renal failure: the role of dietary polyunsaturated fatty acids, *Proc NAVC*, Orlando, Fla, 5-8, 1998.

388. Fries JWU, Sandstrom DJ, Meyer TW, and others: Glomerular hypertrophy and epithelial cell injury modulate progressive glomerulosclerosis in the rat, *Lab Invest* 60:205-218, 1989.

389. Barcelli U, Miyata J, Ito Y, and others: Beneficial effects of polyunsaturated fatty acids in partially nephrectomized rats, *Prostaglandins* 32.211 219, 1986.

390. Clark WF, Parbani A, Philbrick DJ, and others: Chronic effects of omega-3 fatty acids (fish oil) in a rat 5/6 renal ablation model, *J Am Soc Nephrol* 1:1343-1353, 1991.

391. Logan JL, Michael UF, Benson B: Dietary fish oil interferes with renal arachidonic acid metabolism in rats: correlation with renal physiology, *Metabolism* 41:382-389, 1992.

392. Donadio JV, Bergstralh EJ, Offord KP, and others: A controlled trial of fish oil in IgA nephropathy, *New Engl J Med* 331:1194-1199, 1994.

393. Clark WF, Parabtani A, Maylor CD, and others: Fish oil in lupus nephritis: clinical findings and methodological implications, *Kidney Int* 44:75-86, 1993.

394. Brown SA: Influence of dietary fatty acids on intrarenal hypertension. In Reinhart GA, Carey DP, editors: *Recent advances in canine and feline nutrition*, vol 2, Iams Nutrition Symposium Proceedings, Wilmington, Ohio, 1998, Orange Frazer Press.

395. Brown SA, Brown CA, Crowell WA, and others: Beneficial effects of chronic administration of dietary omega-3 polyunsaturated fatty acids in dogs with renal insufficiency, *J Lab Clin Med*, 131:447-455, 1998.

396. Bauer J, Crocker R, Markwell P, and others: Dietary n-6 fatty acid supplementation improves ultrafiltration in spontaneous canine chronic renal failure (abstract), *J Vet Int Med* 11:2, 1997.

397. Dworkin L, Benstein J, Tolbert E, and others: Salt restriction inhibits renal growth and stabilizes injury in rats with established renal disease, *J Am Soc Nephrol* 7:437-442, 1996.

398. Lulich J, Osborne C, O'Brien T, and others: Feline renal failure: questions, answers, questions, *Compend Cont Edu Pract Vet* 14:127-152, 1992.

399. Dow SW, Fettman MJ, Smith KR, and others: Effects of dietary acidification and potassium depletion on acid-base balance, mineral metabolism, and renal function in adult cats, *J Nutr* 120:569-578, 1990.

400. Finco DR: Chronic renal failure: dietary protein and phosphorus, *Proc NAVC*, Orlando, Fla, 9-10, 1998.

401. Carey DP: Clinical assessment of chronic renal failure. In Reinhart GA, Carey DP, editors: *Recent advances in canine and feline nutrition*, vol 2, Iams Nutrition Symposium Proceedings, Wilmington, Ohio, 1998, Orange Frazer Press.

402. Hansen B, Dibartola SP, Chew DJ, and others: Clinical and metabolic findings in dogs with chronic renal failure fed two diets, *Am J Vet Res* 53:326-334, 1992.

403. National Research Council: *Nutrient requirements of dogs*, Washington, DC, 1974, National Academy of Sciences.

404. Polzin DJ, Osborne CA: Update—conservative medical management of chronic renal failure. In Kirk RW, editor: *Current veterinary therapy VI*, Philadelphia, 1986, WB Saunders.

405. Polzin DJ, Osborne CA: Current progress in slowing progression of canine and feline chronic renal failure, *Comp Anim Pract* 3:52-62, 1988.

406. Bovee KC: Diet and kidney failure. In *Kal Kan Symposium for the Treatment of Dog and Cat Diseases*, Vernon, Calif, 1977, Kal Can Foods.

407. Polzin DJ, Osborne CA, Stevens JB, and others: Influence of modified protein diets on the nutritional status of dogs with induced chronic renal failure, *Am J Vet Res* 44:1694-1702, 1983.

408. Devaux C, Polzin DJ, Osborne CA: What role does dietary protein play in the management of chronic renal failure in dogs? *Vet Clin North Am Small Anim Pract* 26:1247-1267, 1996.

409. Kronfeld DS: Dietary management of chronic renal disease in dogs: a critical appraisal, *J Small Anim Pract* 34:211-219, 1993.

410. Harte J, Markwell P, Moraillion R, and others: Dietary management of naturally occurring chronic renal failure in cats, *J Nutr* 124:2660S-2662S, 1994.

411. Polzin DJ, Osborne CA, Lulich JP: Diet therapy guidelines for cats with chronic renal failure, *Vet Clin North Am Small Anim Pract* 26:1269-1275, 1996.

412. Keane WF, Kasiske BL, O'Donnell MP: Hyperlipidemia and the progression of renal disease, *Am J Clin Nutr* 47:157-160, 1987.

413. Brown SC, Brown CA, Crowell WA, and others: Does modifying dietary lipids influence the progression of renal failure?, *Vet Clin North Am Small Anim Pract* 26:1277-1285, 1996.

414. Kaplan MA, Canterbury JM, Bourgoignie JJ: Reversal of hyperparathyroidism in response to dietary phosphorus restriction in the uremic dog, *Kidney Int* 15:43-48, 1979.

415. Nagode LA, Chew DJ, Podell M: Benefits of calcitriol therapy and serum phosphorus control in dogs and cats with chronic renal failure, *Vet Clin North Am Small Anim Pract* 26:1293-1331, 1996.

416. Titens I, Livesey G, Eggum BO: Effects of the type and level of dietary fibre supplements on nitrogen retention and excretion patterns, *Brit J Nutr* 75:461-469, 1996.

417. Younes H, Remesey C, Behr S, and others: Fermentable carbohydrate exerts a urea-lowering effect in normal and nephrectomized rats, *Am J Physiol* 272:G515-G525, 1997.

418. Assismon SA, Stein TP: Digestible fiber (gum arabic), nitrogen excretion and urea cycling in rats, *Nutr* 10:544-550, 1994.

419. Bliss DZ, Stein TP, Schleifer CR, and others: Supplementation with gum arabic fiber increases fecal nitrogen excretion and lowers serum urea nitrogen concentration in chronic renal failure patients consuming a low-protein diet, *Am J Clin Nutr* 63:392-398, 1996.

420. Howard MD, Sunvold GD, Reinhart GA, and others: Effect of fermentable fiber consumption by the dog on nitrogen balance and fecal microbial nitrogen excretion, *FASEB J* 10:A257, 1996.

421. Sunvold GD, Fahey GC Jr, Merchen NR, and others: Dietary fiber for dogs. IV. In vitro fermentation of selected fiber sources by dog fecal inoculum and in vivo digestion and metabolism of fiber-supplemented diets, *J Anim Sci* 73:1099-1109, 1995.

422. Hallman JE, Moxley RA, Reinhart GA, and others: Cellulose, beet pulp and pectin/gum arabic effects on canine colonic microstructure and histopathology, *J Vet Clin Nutr* 2:137-142, 1995.

423. Howard MD, Kerley MS, Mann FA, and others: Dietary fiber sources alter colonic blood flow and epithelial cell proliferation of dogs, *J Anim Sci* 75:170, 1997.

424. Muir HE, Murray SM, Fahey GC Jr, and others: Nutrient digestion by ileal cannulated dogs as affected by dietary fibers with various fermentation characteristics, *J Anim Sci* 74:1641-1648, 1996.

425. Brown SA, Reinhart GA, Haag M, and others: Influence of dietary fermentable fiber on nitrogen excretion in dogs with chronic renal insufficiency. In Reinhart GA, Carey DP, editors: *Recent advances in canine and feline nutrition*, vol 2, Iams Nutrition Symposium Proceedings, Wilmington, Ohio, 1998, Orange Frazer Press.

426. Tetrick MA, Sunvold GD, Reinhart GA: Clinical experience with canine renal patients fed a diet containing a fermentable fiber blend. In Reinhart GA, Carey DP, editors: *Recent advances in canine and feline nutrition*, vol 2, Iams Nutrition Symposium Proceedings, Wilmington, Ohio, 1998, Orange Frazer Press.

427. Sunvold GD, Fahey Jr GC, Merchen NR, and others: Dietary fiber for cats: in vitro fermentation of selected fiber sources by cat fecal inoculum and in vivo utilization of diets containing selected fiber sources and their blends, *J Anim Sci* 73:2329-2339, 1995.

428. Smith RC, Haschem T, Hamlin RL, and others: Water and electrolyte intake and output and quantity of feces in the healthy dog, *Vet Med Small Anim Clin* 59:743-748, 1964.

429. Mitchell AR: Salt intake, animal health and hypertension: should sleeping dogs lie? In Burger IH, Rivers JPW, editors: *Nutrition of the dog and cat*, New York, 1989, Cambridge University Press.

430. Hubbard BS, Vulgamott JC: Feline hepatic lipidosis, *Comp Cont Ed Pract Vet* 14:459-464, 1992.

431. Zawie D, Garvey M: Feline hepatic disease, *Vet Clin North Am Small Anim Pract* 14:1201-1230, 1984.

432. Dimski DS, Taboada J: Feline idiopathic hepatic lipidosis, *Vet Clin North Am Small Anim Pract* 25:357-373, 1995.

433. Center SA, Crawford MA, Guida L, and others: A retrospective study of 77 cats with sever hepatic lipidosis, *Am J Vet Res* 5:724-731, 1993.

434. Biourge V, Pion P, Lewis J, and others: Spontaneous occurrence of hepatic lipidosis in a group of laboratory cats, *J Vet Int Med* 7:194-197, 1993.

435. Center SA: Feline hepatic lipidosis, *Vet Ann* 33:244-254, 1993.

436. Thornburg LP, Simpson S, Digilo K: Fatty liver syndrome in cats, *J Am Anim Hosp Assoc* 18:397-400, 1982.

437. Hall JA, Barstad LA, Voller BE, and others: Lipid composition of liver and adipose tissues from normal cats and cats with hepatic lipidosis (abstract), *J Vet Int Med* 6:127, 1992.

438. Hall JA, Barstad LA, Connor WE: Lipid composition of hepatic and adipose tissues from normal cats and cats with idiopathic hepatic lipidosis, *J Vet Int Med* 11:238-242, 1997.

439. Biourge V: Sequential findings in cats with hepatic lipidosis, *Fel Pract* 21:25-28, 1993.

440. Biourge V, Groff JM, Munn R, and others: Experimental induction of feline hepatic lipidosis, *Am J Vet Res* 55:1291-1302, 1994.

441. Hardy PM: Diseases of the liver and their treatment. In Ettinger SJ, editor: *Textbook of veterinary internal medicine*, Philadelphia, 1989, WB Saunders.

442. Alpers DH, Sabesin SM: Fatty liver: biochemical and clinical aspects: In Schiff L, Schiff ER, editors, *Diseases of the liver*, ed 6, Philadelphia, 1987, Lippincott.

443. Biourge VC, Massat B, Groff JM, and others: Effects of protein, lipid, or carbohydrate supplementation on hepatic lipid accumulation during rapid weight loss in obese cats, *Am J Vet Res* 55:1405-1415, 1994.

444. Chapoy PR, Angelini C, Brown WJ: Systemic carnitine deficiency—a treatable inherited lipid storage disease presenting as Reye's syndrome, *N Engl J Med* 303:1389-1394, 1980.

445. Jacobs G, Cornelius L, Keene B, and others: Comparison of plasma, liver, and skeletal muscle carnitine concentrations in cats with idiopathic hepatic lipidosis and in healthy cats, *Am J Vet Res* 51:1349-1351, 1991.

446. Jacobs G, Cornelius L, Allen S, and others: Treatment of idiopathic hepatic lipidosis in cats: 11 cases (1986-1987), *J Am Vet Med Assoc* 195:635-638, 1989.

447. Biourge V: Feline hepatic lipidosis. In *Proceedings of the Petfood Forum*, Chicago, 1996, Watts Publishing.

448. Cornelius LM, Rogers K: Idiopathic hepatic lipidosis in cats, *Mod Vet Pract* 66:377-380, 1985.

449. Bauer JE, Schenck P: Nutritional management of hepatic disease, *Vet Clin North Am Small Anim Pract* 19:513-527, 1989.

450. Barsanti J, Jones B, Spano J, and others: Prolonged anorexia associated with hepatic lipidosis in three cats, *Fel Pract* 7:52-57, 1977.

451. Evans KL, Cornelius LM: Dietary management of feline idiopathic hepatic lipidosis, *Fel Pract* 18:5-10, 1990.

452. Armstrong P, Hand M, Frederick G: Enteral nutrition by tube, *Vet Clin North Am Small Anim Pract* 20:237-275, 1990.

453. Biourge B, MacDonald M, King L: Feline hepatic lipidosis: pathogenesis and nutritional management, *Compend Contin Educ Pract Vet* 12:1244-1258, 1990.

454. Center S: Feline liver disorders and their management, *Compend Contin Educ Pract Vet* 8:889-902, 1986.

455. Wolf AM: Hepatic lipidosis, *Vet Med Rep* 1:67-70, 1988.

456. Crossley DA: Survey of feline dental problems encountered in a small animal practice in NW England, *Brit Vet Dent Assoc J* 2:2, 1991.

457. Harvey CE, Emily PP: Periodontal disease. In Harvey CE, Emily PP, editors: *Small animal dentistry*, St Louis, 1993, Mosby.

458. DeBowes LJ, Mosier D, Logan E, and others: Association of periodontal disease and histologic lesions in multiple organs from 45 dogs, *J Vet Dent* 13:57-60, 1996.

459. Watson ADJ: Diet and periodontal disease in dogs and cats: part 2, *Vet Clin Nutr* 5:11-13, 1998.

460. Okuda A, Harvey CE: Etiopathogenesis of feline dental resorptive lesions, *Vet Clin North Am Small Anim Pract* 22:1385-1404, 1992.

461. Lyon KF: Subgingival odontoclastic resorptive lesions: classification, treatment, and results in 58 cats, *Vet Clin North Am Small Anim Pract* 22:1417-1432, 1992.

462. Watson ADJ: Diet and periodontal disease in dogs and cats: part 1, *Vet Clin Nutr* 4:135-137, 1997.

463. Rosenberg HM, Rehfeld CE, Emmering TE: A method for the epidemiologic assessment of periodontal health-disease state in a Beagle hound colony, *J Periodontal* 37:208-213, 1966.

464. Lindhe J, Hamp SE, Loe H: Plaque induced periodontal disease in Beagle dogs: a 4-year clinical, roentgenographical and histometrical study. *J Periodontal Res* 10:243-255, 1975.

465. Golden AL, Stoller N, Harvey CE: A survey of oral and dental diseases in dogs anaesthetized at a veterinary hospital, *J Am Anim Hosp Assoc* 18:891-899, 1982

466. Hennet PR, Delille B, Favot JL: Oral malodor measurements of a tooth surface of dogs with gingivitis, *Am J Vet Res* 59:255-257, 1998.

467. Lund EM, Bohacek LK, Dahlke JL: Prevalence and risk factors for odontoclastic resorptive lesions in cats, *J Am Vet Med Assoc* 212:392-395, 1998.

468. Van Wessum R, Harvey CE, Hennet P: Feline dental resorptive lesions: prevalence patterns, *Vet Clin North Am Small Anim Pract* 22:1405-1417, 1992.

469. Perez G: Results from a home audit survey of pets and their care, *Watham Centre Pet Nutr Data*, 1996.

470. Spouge JD: Halitosis: a review of its cause and treatment, *Dent Pract Dent Rec* 15:307-317, 1964.

471. Attia EL, Marshall KG: Halitosis, *Can Med Assoc J* 126:1281-1285, 1982.

472. Tonaetich J, Carpenter PAW: Production of volatile sulfur compounds from cysteine, cystine and methionine by human dental plaque, *Arch Oral Biol* 16:599-601, 1971.

473. Rosenberg, M: Clinical assessment of bad breath: current concepts, *J Am Dent Assoc* 127:475-482, 1996.

474. McNamara TF, Alexander FE, Lee M: The role of microorganisms in the production of oral malodor, *Oral Surg* 34:41-48, 1972.

475. DeBoever EH, Deuzeda M, Losche WJ: Relationship between volatile sulfur compounds, BANA-hydrolyzing bacteria and gingival health in patients with and without complaints of oral malodor, *J Clin Dent* 4:114-119, 1994.

476. Culham N, Rawlings JM: Oral malodor and its relevance to periodontal disease in the dog, *J Vet Dent* 15:165-168, 1998.

477. Hennet PR, Delille B, Davor JL: Oral malodor measurements on a tooth surface of dogs with gingivitis, *Am J Vet Res* 59:255-257, 1998.

478. Culham N, Rawlings JM: Studies of oral malodor in the dog, *J Vet Dent* 15:169-173, 1998.

479. Marsh P, Martin M. In *Oral microbiology*, London, 1992, Chapman and Hall.

480. Kleinberg I, Westbay G: Oral malodor, *Crit Rev Oral Bio Med* 1:247-260, 1990.

481. Ng W, Tonzetich J: Effect of hydrogen sulfide and methyl mercaptan on the permeability of oral mucosa, *J Dent Res* 63:994-997, 1984.

482. Black AP, Crichlow AM, Saunders JR. In *J Am Anim Hosp Assoc* 16:611, 1980.

483. Harari J, Gustafson SB, Meinkoth K. In *Feline Pract* 19:27, 1991.

484. Colmery B, Frost P: Periodontal disease: etiology and pathogenesis, *Vet Clin North Am Small Anim Pract* 16:817-834, 1986.

485. Hamlin RL: Identifying the cardiovascular and pulmonary diseases that affect old dogs, *Vet Med* 483-497, 1990.

486. Calvert CA, Greene CE: Bacteremia in dogs: diagnosis, treatment and prognosis, *Comp Cont Ed Pract Vet* 8:179-186, 1986.

487. Harvey CE: Feline dental resorptive lesions, *Semin Vet Med Small Anim* 8:187-196, 1993.

488. Okuda A, Harvey CE: Etiopathogenesis of feline dental resorptive lesions, *Vet Clin North Am Small Anim Pract* 22:1385-1401, 1992.

489. Reichart PA, Durr UM, Triadan H, and others: Periodontal disease in the domestic cat: a histopathologic study, *J Periodontal Res* 19:67-75, 1984.

490. Schneck GW: Neck lesions in teeth of cats, *Vet Rec* 99:100-107, 1976.

491. Page RC, Schroeder HE: *Periodontitis in man and other animals*, Basel, 1982, Verlag Karger.

492. Zetner K, Steurer I: The influence of dry food on the development of feline neck lesions, *J Vet Dent* 9:4-6, 1992.

493. Holstrom SE: External osteoclastic resorptive lesions, *Feline Pract* 20:7-11, 1992.

494. Okuda A, Asari M, Harvey CE: Challenges in treatment of external odontoclastic resorptive lesions in cats, *Compend Cont Ed Pract Vet* 17:1461-1469, 1995.

495. Lyon KF: Subgingival odontoclastic resorptive lesions: classification, treatment and results in 58 cats, *Vet Clin North Am Small Anim Pract* 22:1417-1432, 1992.

496. Hamp SF, Lindhe J, Loe H: Long-term effect of chlorhexidine on developing gingivitis in the Beagle dog, *J Periodont Res* 8:63-70, 1973.

497. Robinson JGA: Chlorhexidine gluconate—the solution for dental problems, *J Vet Dent* 12:29-31, 1995.

498. Burwasser P, Hill TJ: The effect of hard and soft diets on the gingival tissues of dogs, *J Dent Res* 18:389-393, 1939.

499. Engelberg J: Local effect of diet on early plaque formation and development of gingivitis in dogs, *Odont Rev* 16:31-50, 1965.

500. Krasse B, Brill N. In *Odont Rev* 11:152. 1960.

501. Japanese Small Animal Veterinary Association: *Survey on the health of pet animals*, 1985.

502. Studer E, Stapley RB: The role of dry foods in maintaining healthy teeth and gums in the cat, *Vet Med Small Anim Clin* 68:1124-1126, 1973.

503. Boyce EN. In *Vet Clin North Am Small Anim Pract* 22:1309, 1982.

504. Harvey CE, Shofer FS, Laster L: Correlation of diet, other chewing activities and periodontal disease in North American client-owned dogs, *J Vet Dent* 13:101-105, 1996.

505. Lage A, Lausen N, Tracy R, and others: Effect of chewing rawhide and cereal biscuit on removal of dental calculus in dogs, *J Am Vet Med Assoc* 197:213-219, 1990.

506. Gorrel C, Rawlings JM: The role of tooth-brushing and diet in the maintenance of periodontal health in dogs, *J Vet Dent* 13:139-143, 1996

507. Gorrel C, Rawlings JM: The role of a "dental hygiene chew" in maintaining periodontal health in dogs, *J Vet Dent* 13:31-34, 1996.

508. Goldstein GS: The effect of rawhide strips on the removal and prevention of plaque and calculus, *Proc Vet Dent*, Auburn, Ala, 1993.

509. Samuelson AC, Cutter GR. In *J Nutr* 121:S162, 1991.

510. Stookey GK, Warrick JM, Miller LL, and others: Hexametaphosphate-coated biscuits significantly reduce calculus formation in dogs, *J Vet Dent* 13:27-30, 1996.

511. Stookey GK, Warrick JM, Miller LL: Sodium hexametaphosphate reduces calculus formation in dogs, *Am J Vet Res* 56:913-918, 1995.

512. Legeros RZ, Shannon IL: The crystalline components of dental calculi: human vs. dog, *J Dent Res* 58:2371-2377, 1979.

513. Jensen L, Logan E, Finney O, and others: Reduction in accumulation of plaque, stain, and calculus in dogs by dietary means, *J Vet Dent* 12:161-163, 1995.

514. Simone A, Jensen L, Setser C, and others: Assessment of oral malodor in dogs, *J Vet Dent* 11:71-74, 1994.

515. Rawlings JM, Gorrel C, Markwell PJ: Effect of two dietary regimens on gingivitis in the dog, *J Small Anim Pract* 38:147-151, 1997.

516. Donoghue S, Scarlett JM, Williams CA, and others: Diet as a risk factor for feline external odontoclastic resorption (abstract), *J Nutr* 124:2693S-2694S, 1994.

517. Zetner K, Steurer I: Role of commercial dry cat food in the pathogenesis of feline neck lesions, *Prakt Tierarzt* 73:289-297, 1992.

518. Hall TJ, Chambes TJ: Optimal bone resorption by isolated rat osteoclasts requires chloride/bicarbonate exchange, *Calcified Tissue Int* 45:378-380, 1989.

519. Dellmann HD, Brown EM. In *Textbook of veterinary histology*, Philadelphia, 1987, Verlag Lea and Febiger.

520. Aller S: Dental home care and preventive strategies, *Sem Vet Med Surg Small Anim* 8:204-212, 1993.

521. Hefferren JJ, Boyce E, Bresnahan ME: Aging and oral health, *Vet Clin Nutr* 3:97-100, 1996.

522. Korman KS: The role of supra gingival plaque in the prevention and treatment of periodontal disease, *J Periodont Res* 16(supp):5-22, 1986.

523. Tromp, JA, van Run LJ, Jansen J: Experimental gingivitis and frequency of tooth brushing in the Beagle dog model: clinical findings, *J Clin Periodont* 13:190-194, 1986.

524. Corba NHC, Jansen J, Pilot T: Artificial periodontal defects and frequency of tooth-brushing in Beagle dogs. I. Clinical findings after creation of the defects, *J Clin Peridont* 13:158-163,1986.

525. Corba NHC, Jansen J, Pilot T: Artificial periodontal defects and frequency of tooth-brushing in Beagle dogs. II. Clinical findings after a period of healing, *J Clin Peridont* 13:186-189,1986.

526. Sanges G: A pilot study on the effect of tooth-brushing on the gingiva of a Beagle dog, *Scand J Dent Res* 84:106-108, 1976.

527. Briner W: Effect of chlorhexidine on plaque, gingivitis, and alveolar bone loss in Beagle dogs after seven years of treatment, *J Periodont Res* 15:390-394, 1980.

528. Tepe JH, Loenard G, Singer R, and others: The long-term effect of chlorhexidine on plaque, gingivitis, sulcus depth, gingival recession and loss of attachment in Beagle dogs, *J Periodont Res* 18:452-458, 1983.

529. Reed JH: A review of the experimental use of antimicrobial agents in the treatment of periodontitis and gingivitis in the dog, *Can Vet J* 29:705-708, 1988.

530. Cummins D, Creeth JE: Delivery of antiplaque agents from dentifrices, gels and mouthwashes, *J Dent Res* 71:1439-1449, 1992.

531. Guilford WG: New ideas for the dietary management of gastrointestinal tract disease, *J Small Anim Pract* 35:620-624, 1994.

532. Reinhart GA, Sunvold GD: The role of diet in the treatment of gastrointestinal disease in dogs, *Proc NAVC,* Orlando, Fla, 23-28, 1996.

533. Williams DA: Malabsorption, small intestinal bacterial overgrowth, and protein-losing enteropathy. In Guilford WG, Center SA, Strombeck DR, and others, editors: *Small animal gastroenterology*, ed 3, Philadelphia, 1996, WB Saunders.

534. Simpson JW: Role of nutrition in aetiology and treatment of diarrhoea, *J Small Anim Pract* 33:167-171, 1992.

535. Rutgers HC, Batt RM, Kelly DF: Lymphocytic-plasmacytic enteritis associated with bacterial overgrowth in a dog, *J Am Vet Med Assoc* 192:1739-1742, 1988.

536. Williams DA: Clinical diagnosis of canine small intestinal disease. In Reinhart GA, Carey DP, editors: *Recent advances in canine and feline nutrition*, vol 2, Iams Nutrition Symposium Proceedings, Wilmington, Ohio, 1998, Orange Frazer Press.

537. Melgarejo T, Williams DA, Setchell KD, and others: Serum total unconjugated bile acids (TUBA) in dogs with small intestinal bacterial overgrowth, *J Vet Int Med* 11:114, 1997.

538. Johnston KL: Small intestinal bacterial overgrowth, *Vet Clin North Am Small Anim Pract* 29:523-551, 1999.

539. Gruffy DD, Jones TJ, Papasouliotis K, and others: The uniqueness of the feline gut and its practical implications. In *Proceedings of the Gastrointestinal Health Symposium: a pre-conference symposium*, 31-35, 1997, World Veterinary Conference.

540. Toskes PP, Donaldson RM Jr: Enteric bacterial flora and bacterial overgrowth syndrome. In Sleisenger MH, Fordtran JS, editors: *Gastrointestinal disease*, ed 5, Philadelphia, 1989, WB Saunders.

541. Rutgers HC, Batt RM, Elwood CM, and others: Small intestinal bacterial overgrowth in dogs with chronic intestinal disease, *J Am Vet Med Assoc* 206:187-193, 1995.

542. Johnston L, Lamport A, Batt RM: Unexpected bacterial flora in the proximal small intestine of normal cats, *Vet Rec* 132:362-363, 1993.

543. Balish E, Cleven D, Brown J, and others: Nose, throat, and fecal flora of Beagle dogs housed in locked or open environments, *Appl Environ Micro* 34:207, 1977.

544. Terada A, Hara H, Kato S, and others: Effects of lactosucrose (4-beta-D-galactosylsucrose) on fecal flora and fecal putrefactive product of cats, *J Vet Med Sci* 55:291-295, 1993.

545. Batt R, Rutgers H, Sancak A: Enteric bacteria: friend or foe?, *J Small Anim Pract* 37:261-267, 1996.

546. Wolin MJ: Volatile fatty acids and the inhibition of *Escherichia coli* growth by rumen fluid, *Appl Microbiol* 17:83-87, 1969.

547. Twedt DC: *Clostridium perfringens* associated diarrhea in dogs, *Proc Ann Conf Vet Intern Med Forum*, 121-125, 1993.

548. Rogers WA, Stradley RP, Sherding RG, and others: Simultaneous evaluation of pancreatic exocrine function and intestinal absorptive function in dogs with chronic diarrhea, *J Am Vet Med Assoc* 177:1128-1131, 1980.

549. Batt RM: Exocrine pancreatic insufficiency, *Vet Clin North Am Small Anim Pract* 23:595-608, 1993.

550. Watson ADJ, Church DB, Middleton DJ, and others: Weight loss in cats which eat well, *J Small Anim Pract* 22:473-482, 1981.

551. Remillard RL, Thatcher CD: Dietary and nutritional management of gastrointestinal disease, *Vet Clin North Am Small Anim Pract* 19:797-816, 1989.

552. Steiner JM, Williams DA: Feline exocrine pancreatic disorders: insufficiency, neoplasia and uncommon conditions, *Compend Cont Ed Pract Vet* 19:836-846, 1997.

553. Rimaila-Parnanen E, Westermarck E: Pancreatic degenerative atrophy and chronic pancreatitis in dogs: a comparative study of 60 cases, *Acta Vet Scand* 23:400-406, 1982.

554. Hill FWG, Osborne AD, Kidder DE: Pancreatic degenerative atrophy in dogs, *J Compar Path* 81:321-330, 1971.

555. Williams DA: Feline exocrine pancreatic insufficiency. In Kirk RW, Bonagura JD, editors: *Current veterinary therapy XII*, Philadelphia, 1995, WB Saunders.

556. Fox JN, Mosley JG, Vogler GA, and others: Pancreatic function in domestic cats with pancreatic fluke infection, *J Am Vet Med Assoc* 178:58-60, 1981.

557. Williams DA, Batt RM, McLean L: Bacterial overgrowth in the duodenum of dogs with exocrine pancreatic insufficiency, *J Am Vet Med Assoc* 191:201-206, 1987.

558. King CE, Toskes PP: Small intestine bacterial overgrowth, *Gastroenterology* 76:1035-1055, 1979.

559. Murdoch DB: Large intestinal disease. In Thomas DA, Simpson JW, Hall EJ, editors: *Manual of canine and feline gastroenterology*, UK, 1996, British Small Animal Veterinary Association.

560. Williams DA, Batt RM: Sensitivity and specificity of radio-immuno-assay of serum trypsin-like immunoreactivity for the diagnosis of canine exocrine pancreatic insufficiency, *J Am Vet Med Assoc* 192:195-201, 1988.

561. Steiner JM, Williams DA: Validation of a radio-immuno-assay for feline trypsin-like immunoreactivity (fTLI) and serum cobalamin and folate concentrations in cats with exocrine pancreatic insufficiency (EPI), *J Vet Intern Med* 9:193, 1995.

562. Simpson JW: Diet and large intestinal disease in dogs and cats, *J Nutr* 128:2717S-2722S, 1998.

563. Richter KP: Lymphocytic-plasmacytic enterocolitis in dogs, *Sem Vet Med Surg Small Anim*, 7:134-144,1992.

564. Johnson SE: Canine eosinophilic gastroenterocolitis, *Sem Vet Med Surg Small Anim* 7:145-152, 1992.

565. Breitschwerdt EB: Immunoproliferative enteropathy of Basenjis, *Sem Vet Med Surg Small Anim* 7:153-161, 1992.

566. Van Kruiningen HJ, Ryan MJ, Shindel NM: The classification of feline colitis, *J Compar Path* 93:275-294 1983.

567. Dimski DS: Therapy for inflammatory bowel disease, In Kirk RW, Bonagura JD: *Current veterinary therapy XII*, Philadelphia, 1995, WB Saunders.

568. Tams TR: Chronic feline inflammatory bowel disorders. II.   Feline eosinophilic enteritis and lymphosarcoma, *Compend Cont Ed Pract Vet* 8:464-471, 1986.

569. Burrows CF: Canine colitis, *Compend Contin Ed Pract Vet* 2:1347-1354, 1992.

570. Magne ML: Pathophysiology of inflammatory bowel disease, *Sem Vet Med Surg Small Anim* 7:112-116, 1992.

571. Simpson JW, Maskell IE, Markwell PJ: Use of a restricted antigen diet in the management of idiopathic canine colitis, *J Small Anim Pract* 35:233-238, 1994.

572. Nelson RW, Dimperio ME, Long GG: Lymphocytic-plasmacytic colitis in the cat, *J Am Vet Med Assoc* 184:1133-1135, 1984.

573. Barnett KC, Joseph EC: Keraconjunctivitis sicca in the dog following 5-amino salicylate administration, *Hum Toxicol* 6:377-383, 1987.

574. Bush BM: Colitis in the dog. In Grunshell CSG, Hill FWG, Raw ME, editors: *The veterinary annual*, UK, 1985, Scientechnia.

575. Batt RM: Diagnosis and management of malabsorption in dogs, *J Small Anim Pract* 33:161-166, 1992.

576. Fossum T: Protein-losing enteropathy, *Sem Vet Med Surg Small Anim* 4:219-225, 1989.

577. Guilford WG: Effect of diet on inflammatory bowel diseases, *Vet Clin Nutr* 4:58-61, 1997.

578. Leib MS, Hay WH, Roth L: Plasmacytic-lymphocytic colitis in dogs. In Bonagura J: *Current veterinary therapy X*, Philadelphia, 1989, WB Saunders.

579. Simpson JW: Management of colonic disease in the dog, *Waltham Focus* 5:17-22, 1995.

580. Nelson RW, Stookey LJ, Kazacos E: Nutritional management of idiopathic chronic colitis in the dog, *J Vet Int Med* 2:133-137, 1988.

581. Guilford WG: Effects of diet on inflammatory bowel disease, *Proc Ann Conf Vet Intern Med Forum*, 50-51, 1996.

582. Bisset SA, Guilford WG, Lawoko CR, and others: Effect of food particle size on carbohydrate assimilation assessed by breath hydrogen testing in dogs, *Vet Clin Nutr* 4:82-88, 1997.

583. Washabau RJ, Strombeck DR, Buffington CA, and others: Evaluation of intestinal carbohydrate malabsorption in the dog by pulmonary hydrogen gas excretion, *Am J Vet Res* 47:1402-1405, 1986.

584. Batt RM, Carter MW, McLean L: Wheat-sensitive enteropathy in Irish Setter dogs: possible age-related brush border abnormalities, *Res Vet Sci*, 39:80-83, 1985.

585. Hall EJ, Batt RM: Development of wheat-sensitive enteropathy in Irish Setters: biochemical changes, *Am J Vet Res*, 51:983-989, 1990.

586. Sherding RG: Diseases of the intestines. In *The cat diseases and their clinical management*, New York, 1989, Churchill Livingstone.

587. Reinhart GA, Sunvold GD: Practical applications of omega-3 and fermentable fiber in gastrointestinal patients.   In *Proceedings of the Gastrointestinal Health Symposium: a pre-conference symposium*, 1997, World Veterinary Congress.

588. Vilaseca J, Salas A, Guarner F, and others: Dietary fish oil reduces progression of chronic inflammatory lesions in a rat model of granulomatous colitis, *Gut* 31:539-544, 1990.

589. Rampton DS, Collins CE: Review article: thromboxanes in inflammatory bowel disease-pathogenic and therapeutic implications, *Ailment Pharmacol Ther* 7:357-367, 1993.

590. O'Moran CA: Nutritional therapy in ambulatory patients, *Digest Dis Sci* 32:95-99, 1987.

591. Aslan AC, Triadafilopoulos G: Fish oil fatty acid: supplementation in active ulcerative colitis; a double blind controlled, cross-over study, *Am J Gastroenterol* 87:432, 1992.

592. Hillier K, Jewel R, Forrell L, and others: Incorporation of fatty acids from fish oil and olive oil into colonic mucosal lipids and effects upon eicosanoid synthesis in inflammatory bowel disease, *Gut* 32:1151, 1991.

593. Stenson WF, Cort D, Rodgers J, and others: Dietary supplementation with fish oil in ulcerative colitis, *Ann Intern Med* 116:609-614,

594. Brown DH: Applications of fructooligosaccharides in human foods. In Carey DP, Norton SA, Bolser SM, editors: *Recent advances in canine and feline nutritional research*, Proceedings of the Iams International Nutrition Symposium, Wilmington, Ohio, 1996, Orange Frazer Press.

595. Reinhart GA, Moxley RA, Clemens ET. Source of dietary fiber and its effects on colonic microstructure, function and histopathology of Beagle dogs, *J Nutr* 24:2701S-2703S, 1994.

596. Clemens ET: Dietary fiber and colonic morphology. In Carey DP, Norton SA, Bolser SM, editors: *Recent advances in canine and feline nutritional research*, Proceedings of the Iams International Nutrition Symposium, Wilmington, Ohio, 1996, Orange Frazer Press.

597. Murdoch DB: Large intestinal disease. In Thomas DA, Simpson JW, Hall EJ, editors: *Manual of canine and feline gastroenterology*, UK, 1996, British Small Animal Veterinary Association.

598. Sunvold GD, Titgemeyer EC, Bourquin LD, and others: Fermentability of selected fibrous substrates by cat fecal microflora. *J Nutr* (suppl):2721S-2722S, 1994.

599. Bergman EN: Energy contributions of volatile fatty acids from the gastrointestinal tract in various species, *Physiol Rev* 70:567-590, 1990.

600. Hague S, Singh B, Parskeva C: Butyrate acts as a survival factor for colonic epithelial cells: further fuel for the *in vivo* versus *in vitro* debate, *Gastroenterology* 112:1036-1040, 1997.

601. Sakata T. Stimulatory effect of short-chain fatty acids on epithelial cell proliferation in the rat intestine: a possible explanation for trophic effect of fermentable fibre, gut microbes and luminal trophic factors, *Br J Nutr* 58:95-103, 1987.

602. Hallman JE, Moxley RA, Reinhart GA, and others: Cellulose, beet pulp and pectin/gum arabic effects on canine colonic microstructure and histopathology, *Vet Clin Nutr* 2:137-142, 1995.

603. Hallman JE, Reinhart GA, Wallace EA, and others: Colonic mucosal tissue energetics and electrolyte transport in dogs fed cellulose, beet pulp or pectin/gum arabic as their primary fiber source, *Nutr Res* 16:303-313, 1996.

604. Clemens ET. Dietary fiber and colonic morphology. In Carey DP, Norton SA, Bolser SM, editors: *Recent advances in canine and feline nutritional research*, Proceedings of the Iams International Nutrition Symposium, Wilmington, Ohio, 1996, Orange Frazer Press.

605. Kripke S, Fox A, Berman J and others: Stimulation of dietary fiber and its effect on colonic growth with intracolonic infusion of short chain fatty acids, *JPEN* 13:109-116, 1988.

606. Koruda M, Rolandelli R, Settle R, and others: Ther effect of short chain fatty acids on the small bowel mucosa, *Am J Clin Nut* 51:685-690, 1990.

607. Kamath PS, Hoepfner MT, Phillips SF: Short-chain fatty acids stimulate motility of the canine ileum, *Am J Physiol* 253:G427-G433, 1987

608. Cherbut C: Effects of short-chain fatty acids on gastrointestinal motility. In Cummins JH, Rombear JL, Sakata T, editors: *Physiological and clinical aspects of short-chain fatty acids*, Cambridge, UK, 1995, Cambridge University Press.

609. Kvietys PR, Granger DN: Effect of volatile fatty acids on blood flow and oxygen uptake by the dog colon, *Gastroenterology* 80:962-969, 1981.

610. Roediger WEW, Rae DA: Trophic effect of short-chain fatty acids on mucosal handling of ions by the defunctioned colon, *Brit J Surg* 69:23-25, 1982

611. Izat AL, Tidwell NM, Thomas RA, and others: Effects of a buffered propionic acid in diets on the performance of broiler chicks and on microflora of the intestine and carcass, *Poultry Sci* 69:818-826, 1990.

612. Kerley MS, Sunvold GD: Favorably modifying gut flora with a novel fiber (FOS). In *Proceedings of the Gastrointestinal Health Symposium: a pre-conference symposium*, 1997, World Veterinary Congress.

613. Blomberg L, Henriksson A, Conway PL: Inhibition of adhesion of *Escherichia coli* K88 to piglet ileal mucus by *Lactobacillus* spp., *Appl Environ Micro* 59:34-39, 1993.

614. Kerley MS, Sunvold GD: Physiological response to short-chain fatty acid production in the intestine. In Carey DP, Norton SA, Bolser SM, editors: *Recent advances in canine and feline nutritional research*, Proceedings of the Iams International Nutrition Symposium, Wilmington, Ohio, 1996, Orange Frazer Press.

615. Buddington RK, Sunvold GD: Fermentable fiber and the gastrointestinal tract ecosystem. In Reinhart GA, Carey DP, editors: *Recent advances in canine and feline nutrition*, vol 2, Iams Nutrition Symposium Proceedings, Wilmington, Ohio, 1998, Orange Frazer Press.

616. Chapman MAS, Grahn MF, Boyle MA, and others: Butyrate oxidation is impaired in the colonic mucosa of suffers of quiescent ulcerative colitis, *Gut* 35:73, 1994.

617. Scheppach WH, Sommer T, Kirchner GM, and others: Effect of butyrate enemas on the colonic mucosa in distal ulcerative colitis, *Gastroenterology* 103:51-56, 1992.

618. Rolandelli RH, Koruda MJ, Settle G, and others: The effect of enteral feedings supplemented with pectin on the healing of colonic anastomoses in the rat, *Surgery* 99:703, 1986.

619. Mitsuoka T, Hidaka H, Eida T: Effect of fructooligosaccharides on intestinal microflora, *Die Nahrung* 31:427-436, 1987.

620. Okazaki M, Fujikawa S, Matumoto N: Effect of xyloogliosaccharide on the growth of bifidobacteria, *Bifidobacteria Microflora* 9:77-86, 1990.

621. Hidaka H, Hirayaa M, Tokunaga T, and others: The effects of indigestible fructooligosaccharides on intestinal microflora and various physiological functions on human health. In Furda I, editor: *New developments in dietary fiber*, New York, 1990, Plenum Press.

622. Hidaka H, Eida T, Takizawa T, and others: Effects of fructooligosaccharides on intestinal flora and human health, *Bifidobacteria Microflora* 10:37-50, 1986.

623. Terada A, Hara H, Oishi T, and others: Effect of dietary lactosucrose on fecal flora and fecal metabolites of dogs, *Micro Ecol Health Dis* 5:87-92, 1992.

624. Gruffydd-Jones TJ, Papasouliotis K, Sparkes AH: Characterization of the intestinal flora of the cat and its potential for modification. In Reinhart GA, Carey DP, editors: *Recent advances in canine and feline nutrition*, vol 2, Iams Nutrition Symposium Proceedings, Wilmington, Ohio, 1998, Orange Frazer Press.

625. Sparkes AH, Papasouliotis K, Sunvold G, and others: The effect of dietary supplementation with fructo-oligosaccharides on the fecal flora of healthy cats, *Am J Vet Res* 59:436-440, 1998.

626. Willard MD, Simpson RB, Delles EK, and others: Effects of dietary supplementation of fructo-oligosaccharides on small intestinal bacterial overgrowth in dogs, *Am J Vet Res* 55:654-659, 1992.

627. Buddington RK, Buddington KK, Sunvold GD: The influence of fermentable fiber on the small intestine of the dog: intestinal dimensions and transport of glucose and proline, *Am J Vet Res* 60:354-358, 1999.

628. Sunvold GD, Reinhart GA: Maintaining gastrointestinal health via colonic fermentation, *Proc World Small Anim Vet Assoc,* 7-12, 1997.

629. Canine Practice: Tumors in dogs, *Canine Pract* 21:30-31, 1996.

630. DeWys WD: Weight loss and nutritional abnormalities in cancer patients: incidence, severity and significance, *Clin Oncol* 5:251-161, 1986.

631. Ogilvie GK, Vail DM: Unique metabolic alterations associated with cancer cachexia in the dog, In Kirk RE, editor: *Current veterinary therapy XI,* Philadelphia, 1992, WB Saunders.

632. Ogilvie GK: Paraneoplastic syndromes. In Ettinger S, Feldman E: *Textbook of veterinary internal medicine,* ed 4, Philadelphia, 1999, WB Saunders.

633. Crow SE, Oliver J: Cancer cachexia, *Compend Cont Ed Pract Vet* 43:2004-2012, 1979.

634. Vail DM, Ogilvie GK, Wheeler SL: Metabolic alterations in patients with cancer cachexia, *Compend Cont Ed Pract Vet* 12:381-387,1990.

635. Kokal WA: The impact of antitumor therapy on nutrition, *Cancer* 55:273-278, 1985.

636. Trant AS, Serin J, Douglass HO: Is taste related to anorexia in cancer patients?, *Am J Clin Nut* 36:45-58, 1982.

637. Bernstein IL: Etiology of anorexia in cancer, *Cancer* 58:1881-1886, 1986.

638. Ogilvie GK: Interventional nutrition for the cancer patient, *Clin Tech Small Anim Pract* 13:224-231, 1998.

639. Vail DM, Ogilvie GK, Wheeler SL, and others: Alterations in carbohydrate metabolism in canine lymphoma, *J Vet Intern Med* 4:8-11, 1990.

640. Zyliez S, Schwantje O, Wagener DJT, and others: Metabolic response to enteral food to different phases of cancer cachexia in rats, *Oncology* 47:87-91, 1990.

641. Hansell DT, Davies JWL, Barns J, and others: The oxidation of body fuel stores in cancer patients, *Ann Surg* 204:637-642, 1986.

642. Heber D, Byerley LO, Chi J, and others: Pathophysiology of malnutrition in the adult cancer patient, *Cancer* 58:1867-1873, 1986.

643. Burt ME, Lowry SF, Gorschboth C, and others: Metabolic alterations in a noncachectic animal tumor system, *Cancer* 47:2138-2146, 1981.

644. Singh J, Grigor MR, Thompson MP: Glucose homeostasis in rats bearing a transplantable sarcoma, *Cancer Res* 40:1699-1706, 1980.

645. Norton JA, Maher M, Wesley R, and others: Glucose intolerance in sarcoma patients, *Cancer* 55:3022-3027, 1984.

646. Inculet RI: Gluconeogenesis in the tumor-influenced rat hepatocyte: importance of tumor burden, lactate, insulin and glucagon, *J Nat Cancer Inst* 79:1039-1046, 1989.

647. Ogilvie GK, Walters LM, Salman MD, and others: Treatment of dogs with lymphoma with adriamycin and a diet high in carbohydrate or high in fat, *Am J Vet Res* 8:95-104, 1994.

648. Kurzer M, Meguid MM: Cancer and protein metabolism, *Surg Clin North Am* 66:969-1001, 1986.

649. Landel AM, Hammong WG, Meguid MM: Aspects of amino acid and protein metabolism in cancer-bearing states, *Cancer* 55:230-237, 1985.

650. Norton JA: The influence of tumor-bearing on protein metabolism in the rat, *J Surg Res* 30:456-462. 1981.

651. Norton JA, Stein TP, Brennan MF: Whole body protein synthesis and turnover in normal and malnourished patients with and without known cancer, *Ann Surg* 194:123-128, 1981.

652. Warren RS, Jeemvanandam M, Brennan MF: Protein synthesis in the tumor-influenced hepatocyte, *Surgery* 98:275-281, 1985.

653. Ogilvie GK, Vail DM, Wheeler SL, and others: Alterations in fat and protein metabolism in dogs with cancer, *Proc Vet Cancer Soc,* Estes Park, Col, 1988.

654. Ogilvie GK, Walters LM, Salman MD: Alterations in select aspects of carbohydrate, lipid and amino acid metabolism in dogs with non-hematopoietic malignancies, *Am J Vet Res* 8:62-66, 1994.

655. Ogilvie GK, Vail DM: Nutrition and cancer: recent developments, *Vet Clin North Am Small Anim Pract* 20:969-985, 1990.

656. McAndrew PF: Fat metabolism and cancer, *Surg Clin North Am* 66:1003-1012, 1986.

657. Alexopoulos CG, Blatsios B, Avgerinos A: Serum lipids and lipoprotein disorders in cancer patients, *Cancer* 60:3065-3070, 1987.

658. Alexander HR: Substrate alterations in a sarcoma-bearing rat model: effect of tumor growth and resection, *J Surg Res* 48:471-475, 1990.

659. Younes RN: Lipid kinetic alteration in tumor-bearing rats: reversal by tumor excision, *J Surg Res* 48:324-328, 1990.

660. Kern KA, Norton JA: Cancer cachexia, *J Parenteral Nut* 12:286-298, 1988.

661. Ford RB, Babineau C, Ogilvie GK, and others: Serum lipid profiles in dogs with lymphoma, *Proc Vet Canc Soc,* Raleigh, NC, 1989.

662. Lowell JA, Parnes HL, Blackburn GL: Dietary immunomodulation: beneficial effects on carcinogenesis and tumor growth, *Crit Care Med* 18:S145-S148, 1990.

663. Ramesh G, Das UN, Koratkar R, and others: Effect of essential fatty acids on tumor cells, *Nutrition* 8:343-347, 1992.

664. Begin ME, Ellis G, Das UN, and others: Differential killing of human carcinoma cells supplemented with n-e and n-6 polyunsaturated fatty acids, *J Nat Cancer Inst* 77:2053-2057, 1986.

665. Plumb JA, Luo W, Kerr DJ: Effect of polyunsaturated fatty acids on the drug sensitivity of human tumor cell lines resistant to either cisplastin or doxorubicin, *Brit J Cancer* 67:728-733, 1993.

666. Tisdale MJ, Brennan RA, Fearon KC: Reduction of weight loss and tumor size in a cachexia model by a high fat diet, *Brit J Cancer* 56:39-43, 1987.

667. Roush GC, Pero RW, Powell J, and others: Modulation of the cancer susceptibility measure, adenosine diphosphate ribosyl transferase (ADPRT), by differences in n-3 and n-6 fatty acids, *Nutr Cancer* 16:197-207, 1991.

668. Daly JM, Lieberman, M, Goldfinc J, and others: Enteral nutrition with supplemental arginine, RNA, and omega-3 fatty acids: a prospective clinical trial, *Proc Amer Con Parenteral Enteral Nut JPEN* 15:19S, 1991.

669. Mauldin GE: Feeding the cancer patient. In Carey DP, Norton SA, Bolser SM, editors: *Recent advances in canine and feline nutritional research*, Proceedings of the Iams International Nutrition Symposium, Wilmington, Ohio, 1996, Orange Frazer Press.

670. Anderson CR, Ogilvie GK, LaRue SM, and others; Effect of fish oil and arginine on acute effects of radiation injury in dogs with neoplasia: a double blind study, *Proc Vet Cancer Soc,* Chicago, Ill, 1997.

671. Del Ray A, Besedovsky H: Interleukin 1 affects glucose homeostasis, *Am J Physiol* 253:R794-R798, 1987.

672. Beutler B, Cerami A: Cachectic tumor necrosis factor: an endogenous mediator of shock and inflammation, *Immunol Res* 5:281-293, 1986.

673. Reinhart GA, Hayek MG: Nutritional support in the critical care patient, *Proc XXI Cong World Small Anim Vet Assoc,* 66-68, 1996.

674. Arbeit JM: Resting energy expenditure in controls and cancer patients with localized and diffuse diseases, *Ann Surg* 199:292-298, 1984.

675. Dempsey DT, Knox LS, Mullen JL, and others: Energy expenditure in malnourished patients with colorectal cancer, *Arch Surg* 121:789-795, 1986.

676. Hansell DT, Davies JWL, Durns HJG: The relationship between resting energy expenditure and weight loss in benign and malignant disease, *Ann Surg* 203:240-245, 1986.

677. Delarue J, Lerebours E, Till H, and others: Effect of chemotherapy on resting energy expenditure in patients with non-Hodgkins lymphoma, *Cancer* 65:2455- 2459, 1990.

678. Ogilvie GK: Energy metabolism in diseased and critically ill dogs: new horizons, *Vet Clin Nutr* 4:138-142, 1997.

679. Ogilvie GK, Walters LM, Fettman MJ, and others: Energy expenditure in dogs with lymphoma fed two specialized diets, *Cancer* 71:3146-3152, 1993.

680. Ogilvie GK, Salman MD, Fettman MJ, and others: Resting energy expenditure in dogs with non-hematopoietic malignancies before and after excision of tumors, *Am J Vet Res* 57:1463-1467, 1996.

681. Rossi-Fanelli F, Cascino A, Muscaritoli M: Abnormal substrate metabolism and nutritional strategies in cancer management, *JPEN* 15:680-683, 1991.

682. Dempsey DT, Mullen JL: Macro nutrient requirements in the malnourished cancer patient, *Ann Surg* 55:290-294, 1985.

683. Shein PS: The oxidation of body fuel stores in cancer patients, *Ann Surg* 204:637-642, 1986.

684. Donahue S: Nutritional support of hospitalized patients, *Vet Clin North Am Small Anim Pract* 19:475-495, 1989.

685. Tachibana K, Mukai K, Hirauka I, and others: Evaluation of the effect of arginine enriched amino acid solution on tumor growth, *JPEN* 9:428-434, 1985.

686. Heyman SN, Rosen S, Silva P, and others: Protective effect of glycine in cisplastin nephrotoxicity, *Kidney Internat* 40:273-279, 1991.

687. Barbul A, Isto DA, Wasserkrug HL, and others: Arginine stimulates lymphocyte immune response in healthy human beings, *Surgery* 90:244-251, 1981.

688. Buffington CAT: Enteral nutritional support, *Vet Clin Nutr* 3:10-13, 1996.

689. Lippert AC, Armstorng PJ: Parenteral nutritional support. In Kirk RW, editor: *Current veterinary therapy X*, Philadelphia, 1989, WB Saunders.

690. Wheeler SL, McGuire BM: Enteral nutritional support. In Kirk RW, editor: *Current veterinary therapy X*, Philadelphia, 1989, WB Saunders.

691. Lippert AC: Total parenteral nutrition in clinically normal cats, *J Am Vet Med Assoc* 194:669-676, 1989.

692. Lippert AC, Fulton RB, Parr AM: A retrospective study of the use of total parenteral nutrition in dogs and cats, *J Vet Int Med* 7:52-64, 1993.

693. Vail DM, Ogilvie GK, Fettman MJ, and others: Exacerbation of hyperlactatemia by infusion of lactated Ringer's solution in dogs with lymphoma, *J Vet Int Med* 4:228, 1990.

APPENDIX

1

ESTIMATED METABOLIZABLE ENERGY REQUIREMENTS OF DOGS

K = activity constant BW = weight in kilograms
K = 99 (inactive adult)
K = 132 (moderately active adult)
K = 160 (highly active adult)

Weight (lbs)	Weight (kg)	Metabolic Body Size (MBS)	Inactive (kcal/day)	Moderate (kcal/day)	Highly Active (kcal/day)
2	0.91	0.94	93.06	123.83	150.10
4	1.80	1.49	147.51	197.03	238.82
6	2.70	1.96	194.04	258.53	313.37
8	3.60	2.37	234.63	313.49	379.99
10	4.50	2.76	264.33	364.04	441.26
12	5.50	3.12	308.88	411.34	498.60
14	6.40	3.46	342.54	456.10	552.84
16	7.30	3.78	374.22	498.78	604.58
18	8.20	4.09	404.91	539.74	654.23
20	9.10	4.39	434.61	579.22	702.08
25	11.40	5.10	504.90	672.62	815.30
30	13.60	5.76	570.24	760.01	921.23
35	15.90	6.38	631.62	842.71	1021.46
40	18.20	6.98	691.02	921.58	1117.06
45	20.50	7.55	747.45	997.25	1208.79
50	22.70	8.11	802.89	1070.19	1297.20
55	25.00	8.64	855.36	1140.76	1382.75
60	27.30	9.16	906.84	1209.24	1465.74
65	29.50	9.67	957.33	1275.86	1546.50
70	31.80	10.16	1005.84	1340.81	1625.22
75	34.10	10.64	1053.36	1404.24	1702.11

Weight (lbs)	Weight (kg)	Metabolic Body Size (MBS)	Inactive (kcal/day)	Moderate (kcal/day)	Highly Active (kcal/day)
80	36.40	11.11	1099.89	1466.29	1777.33
85	38.60	11.57	1145.43	1527.08	1851.00
90	40.90	12.02	1189.98	1586.69	1923.27
95	43.20	12.46	1233.54	1645.23	1994.21
100	45.50	12.90	1277.10	1702.75	2063.94
105	47.70	13.33	1319.67	1759.33	2132.52
110	50.00	13.75	1361.25	1815.03	2200.04
115	52.30	14.17	1402.83	1869.90	2266.54
120	54.50	14.58	1443.42	1923.99	2332.11
125	56.80	14.98	1483.02	1977.34	2396.77
130	59.10	15.38	1522.62	2029.98	2460.59
135	61.40	15.77	1561.23	2081.97	2523.60
140	63.60	16.16	1599.84	2133.32	2585.85

Based upon MBS: kcal required $= K(BW_{kg})^{0.67}$

APPENDIX

2

STANDARD WEIGHTS FOR AKC DOG BREEDS (lbs)

Group 1: Sporting

Breed	Male	Female
Brittany	35-40	30-40
Pointer	55-75	45-64
German Shorthaired Pointer	55-70	45-60
German Wirehaired Pointer	60-75	50-65
Chesapeake Bay Retriever	65-80	55-70
Curly-Coated Retriever	65-70	65-70
Flat-Coated Retriever	50-65	45-60
Golden Retriever	65-75	55-65
Labrador Retriever	65-80	55-70
English Setter	60-75	55-65
Gordon Setter	55-80	45-70
Irish Setter	~70	~60
American Water Spaniel	28-45	25-40
Clumber Spaniel	70-85	55-70
Cocker Spaniel	25-30	20-25
English Cocker Spaniel	28-34	26-32
English Springer Spaniel	49-54	40-45
Field Spaniel	35-50	35-50
Irish Water Spaniel	55-65	45-58
Sussex Spaniel	35-45	35-45
Welsh Springer Spaniel	35-45	30-40
Vizsla	45-55	40-50
Weimaraner	60-75	55-70
Wirehaired Pointing Griffon	55-65	50-60

Group 2: Hounds

Breed	Male	Female
Afghan Hound	~60	~50
Basenji	~24	~22
Basset Hound	65-75	50-65
Beagle, 13"	13-18	13-16
Beagle, 15"	17-22	15-20
Black and Tan Coonhound	70-85	55-70
Bloodhound	90-110	80-100
Borzoi	75-105	70-90
Dachshund, Miniature	~10	~10
Dachshund, standard	16-22	16-22
American Foxhound	65-75	55-65
English Foxhound	65-75	50-70
Greyhound	65-70	60-65
Harrier	40-50	35-45
Ibizan Hound	~50	~45
Irish Wolfhound	~120	~105
Norwegian Elkhound	~55	~48
Otter Hound	75-115	65-100
Petit Basset Griffon Vendeen	40-45	40-45
Pharaoh Hound	55-70	50-65
Rhodesian Ridgeback	~75	~65
Saluki	50-70	45-65
Scottish Deerhound	85-110	75-95
Whippet	20-28	18-23

Group 3: Working

Breed	Male	Female
Akita	70-85	65-75
Alaskan Malamute	85-95	75-85
Bernese Mountain Dog	75-90	65-80
Boxer	55-70	50-60
Bullmastiff	110-130	100-120
Doberman Pinscher	65-80	55-70
Giant Schnauzer	70-85	60-75
Great Dane	120-180	100-130
Great Pyrenees	100-125	85-115
Komondor	100-130	80-110
Kuvasz	100-115	70-90
Mastiff	75-190	160-180
Newfoundland	130-150	100-120
Portuguese Water Dog	42-60	35-50
Rottweiler	80-95	70-85

Saint Bernard	130-180	120-160
Samoyed	50-65	45-60
Siberian Husky	45-60	35-50
Standard Schnauzer	30-40	25-35

Group 4: Terrier

Breed	Male	Female
Airedale Terrier	45-60	40-55
American Staffordshire Terrier	45-55	40-50
Australian Terrier	12-14	12-14
Bedlington Terrier	17-23	17-23
Border Terrier	13-15	11-14
Bull Terrier	52-62	45-55
Cairn Terrier	~14	~13
Dandie Dinmont Terrier	13-24	18-24
Fox Terrier, Smooth	17-19	15-17
Fox Terrier, Wire	17-19	15-17
Irish Terrier	~27	~25
Kerry Blue Terrier	33-40	30-38
Lakeland Terrier	~17	~17
Manchester Terrier, Standard	12-22	12-22
Miniature Bull Terrier	15-20	15-20
Miniature Schnauzer	16-18	12-16
Norfolk Terrier	11-12	11-12
Norwich Terrier	11-12	11-12
Scottish Terrier	19-22	18-21
Sealyham Terrier	23-24	21-23
Skye Terrier	25-30	20-25
Soft-Coated Wheaten Terrier	35-40	30-35
Staffordshire Bull Terrier	28-28	24-34
Welsh Terrier	18-22	16-18
West Highland White Terrier	12-14	11-13

Group 5: Toy

Breed	Male	Female
Affenpinscher	7-8	7-8
Brussels Griffon	10-12	8-10
Chihuahua	2-5.75	2-5.75
English Toy Spaniel	8-14	8-14
Italian Greyhound	8-15	5-15
Japanese Chin	4-20	4-20
Maltese	4-6	4-6
Manchester Terrier	7-12	7-11
Miniature Pinscher	10-12	9-11
Papillon	8-10	7-9

Group 5: Toy—cont'd

Breed	Male	Female
Pekingese	10-14	10-14
Pomeranian	4-7	3-5
Toy Poodle	7-10	7-10
Pug	14-18	14-18
Shih Tzu	12-17	10-15
Silky Terrier	8-10	8-10
Yorkshire Terrier	4-6.75	3-6

Group 6: Nonsporting

Breed	Male	Female
Bichon Frise	9-12	9-12
Boston Terrier	15-24	15-24
Bulldog	45-55	40-50
Chinese Shar Pei	45-55	35-45
Chow Chow	45-60	40-50
Dalmatian	50-65	45-55
Finnish Spitz	25-35	25-30
French Bulldog	20-28	20-28
Keeshond	40-50	40-50
Lhasa Apso	13-15	13-15
Poodle, Standard	50-60	45-55
Poodle, Miniature	17-20	15-20
Schipperke	12-18	12-16
Tibetan Spaniel	9-15	9-15
Tibetan Terrier	18-30	18-30

Group 7: Herding

Breed	Male	Female
Australian Cattle Dog	35-45	35-45
Australian Shepherd	45-65	45-65
Bearded Collie	55-65	50-60
Belgian Malinois	60-70	43-55
Belgian Sheepdog	60-70	43-55
Belgian Tervuren	60-70	43-55
Bouvier des Flanders	70-90	70-90
Briard	65-75	60-70
Collie	65-75	50-65
German Shepherd Dog	75-90	65-80
Old English Sheepdog	60-70	60-70
Puli	29-33	29-33
Shetland Sheepdog	16-22	14-18
Welsh Corgi, Cardigan	30-38	25-34
Welsh Corgi, Pembroke	27-30	25-28

3

AAFCO NUTRIENT PROFILES: DOG FOODS*

Nutrient	Units DMB†	Growth and Reproduction (Minimum)	Adult Maintenance (Minimum)	Maximum
Protein	%	22.00	18.00	
Arginine	%	0.62	0.51	
Histidine	%	0.22	0.18	
Isoleucine	%	0.45	0.37	
Leucine	%	0.72	0.59	
Lysine	%	0.77	0.63	
Methionine-cystine	%	0.53	0.43	
Phenyalanine-tyrosine	%	0.89	0.73	
Threonine	%	0.58	0.48	
Tryptophan	%	0.20	0.16	
Valine	%	0.48	0.39	
Fat	%	8.0	5.0	
Linoleic acid	%	1.0	1.0	
Minerals				
Calcium (Ca)	%	1.0	0.6	2.5
Phosphorus (P)	%	0.8	0.5	1.6
Ca:P ratio		1:1	1:1	2:1
Potassium	%	0.6	0.6	
Sodium	%	0.3	0.06	
Chloride	%	0.45	0.09	
Magnesium	%	0.04	0.04	0.3
Iron	mg/kg	80.0	80.0	3000.0
Copper	mg/kg	7.3	7.3	250.0
Manganese	mg/kg	5.0	5.0	
Zinc	mg/kg	120.0	120.0	1000.0
Iodine	mg/kg	1.5	1.5	50.0
Selenium	mg/kg	0.11	0.11	2.0

Nutrient	Units DMB[†]	Growth and Reproduction (Minimum)	Adult Maintenance (Minimum)	Maximum
Vitamins				
Vitamin A	IU/kg	5000.0	5000.0	250,000.0
Vitamin D	IU/kg	500.0	500.0	5000.0
Vitamin E	IU/kg	50.0	50.0	1000.0
Thiamin	mg/kg	1.0	1.0	
Riboflavin	mg/kg	2.2	2.2	
Pantothenic acid	mg/kg	10.0	10.0	
Niacin	mg/kg	11.4	11.4	
Pyridoxine	mg/kg	1.0	1.0	
Folic acid	mg/kg	0.18	0.18	
Vitamin B_{12}	mg/kg	0.022	0.02	
Choline	mg/kg	1200.0	1200.0	

Reprinted with permission from the 2000 *AAFCO Official Publication*. Copyright 2000 by the Association of American Feed Control Officials.

*Presumes an energy density of 3.5 kcal ME/g of dry matter.

[†]DMB = dry-matter basis.

4

AAFCO NUTRIENT PROFILES: CAT FOODS*

Nutrient	Units DMB†	Growth and Reproduction (Minimum)	Adult Maintenance (Minimum)	Maximum
Protein	%	30.0	26.0	
Arginine	%	1.25	1.04	
Histidine	%	0.31	0.31	
Isoleucine	%	0.52	0.52	
Leucine	%	1.25	1.25	
Lysine	%	1.20	0.83	
Methionine-cystine	%	1.10	1.10	
Methionine	%	0.62	0.62	1.5
Phenylalanine-tyrosine	%	0.88	0.88	
Phenylalanine	%	0.42	0.42	
Taurine (extruded)	%	0.10	0.10	
Taurine (canned)	%	0.20	0.20	
Threonine	%	0.73	0.73	
Tryptophan	%	0.25	0.16	
Valine	%	0.62	0.62	
Fat‡	%	9.0	9.0	
Linoleic acid	%	0.5	0.5	
Arachidonic acid	%	0.02	0.02	
Minerals				
Calcium	%	1.0	0.6	
Phosphorus	%	0.8	0.5	
Potassium	%	0.6	0.6	
Sodium	%	0.2	0.2	
Chloride	%	0.3	0.3	
Magnesium§	%	0.08	0.04	
Iron‖	mg/kg	80.0	80.0	
Copper (extruded)	mg/kg	15.0	5.0	

Nutrient	Units DMB[†]	Growth and Reproduction (Minimum)	Adult Maintenance (Minimum)	Maximum
Minerals—cont'd				
Copper (canned)	mg/kg	5.0	5.0	
Iodine	mg/kg	0.35	0.35	
Zinc	mg/kg	75.0	75.0	2000.0
Manganese	mg/kg	7.5	7.5	
Selenium	mg/kg	0.1	0.1	
Vitamins				
Vitamin A	IU/kg	9000.0	5000.0	75000.0
Vitamin D	IU/kg	750.0	500.0	10000.0
Vitamin E[¶]	IU/kg	30.0	30.0	
Vitamin K[#]	mg/kg	0.1	0.1	
Thiamin[**]	mg/kg	5.0	5.0	
Riboflavin	mg/kg	4.0	4.0	
Pyridoxine	mg/kg	4.0	4.0	
Niacin	mg/kg	60.0	60.0	
Pantothenic acid	mg/kg	5.0	5.0	
Folic acid	mg/kg	0.8	0.8	
Biotin[††]	mg/kg	0.07	0.07	
Vitamin B_{12}	mg/kg	0.02	0.02	
Choline[‡‡]	mg/kg	2400.0	2400.0	

Reprinted with permission from the 2000 *AAFCO Official Publication*. Copyright 2000 by the Association of American Feed Control Officials.

*Presumes an energy density of 4 kcal/g ME, based on the "modified Atwater" values of 3.5, 8.5 and 3.5 kcal/g for protein, fat and carbohydrate (nitrogen-free extract, NFE), respectively. Rations greater than 4.5 kcal/g should be corrected for energy density; rations less than 4.0 kcal/g should not be corrected for energy.

[†]DMB = dry matter basis.

[‡]Although a true requirement for fat per se has not been established, the minimum level was based on recognition of fat as a source of essential fatty acids and as a carrier of fat-soluble vitamins, to enhance palatability, and to supply an adequate caloric density.

[§]If the mean urine pH of cats fed as libitum is not below 6.4, the risk of struvite urolithiasis increases as the magnesium content of the diet increases.

[‖]Because of very poor bioavailability, iron from carbonate or oxide sources that are added to the diet should not be considered as components in meeting the minimum nutrient level.

[¶]Add 10 IU of vitamin E above minimum level per g of fish oil per kg of diet.

[#]Vitamin K does not need to be added unless diet contains greater than 25% fish on a DMB.

[**]Because processing may destroy up to 90% of the thiamin in the diet, allowances in formulation should be made to ensure the minimum nutrient level is met after processing.

[††]Biotin does not need to be added unless diet contains antimicrobial or antivitamin compounds.

[‡‡]Methionine may substitute for choline as a methyl donor at a rate of 3.75 parts for 1 part choline by weight when methionine exceeds 0.62%.

5

NRC MINIMUM REQUIREMENTS FOR GROWING DOGS

Nutrient	Per 1000 kcal ME	Dry Basis (3.67 kcal ME/g)
Protein*		
Indispensable amino acids		
Arginine	1.37 g	0.50%
Histidine	0.49 g	0.18%
Isoleucine	0.98 g	0.36%
Leucine	1.59 g	0.58%
Lysine	1.40 g	0.51%
Methionine-cystine	1.06 g	0.39%
Phenylalanine-tyrosine	1.95 g	0.72%
Threonine	1.27 g	0.47%
Tryptophan	0.41 g	0.15%
Valine	1.05 g	0.39%
Dispensable amino acids	17.07 g	6.26%
Fat	13.6 g	5.0%
Linoleic acid	2.7 g	1.0%
Minerals		
Calcium	1.6 g	0.59%
Phosphorus	1.2 g	0.44%
Potassium	1.2 g	0.44%

Nutrient	Per 1000 kcal ME	Dry Basis (3.67 kcal ME/g)
Minerals—cont'd		
Sodium	0.15 g	0.06%
Chloride	0.23 g	0.09%
Magnesium	0.11 g	0.04%
Iron	8.7 mg	31.9 mg/kg
Copper	0.8 mg	2.9 mg/kg
Manganese	1.4 mg	5.1 mg/kg
Zinc[†]	9.7 mg	35.6 mg/kg
Iodine	0.16 mg	0.59 mg/kg
Selenium	0.03 mg	0.11 mg/kg
Vitamins		
Vitamin A	1,011.0 IU	3,710.0 IU/kg
Vitamin D	110.0 IU	404.0 IU/kg
Vitamin E[‡]	6.1 IU	22.0 IU/kg
Vitamin K[§]	—	—
Thiamin[‖]	0.27 mg	1.0 mg/kg
Riboflavin	0.68 mg	2.5 mg/kg
Pantothenic acid	2.7 mg	9.9 mg/kg
Niacin	3.0 mg	11.0 mg/kg
Pyridoxine	0.3 mg	1.1 mg/kg
Folic acid	0.054 mg	0.2 mg/kg
Biotin[§]	—	—
Vitamin B_{12}	7.0 μg	26.0 μg/kg
Choline	340 mg	1.25 g/kg

Reprinted with permission from the 2000 *AAFCO Official Publication*. Copyright 2000 by the Association of American Feed Control Officials.

*Quantities sufficient to supply the minimum amounts of available indispensable and dispensable amino acids as specified below. Compounding practical foods from natural ingredients (protein digestability ± 70%) may require quantities representing an increase of 40% or greater than the sum of the amino acids listed below, depending upon ingredients used and processing procedures.

[†]In commercial foods with natural ingredients resulting in elevated calcium and phytate content, borderline deficiencies were reported from feeding foods with less than 90 mg zinc per kg (Sanecki et al: *Am J Vet Res* 43:1642, 1982).

[‡]A five-fold increase may be required for foods of high PUFA content.

[§]Dogs have a metabolic requirement, but a dietary requirement was not demonstrated when foods from natural ingredients were fed.

[‖]Overages must be considered to cover losses in processing and storage.

APPENDIX

6

NRC MINIMUM REQUIREMENTS FOR GROWING CATS*

Nutrient	Unit	Amount
Fat†		
Linoleic acid	g	5.0
Arachidonic acid	mg	200.0
Protein‡ (N × 6.25)	g	240.0
Arginine	g	10.0
Histidine	g	3.0
Isoleucine	g	5.0
Leucine	g	12.0
Lysine	g	8.0
Methionine plus cystine (total sulfur amino acids)	g	7.5
Methionine	g	4.0
Phenylalanine plus tyrosine	g	8.5
Phenylalanine	g	4.0
Taurine	mg	400.0
Threonine	g	7.0
Tryptophan	g	1.5
Valine	g	6.0
Minerals		
Calcium	g	8.0
Phosphorus	g	6.0
Magnesium	mg	400.0
Potassium§	g	4.0

Nutrient	Unit	Amount
Minerals—cont'd		
Sodium	mg	500.0
Chloride	g	1.9
Iron	mg	80.0
Copper	mg	5.0
Iodine	μg	350.0
Zinc	mg	50.0
Manganese	mg	5.0
Selenium	μg	100.0
Vitamins		
Vitamin A (retinol)	mg	1.0 (333 IU)
Vitamin D (cholecalciferol)	μg	12.5 (500 IU)
Vitamin E‖ (α-tocopherol)	mg	30.0 (30 IU)
Vitamin K¶ (phylloquinone)	μg	100.0
Thiamin	mg	5.0
Riboflavin	mg	4.0
Vitamin B$_6$ (pyridoxine)	mg	4.0
Niacin	mg	40.0
Pantothenic acid	mg	5.0
Folacin (folic acid¶)	μg	800.0
Biotin¶	μg	70.0
Vitamin B$_{12}$ (cyanocobalamin)	μg	20.0
Choline#		2.4
Myo-inositol**	g	—

Reprinted with permission from the 2000 *AAFCO Official Publication*. Copyright 2000 by the Association of American Feed Control Officials.

*Units per kg of diet on a dry basis; based on a diet with an ME concentration of 5 kcal/g dry matter fed to 10- to 20-week-old kittens. If dietary energy is greater or lesser, it is assumed that these requirements should be increased or decreased proportionately. Nutrient requirement levels have been selected based on the most appropriate optional response (i.e., growth, nitrogen retention, metabolite concentration or excretion, lack of abnormal clinical signs) of kittens fed a purified diet. Some of these requirements are known adequate amounts rather than minimum requirements. Since diet processing (such as extruding or retorting) may destroy or impair the availability of some nutrients, and since some nutrients, especially the trace minerals, are less available from some natural feedstuffs than from purified diets, increased amounts of these nutrients should be included to ensure that the minimum requirements are met. The minimum requirements presented in this table assume availabilities similar to those present in purified diets.

†No requirement for fat is known apart from the need for essential fatty acids and as a carrier of fat-soluble vitamins. Some fat normally enhances the palatability of the diet.

‡Assuming that all the minimum essential amino acid requirements are met.

§The minimum potassium requirement increases with protein intake.

‖This minimum should be adequate for a moderate to low-fat diet. It may be expected to increase three- to fourfold with a high PUFA diet, especially when fish oil is present.

¶These vitamins may not be required in the diet unless antimicrobial agents or antivitamin compounds are present in the diet.

#Choline is not essential in the diet, but if this quantity of choline is not present, the methionine requirement would be increased to provide the same quantity of methyl groups.

**A dietary requirement for myo-inositol has not been demonstrated for the cat. However, almost all published studies in which purified diets have been used have included myo-inositol at 150 to 200 mg/kg diet and no studies have tested a myo-inositol-free diet.

NOTE: The minimum requirements of all the nutrients are not known for the adult cat at maintenance. It is known that these levels of nutrients are adequate and that protein and methionine can be reduced to 140 and 3 g/kg diet, respectively. It is likely that the minimum requirements of all the other nutrients are also lower for maintenance than for the growing kitten. The minimum requirements of all the nutrients are not known for reproduction for the adult male or female cat. It is known that with the following modifications the nutrient allowances as recommended in the 1978 NRC report are adequate for gestation and lactation (in units/kg purified diet, note these recommendations are based on 4 kcal/g dry diet): arachidonate, 200 mg; zinc, 40 mg; vitamin A, 5500 IU; and taurine 500. It is probably that the minimum requirements for growing kittens in this table would satisfy all requirements for reproduction if the following were modified as shown: vitamin A, 6000 IU/kg diet, and taurine, 500 mg/kg diet.

GLOSSARY

acanthosis nigricans diffuse hyperplasia of the spinous layer of the skin, with gray, brown, or black pigmentation.

accretion growth by addition of material.

acrodermatitis severe skin lesions.

adipocyte hyperplasia an increase in the number of fat cells, occurring normally during certain developmental periods such as early growth and, occasionally, puberty.

adipocyte specialized cells that store large amounts of triglyceride.

alopecia the absence of hair from the skin areas where it is normally present.

anabolism any process by which organisms convert substances into other components of the organism's chemical architecture.

anorexia lack or loss of the appetite for food.

ascites effusion and accumulation of serous fluid in the abdominal cavity.

ataxia failure of muscular coordination; irregularity of muscular action.

azotemia an excess of urea or other nitrogenous compounds in the blood.

bone meal the dried, ground, and sterilized product from undecomposed bones.

BUN blood urea nitrogen.

byproduct secondary products in addition to the principle product; the parts that are left after the economically valuable pieces are harvested.

calculolytic pertaining to the destruction or decomposition of a calculus.

calorie the amount of heat energy that is necessary to raise the temperature of 1 gram of water from 14.5° C to 15.5° C. Because the calorie is such a small unit of measure, the kilocalorie, equal to 1000 calories, is most often used in the science of animal nutrition.

carnivorous eating or subsisting on primarily animal material.

carpus the joint between the paw and the forelimb (the wrist in humans).

cation an ion carrying a positive charge owing to a deficiency of electrons; in an electrochemical cell, cations migrate toward the cathode.

cellulose an unbranched, long-chain polysaccharide that is a component of dietary fiber; forms the skeleton of most plant structures and plant cells.

chylomicron a class of lipoproteins responsible for the transport of exogenous cholesterol and triglycerides from the small intestine to tissues after meals.

colostrum the first product of the mammary gland following parturition.

coprophagy the ingestion of dung or feces.

corn gluten meal the dried residue from corn after the removal of the larger part of the starch and germ and the separation of the bran.

costochondral pertaining to a rib and its cartilage.

creatinine the end product of creatine metabolism, found in muscle and blood and excreted in the urine.

crystalluria excretion of crystals in the urine, in some cases producing urinary tract irritation.

cyanosis a bluish discoloration of the skin and mucous membranes as a result of excessive concentration of reduced hemoglobin in the blood.

cystitis inflammation of the urinary bladder.

cystocentesis perforation or tapping, as with an aspirator, trocar, or needle, to remove urinary bladder contents.

demodicosis skin disease caused by the mange mite Demodex canis in dogs.

deoxyribonucleic acid (DNA) a nucleic acid that constitutes the genetic material of all cellular organisms.

dietary thermogenesis Also called the *specific dynamic action of food*, the energy needed by the body to digest, absorb, and assimilate nutrients.

duodenum the first or proximal portion of the small intestine extending from the pylorus to the jejunum.

dystocia abnormal labor or birth.

eicosanoids biologically active substances that are metabolites of 20-carbon fatty acids; includes prostaglandins, leukotrienes, prosacyclins, and thromboxanes.

endogenous developing or originating within the organism or arising from causes within the organism.

energy density For a pet food, refers to the number of calories provided by the food in a given weight or volume. In the United States it is expressed as kilocalories of metabolizable energy per kilogram or pound of diet; in Europe, kilojoule per kilogram is used.

energy imbalance occurs when an animal's daily energy consumption is either greater or less than its daily requirement, leading to changes in growth rate, body weight, and body composition.

enterohepatic pertaining to the intestine (*entero*) and the liver (*hepatic*).

epiphysis the expanded articular end of a long bone, developed from a secondary ossification center.

erythropoiesis the production of erythrocytes (red blood cells).

essential nutrients nutrients that cannot be synthesized by the body at a rate adequate to meet body needs and must be supplied in the diet.

estrus the recurrent, restricted period of sexual receptivity in female mammals.

exogenous developing or originating outside the organism.

extravasation a discharge or escape, as of blood from a vessel into the tissues.

germ As in wheat germ, the plant embryo found in seeds and frequently separated from the bran (outer coat of a seed) and starch endosperm during milling.

glomerulosclerosis fibrosis and scarring that result in senescence of the renal glomeruli.

gluconeogenesis the formation of glucose from molecules that are not carbohydrates, as from amino acids, lactate, and the glycerol portion of fats.

gluten the tough, thick, proteinaceous substance that remains when the flour, wheat, or other grain is washed to remove the starch.

glycosuria the excretion of an abnormal concentration of glucose in the urine.

grain the seed from cereal plants (e.g., wheat, rice, barley, oats).

Heinz bodies coccoid inclusion bodies resulting from oxidative injury to and precipitation of hemoglobin, seen in the presence of certain abnormal hemoglobins and erythrocytes with enzyme deficiencies.

hematocrit the ratio of the total red cell volume to the total blood volume.

hemicellulose a heterogenous group of branched-chain polysaccharides that, together with pectin, forms the matrix of plant cells within which cellulose fibers are enmeshed.

hemolytic anemia anemia as a result of intravascular fragmentation of red blood cells.

hepatic lipidosis an abnormal accumulation of fats and fatlike substances in the liver.

hepatomegaly enlargement of the liver.

homeostasis the maintenance of stability in the body's internal environment, achieved by a system of control mechanisms activated by negative feedback.

hydrolysis the splitting of a compound into fragments by the addition of water. The hydroxyl group is incorporated in one fragment and the hydrogen atom in the other.

hydroxyapatite an inorganic compound, found in the matrix of bone and the teeth, that is composed of calcium, phosphorous, hydrogen, and oxygen and provides rigidity.

hypercalcemia increased calcium concentration in the blood.

hyperlipidemia a general term for elevated concentrations of triglyceride and/or cholesterol in the plasma of fasted animals.

hyperphagia ingestion of a greater than optimal quantity of food.

hyperplasia increase in cell number.

hypertrophy increase in cell size.

hypophosphatemia decreased phosphorous concentration in the blood.

hypothalamus gland located in the brain that exerts control over the function of a portion of the pituitary gland. Its nuclei comprise part of the mechanism that activates, controls, and integrates the peripheral autonomic mechanisms, which include a general regulation of water balance, body temperature, sleep, and food intake.

iatrogenic any adverse condition occurring as the result of treatment, especially infections acquired during the course of treatment.

icterus jaundice.

idiopathic self-originated or of unknown causation.

inappetence lack of appetite.

indole a compound that is produced by the decomposition of tryptophan in the intestine; it is partly responsible for the peculiar odor of the feces.

jejunum the portion of the small intestine that extends from the duodenum to the ileum.

keratin a scleroprotein that is the principal constituent of epidermis, hair, nails, horny tissues, and the organic matrix of the enamel of teeth.

keratinization the development of or conversion into the structural protein keratin.

kilojoule the amount of mechanical energy that is required for a force of 1 newton to move a weight of 1 kilogram a distance of 1 meter. To convert kilocalories to kilojoule, the number of kilocalories is multiplied by 4.184.

lactic acid an end product of glycolysis that provides energy anaerobically in skeletal muscle during heavy exercise. It can be oxidized aerobically in the heart for energy production or can be converted back to glucose (gluconeogenesis) in the liver.

leukotriene one of a group of biologically active compounds formed from 20-carbon fatty acids that function as regulators of allergic and inflammatory reactions.

ligand a molecule that binds to another molecule; commonly refers to a small molecule that binds specifically to a larger molecule.

lipemia retinalis a milky appearance of the veins and arteries of the retina, occurring as a result of hyperlipidemia.

lipidosis a term for several of the lysosomal storage diseases in which there is an abnormal accumulation of lipids in the reticuloendothelial cells. Also called *lipid storage disease*.

lipogenesis the formation of fat; the transformation of nonfat food materials into body fat.

lipoid granuloma a small, nodular, delimited aggregation of lipid cells; a xanthoma.

lumen the cavity or channel within a tube or tubular organ (e.g., the intestine).

meal an ingredient that has been ground or otherwise reduced in particle size.

meat and bone meal the same as meat meal, except that meat and bone meal can contain a great deal more bone (raising the ash content and lowering the protein quality).

meat byproducts the nonrendered, clean parts, other than meat, derived from slaughtered mammals; include, but are not limited to, lungs, spleen, kidneys, brain, liver, blood, bone, and stomach/intestine, without their contents.

meat meal the rendered product from mammal tissues exclusive of blood, hair, hoof, horn, hide trimmings, manure, stomach, and rumen contents, except in such amounts as may occur unavoidably in good processing practices.

metabolism the sum of all the physical and chemical processes by which living, organized substance is produced and maintained (anabolism); also the transformation by which energy is made available for the uses of the organism (catabolism).

metabolizable energy (ME) the amount of energy that is ultimately available to the tissues of the body after losses in the feces and urine have been subtracted from the gross energy of food. It is the value that is most often used to express the energy content of pet food ingredients and commercial diets.

metaphysis the wider part at the extremity of the shaft of a long bone, adjacent to the epiphyseal disk. During development it contains the growth zone and consists of spongy bone; in the adult it is continuous with the epiphysis.

methemoglobinemia the presence of methemoglobin in the blood, resulting in cyanosis.

necrosis cell and tissue death.

neoplasia the progressive multiplication of cells under conditions that would not elicit or would cause cessation of multiplication of normal cells; may be malignant or benign.

nephrosclerosis sclerosis (invasion of connective tissue at the expense of active tissue) of the kidney.

neuropathies general term denoting functional disturbances and/or pathological changes in the peripheral nervous system.

nonessential nutrients nutrients that can be synthesized by the body at a level sufficient to meet body needs; can be obtained either through de novo synthesis or from the diet.

omnivorous subsisting on both plants and animals.

os penis a heterotopic bone developed in the fibrous septum between the corpora cavernosa and above the urethra, forming the skeleton of the penis.

osmosis the passage of pure solvent from a solution of lesser to one of greater solute concentration when the two solutions are separated by a membrane that selectively prevents the passage of solute molecules but is permeable to the solvent.

osteochondrosis a disease of the growth or ossification centers of bones that begins as a degeneration or necrosis, followed by regeneration or recalcification.

parturition the act or process of giving birth

pearled barley dehulled barley grain.

periosteum a specialized connective tissue covering all bones of the body and possessing bone-forming potentialities.

peristalsis rhythmic movements produced by the functioning longitudinal and circular muscle fibers of the small intestine to propel food forward.

phylogeny the evolutionary history of a group of organisms.

polydipsia chronic excessive thirst.

polyphagia excessive eating.

polyuria the passage of a large volume of urine in a given period of time.

postprandial occurring after a meal.

poultry meal (also includes chicken meal if the origin is strictly chicken) the dry rendered product from a combination of clean flesh and skin, with or without the accompanying bone, derived from the parts of whole carcasses of poultry exclusive of feathers, heads, feet, and entrails.

poultry byproduct meal ground, rendered, clean parts of the carcasses of slaughtered poultry such as necks, feet, undeveloped eggs, and intestines, exclusive of feathers except in such amounts as might occur unavoidably in good processing practices.

poultry byproducts nonrendered, clean parts of carcasses of slaughtered poultry such as heads, feet, and viscera free from fecal content and foreign matter except in such trace amounts as might occur unavoidably in good processing practices.

prepuce a covering fold of skin over the penis.

proprioception perception/awareness of position provided by sensory nerve terminals that give information concerning movements and position of the body.

prostacyclin a prostaglandin synthesized by endothelial cells lining the cardiovascular system; a physiological antagonist of thromboxane.

prostaglandins any of a group of components derived from unsaturated 20-carbon fatty acids, primarily arachidonic acid.

pruritus descriptive of any of various conditions marked by itching.

purulent consisting of or containing pus.

pylorus the distal opening of the stomach surrounded by a strong band of circular muscle through which the stomach contents are emptied into the duodenum.

pyoderma any purulent skin disease.

pyrexia a fever or febrile condition; abnormal elevation of body temperature.

senescence the process or condition of growing old, especially the condition resulting from the transitions and accumulations of the deleterious aging processes.

skatole a crystalline amine with a strong characteristic odor, found in feces; produced by the decomposition of proteins in the intestine and directly from the amino acid tryptophan by decarboxylation.

stenosis narrowing or stricture of a duct or canal.

struvite a urinary calculus composed of magnesium ammonium phosphate.

subluxation an incomplete or partial dislocation; in the case of canine hip dysplasia, the head of the femur partially dislodges from the cup (acetabulum) of the pelvic bone.

suppuration the formation of pus.

taurine a beta-amino acid that contains a sulfonic group rather than a carboxylic group and so cannot form a peptide bond. It is an essential amino acid for cats, but not for dogs.

theobromine a methylxanthine contained in chocolate; has physiological properties similar to those of caffeine.

thermogenesis the production of heat by physiological processes.

thromboxane an extremely potent inducer of platelet aggregation and platelet-release reactions; also a vasoconstrictor; it is a physiological antagonist of prostacyclin.

urethritis inflammation of the urethra.

urolithiasis the disease condition associated with the presence of urinary calculi or stones.

villi multitudinous, threadlike projections that cover the surface of the mucosa of the small intestine and serve as the sites of absorption (by active transport and diffusion) of fluids and nutrients.

vulva the region of the external genital organs of the female.

xanthoma a tumor composed of lipid-laden foam cells.

INDEX

Amino acid—cont'd
  limiting, 27
  nutrient absorption and, 58
  protein quality and, 101-102
  protein requirement and
    for cats, 105, 106
    for dogs, 104
  renal failure and, 463
  struvite urolithiasis and, 416
  synthesis of protein and, 24-25
  taurine requirements in cat and, 110
Amino peptidase, 56
Ammonium chloride, 415
Ammonium in struvite urolithiasis, 412, 413
Amyloid, 398
Anaerobic bacteria
  intestinal overgrowth with, 490
  periodontitis and, 479-480
Analysis, guaranteed, 153-155
Anemia
  copper and, 47
  iron deficiency, 46-47
Animal fat, 178-179, 355; *see also* Fat
Anion, 51
Anorexia
  in elderly animal, 281
  feline hepatic lipidosis and, 474-475
Antihistamine, 441
Antiinflammatory agent, 492
Antioxidant
  action of, *181*
  natural-derived, 182-183
  synthetic, 183-184
  types of, 181-184
  vitamin E as, 35
Apatite, 427
Appetite
  estrus affecting, 226
  food intake and, 79-80
Appetite stimulant, in cancer, 512-513
Arachidonic acid
  in cat, 94-95
  function of, 21
  sources of, 22
  structure of, *20*
Arginine
  cancer and, 508, 511
  cats' need for, 107-108, 108t
  deficiency of, 130
  feline hepatic lipidosis and, 474
Arsenic, 50
Arthritis, 304
Ascorbic acid, 40
  supplementation with, 343-344

Ash, 10
Association of American Feed Control Officials
  brand name regulations of, 150
  calcium and phosphorus requirements of, 124
  calcium supplementation and, 337
  caloric content statement and, 151
  current regulations of, 149
  descriptive terms, regulations about, 151
  evaluation of pet food and, 200, 204
  fat requirements and, 95
  function of, 145t, 146
  ingredient list on label and, 155
  label changes and, 158-160
  label claims and, 157-158
  protein requirements and, 104
  standards of, 69
  struvite urolithiasis and, 414
  vitamin A requirement and, 118
  vitamin D and, 121
Athlete; *see* Performance
Atwater factor, 6-7
  modified, 7
    energy density and, 9
Autoimmune disease, 365-366
Avidin, 350
Azotemia, 452

B

B complex vitamins; *see* Vitamin B complex
Bacteria
  feline odontoclastic resorptive lesions and, 480
  fermentable fiber and, 500
  fiber fermentation and, 16-17, 17t, 59
    renal failure and, 467, *468,* 469
  intestinal overgrowth with, 490-491
  oral malodor and, 478
  periodontitis and, 479-480
  vitamin K and, 36
Bacteroides, 490
Balance
  nitrogen
    aging and, 283
    calculation of, 99
    states of, 100t
  water, 12-13
    struvite urolithiasis and, 416-417
Balanced pet food, 200
Barley, 402, 403
Beagle
  aging in, 278-279
  endurance performance in, 269-270
  renal function and aging in, 279-280
Bedlington Terrier, 387-388

Beet pulp, 17, 18, 178, 467
Behavior
  aging and, 281-282
  normal feeding
    in cats, 219
    in dogs, 217-219
Behavior modification for obesity, 318, 320
Beta-bond in plant fiber, 16
Beta-carotene, 31, *32*
Bicarbonate
  overacidification of urine and, 421
  renal failure and, 461, 471
Bifidobacterium, 501
Bile
  copper metabolism and, 126-127
  digestion and, 57
Biological value of protein, 28
Biotin, 38
  deficiency of, 349-350
Biscuit, 187
  oral care, 484
Bitch
  amount to feed, 86
  calcium requirements of, 125
  carbohydrate requirement and, 89
  feeding of, during pregnancy, 226, 227-229
  lactating, 230-231
Bloat, 361-362
Blood
  calcium levels of, 43
  iron and, 46-47
  proteins in, 23-24
Blood clotting, 36, 122-123
Blood flow, renal, 451
Blood urea nitrogen
  protein restriction and, 463
  renal failure and, 452-453
Body composition, aging and, 277, 278t
Body condition
  assessment of, *257, 258, 315, 316*
  early-age neutering and, 309
  obesity and, 313-317, *315, 316*
Body weight; *see* Weight
Bolus feeding in cancer, 513
Bombesin, 79
Bone
  calcium and phosphorus in, 43
  calcium supplementation and, 338
  deforming cervical spondylosis and, 346-349
  growth rate and, 334-335
  overacidification of urine and, 421
  as protein source, 176
  vitamin A and, 31
  vitamin D and, 33, 121

Bran, 178
Brand name, 150
Brand of pet food, 193-196
Breath malodor, 478-479
Breed
  of cat, struvite urolithiasis and, 410
  of dog
    growth and, 245
    obesity and, 310
    struvite urolithiasis and, 410, 422
Breeding, feeding and care before, 225-226
Breed-specific nutrition, 246-248, *247*
Brewer's yeast, 357
Brush border of small intestine, 57
Brushing, tooth, 487
Bull Terrier
  lethal acrodermatitis in, 432
  zinc malabsorption in, 388
Butylated hydroxyanisole, 183-184
Butylated hydroxytoluene, 183-184
Byproduct, definition of, 176

C
C cell, 338
Cachexia in cancer, 505-510
Cafeteria feeding, 83, 129
Calcitonin, 43-44
Calcitonin-producing C cell, 338
Calcium, 42t, *44*
  calcium oxalate urolithiasis and, 423-427
  gestation and lactation and, 232
  growth and, 250, 289, 337-339
  sources and functions of, 41-45, 42t, *44*
  supplementation of, 337-343, *341,* 370
    in gestation and lactation, 342-343
    during growth, 337-339
    for large and giant breeds, 336-340, 340t, *341,* 342
  vitamin D and, 33, 119-121
Calcium oxalate urolithiasis
  in cats, 423-426
    incidence of, 411
  in dogs, 426-427
  overacidification of urine and, 421
Calcium phosphate, 427, 428
Calculation
  of energy, 6-7
    of cat, 87
    for dog, 84
    of dog, 84
    metabolizable, 169-170
  of nitrogen balance, 99
  of nutrient content, 166-167
Calculus; *see* Urolithiasis

Maillard products, 111
Maintenance diet, 255-256
  amount to feed for, 223-224
  for dental health, 486-488
  for growing puppy, 253
  struvite urolithiasis prevention and, 419-420
  weight loss and, 324, 329
Malabsorption
  of fat, 495
  pancreatic insufficiency and, 491
  of vitamin B₁₂, in Giant Schnauzers, 386
Malamute, lethal acrodermatitis in, 432
Malignancy, 505-514; *see also* Cancer
Malnutrition, protein/calorie, 114-115
Malodor, oral, 478-479
Mammary gland, development of, 228-229
Mandibular premolar, in feline odontoclastic re-
    sorption, 480
Manganese, 42t, 48
Manufacturer, reputation of, 206-207
Marketing of pet food, 160-163
Mastication, 53
Meal
  dry, 187-188
  feeding of, 222
  history of pet food and, 143-144
  as protein source, 176-177
  timing of, in diabetes mellitus, 408
Meal-induced thermogenesis, 76, 306
  frequency of meals and, 82
Measurement of energy, 4-8
Meat
  dermatosis and, 430
  myths about, 353
  as protein source, 176
  semimoist food resembling, 192
Mechanical digestion in small intestine, 56
Medial paraventricular nucleus, 79
Menaquinone, 35
Menhaden fish oil, 460, *460*
Metabolic acidosis, renal failure and, 471
Metabolic acidosis in renal failure, 461
Metabolic body weight, 83-84
Metabolic disorder, inherited, 385-396, 385t
  copper-storage disease as, 387-388
  hyperlipidemia as, 389-394
  purine, in Dalmatians, 394-396
  vitamin B₁₂ malabsortion, 386
  zinc malabsorption as, 388-389, *389*
Metabolic rate
  early-age neutering and, 309
  resting, 75-76
    aging and, 277
    obesity and, 305

Metabolic stress, skeletal disorder and, 334-335
Metabolic water, 13
Metabolism
  in cancer, 505-510
  carbohydrate, 89-92
  endurance and, 260
  of omega-3 and omega-6 fatty acids, *437*
  protein's function in, 23
Metabolizable energy, 289
  calculation of, 7-8
  definition of, 5
  determination of, 61, 169-170
  of pet food, 205-206
  of protein, 26
  protein requirements of dogs and, 103
Methane gas, 60
Methionine, 112-113
Metoclopramide, 512
Microbe; *see* Bacteria
Micromineral, 41
Microvillus, 57
Milk
  amount produced, 236
  colostrum, 233-234, 288
  composition of, 233-235, 235t, 239t
  digestibility, 91, 129
  myths about, 354-355
Milk replacer, 239-240, 241t, 288-289
Minature Schnauzer, vitamin A–responsive der-
    matosis in, 431
Mineral, 41-51, 42t, 63
  absorption of, 58
  aging and, 284-285
  calcium
    function and sources of, 41-45
    requirements for, 124-126
  chromium, 49
  cobalt, 49
  copper
    function and sources of, 47
    requirements for, 126-127
  iodine, 48-49
  iron, 46-47
  labeling and, 159
  magnesium
    function and sources of, 45
    requirements for, 126
  manganese, 48
  phosphorus
    function and sources of, 41-45
    requirements for, 124-126
  in protein source, 176
  requirement for, 123-128
  selenium, 48-49

Renal failure, chronic,—cont'd
  dietary factors in, 455-461
    fat and, 459-461, *461*
    phosphorus and, 458
    protein and, 455-458
    sodium and, 461
  management of, 462-471
    fat and, 465-466
    fiber and, 467, *468,* 469-471, *470*
    phosphorus and, 466-467
    protein and, 462-465
  metabolic acidosis and, 461
  progressive nature of, 454
Renal function
  aging and, 279-280, 284
  protein and, 115-116, 130, 284
  purine metabolism and, 394-395
  vitamin D and, 33
Repellent, flea, 357
Replacer, milk, 239-240, 288-289
Repletion, glycogen, 267-269, *268*
Reproductive status, obesity and, 308-309
Reputation of pet food manufacturer, 206-207
Resistance, insulin, 398-399
Resorptive lesion, feline odontoclastic, 480, 485-486
Resting metabolic rate, 75-76
  aging and, 277
  cachexia of cancer and, 509-510, 511
  energy expenditure and, 77-78
  obesity and, 305
Retina
  taurine and, 110
  vitamin A and, 29-30
Retinal, 117
Retinoid, 431
Retinol, 29, 117
Retinyl palmitate, 119
Retorting, 190
Rhabdomyolysis, external, 262
Rhodopsin, 29-30
Riboflavin, 37
Rice, 402-403
Rickets, 121
Rosemary extract, 182-183

S
Safety of pet foods, 180
Saliva
  breath malodor and, 478-479
  coat color change and, 360-361
  feline odontoclastic resorptive lesion and, 486
Salmonella, 501
Salt, 128

Satiety, 79-80
Saturated fatty acid, 19, *20*
Scaling, dental, 487
Schnauzer
  Giant, 386
  Miniature, 391-392
Sebaceous adenitis, vitamin A–responsive, 431-432
Seborrhea, 431
Secretin, 57
Secretion, gastric, 55
Selenium
  functions and sources of, 42t, 48-49
  vitamin E and, 121
Semimoist food, 192, 400-401
Semisolid food, introduction to, 237
Sensory function in aging, 281
Serotonin, 79
Sexual status, obesity and, 308-309
Shampoo, coat color change and, 360
Short-chain fatty acid, fiber and, 16-17, 59
  gastrointestinal disorder and, 499-501
Siberian Husky
  lethal acrodermatitis in, 432
  zinc malabsorption in, 388-389, *389*
Silica urolithiasis, 428
Silicon, 50
Single nephron glomerular filtration rate, 454
Single-meal feeding, 363
Skatole, 59
Skeletal development, exercise and, 253
Skeletal disorder, 370
  deforming cervical spondylosis and, 346-349
  obesity affecting, 304
  overnutrition and, 331-333
  supplements and, 252, 289
Skin
  aging and, 278
  dermatosis of, 429-450; *see also* Dermatosis
  vitamin E deficiency and, 122
  zinc deficiency and, 48, 389, *389*
Sled dog, 259
  energy requirements of, 265-266
  water and electrolytes for, 266-267
Slow-twitch muscle fiber, 260-261
Small breed of dog, growth of, 248
Small intestine, 56-58
Snacks and treats, 193
Social facilitation in dogs
  aging and, 281
  food intake and, 81, 218
  obesity and, 311
Sodium
  aging and, 285
  nutrient absorption and, 58

Z

Zero nitrogen balance, 100

Zinc

    functions and sources of, 42t, 47-48

    malabsorption of, 388-389, *389*

Zinc-responsive dermatosis, 433-435